(

Polycyclic aromatic hydrocarbons, many of which have been identified as potent human carcinogens, occur widely in the environment as a result of incomplete combustion of fossil fuels and other organic matter. Major sources of emissions arise from wood and coal burning, automobiles, heat and power plants, and refuse burning.

Their widespread occurrence in the air and in food and water underlines the importance of understanding their role as causes of human cancer.

This is the first volume to review the chemical properties of these carcinogens and to relate their carcinogenic activity to their metabolic by-products within the body. The emphasis throughout is on those recent findings, newer methods and techniques which illuminate the process of carcinogenesis.

The volume is suitable for anyone with a professional interest in the chemistry and metabolism of polycyclic aromatic hydrocarbons, environmental chemistry and chemical carcinogenesis.

Cambridge Monographs on Cancer Research

Polycyclic aromatic hydrocarbons

Cambridge Monographs on Cancer Research

Scientific Editors
M. M. Coombs, Imperial Cancer Research Fund Laboratories, London
J. Ashby, Imperial Chemical Industries, Macclesfield, Cheshire
R. M. Hicks, United Biscuits (UK) Ltd, Maidenhead, Berkshire

Executive Editor
H. Baxter, formerly at the Laboratory of the Government Chemist, London

Books in this Series

Martin R. Osborne and Neil T. Crosby *Benzopyrenes*

Maurice M. Coombs and Tarlochan S. Bhatt
Cyclopenta[a]phenanthrenes

M. S. Newman, B. Tierney and S. Veeraraghavan *The chemistry and biology of benz[a]anthracenes*

Jürgen Jacob *Sulfur analogues of polycyclic aromatic hydrocarbons (thiaarenes)*

Forthcoming Volumes

John Higginson, Calum S. Muir and Nubia Muñoz *Human cancer: epidemiology and environmental causes*

W. Lijinsky *The chemistry and biology of* N-*nitroso compounds*

W. F. Karcher *Dibenzanthracenes and environmental carcinogenesis*

Polycyclic aromatic hydrocarbons: chemistry and carcinogenicity

RONALD G. HARVEY

The Ben May Institute
University of Chicago

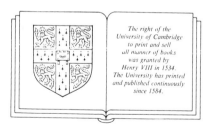

CAMBRIDGE UNIVERSITY PRESS

Cambridge

New York   Port Chester   Melbourne   Sydney

Published by the Press Syndicate of the University of Cambridge
The Pitt Building, Trumpington Street, Cambridge CB2 1RP
40 West 20th Street, New York, NY 10011–4211, USA
10 Stamford Road, Oakleigh, Melbourne 3166, Australia

First published 1991

Printed in Great Britain at the University Press, Cambridge

British Library cataloguing in publication data

Harvey, R. G.
    Polycyclic aromatic hydrocarbons.
    1. Man. Cancer. Pathogens: Polycyclic aromatic
    hydrocarbons
    I. Title
    616.994071

Library of Congress cataloguing in publication data

Harvey, Ronald G., 1927–
    Polycyclic aromatic hydrocarbons: chemistry and carcinogenicity
R. G. Harvey.
        p.   cm. – (Cambridge monographs on cancer research)
    Includes index.
    ISBN 0-521-36458-2 (hardback)
    1. Polycyclic aromatic hydrocarbons–Carcinogenicity.
    2. Polycyclic aromatic hydrocarbons.   I. Title.   II. Series.
    RC268.7.P64H37   1991
    616.99'4071–dc20   90-26905   CIP

ISBN 0 521 36458 2 hardback

This book is dedicated to my wife Helene in appreciation of her many fine qualities and for her loving support and encouragement during the writing of this book.

Contents

Preface

Polyarenes (i.e. polycyclic aromatic hydrocarbons) and their derivatives represent one of the major classes of organic molecules. Their unique chemical properties and the nature of their aromaticity has long intrigued scientists. Although the number of theoretically possible polyarenes is very large, only a small percentage of these have been synthesized in the laboratory, and research in this field has been mainly confined to the smaller polyarene ring systems.

A resurgence of interest in polyarenes has been stimulated by growing awareness that compounds of this class, including a number of relatively potent carcinogens, are prevalent in the human environment and may play an important role in the causation of cancer. Extensive epidemiological studies by the World Health Organization and other organizations support the view that a high percentage of human cancer, as much as 80%, has its origin in lifestyle, diet, and other environmental factors. Research interest has focused on the polyarenes because of their widespread environmental prevalence and the high carcinogenic potency of some members of this class. Polyarenes are formed as products of incomplete combustion of fossil fuels and other organic matter. Major sources include emissions from wood and coal burning, automobiles, heat and power plants, and refuse burning. Polyarenes are also present in many common foods and are significant components of tobacco smoke. Inhalation of cigarette smoke has been implicated as the principal cause of lung cancer in human populations. We are all exposed daily to significant levels of polyarenes in the air we breathe, the water we drink, and the food we eat.

Recent research has led to recognition that most carcinogens are metabolized to reactive intermediates which become covalently bound to proteins and nucleic acids. Binding of carcinogen metabolites to nucleic acids, particularly DNA, is now generally accepted to be a critical event which leads ultimately to tumor induction. Metabolic transformation of polyarenes furnishes a complex pattern of isomeric quinones, phenols, dihydrodiols, and other oxidized metabolites, which varies from hydrocarbon to hydrocarbon. While the majority of these are excreted as such or in the form of their glucuronic acid and glutathione conjugates, a significant percentage are covalently bound to nucleic acids. Studies of the metabolism and DNA binding of benzo[a]pyrene conducted in the mid-1970s by several groups of investigators, particularly Brookes, Conney, Gelboin, Harvey, Jerina, Sims, Weinstein and their associates, led to identification of a chemically reactive diol epoxide metabolite as the principal DNA-bound form of this carcinogen. This finding stimulated a major expansion of research activity, and analogous diol epoxide intermediates were implicated subsequently as the active forms of numerous other alternant polyarenes. While many questions remain to be answered, there is increasing confidence that the way is now open to eventual understanding of the mechanism of cancer induction by this class of carcinogens at the molecular–genetic level.

This book is written to fill the need for a volume on the chemistry of the polyarenes and their oxidized metabolites in relation to their carcinogenic properties. In the opening chapters an introduction is provided to the environmental occurrence of polyarenes and modern concepts of their metabolic activation and mechanisms of carcinogenesis. Following this, the molecular structural properties of polyarenes and their modes of chemical reactivity are surveyed, integrating purely descriptive facts, in so far as possible, into a unifying theoretical framework. In the next section of the book, general methods for the synthesis of polycyclic aromatic hydrocarbons are reviewed, with emphasis on modern synthetic approaches. This is followed by a series of chapters which survey the synthesis and properties of individual polyarenes. In order to restrict this work to a reasonable length, only polycyclic ring systems with four to seven fused aromatic rings, including nonalternant as well as alternant polyarenes, are covered. This includes virtually all the known carcinogenic hydrocarbons. Excluded are smaller inactive molecules, such as anthracene, naphthalene, fluorene, and large high molecular weight molecules, such as coronene, and linked polybenzenoid hydrocarbons, such as terphenyl, in which the aromatic rings are not fused. These types of polyarenes tend to be biologically inactive and are only of peripheral interest from the viewpoint of carcinogenesis research. Also excluded, in order to keep the size of this volume within reasonable bounds, are the heterocyclic analogs of the polyarenes, many of which are active as carcinogens and mutagens. It has not been attempted to provide encyclopedic coverage of the older literature. This is reviewed comprehensively in Clar's excellent two-volume treatise. Instead, the emphasis is on more recent findings and newer methods and techniques. The remainder of the book is devoted to a survey of the synthesis and properties of the oxidized metabolites and related derivatives of polyarenes. This is a rapidly expanding field never before reviewed in its entirety.

The coverage of this book is as comprehensive as possible through 1989. In order to keep the number of references within practical limits, citation is restricted in so far as practical, to leading references and review articles. This book complements the other volumes in this series that deal with individual polyarenes and the earlier book *Polycyclic Hydrocarbons and Carcinogenesis* (1985) Symp. Monograph No. 283, American Chemical Society: Washington, DC, edited by the author, that deals with mechanisms of carcinogenesis and binding to nucleic acids of this class of molecules.

This book may be read with profit by anyone interested in the chemistry of polyarenes, environmental analysis, chemical carcinogenesis, and the prevention of cancer in human populations. It is also intended to serve as a reference source for all aspects of the chemistry of polyarenes and their oxidized metabolites and a text for graduate level courses of instruction in environmental chemistry and chemical carcinogenesis. Since errors and omissions are likely in a work of this scope, the author will welcome any suggestions from interested readers for changes or corrections.

I would like to express my gratitude to Charles B. Huggins, the first director of the Ben May Institute, who stimulated my interest in research in this field by his encouragement and enthusiasm. I would also like to thank the many postdoctoral fellows, graduate students, and research technicians who contributed their efforts to carry out so much difficult but rewarding research in my laboratories. In particular, I would like to cite Fred Beland, Bongsup Cho, Cecilia Cortez, Pasquale Di Raddo, Peter Fu, Swee Hock Goh, Maria Konieczny, Hongmee Lee, Peter Rabideau, and Robert Young. It is also my pleasure to acknowledge the numerous colleagues and collaborators who contributed importantly to the success of our research program through numerous stimulating discussions and research collaborations. These include William Baird, Peter Brookes, John DiGiovanni, Anthony Dipple, Nickolas Geacintov, Jenny Glusker, Stephen Hecht, Charles Heidelberger, Alan Jeffrey, John Pataki, Thomas Slaga, Bernard Weinstein, and Samuel Weiss. I would also like to express my thanks to Robert Young for his helpful critical reading of most of the manuscript. Finally, I would also like to acknowledge the generous financial support of the American Cancer Society, the National Cancer Institute, the National Institute for Environmental Health Sciences, and the Council for Tobacco Research for our research program over the years.

Ronald G. Harvey

1

Nomenclature

1.1 Polyarenes (polycyclic aromatic hydrocarbons)

Various systems of nomenclature have been employed in the past to designate the molecular structures of *polycyclic aromatic hydrocarbons*, also referred to herein by the shorter more convenient name *polyarenes*. The older terminology *polynuclear aromatic hydrocarbons* is less accurately descriptive and is not recommended. The IUPAC nomenclature rules (1979) are now the currently accepted international standard and will be employed throughout this book. Prior to the introduction of the IUPAC system, different peripheral numbering systems were employed by American and European scientists, leading to considerable confusion. Unfortunately, some confusion persists, since the older names and ring numbering systems are encountered in the classic, and still relevant, papers of Fieser, Badger, Cook, Bachmann, Newman, and other pioneers in the field. They are also found in Clar's (1964) two-volume treatise on polycyclic hydrocarbon chemistry as well as in some current chemical catalogs.

In the IUPAC system, trivial names are retained for several ring systems. Some of those encountered frequently are indicated in Table 1.1. For the purpose of numbering, the polycyclic ring system is oriented so that (a) the maximum number of rings lie in a horizontal row, and (b) as many rings as possible are above and to the right of the horizontal row (upper right quadrant). If two or more orientations meet these requirements, the one having as few rings as possible in the lower left quadrant is chosen. These rules are illustrated for benzo[a]pyrene in Fig. 1.1. Numbering commences with the carbon atom in the most counter-clockwise position in the upper-most ring farthest to the right, and proceeds in a clockwise direction (Fig. 1.2). Atoms at ring junctures are designated by adding letters to the number of the position immediately preceding. Interior atoms follow the highest number in clockwise sequence.

Table 1.1. *Names and numbering of common polycyclic aromatic ring systems*

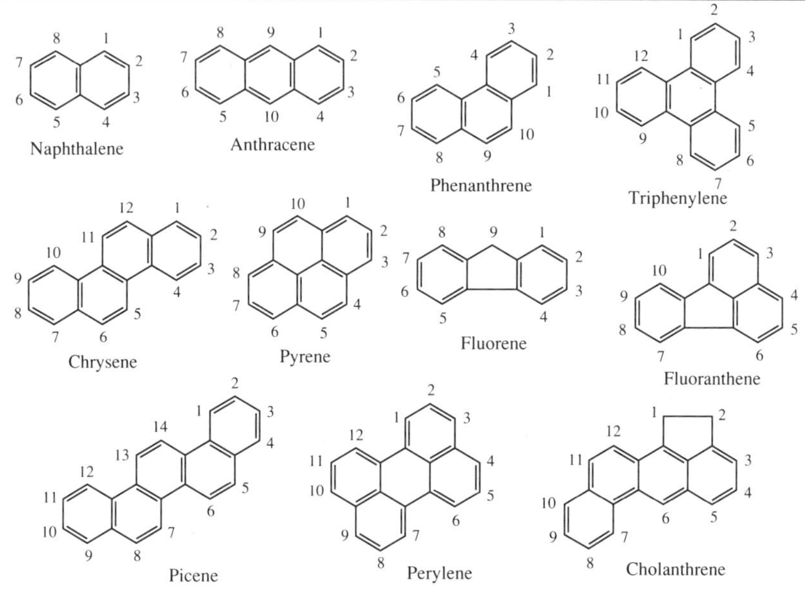

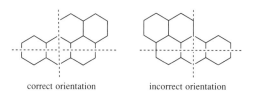

The names of fused ring structures which lack trivial names are obtained by prefixing to the name of a component ring system (the base component) the name(s) of the additional component ring system(s). The base component should contain as many rings as possible, while the attached components should be as simple as possible. Isomers are then distinguished

Fig. 1.1. Orientation of polycyclic ring systems for numbering.

correct orientation   incorrect orientation

Fig. 1.2. Method of numbering and lettering of polycyclic rings.

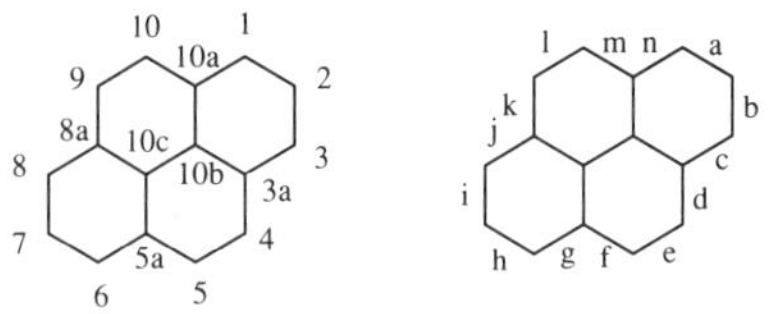

Table 1.2. *Examples of complex polycyclic aromatic ring systems*

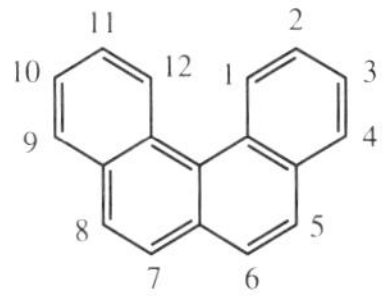

Benzo[c]phenanthrene

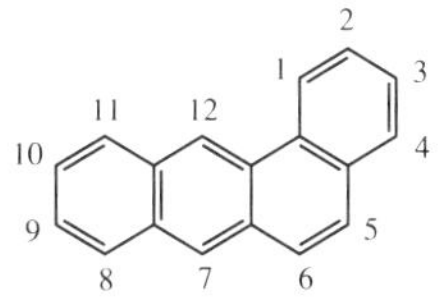

Benz[a]anthracene

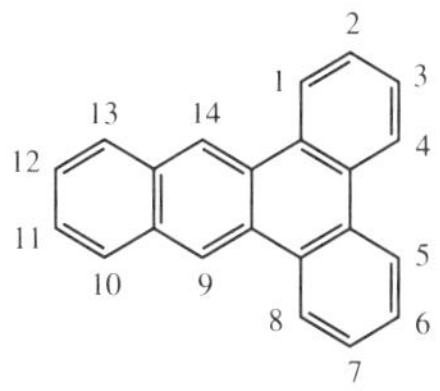

Dibenz[a,c]anthracene

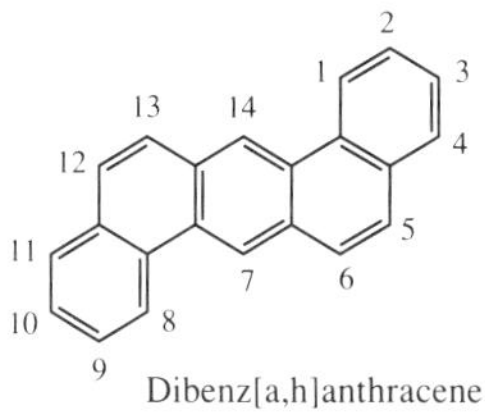

Dibenz[a,h]anthracene

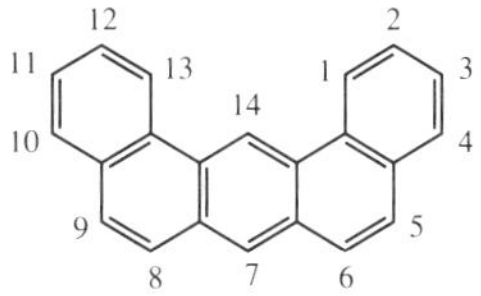

Dibenz[a,j]anthracene

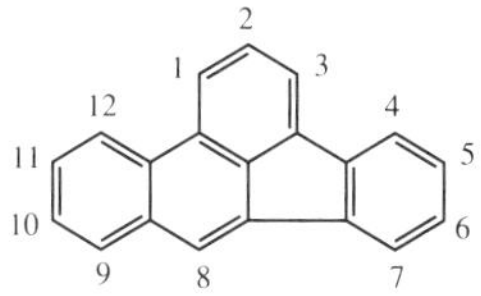

Benz[e]acephenanthrylene

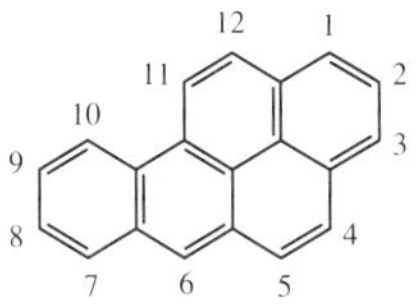

Benzo[a]pyrene

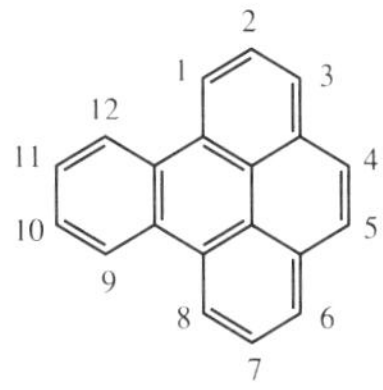

Benzo[e]pyrene

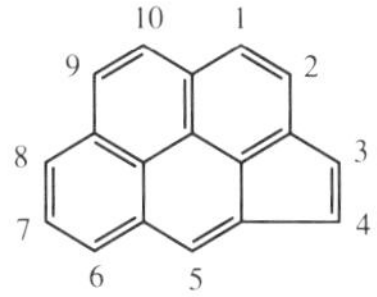

Cyclopenta[c,d]pyrene

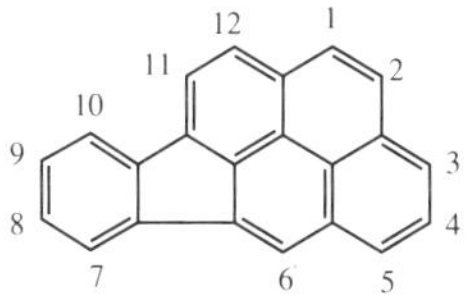

Indeno[1,2,3-cd]pyrene

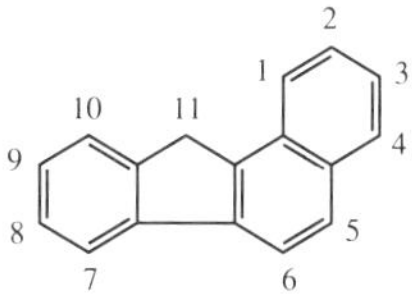

11H-Benzo[a]fluorene

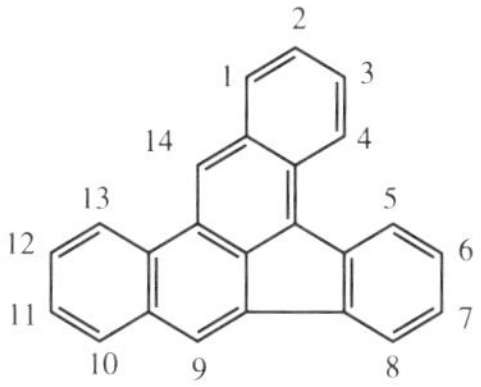

Dibenzo[a,e]fluoranthene

by lettering the sides of the base component a,b,c, etc., beginning with 'a' for the 1,2-side and lettering every side around the periphery. Sides where fusion occur are then designated by a letter as early in the alphabet as possible. The letters are enclosed in brackets and placed immediately after the prefix specifying the attached component. The latter are designated as benzo-, naphtho-, etc., except that the final 'o' is dropped where the base component begins with a vowel. The entire structure is then renumbered according to the rules specified in previous paragraphs. Examples of the names and numbering of some common polycyclic aromatic ring systems are shown in Table 1.2. These relatively simple rules suffice to designate the structures and numbering systems of virtually all of the polyarenes discussed herein.

Certain polyarenes are classed as *acenes* and *phenes,* depending upon whether the rings are *kata*-annealated (i.e. fused linearly), e.g. anthracene, naphthacene (tetracene), pentacene, etc., or *peri*-fused in an angular arrangement, e.g. phenanthrene, benz[a]anthracene (tetraphene), pentaphene, etc. Another class of polyarenes, the helicenes, e.g. hexahelicene, are characterized by a repeating peri-fused arrangement which results in twisting of the ring system out of planarity into a helical corkscrew structure (Fig. 1.3).

Polyarenes may also be classified as *alternant* or *nonalternant.* The common fused aromatic ring systems which contain only benzenoid and fused-benzenoid rings are alternant. These include the arenes and phenes and linear molecules, such as biphenyl and terphenyl. In molecules of this type the conjugated atoms can be divided into two groups, such that each atom is directly linked only to atoms of the opposite group. Conjugate molecules of this type are readily dealt with by perturbational molecular orbital theory (Dewar & Dougherty, 1975). Nonalternant polyarenes, on the other hand, contain odd-numbered rings and are not amenable to treatment by the simple perturbational MO method. Examples of nonalternant hydrocarbons are phenalene, fluoranthene, and cyclopenta[c,d]pyrene (Fig. 1.4).

1.2   Specialized nomenclature in common use

Carcinogenesis research, like all specialized fields, has engendered a specialized terminology outside the formal rules. Thus, certain molecular

Fig. 1.3. Examples of *acene* and *phene* hydrocarbons.

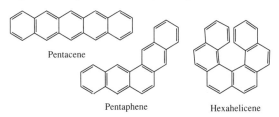

Pentacene

Pentaphene   Hexahelicene

Fig. 1.4. Examples of nonalternant polyarenes.

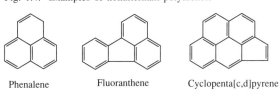

Phenalene   Fluoranthene   Cyclopenta[c,d]pyrene

regions of polyarenes are commonly designated as K-, L-, or M-regions (Fig. 1.5). These terms derive from the quantum mechanical theories of carcinogenesis developed by the Pullmans (1955) and others reviewed in Chapter 4. The *K-region* is a bond, typified by the 9,10-bond of phenanthrene, which is formed by angular fusion of two aromatic rings on a benzene ring. Excision of a *K-region* bond leaves a fully conjugated polyarene. Such bonds tend to be more olefinic, i.e. possess more double bond character, than other bonds in the fused aromatic ring system. Structure–activity studies show that carcinogenic polyarenes generally possess a *K-region*. An *L-region* is a meso molecular region, typified by the 9,10-positions of anthracene or the 7,12-positions of benz[a]anthracene. The term *M-region* was at one time employed to designate molecular sites, such as the 3,4-positions of benz[a]anthracene, where it was thought that metabolism to oxidized products took place selectively. This term was abandoned with the realization that metabolism occurs at numerous structurally diverse molecular sites.

The term '*bay region*', derived from NMR spectroscopy, refers to a molecular region between two angularly fused aromatic rings, typified by the 4,5-positions of phenanthrene. A bay region often accompanies a K-region and is sometimes referred to as 'the back door' of the K-region. Bay region protons are sterically crowded and show characteristic NMR downfield shifts (Jones & Bartle,1972; Memory & Wilson, 1982). Protons in '*fjord regions*', such as the 1,12-positions of benzo[c]phenanthrene, are even more severely hindered and exhibit even greater downfield shifts.

Since the names of the polyarenes are often cumbersome, abbreviations are commonly employed in the biological literature. The following abbreviations are frequently encountered; other abbreviations are given at appropriate points in the text:

BA: benz[a]anthracene
DMBA: 7,12-dimethylbenz[a]anthracene
3-MC: 3-methylcholanthrene
BaP: benzo[a]pyrene

Fig. 1.5. Special molecular regions of polyarenes.

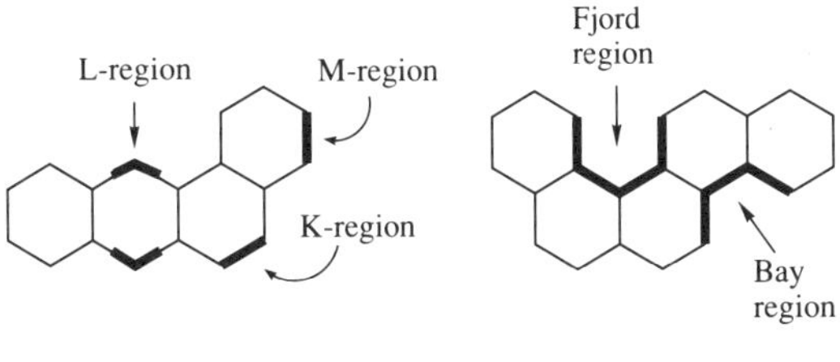

BeP: benzo[e]pyrene
DBahA: dibenz[a,h]anthracene
DBajA: dibenz[a,j]anthracene
PAH(s): polycyclic aromatic hydrocarbon(s)

Finally, it is often convenient for purposes of discussion to letter the rings of polyarenes with capital letters in sequence following the IUPAC ring numbering system. One can then discuss, for example, metabolism in the A-ring or the D-ring without having to employ complicated names.

1.3   Nomenclature of polyarene metabolites

There is currently considerable confusion in the literature in the names employed for polyarene metabolites. The situation is further complicated by the fact that the names used by Chemical Abstracts are in many cases more suited for ease of computer retrieval of information than for facilitation of communication between chemists. Consequently, they frequently differ from those commonly used by the majority of investigators.

According to the IUPAC recommendations, three types of nomenclature systems may be employed: *substitutive, additive,* and *fusion.* The application of these systems to polyarene metabolites is discussed by Loening & Merritt (1988).

In the *substitutive* method, functional groups are cited as prefixes or as suffixes according to their rank in an established order of precedence of functions. For example, phenols may be named with the prefix *hydroxy-* or the suffix *-ol* attached to the name of the hydrocarbon, e.g. 3-hydroxybenzo[a]pyrene or benzo[a]pyren-3-ol. When multiple groups are present as prefixes, they are arranged in alphabetical order among themselves; hydro-prefixes may be treated as detachable and arranged in alphabetical order, or they may be treated as non-detachable and affixed to the name of the parent molecule. When a group is cited as a prefix, it is formally considered to substitute for one or more hydrogen atoms of the parent molecule. According to this concept, arene oxides are considered to be products of substitution of the corresponding dihydroaromatic hydrocarbons by the '*epoxy*' group. Thus, the arene oxide produced by metabolism of benz[a]anthracene in the 3,4-position would be designated as 3,4-epoxy-3,4-dihydrobenz[a]anthracene (Fig. 1.6). In this system, the related dihydrodiol of benz[a]anthracene might be named 3,4-dihydroxy-3,4-dihydrobenz[a]anthracene or 3,4-dihydrobenz[a]anthracene-3,4-diol. However, neither of these names specifies the stereochemistry of the molecule. The relative steric relationship of the hydroxyl groups is commonly designated by the prefix *cis* or *trans*; however, this is not approved nomenclature. Each of the *cis/trans* stereoisomers may exist as pairs of (+) and (-) enantiomers. The nomenclature for optical isomers is discussed in later paragraphs.

In the *additive* nomenclature, atoms are considered to simply add to the parent structure, leaving the total number of hydrogen atoms unchanged. In this system, the name of the attached group (except for hydro prefixes) is placed after that of the parent compound. Although it is useful in some cases, this method of nomenclature is generally discouraged. In the additive system, the benz[a]anthracene derivatives in the previous paragraph would be named benz[a]anthracene 3,4-oxide and 3,4-dihydrobenz[a]anthracene 3,4-diol, respectively.

The *fusion* method of nomenclature is documented in IUPAC Rule A-21.3, and its application to polycyclic aromatic hydrocarbons and their heterocyclic analogs is discussed in detail by Loening & Merritt (1983). In this method, rings containing the maximum number of non-cumulative double bonds are fused, and the structure is then oriented and renumbered. The naming of the arene oxide derivative of benz[a]anthracene by the fusion nomenclature is shown in Fig. 1.6. This method is used by Chemical Abstracts, but has not gained acceptance by investigators in the field of hydrocarbon carcinogenesis research.

The specification of the stereochemistries of polyarene metabolites is one of the more difficult and confusing features of their nomenclature. Both the relative and absolute stereochemical configurations must be considered. Metabolic transformation of hydrocarbons tends to proceed with high stereoselectivity (Chap. 4). The dihydrodiol metabolites produced by mammalian cells are generally the *trans* isomers in which the hydroxyl

Fig. 1.6. Examples of the IUPAC nomenclature systems illustrated for two benz[a]anthracene (BA) derivatives.

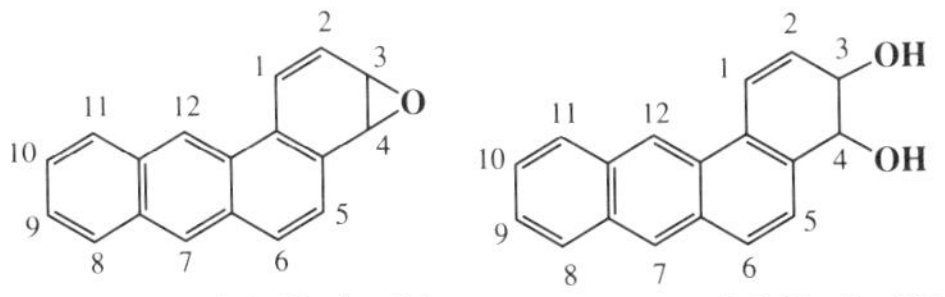

Substitutive: 3,4-Epoxy-3,4-dihydro-BA   3,4-Dihydroxy-3,4-dihydro-BA

Additive: BA 3,4-oxide   3,4-Dihydro-BA-3,4-diol

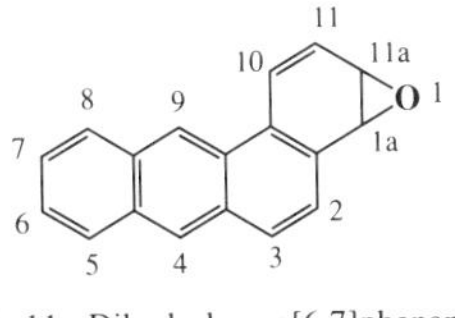

Fusion: 1a,11a-Dihydrobenzo[6,7]phenanthro[1,2-<u>b</u>]oxirene

groups are on opposite faces of the planar hydrocarbon molecule, whereas metabolism by bacteria affords exclusively the *cis* isomers. In both cases strong preference for formation of a particular enantiomer is generally observed.

In the most popular nomenclature, the relative orientation of the hydroxyl groups in the dihydrodiols is designated by the prefixes *cis* or *trans*. The Greek symbols α and ß are also often used to indicate relative stereochemistry, and this usage is sanctioned by *Chemical Abstracts*. The IUPAC rules introduce the use of two new symbols, *R** and *S** for describing relative configurations. These symbols are assigned by the same sequence procedure used in the Cahn–Ingold–Prelog Sequence Rule for the assignment of absolute stereochemistries. According to this rule, assignment of the absolute terms *R* and *S* depends upon the priority of ranking of atoms or groups attached to the chiral center being considered. The ranking depends upon the descending order of atomic number of the atoms directly attached to

Fig. 1.7. Assignment of the stereodescriptors R and S.

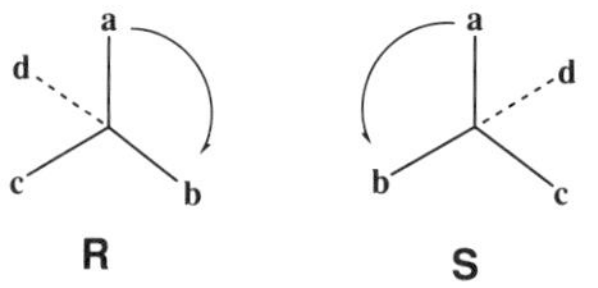

Fig. 1.8. Nomenclature of the racemic benz[a]anthracene diol epoxide (BADE).

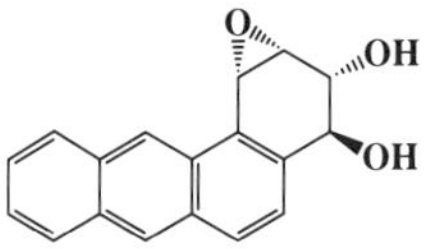

Common usage: A. 1α,2α -epoxy-3α,4ß-dihydroxybenz[a]anthracene
  B. trans-3,4-dihydroxy-anti-1,2-epoxy-1,2,3,4-tetrahydro-BA
  C. anti- or anti-BADE

IUPAC (substitutive): 1R*,2S*,3S*,4R*-1,2-epoxy-1,2,3,4-tetrahydro-BA-3,4-diol

Fig. 1.9. Absolute configurations of the benzo[a]pyrene diol epoxides.

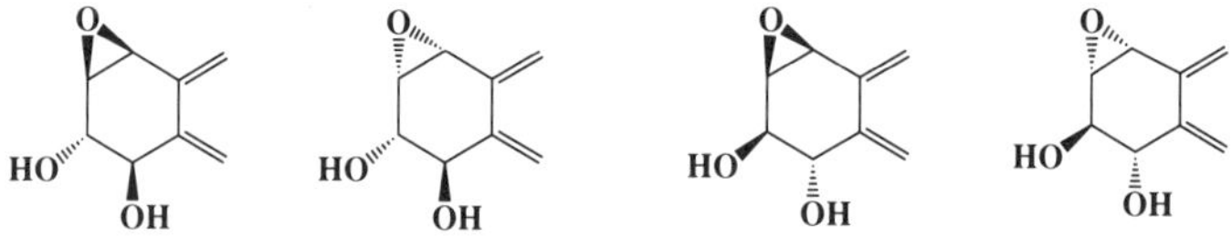

| (-)-(7R,8S,9R,10S) | (+)-(7R,8S,9S,10R) | (-)-(7S,8R,9R,10S) | (+)-(7S,8R,9S,10R) |
| (-)-Syn | (+)-Anti | (-)-Anti | (+)-Syn |

the chiral center and the size of the groups attached. This sequence may be represented by the letters *a, b, c, d* in Fig. 1.7. The least preferred atom or group *d* is considered to lie below the plane of the paper, while *a, b, c* may be imagined to project toward the viewer. The clockwise sequence *a, b, c* is assigned the descriptor *R*, while the counterclockwise sequence is designated as *S*. The symbols *R** and *S** may be used to specify relative configuration by arbitrary assignment of *R** to the center of chirality with the lowest locant. However, these latter symbols have not as yet gained acceptance in the polyarene field.

The nomenclature of the biologically important diol epoxide metabolites offers the greatest potential for confusion. Two diastereomers are possible for the diol epoxides formed from the vicinal *trans* dihydrodiols. These differ in whether the epoxide oxygen atom is on the same or the opposite face of the molecule relative to the benzylic hydroxyl group. Since each diastereomer may exist as a pair of enantiomers, four stereoisomers are possible. The relative configurations of the diastereomers are most commonly specified by the Greek letters α and β or by the terms *anti* and *syn* (Fig. 1.8). In the latter terminology, the *anti* diastereomer is the one in which the epoxide oxygen atom is on the opposite face of the molecule as the benzylic hydroxyl group, while in the *syn* isomer these groups are on the same face of the molecule (Beland & Harvey, 1960). While these terms have no official IUPAC status, they offer considerable convenience and simplicity for communication and are widely employed. In the IUPAC system, the relative configuration of the diol epoxides are specified by the symbols R* and S* (Fig. 1.8). Finally, the arbitrary names *diol epoxide* **1** and **2** are also sometimes used to designate the *syn* and *anti* isomers, but these terms offer no advantage and are not recommended. In all of these nomenclature methods, optical activity or its lack is ordinarily indicated by the symbols (+)(-) or ($\pm$) placed before the name. The absolute configurations of diol epoxide molecules are unambiguously specified by the R,S system. The absolute configurations and names of the diol epoxide isomers of benzo[a]pyrene are shown in Fig. 1.9.

1.4   References

Beland, F. & Harvey, R. G. (1976). The isomeric 9,10-oxides of *trans*-7,8-dihydroxy 7,8-dihydrobenzo[a]pyrene. *J. Chem. Soc. Chem. Commun*, 84-5.

Clar, E. (1964). *Polycyclic Hydrocarbons*. New York: Academic Press.

Dewar, M. J. S. & Dougherty, R. C. (1975). *The PMO Theory of Organic Chemistry*. New York: Plenum.

IUPAC (1979). *Nomenclature of Organic Chemistry*, Sections A to H, p. 559. Oxford: Pergamon.

Jones, D. W. & Bartle, K. D. (1972). The application of proton magnetic spectroscopy to structure identification in polycyclic aromatic molecules. In *Advances in Organic Chemistry*, ed. E. C. Taylor, pp. 317-423. New York: Wiley-Interscience.

Loening, K.L. & Merritt, J. E. (1983). Some aids for naming polycyclic aromatic hydrocarbons and their heterocyclic analogs. In *Polynuclear Aromatic Hydrocarbons*, eds. M. Cooke & A. J. Dennis, pp. 819-43. Columbus, OH: Battelle Press.

Loening, K.L. & Merritt, J. E. (1988). Nomenclature of metabolic products of PAH. In *Polynuclear Aromatic Hydrocarbons*, eds. M. Cooke & A. J. Dennis, pp. 535-54. Columbus, OH: Battelle Press.

Memory, J. D. & Wilson, N. K. (1982). *NMR of Aromatic Compounds*. New York: Wiley-Interscience.

Pullman, A. & Pullman, B. (1955). Electronic structure and carcinogenic activity of aromatic molecules. In *Advances in Cancer Research*, Vol. III, ed. J. P. Greenstein & A. Haddow, pp. 117-69. Wiley-Interscience: New York.

2

Environmental occurrence and cancer

Polyarenes are probably the most widely distributed class of potent carcinogens present in the human environment. Significant levels of polyarenes are found in the air we breathe, the food we eat, and the water we drink.

In this chapter we will survey briefly current information on the occurrence and sources of polyarenes in the environment and the history and methods of experimental polyarene carcinogenesis research. The following chapter will review structure–activity relationships, metabolic activation and current concepts of the mechanism(s) of polyarene carcinogenesis.

2.1   Environmental occurrence

The principal sources of PAHs in the atmosphere are combustion of fossil fuels in heat and power generation, refuse burning, and coke ovens, together contributing over 50% of the total estimated nationwide emission of the carcinogenic hydrocarbon benzo[a]pyrene (BaP). Vehicle emissions, though less significant as a percentage of the total worldwide, may account for as much as 35% of the total PAH emissions in the United States (Bjorseth & Ramdahl, 1985). Emissions from this source are major contributors to urban environmental contamination, particularly in areas adjacent to highways and airports. Although there are natural sources of PAHs (e.g. volcanic activity and forest fires), the anthropogenic sources are considered to be by far the most important for air pollution (Grimmer, 1983). According to recent estimates, the annual emission of BaP into the atmosphere of the United States is approximately 1300 tonnes!

Polyarenes can be formed by the combustion or pyrolysis of virtually all organic materials. Pioneering contributions to understanding the mechanisms of formation of PAHs under pyrolysis conditions were made by Badger (1965). The principal mechanistic pathways are thought to involve free radical pathways. While there is evidence for alternative modes of formation, e.g. polymerization of acetylene or Diels–Alder reactions of butadiene, they appear to be of lesser importance. The patterns of polyarenes produced by pyrolysis vary markedly with temperature (Blumer, 1976). At high temperatures, as in the coking of coal, the products consist of relatively simple mixtures of unsubstituted polyarenes; under these conditions the less stable alkyl bonds are rapidly cleaved. At intermediate temperatures, as in the smoldering of wood, complex mixtures of unsubstituted and alkyl-substituted polyarenes are formed, with the former predominating. At low temperatures, aromatization also proceeds given enough time. Crude oils formed by the decay of plants over millions of years exhibit characteristic patterns of aromatic hydrocarbons in which alkyl-substituted polyarenes far exceed unsubstituted polyarenes. Evidently, the temperature is too low for fragmentation of the carbon–carbon bonds in the alkyl chains to occur. Crude petroleum is also distinguished by the relatively high ratio of compounds with saturated five-membered rings and the presence of highly strained molecules, such as 4,5-methylenephenanthrene, having a methylene bridge between aromatic rings (Blumer, 1976).

Urban atmospheric polyarene levels are dependent upon season, meteorological conditions, and the density and types of local emission sources. Because of the complexity of the mixtures present and the limitations of the analytical techniques, BaP was the only PAH determined in many older investigations. Data compiled by Sawicki *et al.* (1962) for several US cities revealed average PAH concentrations of 14.3 and 2.6 ng/m^3 in winter and summer, respectively, during 1958–9. The higher concentrations observed during the winter season reflect the increase in fossil fuel consumption during the colder months. The PAH concentrations in urban air are less related to city size than to types of industries and other sources present. As might be anticipated, high levels are associated with heavy coal burning industry (e.g. in the cities of Birmingham and Pittsburg). In recent years these levels have exhibited a downward declining trend in both coke oven and noncoke oven population centers.

Although BaP is often employed as an index of airborne PAH levels, its concentration may vary widely relative to the numerous other polyarenes present. Other polyarenes (with four or more rings) commonly present in significant concentrations include: pyrene, fluoranthene, benz[a]anthracene, chrysene, 5-methylchrysene, benzo[e]pyrene, benzo[b]fluoranthene, benzo[j]fluoranthene, benzo[k]fluoranthene, benzo[g,h,i]fluoranthene, dibenz[a,h]anthracene, cyclopenta[c,d]pyrene, anthanthrene, benzo[g,h,i]-perylene, and coronene.

Many of the airborne polyarenes are associated with or adsorbed on particulate matter. In general, the PAHs remain in the gas phase at temperatures above 150 °C but rapidly condense onto fly-ash particles below that temperature (Schure & Natusch, 1982). At typical ambient temperatures, PAHs exist primarily in the particle phase. In a Canadian study of urban airborne particulates it was found that 85% of the PAHs were associated with particles less than 5 μm in diameter (Albagli *et al.*, 1974). Particles less than 5 μm are defined to be 'respirable particles' because they can penetrate through the upper respiratory airways to the lower airways and even to the alveoli. Thus, it appears that the majority of PAHs in the atmosphere may contribute to the health risk.

Atmospheric polyarenes, free or in the form of particulates, are subject to a variety of chemical and photochemical transformations. Among the major pathways for PAH degradation in the atmosphere are reactions with the oxides of nitrogen and sulfur, photochemical reactions with oxygen, and reactions with secondary air pollutants produced by photolysis, such as ozone, peroxyacetylnitrate, and hydroxyl and peroxyl radicals. These chemical processes have been reviewed (Lane, 1989; Van Cauwenberghe,1985). While the majority of these reaction pathways result in formation of products exhibiting diminished bioactivity, mutagenicity assays of environmental samples have revealed the presence of direct-acting mutagens not accounted for by the polyarenes present (Wang, 1978). Evidence that some of these might be nitro derivatives was provided by the observation by Pitts *et al.* (1978) that direct-acting mutagenic nitropolyarenes were formed in model atmospheres containing PAHs, nitrogen oxide, and traces of nitric acid. In this system BaP underwent 60% conversion into three isomeric mononitro derivatives in 8 hours. More direct evidence was provided by detection of 6-nitro-BaP as an air pollutant by Jager (1978). Since these initial reports, numerous papers have appeared which show that nitropolyarenes are widespread environmental contaminants which may pose a significant human health hazard. The formation of nitropolyarenes and their biological properties have been reviewed by Van Cauwenberghe (1985) and Beland *et al.* (1985), respectively.

Not surprisingly, significant levels of polyarenes are also found in the earth in all regions of the planet. Concentrations in urban and industrial areas are 10–100 times higher than in nonurban areas. Forest fires and airborne pollution account for a significant percentage of the PAH levels in remote regions. Biosynthesis has been suggested as another potentially important source. Experimental evidence for the biosynthesis of BaP by bacteria, algae, and various higher plants (rye, wheat, lentils) grown in PAH-free environments has been reviewed by Baum (1978). However, Grimmer & Duvel (1970) were unable to confirm the biosynthetic formation of PAHs in

Table 2.1. *Levels of polyarenes in foods*[a]

Food type	Benz[a]anthracene	Chrysene	Benzo[a]pyrene
Cereals	0.4–6.8	0.8–14.5	0.25–0.84
Salad	4.6–15.4	5.7–26.5	2.8–5.3
Spinach	16.1	28.0	7.4
Tomatoes	0.3	0.5	0.2
Cooking oil	0.5–13.5	0.5–129	0.9–1
Broiled meat or fish	0.2–31	0.5–25	0.2–11
Smoked meat or fish	0.02–189	0.3–123	
Roasted coffee	0.5–14	0.6–19	0.1–4
Tea		4.6–6.3	3.9–21

[a]Data are from Baum (1978) and are expressed as μg PAH/kg dried material.

higher plants. More extensive experimental investigations with a wider range of plant species will be required to settle this question. The PAHs present in recent sediments and soils outside of industrial areas consist mainly of unsubstituted polyarenes. They are accompanied by methyl and alkyl-substituted analogs and derivatives containing five-membered rings. Sulfur-containing analogs are also present. Blumer (1976) has noted that this pattern corresponds to that found for medium temperature pyrolysis and suggests that the major source of PAHs in soils uncontaminated by anthropogenic sources is from natural fires.

The polyarenes in fresh water may originate from fallout of particulate matter transported through the air, from runoff of polluted ground sources, as well as from direct pollution of rivers and lakes by municipal and industrial effluents. In fact, PAHs are widely distributed throughout the waters of the earth and enter the food chain by being taken up by plankton, mollusks, and fish. Since some of these PAHs are only slowly degraded, they represent a potential health hazard to man through drinking water. The average level of BaP in drinking water is estimated to be about 0.01 μg/l which is of a similar order to that from breathing reasonably clean air (Baum, 1978). Treatment of water with chlorine or ozone reduces PAH levels (Radding *et al.*, 1976). The PAH profiles of marine sediments uncontaminated from anthropogenic sources contain relatively high ratios of terpene-derived hydrocarbons, such as alkylated-tetrahydrophenanthrenes, indicative of early fossilization (diagenetic) origin (Laflamme & Hites, 1979; Wakeham *et al.*, 1980). However, the PAH concentrations in marine sediments tends to reflect the industrial situation in the surrounding land area.

Contamination of foods with polyarenes is also widespread. The levels of several PAHs in various foods are summarized in Table 2.1. Highest levels of

PAHs are found in leafy plants, such as lettuce, spinach, tea, and tobacco, and in smoked meats and fish. The relatively high concentrations in leafy vegetables apparently reflects contamination from the atmosphere. However, only a small portion (10%) is removable by washing (Grimmer, 1968). Apparently substantial absorption of the deposited polyarenes into the leaf tissues takes place. Polyarenes are present not only in broiled and smoked fish and meats, but also in fresh meats and seafood. In the latter cases, the PAH contamination may derive from air and water pollution as well as from animal feed. Cooking of meat increases the total PAH burden through pyrolysis and contamination by smoke.

Another potentially important source of exposure of human populations to PAHs is through mineral oils and refined petroleum products used in cosmetics and medicinal products (IARC, 1983). Refined petroleum products with potential traces of PAHs are ingredients of many cosmetic preparations (e.g. cold creams, suntan oils, baby lotions). Some cosmetics prepared from vegetable oils may also contain trace amounts of BaP and other PAHs.

While public attention has focused primarily on industrial sources of environmental contamination, there is substantial evidence that personal habits and lifestyle contribute more importantly to individual risk. The greatest increase in cancer mortality in the USA over the past 30 years is in lung and other tobacco-related cancers. Numerous studies both in the USA and abroad have concluded that cigarette smoking is by far the most important single factor contributing to an increased risk of developing cancer of the respiratory tract (Loeb *et al.*, 1984). Tobacco smoke is a complex mixture in which the gas phase is estimated to contain at least 150 compounds, and more than 2000 components have been identified in the particulate phase (Hoffmann *et al.*, 1978). Among the latter are numerous polyarenes, including many having tumorigenic properties (Table 2.2). Although less is known about marijuana smoke, recent studies indicate that marijuana smoke condensates exhibit mutagenic activity near the same range as that of tobacco smoke condensates (Busch *et al.*, 1979).

It is evident from the foregoing brief summary that human populations are chronically exposed to a wide diversity of polyarenes many of which are carcinogenic. The relative extent of exposure of an individual is dependent upon a range of factors including geographical location, occupation, diet, and lifestyle.

2.2   Experimental carcinogenesis

Research in chemical carcinogenesis has its foundation in the astute observation of the British surgeon Sir Percival Pott (1775), of an association between the incidence of scrotal cancer in chimney sweeps and their

Table 2.2. *Polyarenes in the particulate phase of tobacco smoke*[a]

Polyarene	Carcinogenic activity	ng/cigarette
benzo[a]pyrene	+++	10–50
5-methylchrysene	+++	0.6
dibenz[a,h]anthracene	++	40
benzo[b]fluoranthene	++	30
benzo[j]fluoranthene	++	60
dibenzo[a,h]pyrene	++	ND[b]
dibenzo[a,i]pyrene	++	ND
indeno[1,2,3-c,d]pyrene	+	4
benzo[c]phenanthrene	+	ND
benz[a]anthracene	+	40–70
chrysene	±	40–60
benzo[e]pyrene	±	5–40
2- and 3-methylchrysene	±	7
1- and 6-methylchrysene	–	10
2-methylfluoranthene	+	34
3-methylfluoranthene	ND	40
dibenz[a,c]anthracene	+	ND

[a]Data are from Hoffmann *et al.* (1978). [b]ND = no data available.

exposure to soot. The modern era of experimental hydrocarbon carcinogenesis research was initiated 140 years later by Yamagiwa and Ichikawa in Japan (1915) who succeeded in inducing skin tumors in the ears of rabbits by repeated applications of coal tar. Shortly thereafter Tsutsui (1918) produced tumors in mice by repeated application of tar to the skin. This assay was quickly adopted by other laboratories and is still in use today.

Subsequent events which led to the identification of specific PAHs as active carcinogenic components of coal tar represent one of the classic tales of scientific discovery. The complete story has been reviewed by Kennaway (1955) who was one of the key participants. Initial studies by Bloch & Dreifuss (1921) in Switzerland established that the carcinogen present in coal tar was high boiling, free of nitrogen and sulfur, formed a stable picrate, and was probably a complex hydrocarbon molecule. Kennaway in London (1925), who conducted a number of notable studies on coal tar, demonstrated that pyrolyses of isoprene and acetylene in an atmosphere of hydrogen gave rise to carcinogenic distillates, providing additional evidence that carcinogenic activity could reside in a compound containing only carbon and hydrogen. A second vital clue was the observation by Mayneord, a physicist working with Kennaway, that the carcinogenic tars exhibited a characteristic fluorescence spectrum. None of the PAHs available at the time had this unique spectral property. The problem was resolved by Cook, Hewett & Hieger (1933) who isolated from two tonnes of coal tar pitch the principal carcinogenic component that exhibited the characteristic fluorescence. This they identified as BaP by comparison with an authentic sample synthesized independently. According to Kennaway, the clue which provided 'the single thread that led all through the labyrinth' was the characteristic strong fluorescence spectrum of the active component. Fluorescence spectroscopy provided the twin advantages of high sensitivity and speed of measurement, whereas carcinogenicity tests required 1–2 years. Prior to the isolation of BaP, Kennaway & Hieger (1930) tested the hydrocarbon dibenz[a,h]-anthracene, synthesized by Clar, and found it to be a carcinogen. Thus, dibenz[a,h]anthracene was actually the first pure hydrocarbon of established molecular structure shown to be a carcinogen.

Almost simultaneous with the isolation and identification of BaP was the finding by Wieland & Dane (1933) that pyrolysis of the bile acid 12-ketocholanic acid in the presence of selenium afforded another carcinogenic hydrocarbon identified as 3-methylcholanthrene. Shortly thereafter, Fieser & Seligman (1935) devised a total synthesis of cholanthrene and its 3-methyl derivative, both of which proved to be carcinogenic. The origin of 3-MC from the bile suggested that carcinogens might be produced *in vivo* by abnormal metabolic processes.

The discovery that hydrocarbon molecules of specific structure induced cancer in experimental animals was a momentous discovery, since it marked a departure from the 'germ theory' of disease. This finding also provided a powerful stimulus for research into the chemistry and biological properties of polyarenes. Chemists on both sides of the Atlantic undertook the synthesis of structurally diverse fused aromatic hydrocarbon molecules in the hope that structure–activity correlations might provide some insight into the mechanism of causation of cancer. Synthetic approaches to numerous types of polyarenes and their substituted derivatives were devised by Cook, Clar, Bachmann, Fieser, Badger, and others in the decade following the discovery of the carcinogenic activity of BaP. From these investigations emerged certain generalizations concerning the structural requirements of molecular size and shape and the influence of substituents as well as steric and electronic factors on biological activity.

2.3 Methods of bioassay

Before proceeding to a discussion of the structure–activity relationships, it is necessary to consider briefly the bioassay systems employed. The most valid test of carcinogenic activity is direct demonstration of tumor induction in experimental animals. However, activity in animals is strongly dependent upon experimental variables, e.g. species and strain, sex, age, site and mode of administration, the purity of the compounds tested, and whether promoters are employed. For this reason, it is invalid to compare literature results obtained using different test systems. More complete surveys of bioassay procedures may be found in reviews by Arcos & Argus (1968) and Weisburger & Williams (1984).

Species differ markedly in their susceptibility to various carcinogens. For example, the skins of rabbits and mice are highly susceptible to induction of tumors by PAHs painted on the surface, while rat epidermis is quite resistant. Conversely, on subcutaneous injection of the same compound the rat is often highly sensitive, while the rabbit is relatively unresponsive. More remarkably, these susceptibilities may be reversed towards a different carcinogen. Thus, 2-aminoanthracene elicits a high incidence of malignant skin tumors in the rat, but not in the mouse. Mice and rats are the predominant species employed for PAH carcinogenesis testing. Their choice is dictated by their short life span, high reproductive rates, small size, low cost, and relatively high susceptibility to PAH carcinogens. Hamsters, cats, guinea pigs, monkeys, and dogs are increasingly more resistant to this class of carcinogens.

Differences in susceptibilities between wild strains and inbred strains are also often large. Genetically homogeneous strains of rats and mice available from commercial sources yield more reproducible results and allow comparison of results from different laboratories. Inbred rat strains in common use are Wistar albino, Sprague–Dawley albino, and Long–Evans hooded. The inbred mouse strains in common use include A (albino), BALB (albino), C (cinnamon), CH3, C57 black, DBA (dilute brown), SWR (Swiss albino), and SENCAR. These strains are selected for their predictable incidences of spontaneous tumor formation in specific tissues. For example, CH3 mice show a high incidence of mammary tumors, whereas C57 black mice exhibit a particularly low incidence of both mammary and lung tumors.

Pronounced sex differences in susceptibility are also frequently observed. These differences were frequently ignored in the older literature, undermining the significance of much of the reported data. In one of the more dramatic examples of sex differences, Huggins *et al.* (1961) showed that administration of 7,12-dimethylbenz[a]anthracene (DMBA) by oral stomach tube (20 mg) elicited mammary cancer in 100% of female Sprague–Dawley rats, whereas in male Sprague–Dawley rats this compound proved highly toxic at the same dosage, and administration of lower dosages resulted in high yields of stem cell leukemias (Huggins *et al.*,1974; Huggins, 1979). The DMBA-induced mammary tumors exhibit hormone dependency, regression of the tumors occurring on ovariectomy, hypophosectomy, or hormonal treatment (Huggins, 1979; Welsch, 1985). Sex differences in administration by skin painting may be partially related to the difference in the amount of skin fat. In female mice, the thickness of the fat layer doubles in the proestrus period and decreases quite suddenly after ovulation.

The mode of administration is another critical factor. The most commonly employed methods in addition to skin painting are oral, subcutaneous, intraperitoneal, intramuscular, implantation, and inhalation. The choice of method is dictated by the susceptibility of the animal to tumor induction by the means selected, the stability and solubility of the compound under the conditions employed, the desire to mimic human exposure conditions, and other factors. Skin painting on mice is the most common method employed. However, many potent carcinogenic PAHs, such as DMBA, undergo photo-oxidation on exposure to air and light, making it essential to observe appropriate precautions to prevent this possibility. It is also important to note that the nature of the carcinogenic response is often dependent upon the route of administration. For example, intravenous administration of an emulsion of DMBA and other PAHs to male Long–Evans rats leads to induction of leukemia (Huggins & Sugiyama, 1966), whereas intramuscular injection of the same PAHs to the same strain of rats produces local sarcomas at the site of injection (Harvey & Dunne, 1978). The pros and cons of the various routes of administration are discussed by Arcos *et al.* (1968).

The age of the animals must also be taken into account. Immature animals exhibit enhanced susceptibility to the effects of carcinogens. This effect is partially a consequence of the greater percentage of their cells undergoing differentiation coupled with the less developed state of their immune systems and detoxifying microsomal enzyme systems. At the opposite end of the age spectrum, older animals also show increased susceptibility to carcinogen-induced tumorigenesis.

Tumor promotion is another important variable in carcinogenesis assays. Tumor promoters are defined as agents that are not in themselves carcinogenic but which significantly increase tumor incidence in animals pretreated with carcinogens. In the classic experiments of Berenblum & Shubik (1947), tumors were elicited in mice by painting on the skin a single subthreshold dose of a PAH insufficient to induce tumors, followed by treatment at weekly intervals with croton oil. The active components of croton oil are the phorbol esters (Fig. 2.1), the chemistry of which has been reviewed by Hecker (1971) and by Van Duuren (1969). Phorbol, the parent alcohol ($R_1 = R_2 = H$), is inactive while 12-o-tetradecanoyl-phorbol-13-acetate (TPA) is the most active ester derivative. The combination of TPA plus an initiating carcinogen is approximately ten times as effective in inducing tumors as the carcinogen alone (Marx, 1978). Other commonly employed promoters are Tween and anthralin. Tobacco smoke contains a number of promoters (Hoffmann *et al.*, 1978).

The mechanism of promotion is not well understood. According to the *two-stage theory of carcinogenesis* proposed by Berenblum (1954), the *initiation* step, which may result in no morphological change, induces latent tumors and is irreversible. The *promotion* step in which the initiated cells undergo conversion to cancer cells is reversible. The time interval between initiation and promotion may influence the latency period but not the overall consequences. While all carcinogens are initiators, some function solely as initiators, e.g. benz[a]anthracene, requiring promotion to elicit the tumorigenic response. The more potent carcinogens, e.g. BaP, act as their own promoters, and are said to be *complete carcinogens*. It is generally assumed by most investigators that initiation involves covalent interaction of an active PAH metabolite with DNA, although alternative mechanisms cannot be ruled out. Understanding of the mechanism of promoter action is complicated by the multiplicity of biological effects observed. Phorbol esters induce hyperplasia, alter the growth properties and morphology of cells in culture, increase phospholipid synthesis, induce plasminogen activator and ornithine decarboxylase, and inhibit cell differentiation. Phorbol esters have also been found to cause gene amplifications, chromosomal aberrations, DNA strand breaks, and the induction of sister chromatid exchange.

Understanding of the mechanisms of tumor promotion has been advanced recently by the discovery (Nishizuka, 1986) that the phorbol ester TPA activates protein kinase C, an enzyme of critical importance in the regulation of cell surface signal transduction and cellular proliferation. Subsequent studies indicate that PKC is the major cellular receptor for TPA (Weinstein, 1988). Several other high affinity but structurally dissimilar PKC activators with tumor promoter activity have also recently been discovered (Sugimura *et al.*, 1983). These and other recent findings suggest that PKC plays a critical role in normal cellular growth control and that it mediates several of the cellular effects of the phorbol ester tumor promoters (Weinstein, 1988). Other mechanistic pathways may also be operative (Blumberg, 1981; Murray *et al.*, 1990).

Fig. 2.1. Structure of the phorbol esters.

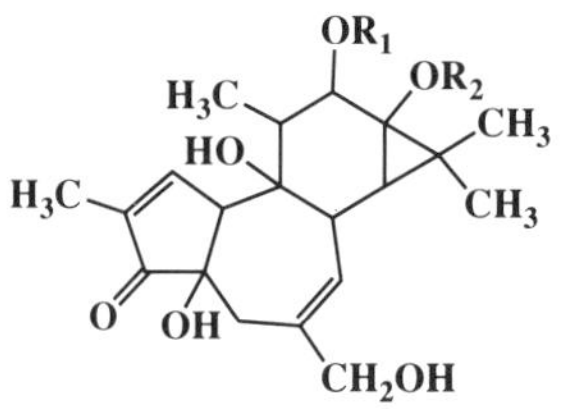

Cocarcinogens and *anticarcinogens* may also influence the outcome of carcinogenesis experiments. Cocarcinogens are agents which when administered simultaneously with a carcinogen to an experimental animal result in a higher incidence of tumors than does either agent alone. Although cocarcinogens are generally thought of as chemical compounds, the definition may be broadened to include viruses and radiation. Many examples of a synergistic enhancement of activity between carcinogens have been reported, but cocarcinogenic activity is also exhibited by noncarcinogens, such a *n*-dodecane and catechol. Since cocarcinogens often occur in the environment with carcinogens, e.g. in tobacco smoke or polluted atmospheres, their potential importance in human cancer cannot be ignored. Cocarcinogenesis has been reviewed by Sivak (1979).

Anticarcinogens, as the name implies, are agents which inhibit carcinogenesis. Lacassagne *et al.* (1945) first showed that combined application of a strong carcinogen, such as 3-methylcholanthrene, and a weak or inactive PAH like 13H-dibenzo[a,g]fluorene, inhibited tumor induction. Huggins *et al.* (1964) subsequently demonstrated that even a highly potent carcinogen, such as DMBA, could act as an anticarcinogen when a subthreshold dose is administered prior to a larger dose of the same or different carcinogen. Astonishingly diverse classes of chemicals exhibit anticarcinogenic properties. These include phenolic antioxidants, ascorbic acid, flavones, coumarins, PAHs, azo dyes such as Sudan III, retinoids, inhibitors of prostaglandin synthesis, anti-inflammatory steroids, protease inhibitors, and various sulfur compounds. The antioxidants BHA (butylated hydroxyanisole) and BHT (butylated hydroxytoluene), which are common food additives, are effective inhibitors of PAH-induced tumor induction (Slaga & Bracken, 1977). Anticarcinogenic coumarin derivatives are constituents of a wide variety of plants, including vegetables such as cabbage and brussel sprouts. The mechanisms of inhibition of carcinogenesis appear to be diverse. Theories advanced to explain the effects of the anticarcinogens include: (1) direct interaction of the anticarcinogen with the carcinogen or its active metabolite; (2) inhibition of enzymatic activation of the carcinogen; and (3) induction of detoxifying microsomal enzymes. Anticarcinogenesis has been reviewed by Wattenberg (1978,1985) and by DiGiovanni & Slaga (1981).

2.4 Short-term *in vitro* bioassays

The standard animal bioassays for the detection of chemical carcinogens require large resources of time and money and necessitate the specialized skills of veterinarians and pathologists. Costs have escalated rapidly in recent years. For these reasons a variety of *in vitro* tests have been developed for the preliminary screening of potential carcinogens (Weisburger & Williams, 1984). Since no single test system is 100% effective, a battery of tests is commonly employed.

The most widely employed short-term bioassay procedures involve bacterial mutagenesis. The popular Ames test measures back mutation to histidine independence of histidine-requiring mutants of *Salmonella typhimurium*. Mammalian enzyme preparations are employed for the metabolic activation of polyarenes and other procarcinogens. The test procedure may be modified to employ bacterial strains that are also repair-deficient, that possess abnormalities in the cell wall that make them permeable to carcinogens, or that carry an R factor that enhances mutagenesis. The validity of the Ames assay has been tested with a large number of compounds and found to be about 80% accurate.

Mutational assays using mammalian cells are also widely employed for screening. The most popular of these entails mutagenesis at the hypoxanthine-guanine phosphotransferase (HGPRT) locus. In this assay, mutants deficient in the purine salvage enzyme are identified by their resistance to toxic purine analogs, such as 8-azaguanine or 6-thioguanine. The target cells employed are usually fibroblast types, such as the Chinese hamster V79 and CHO cell lines. While fibroblast lines lack the ability to metabolize all potential carcinogens to active species, they are able to activate polyarenes. HGPRT mutagenesis can also be measured in human cells that can be combined with hepatocytes for bioactivation. Such systems provide direct evidence of effects on the human genome.

Bioassay procedures involving mutagenesis are based on the assumption that most carcinogens act by damaging DNA. While most carcinogens are mutagens with appropriate metabolic activation, the inverse does not follow. Some agents, such as azo dyes that intercalate into DNA, exhibit mutagenic activity but are not carcinogens in animal species. Another problem with such assays concerns the validity of the rat liver enzyme systems commonly employed for activation, particularly with application to polyarenes. Liver tumors are rarely seen in experimental animals exposed to carcinogenic polyarenes. The S-9 fraction possesses different ratios of specific metabolizing enzymes than the tumor susceptible tissues and is deficient in enzymes that yield conjugated metabolites. Despite their inadequacies, mutational assays provide useful procedures for the preliminary screening of potential carcinogenic hydrocarbons.

Chromosome tests reveal genetic damage at a higher level than do mutagenesis assays. Measurement of sister chromatid exchanges (SCE) is relatively convenient to carry out and has shown sensitivity to a wide range of carcinogens. The determination of SCEs is usually carried out in V79 or

CHO cells in the presence of an exogenous metabolizing system, as required. The assessment of SCEs can also be monitored in the peripheral lymphocyctes of exposed human populations.

Further information on *in vitro* bioassay methods may be found in the review by Weisburger & Williams (1984).

2.5   References

Albagli, A., Oja, H. & Dubois, L. (1974). Size-distribution pattern of PAHs in airborne particulates. *Environ. Lett.* **6**, 241-51.

Arcos, A. C. & Argus, M. F. (1974). *Chemical Induction of Cancer*, IIA. New York: Academic Press.

Arcos, A. C., Argus, M. F. & Wolf, G. (1968). *Chemical Induction of Cancer*, Vol. I. New York: Academic Press.

Badger, G. M. (1965). Pyrolysis of hydrocarbons. *Progr. Phys. Org. Chem.* **3**, 1–40.

Baum, E. J. (1978). Occurrence and surveillance of polycyclic aromatic hydrocarbons. *Polycyclic Hydrocarbons and Cancer*, Vol. I., eds H. V. Gelboin & P. O. P. Ts'o, pp. 45–70. New York: Academic Press.

Beland, F. A., Heflich, R. H., Howard, P. C. & Fu, P. P. (1985). The *in vitro* metabolic activation of nitro polycyclic aromatic hydrocarbons. *Polycyclic Hydrocarbons and Carcinogenesis.* Amer. Chem. Soc. Monogr. 283, ed. R. G. Harvey, 371–6. Washington, DC: American Chemical Society.

Berenblum, I. (1954). A speculative review: The probable nature of promoting action and its significance in the understanding of the mechanism of carcinogenesis. *Cancer Res.* **14**, 471–7.

Berenblum, I. & Shubik, P. (1947). A new quantitative approach to the study of the stages of chemical carcinogenesis in the mouse's skin. *Brit. J. Cancer*, **1**, 383–91.

Bjorseth, A. & Ramdahl, T. (1985). Sources and emissions of PAH. *Handbook of Polycyclic Aromatic Hydrocarbons*. 2. A. Bjorseth & T. Ramdahl, 1–20. New York: Marcel Dekker.

Bloch, B. & Dreifuss, W. (1921). Ueber die experimentelle erzeugung von carcino men mit Lymphdriisen und Lungenmetastasen durch Tierbestandteile. *Schweiz. Med. Wochenschr.* **51**, 1033–7.

Blumberg, P. (1981). In vitro studies on the mode of action of the phorbol esters, potent tumor promoters, part 2. *CRC Crit. Rev. Toxicol.* **9**, 199–234.

Blumer, M. (1976). Polycyclic aromatic hydrocarbons in nature. *Sci. Am.* **234 (10)**, 35–45.

Busch, F. W., Seid, D. A. & Wei, E. T. (1979). Mutagenic activity of marihuana smoke condensates. *Cancer Lett.* **6**, 319–24.

Buu-Hoi, N. P. (1964). New developments in chemical carcinogenesis by polycyclic hydrocarbons and related heterocycles: A review. *Cancer Res.* **24**, 1511–23.

Cook, J. W., Hewett, C. L. & Hieger, I. (1933). The isolation of a cancer-producing hydrocarbon from coal tar. *J. Chem. Soc.* 395–405.

DiGiovanni, J., Diamond, L., Harvey, R. G. & Slaga, T. J. (1983). Enhancement of the skin tumor-initiating activity of polycyclic aromatic hydrocarbons by methyl substitution of nonbenzo 'bay region' positions. *Carcinogenesis*, **4**, 403–7.

DiGiovanni, J. & Slaga, T. J. (1981). Modification of polycyclic aromatic hydrocarbon carcinogenesis. *Polycyclic Hydrocarbons and Cancer*, Vol. 3., eds H. V. Gelboin & P. O. P. Ts'o, pp. 259–92. New York: Academic Press.

Fieser, L. F. & Seligman, A. M. (1935). Synthesis of methylcholanthrene. *J. Amer. Chem. Soc.* **57**, 228–9, 942–6.

Fieser, L. F. & Seligman, A. M. (1935a). Cholanthrene and related hydrocarbons. *J. Amer. Chem. Soc.* **57**, 2174–6.

Grimmer, G. (1968). Carcinogenic hydrocarbons in the human environment. *Dtsch. Apoth. Ztg.* **108**, 529.

Grimmer, G. (1983). *Environmental Carcinogens: Polycyclic Aromatic Hydrocarbons, Chemistry, Occurrence, Biochemistry, Carcinogenicity.* Boca Raton, Fla: CRC Press.

Grimmer, G. & Duvel, D. (1970). Biosynthetic formation of polycyclic hydrocarbons in higher plants. VIII. Carcinogenic hydrocarbon in the human environment. *Z. Natur. Forsch. B.* **25** (**10**), 1171–5.

Harvey, R. G. & Dunne, F. B. (1978). Evidence for multiple regions of activation of carcinogenic hydrocarbons. *Nature(Lond.)* **273**, 566–7.

Hecker, E. (1971). Isolation and characterization of the co-carcinogenic principles from croton oil. *Methods in Cancer Res.* **6**, 439–84.

Hecker, E. (1978). Structure–activity relationships in diterpene esters irritant and cocarcinogenic to mouse skin. *Carcinogenesis – A Comprehensive Survey*, eds T. J. Slaga, R. K. Sivak & R. K. Boutwell, pp. 11–48. New York: Raven Press.

Hoffmann, D., Schmeltz, I., Hecht, S. S. & Wynder, E. L. (1978). Tobacco carcinogenesis. *Polycyclic Hydrocarbons and Cancer*, Vol. 1., eds H. V. Gelboin & P. O. P. Ts'o, pp. 85–117. New York: Academic Press.

Huggins, C., Grand, L. C. & Brillantes, F. P. (1961). Mammary cancer induced by a single feeding of polynuclear hydrocarbons and its suppression. *Nature(Lond.)* **189**, 204–7.

Huggins, C. B. (1979). *Experimental Leukemia and Mammary Cancer*, Chicago, IL: University of Chicago Press.

Huggins, C. B., Grand, L. & Fukunishi, R. (1964). Aromatic influences on the yields of mammary cancers following administration of 7,12-dimethylbenz[a]anthracene. *Proc. Natl. Acad. Sci. USA.* **51**, 737–42.

Huggins, C. B. & Sugiyama, T. (1966). Induction of leukemia in rat by pulse-dose of 7,12-dimethylbenz[a]anthracene. *Proc. Natl. Acad. Sci. USA*, **55**, 74–81.

Huggins, C. B., Yoshida, H. & Bird, C. C. (1974). Hormone-dependent stem-cell rat leukemia evoked by a series of feedings of 7,12-dimethylbenz[a]anthracene. *J. Natl. Cancer Inst.* **52**, 1301–5.

IARC. (1983). *IARC Monographs on the Evaluation of the Carcinogenic Risk of Chemicals to Humans: Polynuclear Aromatic Compounds, Part 1, Chemical, Environmental and Experimental Data*, vol. 32, Lyon, France: Internat. Agency Res. Cancer.

Jager, J. (1978). Detection and characterization of nitro derivatives of some polycyclic aromatic hydrocarbons by fluorescence quenching after thin-layer chromatography: application to air pollution analysis. *J. Chromatogr.* **152**, 575–8.

Kennaway, E. (1925). Experiments on cancer-producing substances. *Br. Med. J.* **2**, 1–4.

Kennaway, E. (1955). The identification of carcinogenic compounds of coal tar. *Br. Med. J.* **ii**, 749–52.

Kennaway, E. & Hieger, I. (1930). Carcinogenic substances and their fluorescence spectra. *Br. Med. J.* **1**, 1044–6.

Lacassagne, A., Buu-Hoi, N. P. & Rudali, G. (1945). Inhibition of the carcinogenic action produced by a weakly carcinogenic hydrocarbon on a highly active carcinogenic hydrocarbon. *Brit. J. Exper. Path.* **26**, 5–12.

Laflamme, R. E. & Hites, R. A. (1979). Tetra- and pentacyclic, naturally-occurring, aromatic hydrocarbons in recent sediments. *Geochim. Cosmochim. Acta.* **43**, 1687–91.

Lane, D. A. (1989). The fate of polycyclic aromatic compounds in the atmosphere during sampling. *Chemical Analysis of Polycyclic Aromatic Compounds*, ed. T. Vo-Dinh, 31–58. New York: Wiley.

Loeb, L. A., Ernester, V. L., Warner, K. E., Abbotts, J. & Laszlo, J. (1984). Smoking and lung cancer: An overview. *Cancer Res.* **44**, 5940–58.

Marx, J. L. (1978). Tumor promoters: Carcinogenesis gets more complicated. *Science.* **201**, 515–18.

Murray, A. W., Edwards, A. M. & Hii, C. S. T. (1990). Tumour promotion: Biology and molecular mechanisms. *Chemical Carcinogenesis and Mutagenesis II*, eds C. S. Cooper & P. L. Grover, 135–57. New York: Springer–Verlag.

Nishizuka, Y. (1986). Studies and perspectives of protein kinase C. *Science*, **233**, 305–12.

Pitts, J. N. J., Van Cauwenberghe, K. A., Grosjean, D., Schmid, J. P., Fitz, D. R., Belser, W. L. J., Knudson, G. B. & Hynds, P. M. (1978). Atmospheric reactions of polycyclic aromatic hydrocarbons: Facile formation of mutagenic nitro derivatives. *Science*. **202**, 515–19.

Pott, P. (1775). *Chirurgical Observations Relative to the Cataract, the Polypus of the Nose, the Cancer of the Scrotum, the Different Kinds of Ruptures, and the Mortification of the Toes and Feet*, London: L. Hawes, W. Clarke & R. Collins

Radding, S. B., Mill, T., Gould, C. W., Liu, D. H., Johnson, H. L., Bomberger, D. C. & Fojo, C. V. (1976). *The Environmental Fate of Selected Polynuclear Aromatic Hydrocarbons*, Final Rep., Task Two, EPA 560/5–75–009. Washington, DC: Environ. Prot. Agency, Office of Toxic Substances.

Sawicki, E., Hauser, T. R., Elbert, W. C., Fox, F. T. & Meeker, J. E. (1962). Polynuclear aromatic hydrocarbon composition of the atmosphere in some large American cities. *Am. Ind. Hyg. Assoc. J.* **23**, 137–44.

Schure, M. R. & Natusch, D. F. S. (1982). The effect of temperature on the association of POM with airborne particles. *Polynuclear Aromatic Hydrocarbons: Physical and Biological Chemistry*, eds M. Cooke, A. J. Dennis & G. L. Fisher, 713–24. Columbus, OH: Battelle.

Sivak, A. (1979). Cocarcinogenesis. *Biochem. Biophys. Acta*, **560**, 67–89.

Slaga, T. & Bracken, W. M. (1977). The effect of antioxidants on skin tumor initiation and aryl hydrocarbons hydroxylase. *Cancer Res.* **37**, 1631–5.

Sugimura, T. & Fujiki, H. (1983). New tumor promoters: indole alkaloids, aplisiatoxins, and palytoxin. *Inst. Natl. Sante Rech. Med.* **117**, 109–29.

Tsutsui, H. (1918). Uber das kunstlich Erzeugte Cancroid bei die Maus. *Gann.* **12**, 21.

Van Cauwenberghe, K. A. (1985). Atmospheric reactions of PAH. *Handbook of Polycyclic Aromatic Hydrocarbons*, Vol. 2, eds A. Bjorseth & T. Ramdahl, 351–384. New York: Marcel Dekker.

Van Duuren, B. L. (1969). Tumor-promoting agents in two-stage carcinogenesis. *Prog. Exp. Tumor Res.* **11**, 31–68.

Wakeman, S. G., Schaffner, C. & Giger, W. (1980). Polycyclic aromatic hydrocarbons in recent lake sediments-II. Compounds derived from biogenic precursors during early diagenesis. *Geochim. Cosmochim. Acta*, **44**, 415–29.

Wang, Y. Y., Rappaport, S. M., Sawyer, R. F., Talcott, R. E. & Wei, E. T. (1978). Direct-acting mutagens in automobile exhaust.

Wattenberg, L. W. (1978). Inhibitors of chemical carcinogens. *Adv. Cancer Res.* **26**, 197–226.

Wattenberg, L. W. (1985). Chemoprevention of cancer. *Cancer Res.* **45**, 1–8.

Weinstein, I. B. (1988). The origins of human cancer: Molecular mechanisms of carcinogenesis and their implications for cancer prevention and treatment. *Cancer Res.* **48**, 4135–43.

Weisburger, J. H. & Williams, G. M. (1984). Bioassay of carcinogenes: In vitro and in vivo tests. *Chemical Carcinogens*, Amer. Chem. Soc. Monogr. 182, ed. C. E. Searle, pp. 1323–73. Washington, DC: American Chemical Society.

Welsch, C. W. (1985). Host factors affecting the growth of carcinogen-induced rat mammary carcinomas: A review and tribute to Charles Brenton Huggins. *Cancer Res.* **45**, 3415–43.

Wieland, H. & Dane, E. (1933). The constitution of the bile acids LII. The place of attachment of the side chain. *Z. Physiol. Chem.* **219**, 240–4.

Yamagiwa, K. & Ichiwawa, K. (1915). Uber die kunstliche Erzeugung von Papillom *V. Jap. Path. Ges.* **5**. 142.

3

Structure–activity relationships

The discovery of the carcinogenic properties of polyarenes stimulated wide-ranging investigations of their structure–activity relationships. Implicit in many of these early studies was the assumption that these compounds were directly active and did not require metabolic transformation. This assumption was based on the general observation that all the isolatable metabolites, which included various isomeric phenols, dihydrodiols, quinones, and their conjugates, were less active in animal tests than the parent compounds. Although it has subsequently been established that metabolic activation is a prerequisite for biological activity, structure–activity correlations still provide an important source of information for understanding the molecular mechanisms of enzymatic activation and the covalent interactions of the active metabolites with their ultimate cellular targets, generally presumed to be nucleic acids.

Polyarenes exhibit a remarkably wide spectrum of carcinogenic activity ranging from inactive to the high levels of potency. This fact coupled with their widespread occurrence as environmental pollutants and their ready detectability at low concentrations by their strong UV absorption and fluorescence makes the PAHs particularly attractive models for carcinogenesis research. A large body of data on the carcinogenic properties of polyarenes and their derivatives is available. In addition to various reviews on this topic (Dipple *et al.*, 1984; Harvey, 1979; Arcos & Argus, 1974; Buu-Hoi, 1964; Badger, 1954), detailed information may be found in the series of volumes entitled *Survey of Compounds which have been Tested for Carcinogenic Activity* (National Cancer Institute, 1985) and in the publications of the International Agency for Research on Cancer (IARC, 1973,1983). Spatial limitations do not allow comprehensive survey of all the published data on the carcinogenic activities of polyarenes and their substituted derivatives. Instead, the general features of the relationship between hydrocarbon molecular structure and carcinogenic activity will be reviewed.

Table 3.1. *Carcinogenic activities of alternant polyarenes with 2-4 rings* [a]

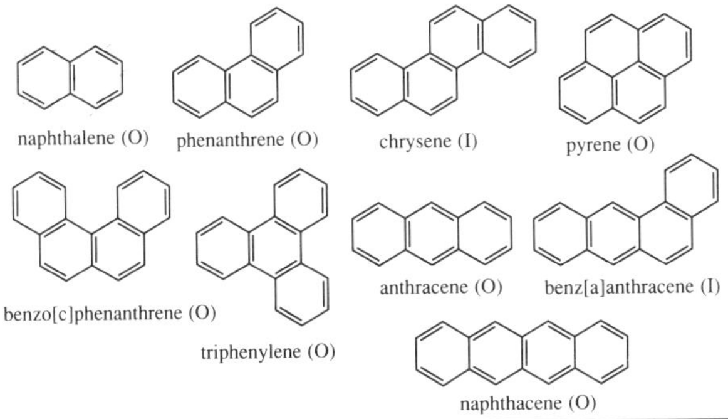

naphthalene (O)   phenanthrene (O)   chrysene (I)   pyrene (O)

benzo[c]phenanthrene (O)   anthracene (O)   benz[a]anthracene (I)

triphenylene (O)

naphthacene (O)

[a]Carcinogenic activity: O= inactive; I = active as initiator. Data are from National Cancer Institute (1985) and Dipple et al. (1984).

3.1   Unsubstituted polyarenes

Most unsubstituted polyarenes having two to four rings (Table 3.1) are inactive as initiators or complete carcinogens. Chrysene and benz[a]anthracene fail to show activity as complete carcinogens, but both exhibit moderate tumor-initiating activity on mouse skin following promotion by TPA.

A number of unsubstituted pentacyclic polyarenes (Table 3.2) exhibit activity as complete carcinogens. In addition to BaP and dibenz[a,h]anthracene, the activities of which have already been mentioned, benzo[c]chrysene and benzo[g]chrysene are moderately active as complete carcinogens and dibenz[a,j]anthracene is a weak carcinogen. The remaining ten pentacyclic isomers are inactive as complete carcinogens, while benzo-[e]pyrene and dibenz[a,c]anthracene are weak tumor initiators on mouse skin.

While larger polyarenes with six or more rings (Tables 3.3 and 3.4) have been less intensively investigated, there is no evidence for an upper size limit on activity. However, the exceedingly low solubility of the high molecular weight PAHs provides a practical upper limitation. Four of the five isomeric dibenzopyrenes tested by subcutaneous injection in mice were found to be exceptionally potent carcinogens; only dibenzo[e,l]pyrene proved to be inactive (Buu-Hoi, 1964). These findings were confirmed by Hoffmann & Wynder (1966). The large naphthacene derivatives naphtho[2,3-a]pyrene, phenanthro[2,3-a]pyrene, dibenzo[a,c]naphthacene, and tribenzo[a,c,j]-naphthacene were also found to be moderately active carcinogens, while the related naphtho[2,3-e]pyrene was inactive (Hoffmann & Wynder, 1966). Benzo[ghi]perylene was weakly active by subcutaneous injection in mice,

Table 3.2. *Carcinogenic activities of pentacyclic alternant polyarenes*[a]

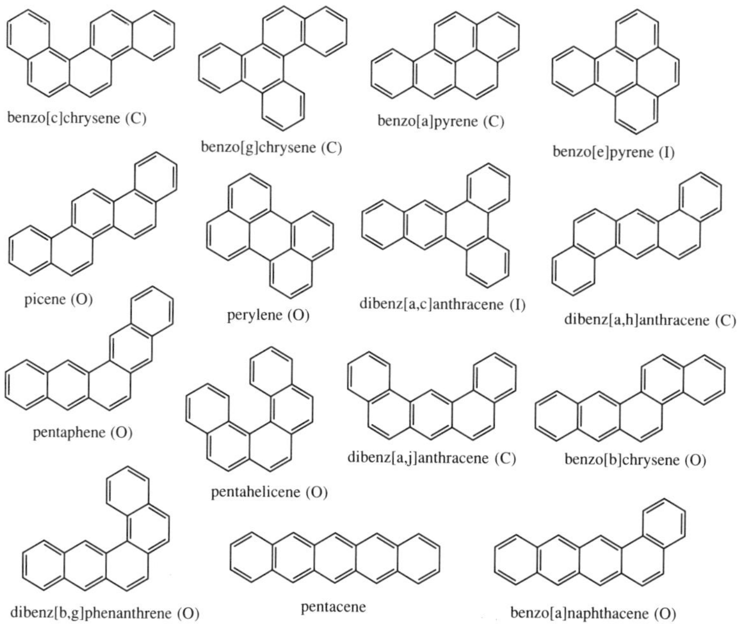

benzo[c]chrysene (C)

benzo[g]chrysene (C)

benzo[a]pyrene (C)

benzo[e]pyrene (I)

picene (O)

perylene (O)

dibenz[a,c]anthracene (I)

dibenz[a,h]anthracene (C)

pentaphene (O)

pentahelicene (O)

dibenz[a,j]anthracene (C)

benzo[b]chrysene (O)

dibenz[b,g]phenanthrene (O)

pentacene

benzo[a]naphthacene (O)

[a]Carcinogenic activity: C = complete carcinogen; O= inactive; I = tumor initiator. Data are from National Cancer Institute (1985), Dipple et al. (1984), Scribner (1973), and Slaga et al. (1980).

but was inactive on mouse skin. The highly symmetrical coronene displayed activity only as an initiator. The heptacyclic hydrocarbons peropyrene and tribenzo[a,e,i]pyrene were moderately active carcinogens, while pyranthrene, benzo[a]coronene, and benzo[e]naphtho[2,3-a]pyrene were all inactive (Lacassagne *et al.*, 1968).

3.2   Effects of substitution

Substitution of polyarenes strongly influences their carcinogenic properties. Benz[a]anthracene has been most thoroughly investigated. In Table 3.5 are summarized data on the carcinogenicity of the monomethylbenz[a]anthracenes for several experimental systems. Essentially similar results were obtained in two-stage initiation-promotion experiments (Wislocki *et al.*, 1982). Methyl substitution in the 6-, 7-, 8-, and 12-positions of BA confers strong activity, independent of the experimental test system. Introduction of two or more methyl groups into these sites gives enhanced activity, while methyl substitution in the benzo ring or the adjacent 5-position tends to diminish or abolish activity (Table 3.6). 3-Methyl-

Table 3.3. *Carcinogenic activities of alternant polyarenes with six rings*[a]

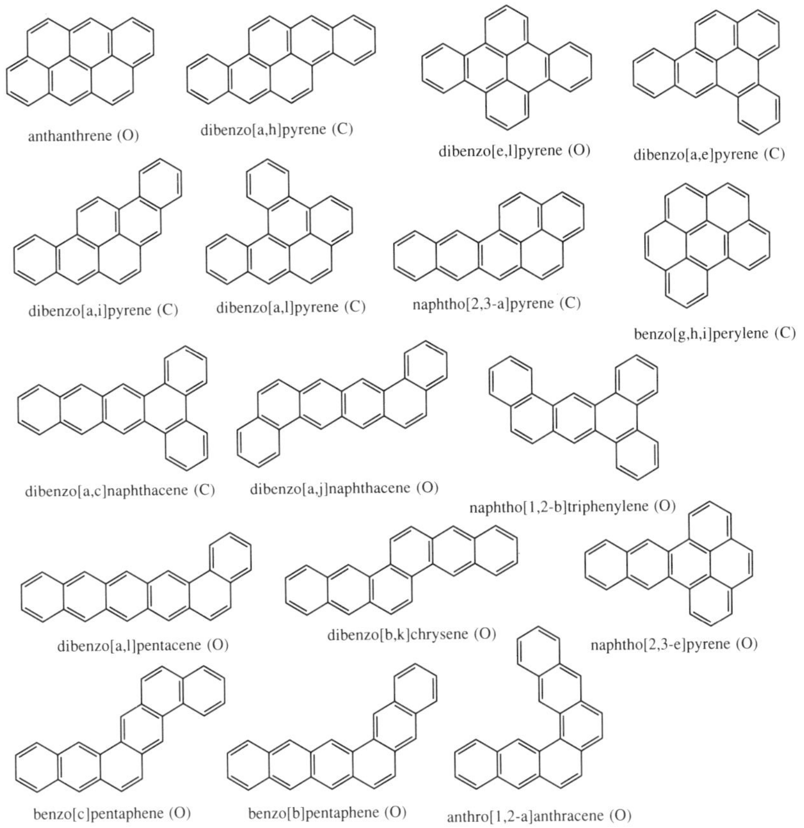

anthanthrene (O)

dibenzo[a,h]pyrene (C)

dibenzo[e,l]pyrene (O)

dibenzo[a,e]pyrene (C)

dibenzo[a,i]pyrene (C)

dibenzo[a,l]pyrene (C)

naphtho[2,3-a]pyrene (C)

benzo[g,h,i]perylene (C)

dibenzo[a,c]naphthacene (C)

dibenzo[a,j]naphthacene (O)

naphtho[1,2-b]triphenylene (O)

dibenzo[a,l]pentacene (O)

dibenzo[b,k]chrysene (O)

naphtho[2,3-e]pyrene (O)

benzo[c]pentaphene (O)

benzo[b]pentaphene (O)

anthro[1,2-a]anthracene (O)

[a]Carcinogenic activity: C = complete carcinogen; O = initiator; I = tumor initiator. Data are from National Cancer Institute (1985), Hoffmann & Wynder (1966), Dipple et al. (1984), and Buu-Hoi (1964).

cholanthrene, which may be considered a 7,8,9-trialkyl-BA derivative, also exhibits strong carcinogenic activity. The parent hydrocarbon cholanthrene is somewhat less active, while 3,6-dimethylcholanthrene, which is a structural analog of DMBA, exhibits twice the activity of 3-MC at the same dosage (DiGiovanni *et al.*, 1983; Sawyer *et al.*, 1988).

Fluoro-substituted derivatives of BA have also been studied on the rationale that the size of the fluorine atom resembles that of hydrogen (Fig. 3.1). However, this assumption is somewhat simplistic, since the strong inductive effect of the halogen atom is likely to seriously distort the electron density of the polyarene ring system, altering its reactivity.

The effects on tumorigenicity of alkyl groups larger than methyl on BA

Table 3.4. *Carcinogenic activities of alternant polyarenes with more than six rings*[a]

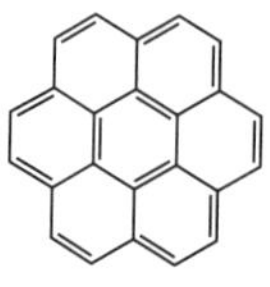

coronene (I)

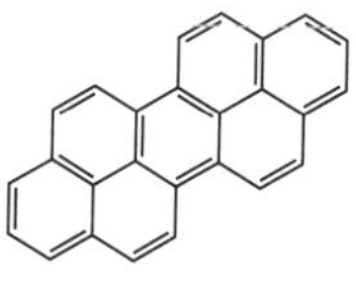

peropyrene (C)

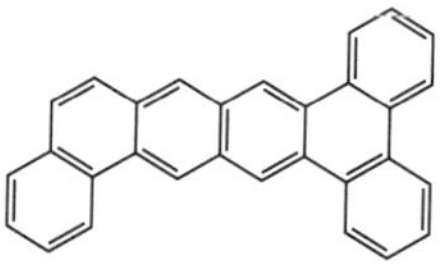

tribenzo[a,c,j]naphthacene (C)

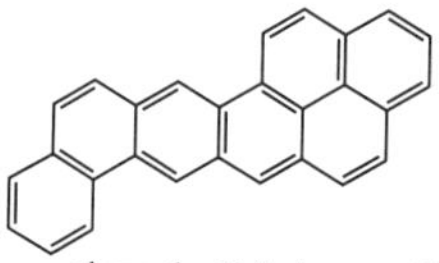

phenanthro[2,3-a]pyrene (C)

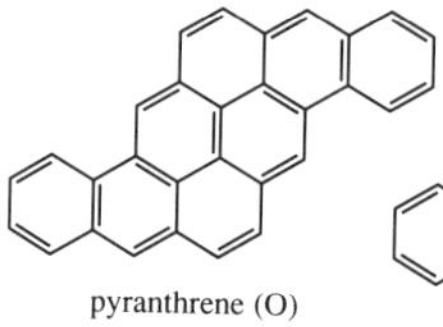

pyranthrene (O)

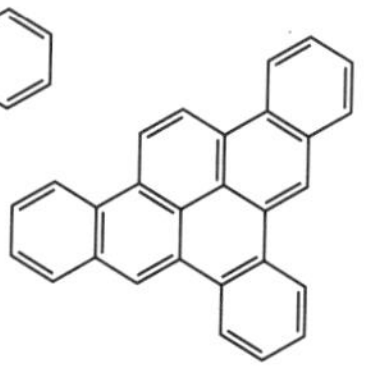

tribenzo[a,e,i]pyrene (C)

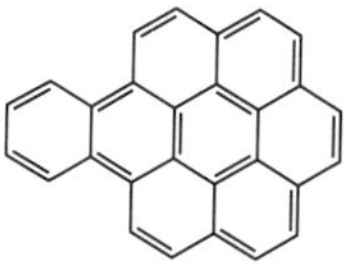

benzo[a]coronene (O)

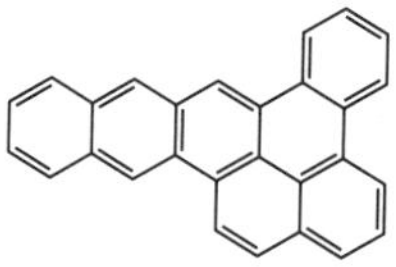

benzo[e]naphtho[2,3-a]pyrene (O)

[a]Carcinogenic activity: C = complete carcinogen; O = inactive; I = initiator. Data are from National Cancer Institute (1985), Lacassagne et al. (1968), and Dipple et al. (1984).

Table 3.5. *Comparative carcinogenicities of monomethylbenz[a]anthracenes*

Methyl isomer	Mode of administration			Methyl isomer	Mode of administration		
	Subcut[a]	Skin[b]	Intramusc[c]		Subcut[a]	Skin[b]	Intramusc[c]
1-	+1	0	0	7-	+4	+4	+4
2-	0	0	0	8-	+3	+3	+3
3-	0	0	0	9-	+1	+1	0
4-	+1	0	0	10-	+1	0	0
5-	+1	0	0	11-	0	+1	0
6-	+3	+3	+3	12-	+3	+3	+3

The data are from [a]Dunning & Curtis (1960), [b]Stevenson & Haarn (1965), and [c]Huggins *et al.* (1967).

have also been extensively investigated (Table 3.7). The 7- and 12-ethyl-BAs exhibit only moderate carcinogenic activity, suggesting that the ethyl group has a lower enhancing effect on bioactivity than the methyl group. One of the most interesting effects of ethyl substitution is the observation of Huggins *et al.* (1967) that both 7-ethyl-12-methyl-BA and 7-methyl-12-ethyl-BA are strongly tumorigenic, while 7,12-diethyl-BA is devoid of activity. It was

Table 3.6. *Carcinogenicities of di- and trimethylbenz[a]anthracenes (DMBA and TMBA)*[a]

DMBA	activity	DMBA	activity	TMBA	activity	TMBA	activity
1,12-	+1	8,9-	+3	1,7,12-	±	6,8,12-	+4
2,9-	0	8,12-	+4	2,7,12-	±	7,8,12-	+4
3,9-	+2	9,10-	+2	3,7,12-	0		
6,7-	+4	4,7-	0	4,7,12-	+4		
6,8-	+4	4,12-	0	5,7,12-	+2		
6,12-	+4	5,12-	0	7,10,11-	+4		
7,12-	+4	7,11-	+4	6,7,8-	+4		
7,8-	+4			6,7,12-	+4		

[a]Data are from the following sources: Harvey (1978); Huggins *et al.* (1967); Dunning & Curtis (1960); Pataki & Huggins (1969); Pataki *et al.* (1971); Lacassagne *et al.* (1962); Heidelberger *et al.* (1962); Huggins *et al.* (1964); Dunning *et al.* (1968); Slaga *et al.* (1979).

suggested that this finding is consistent with a mechanism involving inter-calation of the PAH (or its active metabolite in modern terms) between the base pairs of the DNA helix. 6,8-Diethyl-BA also exhibited strong carcinogenic activity (Pataki & Balick, 1972). Activity falls off rapidly with groups larger than ethyl. The effects of a wide range of other groups on the activity of BA have also been investigated (Badger, 1954; National Cancer Institute, 1972–73; Dipple *et al.*, 1984), and no obvious pattern of structure–activity relationships has emerged. Both electron-donating and electron-accepting groups can enhance carcinogenicity. The only apparent rule is that highly polar groups, such as OH, CO_2H, OCH_2CO_2H, and SO_3H, in

Fig. 3.1. Carcinogenic activities of fluoro-substituted benz[a]anthracenes expressed in a scale of 0 to +4. Data are combined from the following sources which use different test conditions: Miller & Miller, 1960, 1963; Harvey & Dunne, 1978; Slaga *et al.*, 1979, 1980.

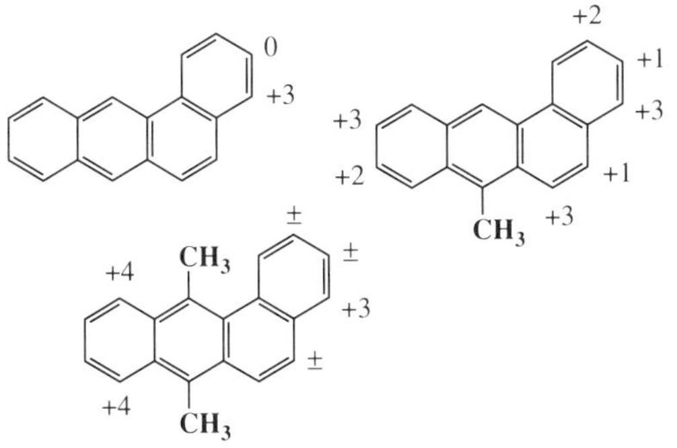

Table 3.7. *Carcinogenic activities of alkyl-substituted benz[a]anthracenes*[a]

Group[b]	Activity[c]	Group[b]	Activity[c]	Group[b]	Activity[c]
7-Et	±	7,8-Et$_2$	0	8-Bu	+2
8-Et	+2	7,9-Et$_2$	0	7-Bu-12-Me	0
12-Et	±	8,12-Et$_2$	+3	7-iBu-12-Me	0
7-Et-12-Me	+3	8-Pr	+1	8-C$_5$H$_{11}$	+2
12-Et-7-Me	+4	8-iPr	+2	8-C$_6$H$_{13}$	+1
7,12-Et$_2$	0	9-iPr	+3	8-C$_7$H$_{15}$	±
6,8-Et$_2$	+4	7-Bu	0		

[a]Data are from Arcos & Argus (1974); National Cancer Institute (1985); Pataki *et al.* (1971); DiGiovanni *et al.* (1983); Charles B. Huggins, personal communication. [b]Et = ethyl; Me = methyl; Pr = n-propyl; iPr = isopropyl; Bu = n-butyl. [c]Activity is expressed in a scale of 0 (inactive) to +4 (highly potent).

Table 3.8. *Carcinogenic activities of mono-, di-, and trimethylbenzo[a]pyrenes*[a]

Methyl isomer	activity	Methyl isomer	activity	Dimethyl isomer	activity	Di- or tri-methyl isomer	activity
BaP	+2	7-	+2(0)	1,2-	+3	4,5-	+3
1-	+3	8-	0	1,3-	+3	7,10-	0
2-	+2	9-	0	1,4-	+3	4,5,7-	+3
3-	+3	10-	±	1,6-	+2	1,3,6-	+1
4-	+3	11-	+3	2,3-	+3		
5-	+2	12-	+3	3,6-	+2		
6-	+2						

[a] Activity is expressed in a scale of 0 (inactive) to +4 (highly potent). Data are from Lacassagne *et al.* (1962a); Dunlap & Warren (1941); Harvey & Dunne (1978); Schurch & Winterstein (1935); and Slaga *et al.* (1980a).

the 7-position abolish activity. This effect may be merely a consequence of the greater water solubility of these polar molecules which facilitates their excretion.

Extensive investigations of the carcinogenic activities of methyl-substituted benzo[a]pyrenes have also been conducted (Table 3.8). The findings indicate that substitution in the benzo ring tends to strongly diminish activity, while substitution elsewhere in the molecule has no effect or enhances activity. Substitution of a wide range of other groups in the 6-position of BaP exhibits a similar pattern of effects as substitution in the analogous 7-position of BA. Thus, the groups OH, Br, CO_2H, and $CONH_2$ negatively influence activity, while the groups CH_2OH, CH_2OSO_3H, CH_2Br, CH_2Cl tend to enhance activity (Badger, 1954; National Cancer Institute, 1972–73; Dewhurst *et al.*, 1972; Cavalieri *et al.*, 1978; Dipple *et al.*, 1984). Particularly notable is the exceptionally high tumorigenicity of the $6\text{-}CH_2OSO_3Na$ derivative of BaP observed by Cavalieri *et al.*, 1978. It has been suggested that this reactive sulfate ester may be an active metabolite of 6-methyl-BaP.

The carcinogenicities of the methylchrysenes have been investigated by Hoffmann *et al.* (1974). 5-Methylchrysene and 5,6-dimethylchrysene were found to be potent carcinogens, while 1-, 2-, 3-, 4-, and 6-methylchrysene were weakly carcinogenic (Fig. 3.2). The 1-, 3-, and 12-fluoro derivatives of 5-methylchrysene proved less active than the parent hydrocarbon, whereas the 6-, 7-, 9-, and 11-fluoro isomers were found to be equipotent with 5-methylchrysene (Hecht *et al.*, 1978).

In the benzo[c]phenanthrene series, five of the six possible monomethyl isomers have been tested. The 3-, 4-, 5-, and 6-methylbenzo[c]phenanthrenes were found to initiate skin tumors in mice on topical application, while the 2-isomer was inactive (Fig. 3.2). The 5-isopropyl- and 5-*n*-propylbenzo-[c]phenanthrenes were also carcinogenic on mouse skin.

Methyl substitution in the meso region of the isomeric dibenzanthracenes,

Fig. 3.2. Carcinogenic activities of (A) methylchrysenes, (B) fluoro-5-methylchrysenes, (C) methylbenzo[c]phenanthrenes, and (D) methyldibenz[a,h]anthracenes expressed in a scale of 0 to +4. Data are from the sources indicated in the text.

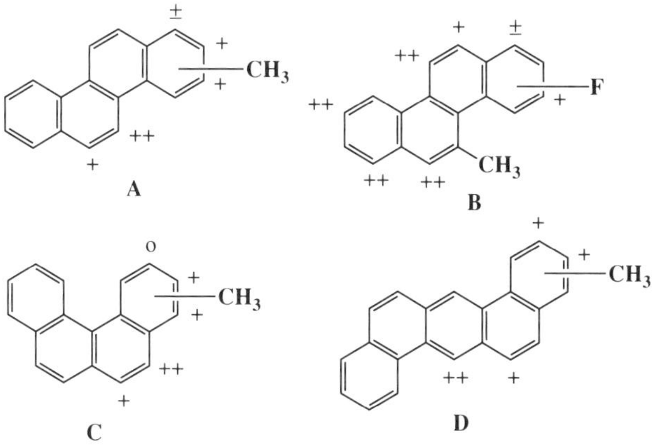

as in benz[a]anthracene, had a dramatic effect on tumorigenicity (Fig. 3.3). While 2-, 3-, and 6-methyldibenz[a,h]anthracene exhibited tumorigenic activity on mouse skin similar to that of the parent hydrocarbon, the 7-methyl isomer showed considerably higher potency, and 7,14-dimethyldibenz- [a,h]anthracene (Fig. 3.3) was strongly carcinogenic towards both the skin and subcutaneous tissues of mice (DiGiovanni *et al.*, 1983; Heidelberger *et al.*, 1962). Methyl substitution in the meso region of the isomeric dibenz[a,j]anthracene also resulted in markedly enhanced carcinogenic activity. While the parent hydrocarbon was only a weak tumor initiator on mouse skin, the 7-methyl derivative showed moderate activity under the same conditions, and 7,14-dimethyldibenz[a,j]anthracene (Fig. 3.3) exhibited a high level of carcinogenic potency, comparable to that of DMBA (DiGiovanni *et al.*, 1983). In contrast, methyl substitution in the same region of dibenz[a,c]anthracene had no effect on activity; 9,14-dimethyldibenz- [a,c]anthracene (Fig. 3.3) exhibited essentially no tumor-initiating activity even at relatively high dosage. This is one of the few exceptions to the rule that substitution of methyl groups in the bay regions of nonbenzo rings enhances carcinogenic activity (DiGiovanni *et al.*, 1983; Hecht *et al.*, 1986).

There are fewer studies of the effects of methyl substitution on the activities of the larger polycyclic aromatic ring systems. Both positive and negative effects on activity are observed. Thus, while benzo[g,h,i]perylene is only weakly active, its 1- and 7-methyl derivatives are moderately potent carcinogens (Lacassagne *et al.*, 1957). Similarly, 6-methylanthanthrene exhibited weak carcinogenic activity and the 6,12-dimethyl compound showed moderate activity, while anthanthrene itself was inactive (Lacassagne

Fig. 3.3.   7,14-Dimethyldibenz[a,h]anthracene (A) and 7,14-dimethyl-dibenz[a,j]anthracene (B) are potent carcinogens, while 9,14-dimethyl-dibenz[a,c]anthracene (C) is noncarcinogenic.

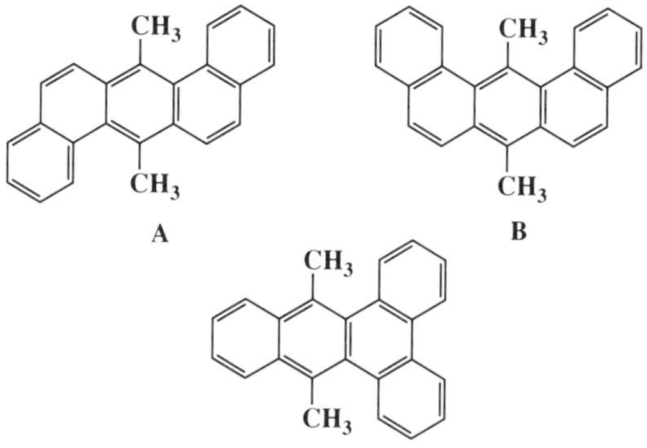

et al., 1958). In contrast, substitution of methyl groups in the dibenzopyrenes in positions corresponding to the meso region of BA results in diminished carcinogenic activity (Lacassagne *et al.*, 1957a, 1958). Thus, 7-methyldibenzo[a,h]pyrene and 5-methyldibenzo[a,i]pyrene are markedly less active than the parent unsubstituted hydrocarbons, while 7,14-dimethyldibenzo[a,h]pyrene and 5,8-dimethyldibenzo[a,i]pyrene are devoid of activity. Methyl substitution in the 5- and 6-positions of dibenzo[a,e]pyrene also results in diminished activity.

3.3 Partially saturated polyarenes

Addition of hydrogen to polyarenes generally alters their chemical and biological properties. The physical effects of hydrogenation include a decrease in the resonance energy of the aromatic ring system, a decrease in molecular planarity and an increase in the molecular thickness, and frequently an improvement in lipid solubility. When hydrogenation occurs in a terminal ring it generally leaves a fully conjugated aromatic ring system. However, when hydrogen addition takes place in a K-region some loss of conjugation may occur due to twisting of the molecule out of planarity. NMR studies of the K-region dihydro derivatives of phenanthrene and related molecules show that molecules of this type exist as an equilibrium mixture of two rapidly interconverting nonplanar conformers (Rabideau *et al.*, 1969; Harvey *et al.*, 1976; Harvey, 1988). The nonplanarity of 5,6-dihydrobenz[a]-anthracenes is also supported by X-ray crystallographic evidence (Zacharias *et al.*, 1977; Glusker, 1978). Addition of hydrogen to the meso region of PAHs with three or more linear rings, such as BA or DBA, interrupts the conjugation of the fused aromatic system leaving two isolated aromatic ring components. NMR studies of molecules of this type indicate that they too exist as mixtures of nonplanar conformers in dynamic equilibrium.

The carcinogenic properties of hydroaromatic polyarenes may be anticipated to resemble those of the analogous dialkyl derivatives of the residual aromatic ring system, if one considers the saturated carbon atoms as alkyl substituents. In agreement with this expectation, 1,2,3,4- and 8,9,10,11-tetrahydro-7-methyl-BA (**1**, **2**) are inactive, and 7,8,9,10-tetrahydro-BP (**3**) and 8,9,10,11-tetrahydro-DMBA (**4**) are only weakly active in comparison with the potent carcinogenic fully aromatic polyarenes (Table 3.9). An interesting exception is 1,2,3,4-tetrahydro-DMBA (**5**) which is reported to be a moderately potent carcinogen on mouse skin (Lijinsky *et al.*, 1983).

The carcinogenic activities of a series of hydrogenated derivatives of dibenz[a,h]anthracene (Table 3.9) on mouse skin were investigated by Lijinsky *et al.* (1965). Saturation of one of the angular benzo rings gave

Table 3.9. *Hydroaromatic derivatives of polyarenes*[a]

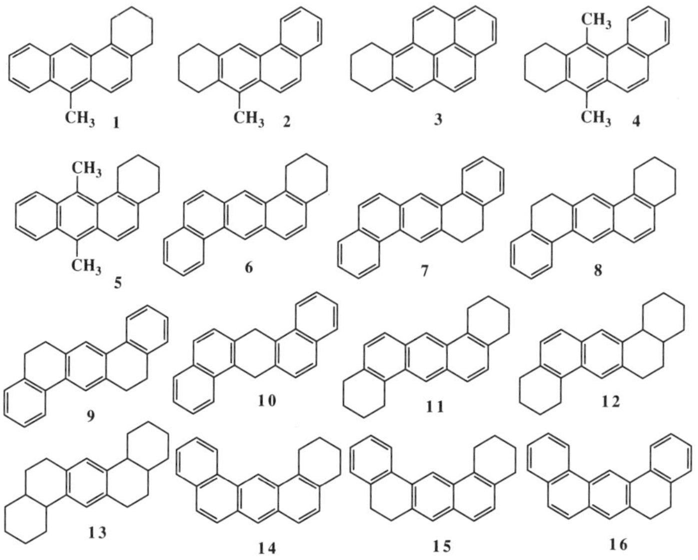

[a]Carcinogenicity data on these compounds may be found in National Cancer Institute (1985) and in references cited in the text.

1,2,3,4-tetrahydro-DBA (**6**) which exhibited activity comparable to that of DBA. Structure **6** is analogous to that of 8,9-dimethyl-BA, a moderately potent carcinogen (Table 3.6). 5,6-Dihydro-DBA (**7**) and 1,2,3,4,12,13-hexa-hydro-DBA (**8**) were both moderately active carcinogens, while 5,6,12,13-tetrahydro-DBA (**9**) was inactive on mouse skin. Addition of hydrogen to the meso region of DBA to afford 7,14-dihydro-DBA (**10**) virtually abolishes carcinogenic activity, and the more extensively hydrogenated DBA derivatives **11**, **12**, and **13** are inactive. In the dibenz[a,j]anthracene series, the tetrahydro and hexahydro derivatives **14** and **15** exhibit activity comparable to that of the parent hydrocarbon, while the 5,6-dihydro derivative **16** showed a fourfold increase in activity. Since these studies were conducted prior to advent of HPLC and other modern analytical methods, it is conceivable that part of the observed activity may derive from small amounts of the parent hydrocarbons which are generally quite difficult to remove. Although there is no direct evidence, it is also conceivable that rearomatization of the hydroaromatic compounds may take place enzymatically in animal tissues (e.g. via benzylic hydroxylation and dehydration).

Additional polyarenes which contain a saturated five or six-membered ring

Table 3.10. *Cyclopentano and cyclohexano-fused polyarenes*[a]

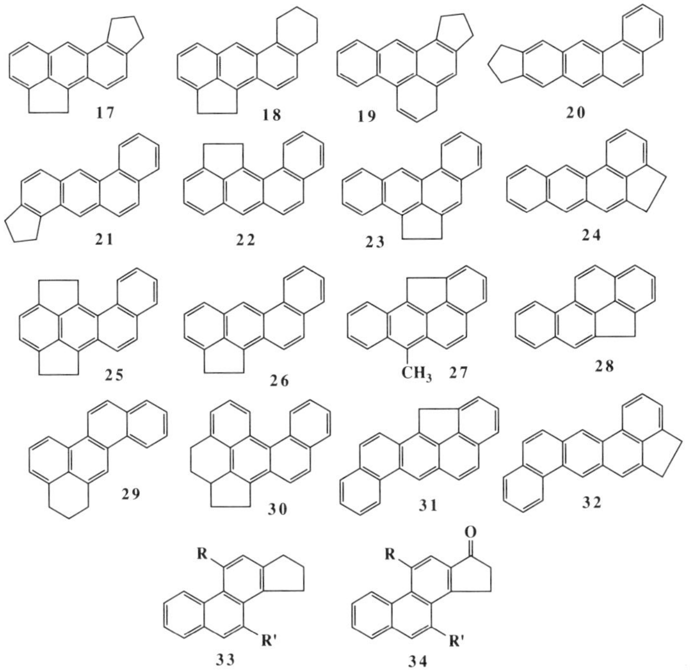

17 18 19 20

21 22 23 24

25 26 CH₃ 27 28

29 30 31 32

R 33 R'   R 34 R' O

a: R = R' = H; b: R = H; R' = CH₃; c: R = CH₃; R' = H

[a]Carcinogenicity data on these compounds may be found in National Cancer Institute (1985) and in references cited in the text.

and exhibit variable levels of carcinogenic activity are listed in Table 3.10. The anthracene derivatives **17–19** show weak to moderate activity on subcut. injection into mice. The cyclopentano derivatives of BA **20–25**, like the isomeric cholanthrene (**26**), are all moderately active carcinogens, while **27** which contains a methylene bridge is only weakly tumorigenic. The chrysene derivatives **28** and **29** are weakly active on subcut. administration to mice. The angular 'stearanthrene' **30**, which may be considered a benzo[c]phenanthrene derivative, was found by Dannenberg (1957) to be equivalent in potency to BaP and 3-MC. Introduction of a methylene bridge into the bay region of DBA to yield **31** had no influence on tumorigenicity, while the cyclopentano DBA derivative **32** was only weakly active. The analogs of **22, 23, 24**, and **26** with a double bond in the cyclopentano ring are active as mutagens in bacterial and rodent cells in the presence of rat liver microsomes, and are therefore potential carcinogens (Nesnow *et al.*, 1984). Interest in PAHs derived from 15,16-dihydro-17H-cyclopenta[a]phenanthrene (**33a**) was originally stimulated by their structural relationship to steroids. These PAHs have been studied extensively by Coombs who has recently reviewed this topic (Coombs & Bhatt, 1987). While the parent hydrocarbon **33a** is inactive as a carcinogen, the 7- and 11-methyl derivatives (**33b,c**) exhibit moderate activity, and the 11-methyl derivative and 11,12-dimethyl derivatives of 15,16-dihydro-17*H*-cyclopenta[a]phenanthren-17-one (**34b,c**) are relatively strong carcinogens.

3.4   Nonalternant polyarenes

In comparison with the alternant polyarenes, the chemical and carcinogenic properties of nonalternant polyarenes are relatively unexplored. Investigations in this area have been hampered by the relative unavailability of nonalternant polyarenes from commercial sources. The potential importance of nonalternant PAHs in human cancer is suggested by their relatively widespread environmental occurrence coupled with the reported tumorigenicity of certain members of this class. Nonalternant polyarenes are of particular interest from the viewpoint of the mechanism of carcinogenesis because of evidence that in some cases they may undergo metabolic activation by different pathways than do alternant PAHs. Three types of nonalternant polyarenes are currently prominent in carcinogenesis research. These are the cyclopenta-fused PAHs and the polycyclic derivatives of fluorene and fluoranthene (Table 3.11), all of which contain a five-membered ring.

Fluorene, which may be considered a methylene-bridged analog of biphenyl, produced no tumors in rats or mice (IARC, 1983). Benzo[a]fluorene (**35**), benzo[c]fluorene (**37**), and dibenzo[c,g]fluorene (**38**) are all reportedly noncarcinogenic, while benzo[b]fluorene (**36**) is a weak tumor-initiator on mouse skin (IARC, 1983), and the dibenzofluorenes **39-41** are all weakly tumorigenic on mouse skin (Buu-Hoi, 1964; Natl. Cancer Inst., 1985).

The polycyclic fluoranthenes are a particularly important class of nonalternant polyarenes due to their environmental prevalence and tumorigenicity. While fluoranthene was found to be a potent mutagen in several assays (Kaden *et al.*, 1979; Thilly *et al.*, 1980), it proved inactive towards the skin and subcutaneous tissues of mice (Buu-Hoi, 1964; Hoffmann *et al.*, 1972). Recently, however, it has been found to be tumorigenic in a newborn mouse lung bioassay (Busby *et al.*, 1984). The benzo analogs benzo[b]fluoranthene (**42**) and benzo[j]fluoranthene (**43**) are moderately active carcinogens (IARC, 1983, LaVoie *et al.*, 1987). In contrast, benzo[k]fluoranthene (**44**) exhibits only borderline activity, and benzo[g,h,i]fluoranthene (**45**) is inactive. Among the dibenzo analogs, dibenzo[a,e]fluoranthene (**46**) is a moderately

Table 3.11. *Fluorenes, fluoranthenes, and cyclopenta-fused polyarenes*

35
36
37
38
39
40
41
42
43
44
45
46
47
48
49
50
52
54
51
53
55

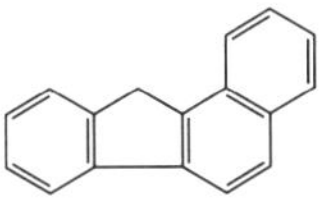

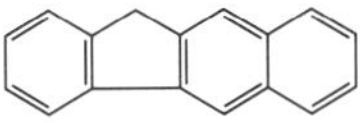

strong carcinogen (IARC, 1983), while the isomer **47** is weakly active and **48** is inactive (Natl. Cancer Inst., 1985). Indeno[1,2,3-cd]pyrene (**49**) is an ubiquitous environmental pollutant which is active as a tumor initiator and complete carcinogen on mouse skin and is carcinogenic in rat lung (Rice *et al.*, 1986).

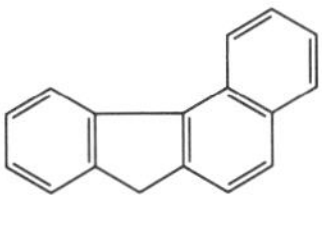

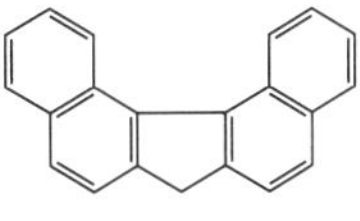

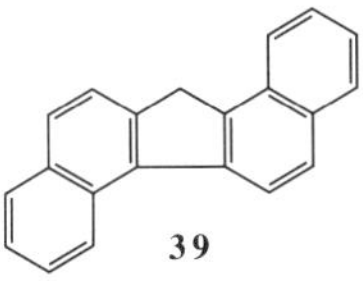

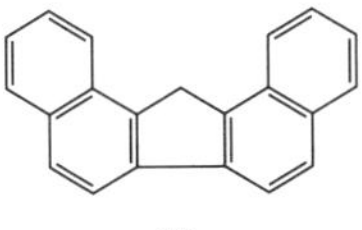

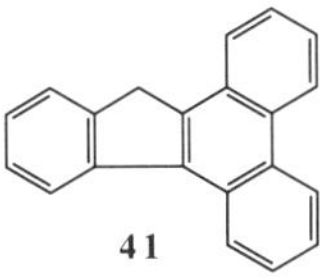

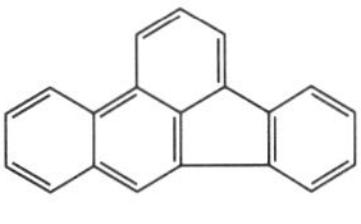

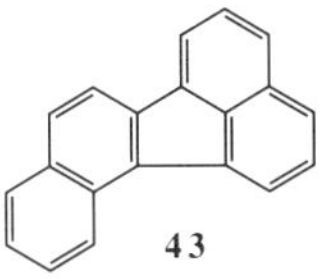

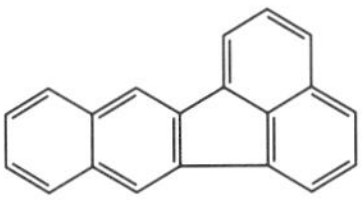

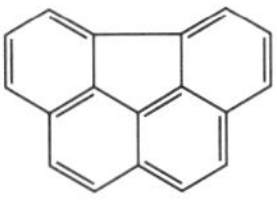

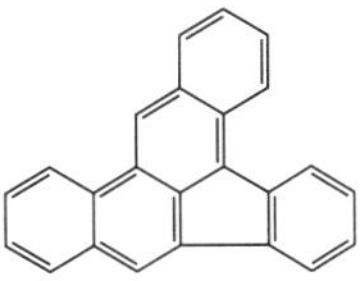

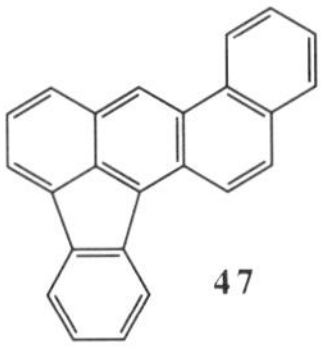

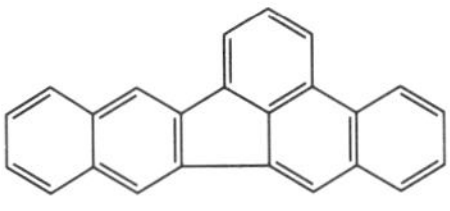

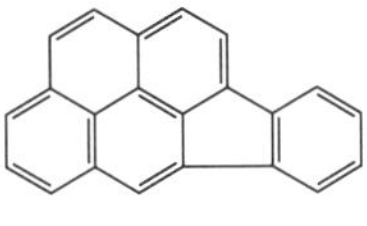

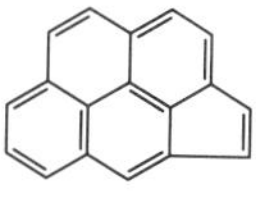

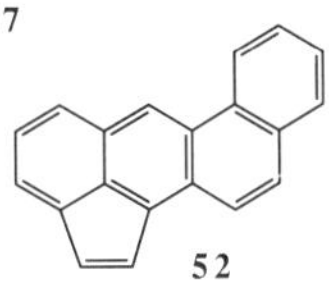

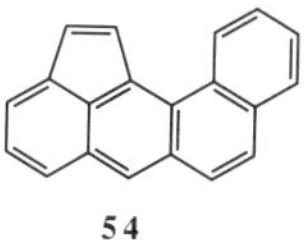

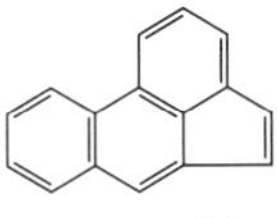

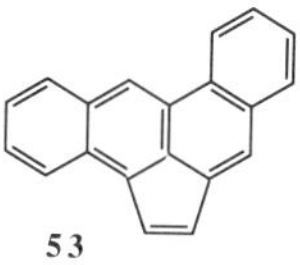

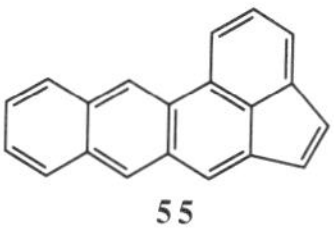

The cyclopenta-fused PAHs, of which cyclopenta[c,d]pyrene (**50**) is the most prominent example, are another potentially important class of nonalternant polyarenes. Cyclopenta[c,d]pyrene has been identified in automobile exhaust, carbon black, ambient air, and cigarette smoke, is mutagenic in bacterial and mammalian cells, and is a tumor initiator on mouse skin and a complete carcinogen (Busby *et al.*, 1988; Cavalieri *et al.*, 1981; Wood *et al.*, 1980). Acephenanthrylene (**51**) has also been identified as an environmental pollutant, but information on its biological properties is not available (Krishnan & Hites, 1981). The four cyclopenta derivatives of benz[a]anthracene **52-5** were all active as mutagens in *Salmonella typhimurium* and in Chinese hamster V79 cells (Nesnow *et al.*, 1984a). Benz[e]aceanthrylene (**53**) and benz[l]aceanthrylene (**54**) are potent tumor initiators on mouse skin (Nesnow *et al.*, 1984); however, no data was available on the tumorigenicity of benz[j]aceanthrylene (**52**) and benz[k]acephenanthrylene (**55**) at the time of writing.

3.5   Minimal structural requirements for activity

Early investigators sought to determine a relationship between molecular structure and oncogenic activity in the hope that this knowledge might provide insight into the mechanism of cancer induction at the molecular level. It was rapidly established that only a small fraction of all PAHs tested exhibited carcinogenic properties, and activity varied widely dependent upon molecular size and shape and other structural features. However, attempts to define precise molecular structural requirements for activity met with only limited success. This is not surprising in the light of more recent research findings that metabolic activation and competing detoxification pathways are intimately involved in the mechanism of PAH carcinogenesis.

Nevertheless, certain broad generalizations relating alternant polyarene structure to activity may be arrived at from consideration of the carcinogenicity data. Thus, the basic minimal requirements for tumorigenic activity appear to be: (1) 4–6 fused aromatic rings; (2) a K-region; and (3) an unsubstituted angular benzo ring. In addition, although not essential, activity is greatly enhanced by the presence of methyl groups in nonbenzo bay region sites (DiGiovanni *et al.*, 1983). The presence of methyl or other groups at other molecular sites may enhance or diminish activity, depending upon the nature of the group and the site of substitution (Hecht *et al.*, 1986). The molecular basis for these substitution effects are only partly understood (Harvey, 1988). They will be discussed in greater detail in Chapter 4 in connection with the discussion of mechanisms of PAH carcinogenesis.

3.6   The relation of chemical properties to activity

Attempts to relate tumorigenicity to some chemical property of the active polyarenes have stimulated numerous investigations. Since no unique mode of chemical reactivity has been uncovered, only a brief survey of these studies will be presented. In one of the earliest reports, Badger (1950) observed increasing reactivity with OsO_4 of a series of hydrocarbons (phenanthrene < pyrene < BA < DBA < BaP < 3-MC < DMBA), correlating with their carcinogenicities. This reaction involves addition exclusively to the K-region bonds to yield on hydrolysis the corresponding *cis*-dihydro-diols. The correlation between osmate reactivity and carcinogenic activity breaks down on extension to a broader range of compounds. However, these studies served to focus attention on the electron-rich K-region which became a key feature of the later electronic theories.

Attempts to relate carcinogenicity to oxidizability by other reagents, such as chromic acid (Cook, 1933), lead tetraacetate (Fieser & Hershberg, 1938a; Fieser & Putnam, 1947), perbenzoic acid (Roitt & Waters, 1949), and ozone (Newman & Otsuka, 1958), have met with even less success. These reactions occur predominantly in molecular regions susceptible to electrophilic attack. The primary oxidation products formed tend to undergo further oxidative transformation to quinones and other more highly oxidized products not usually found as metabolites.

Oxidation of PAHs to radical cations has also been postulated to be involved in tumor induction (Fried & Schumm, 1967; Cavalieri & Rogan, 1985). The ease of formation of radical cations by one-electron oxidants such as iodine or $Mn(OAc)_3$ is related to the ionization potential (IP) of the PAH. According to Cavalieri and Rogan (1985), only polyarenes with low IPs (below 7.35 eV) can be biologically activated to radical cations by one-elec-tron oxidation. According to these investigators, stabilization of the radical cation intermediate by delocalization of its charge tends to favor its reaction with the cellular target. However, correlation between IP and carcinogenicity has a number of exceptions, particularly for methyl-substituted PAHs. For example, 5-methylchrysene whose IP is relatively high (7.7 eV) is a potent carcinogen on mouse skin, while perylene whose IP is low (7.06 eV) is essentially inactive. Also, there is no obvious correlation between the experimentally determined IPs of the methyl-substituted BAs and their carcinogenic properties (Akiyama *et al.*, 1981). Discrepancies of this type may be partly due to dual mechanistic pathways involving one-electron oxidation and diol epoxide intermediates (see **4.3**). However, these mechanisms predict formation of different DNA adducts (assuming nucleic acids are the critical target), and current evidence indicates that the adducts formed with DNA *in vivo* are predominantly those expected to arise by the diol epoxide pathway.

Diels–Alder cycloaddition is another typical reaction of polyarenes which has been considered to be potentially relevant to bioactivity. However, Newman & Otsuka (1958) investigated the rates and equilibrium constants for formation of adducts with maleic anhydride of a series of methylbenz-anthracenes and found no correlation with carcinogenicity.

Polyarenes form complexes with various inorganic and organic compounds as well as with cellular constituents, such as proteins and purines. In one of the earliest studies, Kofahl & Lucas (1954) measured the equilibrium constants for coordination of silver ions with a series of polyarenes. Moderately good correlation between the argentation constants and carcinogenic potency was found. However, the observed range of values was relatively narrow, and these studies were never extended to a broader range of compounds. If, as suggested by Kofahl, coordination with Ag^+ occurs in the electron-rich K-region, complexation with Ag^+ provides an experimental measure of electron density in this region.

Polyarenes form donor–acceptor complexes with a wide variety of molecules substituted with electron-withdrawing groups (Foster, 1969). These noncovalent complexes, which are usually colored, exist as molecular sandwiches stabilized by electronic interactions, hydrogen bonding, and Van der Waals interactions. Although they are often referred to as 'charge-transfer complexes', the term is a misnomer, since charge-transfer forces are generally only a minor component of the binding forces involved. Donor strength is directly related to the number of fused aromatic rings and is enhanced by methyl, alkoxy, amino, and other electron-donating groups in suitable sites and is diminished by electron-withdrawing groups. Conversely, acceptor strength is enhanced by nitro, halo, cyano, carbonyl, and other similar groups. Bulky substituents which interfere sterically with close face-to-face approach of either component retard complexation.

An apparent parallelism between the ability of polyarenes to serve as donors in noncovalent complexes and their carcinogenic activity has intrigued numerous investigators (Mason, 1958; Szent-Gyorgi *et al.*, 1960; Huggins & Yang, 1962). It is striking that the most potent carcinogenic PAHs tend to be strong donors. With 2,4,7-trinitrofluorenone the carcinogenic PAHs BaP, DMBA, and 3-MC afford deeply colored, brown or black complexes, while inactive PAHs generally furnish yellow or orange complexes. However, no correlation between the dissociation constants for TNF complexation and the carcinogenicity of a series of PAHs was found (Takemura *et al.*, 1953; Harvey & Halonen, 1966). In other studies, Allison & Nash (1963) measured the comparative electron donating abilities of a series of PAHs with *o*-chloranil and 1,3,5-trinitrobenzene, and inferred from the results that the carcinogens might act as either electron-donors or electron-acceptors with a cellular receptor. Subsequent studies by other investigators have failed to reveal any clearcut correlation between complexation and biological activity. However, these findings may be irrelevant, since the compounds employed as model acceptors are not the specific cellular receptor involved in the mechanism of carcinogen action.

Complexation of polyarenes with nucleosides and other biologically important compounds was investigated by Harvey & Halonen (1968) utilizing the technique of 'charge-transfer chromatography'. They found the capacity of nucleosides to serve as acceptors follow the order: adenosine > thymidine > uridine > guanosine, with the extent of binding to polyarenes related more directly to the number of fused rings than to carcinogenic activity.

The solubilization of polyarenes by purines and pyrimidines is another closely related phenomenon. Solubilization of BaP in neutral aqueous media by caffeine, xanthine, theobromine, and theophylline was first noted by Brock *et al.* (1938) and extended to other polyarenes and investigated in greater detail by Weil-Malherbe (1946) and Boyland & Green (1962). Relatively high ratios of purines were required for solubilization, and solubility was found to decrease with the number of condensed rings. For example, approximately 1000 molecules of caffeine were needed to solubilize 1 molecule of BaP or 15 molecules of pyrene in a 0.7 M caffeine solution. The solubilizing power of purine and pyrimidines for BaP was in the order: tetramethyluric acid > caffeine > 6-dimethylaminopurine > guanine > adenine > hypoxanthine. The nucleosides were somewhat less effective than the parent purine bases, and the pyrimidines (thymidine, cytidine, and uracil) were ineffectual.

Boyland & Green (1962a) were the first to show that polyarenes and their heterocyclic analogs are solubilized by DNA. They proposed that polyarenes are intercalated between the base pairs of the DNA helix (Boyland *et al.*, 1964). Their findings were confirmed and extended by Liquori *et al.* (1962). In other related studies, Lerman (1964) observed enhancement of the viscosity of dilute solutions of DNA by acridine dyes and polyarenes which he interpreted in terms of an intercalation model. Solubilization of polyarenes is accompanied by bathochromic shifts of the absorption spectra and fluorescence quenching. These effects are abolished on heat denaturation or treatment of the DNA complexes with ethylene glycol or formamide which disrupt the hydrogen bonding critical to the helical structure. RNA exhibits lower solubilizing power consistent with its minimal helical structure. Additional evidence for complexation is found in the ability of hydrocarbons to increase the median melting temperature (T_m) of calf thymus DNA (Boyland, 1964), and from flow dichroism (Nagata *et al.*, 1966), fluorescence quenching (Geacintov *et al.*, 1976, 1980), triplet flash photolysis (Geacintov *et al.*, 1980), electric linear dichroism (Geacintov *et al.*, 1980), and photoelectron (Shabbaz *et al.*, 1983) experiments.

The relative extent of binding of various polyarenes to DNA appears to be dependent on the size and shape of the hydrocarbon molecule with no obvious relationship to bioactivity. Thus, the binding constants for BaP and its noncarcinogenic isomer BeP were identical and four- to five-fold greater than those for DBA and its noncarcinogenic isomer dibenz[a,c]anthracene which were also identical (Lesko *et al.*, 1968). The greater binding efficiency of the benzopyrene isomers appears to be mainly due to the fact that they are more nearly isosteric with the DNA base pairs than are the more extended dibenzanthracenes.

The intercalated PAH–DNA complexes undergo covalent bonding under certain circumstances. On irradiation of the BaP–DNA complex in the absorbance range of BaP (350–390 nm) where absorption by DNA is minimal, covalent binding takes place (Ts'o *et al.*, 1969). Covalent binding of BaP and other polyarenes also occurs under X-irradiation and in the presence of chemical oxidants, such as iodine, peroxides, and ascorbic acid–EDTA–Fe^{2+}. In the iodine-induced reactions, the potent carcinogens BaP, 3-MC, and DMBA react to greater extent with DNA than BA, BeP, and other less active polyarenes, and covalent binding takes place predominantly on guanine (Ts'o *et al.*, 1969; Hoffmann *et al.*, 1970). Predominant attack on guanine also occurs in X-ray induced (Hoffmann & Muller, 1969) and photo-induced (Wilk & Girke, 1972) covalent binding to nucleic acids. In contrast, the Fe^{2+}–H_2O oxidation system exhibits equal reactivity towards guanine and adenine (Hoffmann *et al.*,1970). Radical cation intermediates are thought to be involved in both the iodine- and photo-induced reactions. BaP reacts with pyridine in the presence of I_2 to yield a 6-benzo[a]pyrenylpyridinium salt (Hoffmann *et al.*, 1970), and analogous reactions of BaP with purines and pyrimidines also afford mainly 6-substituted derivatives (Wilk & Gerke, 1972). Similar products have also been identified from both the X-ray and photo-induced binding of BaP to DNA (Hoffmann & Muller, 1969; Wilk & Gerke, 1972). Any relevance to carcinogenesis of these modes of binding of polyarenes to DNA appears unlikely, since the DNA adducts formed in these *in vitro* chemical processes generally do not correspond to those formed by metabolism *in vivo*.

3.7   References

Akiyama, I., Harvey, R. G. & LeBreton, P. R. (1981). Ultraviolet photoelectron studies of methyl-substituted benz[a]anthracenes. *J. Am. Chem. Soc.* **103**, 6330–2.

Allison, A. C. & Nash, T. (1963). Electron donation and acceptance by carcinogenic compounds. *Nature (Lond.)* **197**, 758–63.

Arcos, A. C. & Argus, M. F. (1974). *Chemical Induction of Cancer*, New York: Academic Press.

Badger, G. M. (1950). The relative reactivity of aromatic double bonds. III. The relation between double bond character and the velocity of addition of osmium tetroxide. *J. Chem. Soc.* 1809–14.

Badger, G. M. (1954). Chemical constitution and carcinogenic activity. *Adv. Cancer Res.* **2**, 73–127.

Boyland, E. (1964). Polycyclic hydrocarbons. *Brit. Med. Bull.* **20**, 121–6.

Boyland, E. & Green, B. (1962). The interaction of polycyclic hydrocarbons and purines. *Brit. J. Cancer*, **16**, 347–60.

Boyland, E. & Green, B. (1962a). The interaction of polycyclic hydrocarbons and nucleic acids. *Brit. J. Cancer*, **16**, 507–17.

Boyland, E., Green, B. & Liu, S. (1964). Factors influencing the interaction of polycyclic hydrocarbons and deoxyribonucleic acid (DNA). *Biochem. Biophys. Acta*, **87**, 653–63.

Brock, N., Druckerey, H. & Hamperl, H. (1938). Mechanism of cancer-producing substances. *Arch. Exp. Path. Pharmakol.* **189**, 709–31.

Busby, W. F. Jr., Goldman, M. E., Newberne, P. M. & Wogan, G. N. (1984). Tumorigenicity of fluoranthene in newborn mouse lung adenoma bioassay. *Carcinogenesis*, **5**, 1311–16.

Busby, W. F. Jr., Stevens, E. K., Kellenbach, E. R., Cornelisse, J. & Lugtenburg, J. (1988). Dose-response relationships of the tumorigenicity of cyclopenta[cd]pyrene, benzo[a]pyrene, and 6-nitrochrysene in a newborn mouse lung adenoma bioassay. *Carcinogenesis.* **9**, 741–6.

Buu-Hoi, N. P. (1964). New developments in chemical carcinogenesis by polycyclic hydrocarbons and related heterocycles: A review. *Cancer Res.* **24**, 1511–23.

Cavalieri, E. & Rogan, E. (1985). One-electron oxidation in aromatic hydrocarbon carcinogenesis. *Polycyclic Hydrocarbons and Carcinogenesis.* Am. Chem. Soc. Monogr. 283, ed. R. G. Harvey, 289–305, Washington, DC: American Chemical Society.

Cavalieri, E., Rogan, E., Toth, B. & Munhall, A. (1981). Carcinogenicity of the environmental pollutants cyclopenteno[cd]pyrene and cyclopentano[cd]pyrene in mouse skin. *Carcinogenesis*, **2**, 277–81.

Cavalieri, E., Roth, R., Grandjean, C., Althoff, J., Patil, K., Liakus, S. & Marsh, S. (1978). Carcinogenicity and metabolic profiles of 6-substituted benzo[a]pyrene derivatives on mouse skin. *Chem.–Biol. Interact.* **22**, 53–67.

Cook, J. W. (1933). Polycyclic aromatic hydrocarbons. Part XII. The orientation of derivatives of 1,2-benzanthracene with notes on the preparation of some new homologues, and on the isolation of 3:4:5:6-dibenzphenanthrene. *J. Chem. Soc.* 1592–7.

Coombs, M. M. & Bhatt, T. S. (1987). *Cyclopenta[a]phenanthrenes.* Monographs on Cancer Research. Cambridge: Cambridge University Press.

Dannenberg, H. (1957). Steranthene, a new connection between steroids and carcinogenic hydrocarbons. *Z. Krebsforsch.* **62**, 217–9.

Dewhurst, F., Kitchen, D. A. & Calcutt, G. (1972). The carcinogenicity of some 6-substituted benzo(a)pyrene derivatives in mice. *Brit. J. Cancer*, **26**, 506–8.

DiGiovanni, J., Diamond, L., Harvey, R. G. & Slaga, T. J. (1983). Enhancement of the skin tumor-initiating activity of polycyclic aromatic hydrocarbons by methyl substitution of nonbenzo 'bay-region' positions. *Carcinogenesis*, **4**, 403–7.

DiGiovanni, J. & Slaga, T. J. (1981). Modification of polycyclic aromatic hydrocarbon carcinogenesis. *Polycyclic Hydrocarbons and Cancer.* 3, eds H. V. Gelboin & P. O. P. Ts'o, 259–2, New York: Academic Press.

Dipple, A., Moschel, R. C. & Bigger, C. A. H. (1984). Polynuclear aromatic carcinogens. *Chemical Carcinogens*, Am. Chem. Soc. Monogr. 182, ed. C. E. Searle, 41–163, Washington, DC: American Chemical Society.

Dunlap, C. E. & Warren, S. (1941). Chemical configuration and carcinogenesis. *Cancer Res.* **1**, 953–4.

Dunning, W. F. & Curtis, M. R. (1960). Relative carcinogenicity of monomethyl derivatives of benz[a]anthracene in Fischer line 344 rats. *J. Natl. Cancer Inst.* **25**, 387–91.

Dunning, W. F., Curtis, M. R. & Stevens, M. (1968). Comparative carcinogenic activity of dimethyl and trimethyl derivatives of benz(a)anthracene in Fischer line 344 rats. *Proc. Soc. Exp. Biol. Med.* **128**, 720–22.

Fieser, L. F. & Hershberg, E. B. (1938a). Substitution reactions and meso derivatives of 1,2-benzanthracene. *J. Am. Chem. Soc.* **60**, 1893–6.

Fieser, L. F. & Hershberg, E. B. (1938b). The oxidation of methylcholanthrene and 3,4-benzpyrene with lead tetraacetate; further derivatives of 3,4-benzpyrene. *J. Am. Chem. Soc.* **60**, 2542–8.

Fieser, L. F. & Putnam, S. T. (1947). Rate of oxidation of aromatic hydrocarbons by lead tetraacetate. *J. Am. Chem. Soc.* **69**, 1041–6.

Foster, R. (1969). *Organic Charge-Transfer Complexes.* New York: Academic Press.

Fried, J. & Schumm, D. (1967). One electron transfer oxidation of 7,12-dimethylbenz-[a]anthracene. *J. Am. Chem. Soc.* **89**, 5508–9.

Geacintov, N. E., Prusik, T. & Khosrofian, J. M. (1976). Properties of benzopyrene-DNA complexes investigated by fluorescence and triplet flash photolysis techniques. *J. Am. Chem. Soc.* **98**, 6444–52.

Glusker, J. P. (1978). X-Ray analysis of polycyclic hydrocarbon metabolite structures. *Polycyclic Hydrocarbons and Carcinogenesis*, Am. Chem. Soc. Monogr. 283, ed. R. G. Harvey, 125–85, Washington, DC: American Chemical Society.

Hartwell, J. L. (1951). *Survey of Compounds which have been Tested for Carcinogenic Activity*, US Public Health Service Publ. No 149. Washington, DC: Superintendent of Documents, US Government Printing Office.

Harvey, R. G. (1979). Carcinogenic hydrocarbons: Metabolic activation and the mechanism of cancer induction. *Safe Handling of Chemical Carcinogens, Mutagens, and Teratogens*, 2, ed. D. B. Walters, 439–68, Ann Arbor, MI: Ann Arbor Science Publishers.

Harvey, R. G. (1989). The conformational analysis of hydroaromatic metabolites of carcinogenic hydrocarbons and the relation of conformation to biological acitivity. *The Conformational Analysis of Cyclohexenes, Cyclohexadienes, and Related Hydroaromatics*, ed. P. W. Rabideau, 267–98, New York: VCH Publishers.

Harvey, R. G. & Dunne, F. B. (1978). Evidence for multiple regions of activation of carcinogenic hydrocarbons. *Nature (Lond.)* **273**, 566–7.

Harvey, R. G., Fu, P. P. & Rabideau, P. W. (1976). Stereochemistry of 1,3-cyclohexadienes: Conformational preferences in 9-substituted 9,10-dihydrophenanthrenes. *J. Org. Chem.* **41**, 3722–5.

Harvey, R. G. & Halonen, M. (1966). Charge-transfer chromatography of aromatic hydrocarbons on thin layers and columns. *J. Chromatog.* **25**, 294–302.

Harvey, R. G. & Halonen, M. (1968). Interaction between carcinogenic hydrocarbons and nucleosides. *Cancer Res.* **28**, 2183–6.

Hecht, S. S., Hirota, N., Loy, M. & Hoffmann, D. (1978). Tumor-initiating activity of fluorinated 5-methylchrysenes. *Cancer Res.* **28**, 1694–8.

Hecht, S. S., Melikian, A. A. & Amin, S. (1986). Methylchrysenes as probes for the mechanism of metabolic activation of carcinogenic methylated polynuclear aromatic hydrocarbons. *Acc. Chem. Res.* **19**, 174–80.

Heidelberger, C., Bauman, M. E., Grisback, L., Ghobar, A. & Vaughan, T. (1962). The carcinogenic activities of various derivatives of dibenzanthracene. *Cancer Res.* **22**, 78–83.

Hoffmann, D., Bondinell, W. E. & Wynder, E. L. (1974). Carcinogenicity of methylchrysenes. *Science*, **183**, 215–17.

Hoffmann, D., Rathkamp, G., Nesnow, S. & Wynder, E. (1972). Fluoranthenes: quantitative determination in cigarette smoke, formation by pyrolysis, and tumor-initiating activity. *J. Natl. Cancer Inst.* **49**, 1165–75.

Hoffmann, D. & Wynder, E. (1966). Beitrag zur carcinogenen wirkung von dibenzopyrenen. *Z. Krebforsch.* **68**, 137–49.

Hoffmann, H. D., Lesko, S. A. & Ts'o, P. O. P. (1970). Chemical linkage of polycyclic hydrocarbons to deoxyribonucleic acids and polynucleotides in aqueous solution and in buffer-ethanol solvent system. *Biochemistry*, **9**, 2594–604.

Hoffmann, H. D. & Muller, W. (1969). Reactions of carcinogens with guanine nucleotides. *Physico-Chemical Mechanisms of Carcinogenesis*, eds E. D. Bergmann & B. Pullman, 183–7, Jerusalem: Israel Acad. Sci.

Huggins, C. B., Pataki, J. & Harvey, R. G. (1967). Geometry of polycyclic aromatic hydrocarbons. *Proc. Natl. Acad. Sci. USA*, **58**, 2253–60.

Huggins, C. B. & Yang, N. C. (1962). Induction and extinction of mammary cancer. *Science*, **137**, 257–62.

IARC (1973). IARC Monographs on the Evaluation of the Carcinogenic Risk of Chemicals to Humans: Polynuclear Aromatic Compounds, Lyon, France: Internat. Agency Res. Cancer.

IARC (1983). IARC Monographs on the Evaluation of the Carcinogenic Risk of Chemicals to Humans: Polynuclear Aromatic Compounds, Part 1, Chemical, Environmental and Experimental Data, Lyon, France: Internat. Agency Res. Cancer.

Ibanez, V., Geacintov, N. E., Gagliano, A. G., Brandimarte, S. & Harvey, R. G. (1980). Physical binding of tetraols derived from 7,8-dihydroxy-9,10-epoxybenzo[a]pyrene to DNA. *J. Am. Chem. Soc.* **102**, 5661–6.

Kaden, D. A., Hites, R. A. & Thilly, W. G. (1979). Mutagenicity of soot and associated polycyclic aromatic hydrocarbons to *Salmonella typhimurium*. *Cancer Res.* **39**, 4152–9.

Kirshnan, F. & Hites, R. A. (1981). Identification of acephenanthrylene in combustion effluents. *Anal. Chem.* **53**, 342–3.

Kofahl, R. E. & Lucas, H. J. (1954). Coordination of polycyclic aromatic hydrocarbons with silver ion; Correlation of equilibrium constants with relative carcinogenic potencies. *J. Am. Chem. Soc.* **76**, 3931–5.

Lacassagne, A., Buu-Hoi, N. P. & Zajdela, F. (1957). Carcinogenic activity of methyl derivatives of perylene and 1,12-perylene. *Compt. rend.* **245**, 991–4.

Lacassagne, A., Buu-Hoi, N. P. & Zajdela, F. (1958). Relation between molecular structure and carcinogenicity in three series of hexacyclic aromatic hydrocarbons. *Compt. rend.* **246**, 1477–80.

Lacassagne, A., Buu-Hoi, N. P., Zajdela, F. & Saint-Ruf, G. (1968). Carcinogenic activity of two seven-ring aromatic hydrocarbons. *Compt. rend.* **266**, 301–4.

Lacassagne, A., Zajdela, F., Buu-Hoi, N. P. & Chalvet, H. (1957a). Carcinogenic action of 3,4,9,10-dibenzopyrene and derivatives. *Compt. rend.* **244**, 273–4.

Lacassagne, A., Zajdela, F., Buu-Hoi, N. P. & Chalvet, O. (1962). Study of carcinogenicity of several methyl derivatives of 1,2-benzanthracene. *Bull. Assoc. Franc. Etude Cancer*, **49**, 312–19.

Lacassagne, A., Zajdela, F., Buu-Hoi, N. P., Chalvet, O. & Daub, G. H. (1962a). Increased carcinogenic activity of mono-, di-, and trimethylbenzo(a)pyrenes. *Int. J. Cancer.* **3**, 238–43.

LaVoie, E., Amin, S., Hecht, S. S., Furuya, K. & Hoffmann, D. (1982). Tumour initiating activity of dihydrodiols of benzo[b]fluoranthene, benzo[j]fluoranthene, and benzo[k]fluoranthene. *Carcinogenesis*, **3**, 49–52.

LaVoie, E. J., Braley, J., Rice, J. E. & Rivenson, A. (1987). Tumorigenic activity of nonalternant polynuclear aromatic hydrocarbons in newborn mice. *Cancer Lett.* **34**, 15–20.

Lerman, L. S. (1964). The combination of DNA with polycyclic aromatic hydrocarbons. *Proceedings of the Fifth National Cancer Conference*, p. 39, Philadelphia: Lippincott.

Lesko, S. A., Smith, A., Ts'o, P. O. P. & Umans, R. S. (1968). Interaction of nucleic acids. IV. The physical binding of 3,4-benzpyrene to nucleosides, nucleotides, nucleic acids, and nucleoproteins. *Biochemistry*, **7**, 434–47.

Lijinsky, W., Garcia, H., Terracini, B. & Saffiotti, U. (1965). Tumorigenic activity of hydrogenated derivatives of dibenz[a,h]anthracene. *J. Natl. Cancer Inst.* **34**, 1–6.

Lijinsky, W., Manning, W. B. & Andrews, A. W. (1983). Skin carcinogenesis tests in mice of derivatives of 7,12-dimethylbenz[a]anthracene. *Carcinogenesis*, **4**, 1221–4.

Liquori, A. M., DeLerma, B., Ascoli, F., Botre, C. & Trasciatti, M. (1962). Interaction between DNA and polycyclic aromatic hydrocarbons. *J. Mol. Biol.* **5**, 521–6.

Mason, R. (1958). A new approach to the mechanism of carcinogenesis. *Brit. J. Cancer*, **12**, 469–79.

Miller, J. & Miller, E. C. (1963). The carcinogenicities of fluoro derivatives of 10-methyl-1,2-benzanthracene. II. Substitution of the K-region and the 3'-, 6-, and 7-positions. *Cancer Res.* **23**, 229–39.

Miller, J. A. & Miller, E. C. (1960). The carcinogenicities of fluoro derivatives of 10-methyl-1,2-benzanthracene. I. 3- and 4'-monofluoro derivatives. *Cancer Res.* **20**, 133-7.

Nagata, C., Kodama, M., Tagashira, Y. & Imamura, A. (1966). Interaction of polynuclear aromatic hydrocarbons, 4-nitroquinoline 1-oxides, and various dyes with DNA. *Biopolymers,* **4**, 409–27.

National Cancer Institute. (1985). *Survey of Compounds which have been Tested for Carcinogenic Activity*, NIH Publication No. 85-2775. Washington, DC: Superintendent of Documents.

Nesnow, S., Gold, A., Sangaiah, R., Triplett, L. L. & Slaga, T. J. (1984). Mouse skin tumor-initiating activity of benz[e]aceanthrylene and benz[l]aceanthrylene in SENCAR mice. *Cancer Lett.* **22**, 263–8.

Nesnow, S., Leavitt, S., Easterling, R., Watts, R., Toney, S. H., Claxton, L., Sangaiah, R., Toney, G. E., Wiley, J., Fraher, P. & Gold, A. (1984a). Mutagenicity of cyclopenta-fused isomers of benz(a)anthracene in bacterial and rodent cells and identification of the major rat liver microsomal metabolites. *Cancer Res.* **44**, 4993–5003.

Newman, M. S. & Otsuka, S. (1958). Rate and equilibrium constants for the reaction of maleic anhydride with the methyl-1,2-benzanthracenes. *J. Natl. Cancer Inst.* **21**, 721–8.

Pataki, J. & Balick, R. (1972). Relative carcinogenicity of some diethylbenz[a]anthracenes. *J. Med. Chem.* **15**, 905–9.

Pataki, J., Duguid, C., Rabideau, P., Huisman, H. & Harvey, R. G. (1971). Carcinogenic and adrenocorticolytic derivatives of benz[a]anthracene. *J. Med. Chem.* **14**, 940–5.

Pataki, J. & Huggins, C. B. (1969). Molecular site of substituents of benz(a)anthracene related to carcinogenicity. *Cancer Res.* **29**, 506–9.

Rabideau, P. W., Harvey, R. G. & Stothers, J. B. (1969). Ring inversion in 9,10-dialkyl-9,10-dihydrophenanthrenes. *J. Chem. Soc. Chem. Commun.* 1005–6.

Rice, J. E., Hosted, T. J., DeFloria, M. C., LaVoie, E. J., Fischer, D. L. & Wiley, J. C. Jr (1986). Tumor-initiating activity of major *in vivo* metabolites of indeno[1,2,3-cd]pyrene on mouse skin. *Carcinogenesis*, **7**, 1761–4.

Roitt, I. M. & Waters, W. A. (1949). The oxidation of some higher aromatic hydrocarbons with perbenzoic acid. *J. Chem. Soc.* 3060–2.

Sawyer, T. W., Baer-Dubowska, W., Chang, K., Crysup, S. B., Harvey, R. G. & DiGiovanni, J. (1988). Tumor-initiating activity of the bay-region dihydrodiols and diol-epoxides of dibenz[a,j]anthracene and cholanthrene on mouse skin. *Carcinogenesis.* **9**, 2203–7.

Schurch, O. & Winterstein, A. (1935). The carcinogenic action of aromatic hydrocarbons. *Z. Physiol. Chem.* **236**, 79–91.

Scribner, H. (1983). Tumor initiation by apparently noncarcinogenic polycyclic aromatic hydrocarbons. *J. Natl. Cancer Inst.* **50**, 1717–19.

Shabbaz, M., Harvey, R. G., Prakash, A. S., Boal, T. R., Zegar, I. S. & LeBreton, P. (1983). Fluorescence and photoelectron studies of the intercalative binding of benz[a]anthracene metabolite models to DNA. *Biochem. Biophys. Res. Commun.* **112**, 1–7.

Slaga, T., Gleason, G. L., Mills, G., Ewald, L., Fu, P. P., Lee, H. M. & Harvey, R. G. (1980). Comparison of the skin tumor-initiating activities of dihydrodiols and diol-epoxides of various polycyclic aromatic hydrocarbons. *Cancer Res.* **40**, 1981–4.

Slaga, T. J., Huberman, E., DiGiovanni, J., Gleason, G. & Harvey, R. G. (1979). The importance of the 'bay-region' diol-epoxide in 7,12-dimethylbenz[a]anthracene skin tumor initiation and mutagenesis. *Cancer Lett.* **6**, 213–20.

Slaga, T. J., Iyer, R. P., Lyga, W., Secrist III, A., Daub, G. H. & Harvey, R. G. (1980a). Comparison of the skin-tumor initiating activities of dihydrodiols, diol-epoxides, and methylated derivatives of various polycyclic aromatic hydrocarbons. *Polynuclear Aromatic Hydrocarbons: Chemistry and Biological Effects*, eds A. Bjorseth & A. J. Dennis, 753–69, Columbus, OH: Battelle Press.

Stevenson, J. L. & Haarn, E. J. (1965). Carcinogenicity of benz(a)anthracene and benzo(c)phenanthrene. *Amer. Ind. Hyg. Assoc. J.* **26**, 475–8.

Szent-Gyorgyi, A., Isenberg, I. & Baird, S. L. (1960). On the electron donating properties of carcinogens. *Proc. Natl. Acad. Sci. USA.* **46**, 1444–9.

Takemura, K. H., Cameron, M. D. & Newman, M. S. (1953). Studies on carcinogenic hydrocarbons: Dissocation constants and free energies of formation of complexes with 2,4,7-trinitrofluorenone. *J. Am. Chem. Soc.* **75**, 3280–2.

Thilly, W. G., DeLuca, J. G., Furth, E. E., Hoppe, H. I., Kaden, D. E., Krolewski, J. J., Liber, H. L., Skopek, T. R., Slapikoff, S. A., Tizard, R. J. & Penman, B. W. (1980). Gene locus mutation assays in diploid human lymphoblast lines. *Chemical Mutagens.* eds F. J. deSerres & A. Hollaender, 331–64, New York: Plenum.

Ts'o, P. O. P., Lesko, S. A. & Umans, R. S. (1969). The physical binding and the chemical linkage of benzpyrene to nucleotides, nucleic acids, and nucleohistones. *Physico-Chemical Mechanisms of Carcinogenesis*, eds E. D. Bergmann & B. Pullman, 106–35, Jerusalem: Israel Acad. Sci.

Weil-Malherbe, H. (1946). The solubilization of polycyclic aromatic hydrocarbons by purines. *Biochem. J.* **40**, 351–63.

Wilk, M. & Gerke, W. (1972). Reaction between benzo[a]pyrene and nucleobases by one electron oxidation. *J. Natl. Cancer Inst.* **49**, 158–9.

Wislocki, P. G., Fiorentini, K. M., Fu, P. P., Yang, S. K. & Lu, A. Y. H. (1982). Tumor-initiating ability of the twelve monomethylbenz[a]anthracenes. *Carcinogenesis*, **3**, 215–17.

Wood, A., Levin, W., Chang, R. L., Huang, M.-T., Ryan, D. E., Thomas, P., Lehr, R. E., Kumar, S., Koreeda, M., Akagi, H., Ittah, Y., Dansette, P., Yagi, H., Jerina, D. M. & Conney, A. H. (1980). Mutagenicity and tumor-initiating activity of cyclopenta(cd)pyrene and structurally related compounds. *Cancer Res.* **40**, 642–9.

Zacharias, D. E., Glusker, J. P., Harvey, R. G. & Fu, P. P. (1977). Molecular structure of the K-region *cis*-dihydrodiol of 7,12-dimethylbenz[a]anthracene. *Cancer Res.* **37**, 775–82.

4

Metabolic activation, DNA binding, and mechanisms of carcinogenesis

The central problem in carcinogenesis research is elucidation of the mechanism(s) whereby molecules of relatively simple structure, such as polyarenes, induce tumors in animal tissues. This chapter reviews historical developments leading to modern concepts of metabolic activation and DNA-binding.

4.1   Steroidogenesis and related theories

The superficial resemblance of some carcinogenic PAHs to steroids has stimulated numerous speculations that certain polyarenes may arise endogenously from steroids via metabolism and/or act by interference with steroid hormone-dependent metabolic pathways.

An early finding was the observation of Wieland & Dane (1933) that reaction of the bile acid 12-ketocholanic acid with selenium at elevated temperature afforded 3-methylcholanthrene, subsequently shown to be a potent carcinogen. Following the suggestion of Bergmann that cholesterol might give rise metabolically to 3,6-dimethylsteranthrene, Dannenberg (1957) synthesized the 'angular steranthrene' (Table 3.10: **30**) which proved to be highly carcinogenic. The closely related F-norsteranthrene (Table 3.10: **25**) was also found to be a potent carcinogen (Lacassagne *et al.*, 1963). Subsequently, Dannenberg (1959) showed that dehydrogenation of cholesterol with chloranil furnished a tumorigenic cyclopentadienophenanthrene compound. In other studies, Nes & Ford (1962) demonstrated conversion of pregnenolone and ergosterol via a series of biomimetic reactions into 4,7-dimethylbenz[a]anthracene, which proved to be inactive.

Renewed interest in the biogenic formation of carcinogenic hydrocarbons has been generated by the finding that cyclopenta[a]phenanthrenes are widely distributed in petroleum, mineral oils, and other natural sources where they are thought to arise from sterols by microbiological dehydrogenation

(Coombs & Bhatt, 1987). There is also evidence that cyclopenta[a]-phenanthrenes, some of which may be carcinogenic, may be formed during cooking by pyrolysis of the sterols present in edible oils. However, unequivocal proof that higher species are able to synthesize polyarenes from steroids is still lacking.

The fact that many spontaneous and PAH carcinogen-induced tumors are hormone dependent (Huggins, 1979) suggests that carcinogenic PAHs may somehow compete with or alter normal steroid hormone dependent functions. Induction of mammary tumors by DMBA is accelerated by estradiol plus progesterone (Huggins & Yang, 1962), polyestradiol phosphate (Huggins, 1979), and anti-estrogen C1628 (DeSombre & Arbogast, 1974). Further evidence is provided by the finding by Jull (1956) that 3-MC, DMBA, BaP, and DBA may mimic certain of the normal physiological reactions produced by steroids. Huggins and Yang (1962) proposed that a steroid-like structure and the ability to form donor–acceptor complexes were essential characteristics of mammary gland PAH carcinogens. However, Pullman (1965) pointed out that there are important electronic and structural differences between carcinogenic polyarenes and steroids which make competition between them at a common receptor site unlikely. In particular, polyarenes are generally planar highly conjugated aromatic structures, while the latter are relatively nonplanar saturated molecules with oxygenated functions. Moreover, there are many carcinogenic PAHs which do not conform to steroidal dimensions (Chap. 3), lending considerable doubt to the significance of this relationship.

4.2   Electronic theories

Attempts to relate carcinogenic activities to the electronic properties of the polyarenes date back to the work of the German physical chemist Otto Schmidt (1941). Using a relatively primitive theoretical approach, Schmidt calculated the electron densities for a series of polyarenes and concluded that regions of high densities, particularly meso regions, were required for bioactivity. This approach was developed further using more refined valence bond methods by Svartholm (1942) who concluded that a reactive phenanthrene-type 9,10-bond was a common feature of the carcinogenic molecules. It was assumed that covalent bonding between this molecular region and a cellular receptor was a critical event in tumorigenesis.

Major development of these ideas took place in France under the leadership of the Daudels and the Pullmans. They applied more sophisticated quantum mechanical theoretical methods (initially valence bond and later molecular orbital methods) to the polyarenes with the aim of developing theoretical indices of reactivity which could be related to carcinogenicity.

This early work has been reviewed by Coulson (1953). The Pullmans introduced the term 'K-region' to designate bonds, such as the 9,10-bond of phenanthrene, known for their high olefinic character. Attention focused initially on this region, since structure–activity studies, chemical reactivity studies, and early theoretical studies all pointed to a correlation between K-region electron density and carcinogenic activity. Exploration of the utility of various theoretical indices, singly or in combination, led A. Pullman (1947) to define the *total charge* on the K-region as the sum of twice the mobile bond order plus the free valence numbers and the net electric charges at the two positions:

$$\text{Total charge} = 2p_{12} + F_1 + F_2 + q_1 + q_2.$$

For unsubstituted hydrocarbons (in which the net electric charge of carbon atoms is zero) this expression simplifies to: $2p_{12} + F_1 + F_2$. This index gave a fair correlation with bioactivity, but there were also numerous exceptions. The concept of *total charge* may also be criticized as an empirical mixture of electronic parameters without clear physical significance.

Subsequently, the Pullmans (1955) proposed to relate carcinogenicity to the reactivities of the polyarenes in both K- and L-regions by a new set of dynamic electronic indices. The 'L-region' was defined as a *meso-anthracenic* region, such as the 7,12-positions of BA (Chap. 1), required to be unreactive for carcinogenic activity. Methyl substitution in the L-region was considered to favor activity by blocking reactions in this region which would deactivate the molecule. In contrast to total charge, which is a static index of π-electron distribution in the isolated molecule, the new set of indices represent the molecule in a dynamic reacting state. These indices, which are based on the *electron localization theory* of Wheland, take into account three types of localization energies (Fig. 4.1).

The *carbon localization energy* (CLE) is defined as the energy required to localize an electron pair on a specific carbon atom, i.e. the difference in resonance energy between the unpolarized parent hydrocarbon and the localized structure. The *bond localization energy* (BLE), also known as the *ortho localization energy*, is the energy to localize a pair of π-electrons

Fig. 4.1. Localization of electrons on polyarenes: (A) carbon localization; (B) bond localization; and (C) para localization.

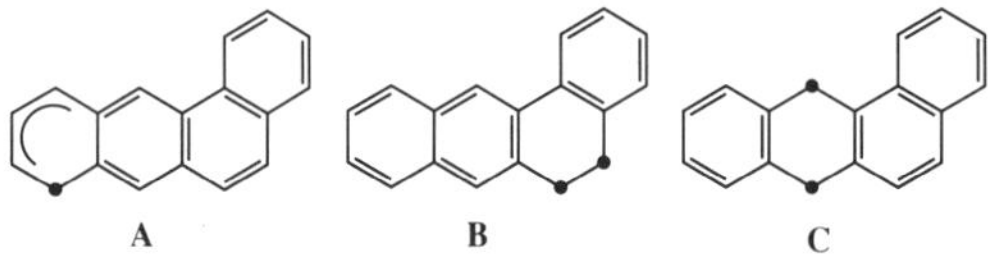

A   B   C

between adjacent carbon atoms unconjugated with the rest of the molecule. For example, the BLE of the K-region of BA would correspond to the difference in resonance energy between BA and 2-phenylnaphthalene. The *para localization energy* (PLE) is defined as the energy to localize simultaneously two individual electrons in positions which are *para* to one another. The PLE of the L-region of BA corresponds to the difference in resonance energy between BA and its 7,12-dihydro derivative. Either the valence-bond or the linear combination of atomic orbitals methods may be used to calculate BLE and PLE. The less laborious LCAO method is usually employed, so that the values of these indices are generally given in ß units. The CLE may be calculated by the more exact procedure of Wheland (1942) or by Dewar's simpler approximation (Dewar & Dougherty, 1975).

The calculated localization energies were utilized by the Pullmans (1955) to derive combined indices to characterize the reactivity of the K- and L-regions of a series of PAHs. The BLE and PLE are appropriate for measuring the ease of electrophilic addition in the K-region and the ease of Diels–Alder addition in an L-region, respectively. However, better agreement with experimental values is obtained when the combinations $BLE + CLE_{min}$ and $PLE + CLE_{min}$ are employed; CLE_{min} is the smaller of the two possible values of CLE. From their study with 50 PAHs, the Pullmans concluded that carcinogenic activity requires the presence of a K-region for which $BLE + CLE_{min} \leq 3.31$ ß. If an L-region is present, then $PLE + CLE_{min} \geq 5.66$ ß is required for carcinogenic activity. Within the limited range of compounds studied a moderately good correlation between the calculated indices and bioactivity was found.

With the aim of improving the correlation, other investigators have developed a number of alternative theoretical models. The *frontier electron* method developed by Nagata *et al.* (1955) is based on the presumption that an electrophile will combine with the electrons in the highest filled orbital in the position where the frontier electron density is maximum, while nucleophilic attack will occur in the region of the lowest unoccupied orbital. They calculated the *frontier electron densities* and another theoretical quantity termed *superdelocalizability* for the K- and L-regions of a relatively small series of unsubstituted PAHs and related these values to carcinogenic activity. This model has been refined by subsequent investigators (Mainster & Memory, 1967; Koutecky & Zahradnick, 1961), and a number of alternative theoretical approaches have also been developed (Hoffman, 1969; Herndon, 1974; Scribner, 1975).

Despite their attractiveness, these quantum mechanical methods suffer from serious shortcomings. In particular, the dramatic effects of substitution on carcinogenic activity are beyond the limits of the theoretical methods. As a consequence, the most potent carcinogenic hydrocarbons, such as DMBA and 3-MC, all of which bear alkyl substituents, are outside the scope of the method. Also excluded from the classical theoretical treatment are nonalternant polyarenes, such as cyclopenta[c,d]pyrene, indeno[1,2,3-cd]pyrene, and the isomeric benzofluorenes, many of which are important environmental pollutants. Even within the limited class of PAHs for which the electronic theories were developed, namely unsubstituted alternant polyarenes, inconsistencies are observed. The exceptions are both positive and negative. Some PAHs predicted theoretically to be active are inactive, while others predicted to be inactive exhibit significant activity. The electronic theories also fail to take into account other differences likely to be important in the mechanism of carcinogenesis. These include differences in solubility, transport from the site of administration to the site of action within the organism (e.g. by association with proteins), differences in susceptibility to enzymatic detoxification, and steric effects on covalent binding of the PAHs or their active metabolites to the cellular receptor.

Recognition of the role of metabolic activation in the mechanism of PAH carcinogenesis rendered obsolete quantum theories based on the assumption that the PAH carcinogens are directly active. However, newer theoretical approaches have been developed which take into account metabolic activation to reactive diol epoxide metabolites which bind covalently to DNA (cf Section 4.4).

4.3   Metabolic activation

It was first recognized by the Millers that most chemical carcinogens must be activated metabolically to electrophilic intermediates capable of reacting covalently with cellular macromolecules, particularly proteins and nucleic acids (Miller, 1978). Elucidation of the specific pathways involved in the metabolism of PAH carcinogens and characterization of the covalently bound adducts are major accomplishments of modern carcinogenesis research. Several reviews on this topic are available (Dipple *et al.*, 1984; Harvey, 1981; Singer & Grunberger, 1983).

The first evidence for the important role of metabolism were the observations that when ^{3}H-labelled PAHs were applied to the backs of mice (Brookes & Lawley, 1964) or were incubated with mouse embryo cells (Duncan *et al.*, 1969), covalently bound adducts to nucleic acids and proteins were formed. The extent of covalent binding to DNA and RNA correlated approximately with carcinogenic potency, and binding was shown to require activation by the P-450 microsomal enzymes (Goshman & Heidelberger, 1967; Grover & Sims, 1968).

Metabolism of PAHs occurs mainly on the microsomes of the endoplasmic reticulum mediated by two groups of enzyme systems sometimes designated as Phase I and Phase II. Phase I enzymes mediate oxidation to introduce polar groups, such as hydroxyl, into the hydrophobic molecules. Phase II enzymes further facilitate removal of the xenobiotic molecules from the cell by conjugation of the primary oxidized products with a polar group and/or further oxidative transformation. The most important Phase I enzyme system is a group of enzymes known as the cytochrome P-450 mixed function oxidases (MFOs) or monooxygenases. The MFOs are an ubiquitous enzyme system found in most mammalian tissues. Although this system is localized primarily in microsomes, it is also present in the nuclei and mitochondria of cells. A principal component of the MFO enzyme system is a family of hemoproteins known as cytochrome P-450 which function together with a flavoprotein known as NADPH-cytochrome P-450 reductase. Phosphatidylcholine is also required for activity. The cytochrome P-450 enzymes catalyze the incorporation of one atom of molecular oxygen into substrates (RH). The overall process can be represented by the equation:

$$RH + O_2 + NADPH + H^+ \rightarrow ROH + H_2O + NADP^+$$

The cytochrome 450 hemoproteins are characterized by a relatively intense absorbance at 450 nm for the CO derivative of the reduced hemoprotein. Multiple cytochrome P-450 isozymes are known, and these are selectively inducible by different substrates. There are two major classes of compounds represented by phenobarbitol (PB) and 3-MC that induce different cytochromes P-450. Liver microsomes isolated from PB-treated animals differ with respect to substrate specificity and the absorption maxima of their reduced CO complex from microsomes prepared from 3-MC-treated animals. 3-MC treatment induces formation of a hemoprotein designated 'cytochrome P448' or 'cytochrome P_1-450'. The existence of multiple forms of cytochrome P-450 that exhibit different, but overlapping, substrate specificities provides an explanation for the remarkably broad substrate specificity of the MFO system. Variations in the levels of individual isozymes can also account for the differences in catalytic activity observed in microsomal preparations from animals of different age, sex, strain, and with the use of different chemical inducers. Differential inhibition of cytochromes is also observed. For example, the 3-MC-induced form of rat liver cytochrome is inhibited by 7,8-benzoflavone, but the PB-induced form is only weakly affected. Thus, induction or inhibition of the MFO system may alter the balance of the metabolic pathways of PAHs.

Recently it has been hypothesized that the differences in the substrate specificity of the two classes of cytochromes is related to their mechanisms of oxygenation (Lewis *et al.*, 1989). The substrates for the cytochromes P-448 tend to be planar molecules with relatively large values of area/depth^2. Their electronic structures are characterized by relatively low values of ΔE, the difference in energy between the frontier orbitals [E(LEMO) – E(HOMO)]. On the other hand, the substrates of other cytochromes P-450 are globular molecules, with relatively low values of area/depth^2 and relatively high values of ΔE. As a consequence, cytochrome P-448 substrates, which are good electron donors, would preferentially accept singlet oxygen, a good electron acceptor, whereas cytochrome P-450 substrates, which are less effective electron donors, would preferentially accept superoxy anion, a good electron donor. It is further proposed that epoxidation involves singlet oxygen, and hydroxylation involves superoxy anion. Several recent reviews on the cytochromes P-450 and their mechanisms of enzymatic action are available (Ioannides & Parke, 1987; Lewis *et al.*, 1987; Ortez de Montellano, 1986).

The metabolic pathways of polyarenes are typified by those of BaP which has been most intensively investigated (Fig. 4.2). The principal primary metabolites are arene oxides arising from epoxidation at various aromatic bonds. These relatively unstable intermediates are subject to further modification by other enzymes present in the endoplasmic reticulum. Principal among these are epoxide hydrolase (also known as epoxide hydrase

Fig. 4.2. Metabolic pathways of polyarenes. In the interest of simplicity, further metabolic transformations, such as P-450-catalyzed oxidation of phenols to phenol-epoxides and conversion of the latter to phenol-dihydrodiols, diphenols, and quinones, are omitted.

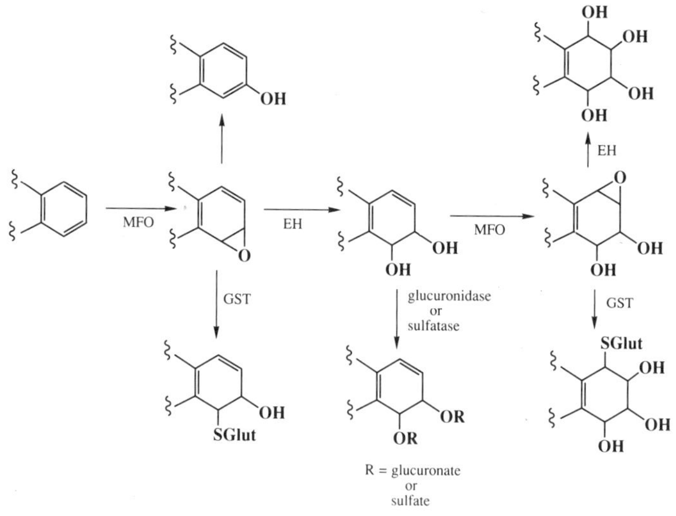

and epoxide hydratase) and glutathione-S-transferase (GST). The former, which catalyzes hydration of epoxides to vicinal *trans*-dihydrodiols, is present in all mammalian tissues. Oesch *et al.* (1984) have provided evidence for multiple forms of microsomal epoxide hydrolase with different substrate specificities. A review on the complex role of this enzyme in the metabolism and carcinogenesis of PAHs is available (Guenther & Oesch, 1983). Although epoxide hydrolase is not induced by 3-MC, the enzyme is effectively induced by *trans*-stilbene oxide.

The second major pathway for the metabolism of PAH oxides is addition of glutathione catalyzed by GST. Multiple forms of GST exhibiting different specific activities have been characterized (Singer & Grunberger, 1983). Although the GST enzymes are components of the endoplasmic reticulum, their highest concentrations are found in the soluble supernatant fraction of the liver. Comparison of the specific activities of GST for various arene oxide substrates reveals that the K-region oxides are superior substrates to the non-K-region oxides (Nemoto, 1981). The levels of GST activity are influenced by inducers, and the response is dependent upon the animal species. For example, rat liver GST activity was increased by 50% of the control by treatment with PB, BaP, and 3-MC. In contrast, 3-MC had no effect on mouse hepatic enzyme activity. The most efficient inducers of GST enzyme activity are antioxidants, such as butylated hydroxyanisole (BHA), which can increase the basal enzyme level in mouse liver up to 11-fold. Most of the glutathione conjugates are preferentially excreted in the bile. In the kidney they undergo biochemical conversion to mercapturic acid conjugates (Fig. 4.3) that are excreted in the urine.

Another important metabolic pathway is isomerization of the arene oxides to phenols. This process is generally assumed to be nonenzymatic. However,

Fig. 4.3. Metabolic degradation of glutathione conjugates to mercapturic acid.

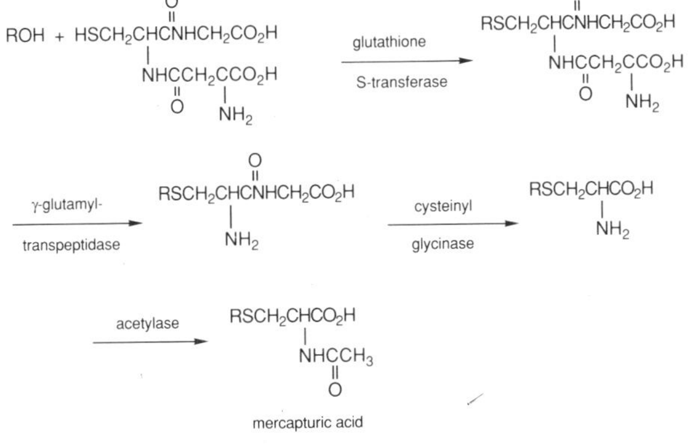

physical chemical studies by Johnson & Bruice (1975) have shown that rearrangement of arene oxides to phenols is susceptible to catalysis by amines, suggesting that similar rearrangements may *in vivo* be catalyzed by the amino or sulfhydryl groups of proteins. Generally a single phenolic isomer tends to be produced predominantly, and the direction of regioselective ring opening is theoretically predictable by molecular orbital methods based on the relative stability of the two possible cationic intermediates (Fu *et al.*, 1978). Thus, 3-hydroxy-BaP, which is a major metabolite of BaP, is produced from ring-opening of BaP 2,3-oxide exclusively in the direction to afford this isomer rather than 2-hydroxy-BaP (Yang *et al.*, 1977) in accord with theoretical prediction. The less stable arene oxides, such as BaP 2,3-oxide, rearrange sufficiently rapidly to prevent their conversion to dihydrodiols. The phenolic products undergo conjugation with glucuronic acid or sulfate to yield water soluble metabolites. Oxidation of the phenols to quinones may also take place under some conditions. Thus, oxidation of 6-hydroxy-BaP by microsomes (Lorenzten *et al.*, 1975) or by arachidonic acid and ram seminal vesicles (Marnett, 1985) produces the 1,6-, 3,6-, and 6,12-quinones as the major products.

The PAH *trans*-dihydrodiols undergo further oxidation by the MFOs to yield diastereomeric *anti-* and *syn*-diol epoxide metabolites, identified as the principal active carcinogenic species. The diol epoxides, as a consequence of their exceptional chemical reactivity, are not normally found as urinary metabolites. Instead, they are detected usually as adducts with nucleic acids and proteins. The diol epoxides appear to be poor substrates for EH (Gozuka *et al.*, 1981). Nonenzymatic hydration of diol epoxides proceeds rapidly in aqueous media in the absence of EH to yield tetraol products arising from both *cis* and *trans* addition. The presence of high levels of EH has little influence on the mutagenicity of diol epoxides, suggesting that EH has minimal activity towards diol epoxides. The detoxification of diol epoxide metabolites is principally through their reaction with glutathione catalyzed by GST (Robertson *et al.*, 1986). The covalent binding to DNA of *anti*-BPDE arising from activation of BaP 7,8-dihydrodiol by the nuclear membrane is inhibited to a small extent by glutathione alone and to a much greater extent by the cytosolic fraction and purified cytosolic GSTs from rat liver. Both the near neutral (μ) and acidic (π) human GSTs are efficient in the conjugation of *anti*-BPDE and in particular the carcinogenic (+)-enantiomer. The basic (α-ε) GSTs show only weak activity. Similar properties may be expected in the detoxification of other PAH diol epoxides, but direct experimental evidence is lacking.

Where alkyl groups are present in a polyarene, e.g. DMBA and 3-MC, hydroxylation frequently occurs at the benzylic sites to yield the corresponding alcohols as well as further oxidized metabolic products. For example, metabolism of DMBA affords the two possible mono-hydroxymethyl derivatives as well as the bishydroxymethyl compound the principal products.

The phenols, dihydrodiols, and other polar metabolites of PAHs undergo conjugation with glucuronic acid and sulfuric acid to more water soluble metabolites. This topic has been reviewed by Nemoto (1981) and Singer & Grunberger (1983). Conjugation of the hydroxylated derivatives with glucuronic acid involves reaction of the PAH compounds with UDP-glucuronic acid catalyzed by UDP-glucuronyltransferase (UGT). The UGT enzyme is localized in endoplasmic reticular membranes, and like other detoxifying enzymes it probably consists of a family of closely related but functionally different enzymes. UGT is present in many tissues including liver, lung, kidney, stomach, and skin. The different forms of the enzyme are differentially induced by 3-MC and PB. The 3-MC inducible form has high activity towards phenols, such as 3-hydroxy-BaP, but low activity towards BaP 7,8-dihydrodiol. The conjugation of oxygenated PAH derivatives with sulfate proceeds via reaction of the substrate with 3'-phosphoadenosine-5'-phosphosulfate catalyzed by sulfotransferase. Sulfate conjugates are major polar metabolites of oxygenated metabolites of BaP (Nemoto, 1981). It has been suggested (Watabe *et al.*, 1982) that the sulfate ester of the hydroxy-methyl metabolite of DMBA may be an active form of this carcinogen capable of alkylating DNA. However, there is minimal evidence that this pathway is important in carcinogenesis.

4.4   Stereochemistry of metabolic activation

Metabolism of PAHs by the P-450 and EH enzymes generally proceeds with high stereoselectivity. Because most aromatic bonds of polyarenes are prochiral, their stereoheterotopic epoxidation catalyzed by P-450 isozymes is likely to result in optically active products. Rapid progress has been made in recent years in elucidating the mechanisms of these transformations. Several reviews are available (Yang, 1988; Yang *et al.*, 1985; Thakker *et al.*, 1985).

The stereochemistry of PAH metabolism may be illustrated by the metabolism of BaP which has been most intensively investigated. Identification and quantification of the full range of BaP metabolites was made possible by development of methods for the synthesis of the various metabolites (McCaustland *et al.*, 1976; Harvey & Fu, 1978; Harvey, 1985, 1986) and HPLC methods for their separation (Selkirk *et al.*, 1974). The primary arene oxide metabolites of BaP are generally not isolated as such due to their instability and strong tendency to undergo further transformation.

Mechanisms of carcinogenesis

Table 4.1. *Enantiomeric composition of epoxides and transdihydrodiols formed in the metabolism of polyarenes by rat liver microsomes*[a]

Isomer	S,R-epoxide (%)			R,R-dihydrodiol (%)		
	Control	PB	3-MC	Control	PB	3-MC
BaP						
4,5-	52	60	95	96	95	>99
7,8-	3	2	1	97	98	>99
9,10-	99	99	99	>99	>99	>99
BA						
3,4-	83	91	90	83	91	90
5,6-	53-75	55-79	97	77	81	84
8,9-	6	10	1	94	90	>99
10,11-	99	95	99	>99	95	>99
chrysene						
1,2-	1	1	1	99	99	99
3,4-	51	41	96	51	41	96
5,6-	32	27	95	86	87	92
benzo[c]phenanthrene						
3,4-	34	54	99	34	54	>99
5,6-	60	58	72	17	20	15
DMBA						
3,4-	57	62	64	57	62	64
5,6-	76	80	97	11	5	6
8,9-	9	4	1	91	96	99
10,11-	91	86	98	91	86	98

[a]The data are from Yang, 1988.

The principal metabolites isolated are the 4,5-, 7,8-, and 9,10-dihydrodiols, the 1-, 3-, 6-, 7-, and 9-phenols, and the 1,3-, 1,6-, and 6,12-quinones. The configuration of the dihydrodiols of BaP and other PAHs appears to be exclusively *trans*, indicating that EH-catalyzed hydration is highly stereoselective.

The enantiomeric composition of the epoxides and *trans*-dihydrodiols formed in the metabolism of BaP is dependent upon whether the microsomes were prepared from untreated, PB-treated, or 3-MC-treated rat liver microsomes (Table 4.1). The 3-MC-inducible cytochrome P-450 isozyme (P-450c) exhibits the highest stereoselectivity in the metabolism of the K-region of BaP, affording predominantly the 4S,5R-oxide enantiomer. Microsomes from untreated and PB-treated rats show considerably lower stereoselectivity. Enzymatic hydration of the enantiomeric BaP 4,5-oxides takes place with preferential attack of water at the S-center of the S,R- and R,S-enantiomers to afford in both cases the (+)-R,R-dihydrodiol (Fig. 4.4). On the other hand, reaction of the BaP 4,5-oxide enantiomers with glutathione mediated by GST takes place preferentially at the carbon atoms with the R-configuration to yield the two corresponding 4S, 5S-glutathionyl adducts (Fig. 4.4).

Metabolism of BaP in the benzo ring also takes place with a high degree of stereoselectivity (Dipple *et al.*, 1984; Yang, 1988). Liver microsomes from rats pretreated with 3-MC oxidize the 7,8-bond of BaP to yield almost exclusively the (+)(7R,8S)-oxide (Fig. 4.5). Each enantiomer of the 7,8-oxide is stereospecifically converted by EH to a different dihydrodiol via reaction involving attack of water at the 8-position. The (+)(7R,8S)-oxide gives rise to the (−)(7R, 8R)-dihydrodiol, while the (−)(7S,8S)-oxide affords the (+)(7S, 8S)-dihydrodiol. Metabolism of BaP with P-450c provides almost exclusively the (−)(7R, 8R)-dihydrodiol enantiomer. This isomer, in turn, is preferentially converted to the (+)-*anti*-diol epoxide which is the most carcinogenic of the four isomeric diol epoxides. Studies of the DNA-bound diol epoxide metabolites formed in rodent, bovine, and human cells (King *et al.*, 1976; Weinstein *et al.*, 1976; Jeffery *et al.*, 1977) show a slightly diminished stereoselectivity for formation of the (+)-anti-diol epoxide. On the other hand, a lower degree of steric preference is observed in some other biological systems. Deutsch *et al.* (1979), who used a reconstituted system of various purified cytochromes P-450 from rabbit liver, have shown that oxidation of the (−)(7R,8R)-dihydrodiol of BaP affords the isomeric diol epoxides in a ratio which ranged from 11:1 to 1.8:1 in favor of the (+)-anti-isomer, dependent upon which purified cytochrome P-450 was used. Similarly, the (+)(7S,8S)-dihydrodiol gave the (+)-*syn* and (−)-*anti*- diol epoxides in a ratio which ranged from 0.4 to 3.0. Since the ratio of P-450 isozymes varies from species to species and from tissue to tissue within a

Fig. 4.4. The enzyme-mediated reactions of BaP 4,5-oxide with water and glutathione proceed with high stereoselectivity. Hydration catalyzed by EH involves preferential attack of water at the S-carbon atom, while the addition of glutathione catalyzed by GST entails preferential attack at the R-carbon atom.

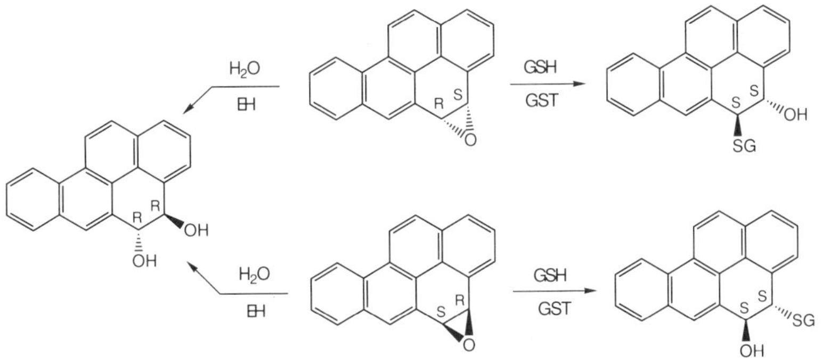

specific organism and these enzymes may be selectively induced or inhibited, these differences in potential for activation may account for much of the differences in susceptibilities between species and between individuals within a species.

Studies similar to those performed with BaP have been conducted with other PAHs, such as BA, 7-MBA, DMBA, DBA, chrysene, 5-methylchrysene, and others. Comparison of the metabolic patterns of PAHs which vary in their carcinogenic potencies provides information to aid in understanding which features of metabolism are associated with biological activity. A brief summary of the findings from metabolic studies of several representative PAHs is presented in the following paragraphs. Further details may be found in the more comprehensive reviews by Sims and Grover, 1981 and Yang, 1988.

Benz[a]anthracene can form five *trans*-dihydrodiols, the 1,2-, 3,4-, 5,6-, 8,9-, and 10,11-dihydrodiols (Fig. 4.6). The main metabolites in liver microsomal fractions from normal and 3-MC-treated rats are the 5,6- and 8,9-dihydrodiols; only small amounts of the 3,4- and 10, 11-dihydrodiols and even smaller amounts of the 1,2-dihydrodiol are formed. Although BA is generally considered to be noncarcinogenic, the synthetic 3,4-dihydrodiol and its *anti*-diol epoxide derivative are highly active in inducing mutations in

Fig. 4.5. Stereochemistry of metabolism of the benzo ring of benzo[a]pyrene.

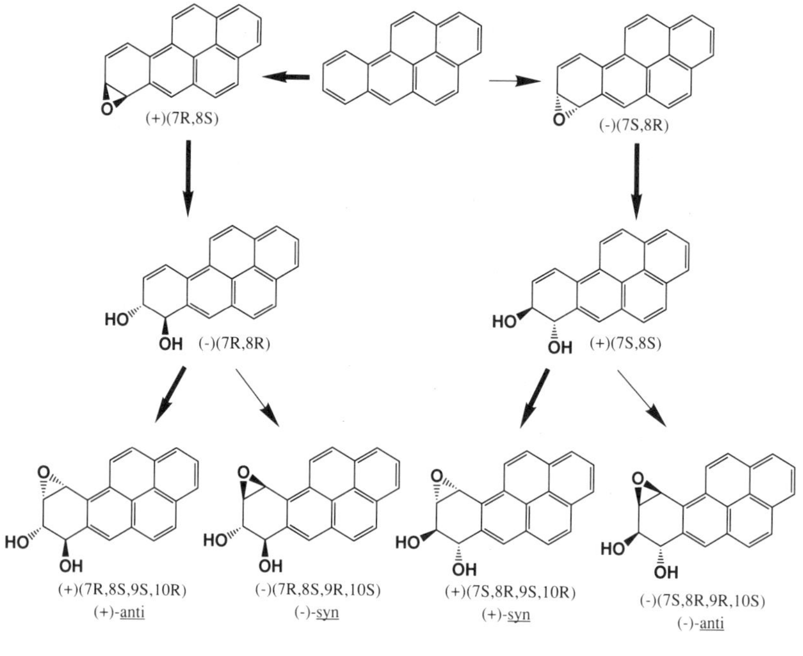

V79 Chinese hamster and bacterial cells. Similarly, the 3,4-dihydrodiol is 10- to 20-fold more active than the isomeric dihydrodiols in producing tumors on mouse skin. These findings indicate that the low carcinogenic activity of BA is probably due to its low level of metabolic activation to the 3,4-dihydrodiol and the corresponding diol epoxide.

7-Methylbenz[a]anthracene can, in principle, form five *trans*-dihydrodiols analogous to those formed by BA (Fig. 4.6). All five dihydrodiols of 7-MBA are detected in liver homogenates and microsomal fractions prepared from rats pretreated with 3-MC; the principal dihydrodiols formed in mouse skin are the 3,4- and 8,9-dihydrodiols. In the induction of malignant transformation in mouse fibroblasts or in mutagenesis tests, the 3,4-dihydrodiol of 7-MBA is the most active dihydrodiol isomer, followed by the 8,9-dihydrodiol, and both dihydrodiol isomers are more active than 7-MBA. The 3,4-dihydrodiol was also more active than the parent hydrocarbon in its ability to initiate skin tumors in mice (Slaga *et al.*, 1980). On the basis of this and other evidence, the 3,4-dihydrodiol is considered to be the proximate carcinogenic form of 7-MBA which is converted metabolically to the corresponding bay region diol epoxide, its ultimate carcinogenic form.

Metabolism of DMBA is complicated by the fact that hydroxylation of the methyl groups is a relatively important pathway. The 7-hydroxymethyl,12-hydroxymethyl, and 7,12-bishydroxymethyl derivatives are among the major metabolites. In microsomal systems from 3-MC-pretreated rats the 3,4-, 5,6-, 8,9-, and 10,11-dihydrodiols are important metabolites. The corresponding dihydrodiol derivatives of DMBA hydroxylated on one or both methyl groups are also found as metabolites. On the other hand, the 1,2-dihydrodiol is not detected among the products of metabolism, probably as a

Fig. 4.6. Metabolism of BA (R = H) and 7-methyl-BA (R = CH₃) can afford five dihydrodiols.

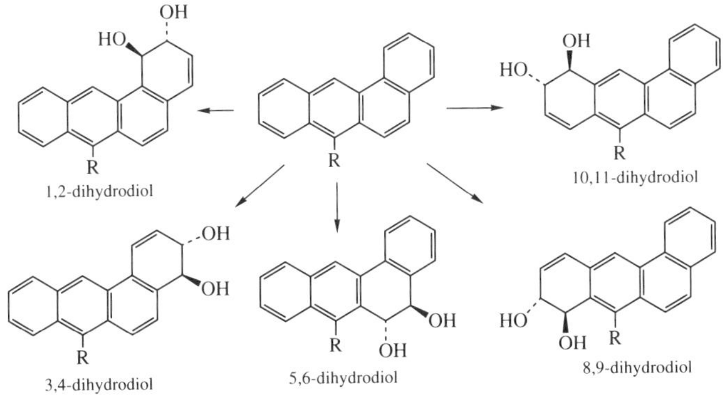

1,2-dihydrodiol

10,11-dihydrodiol

3,4-dihydrodiol

5,6-dihydrodiol

8,9-dihydrodiol

consequence of the steric crowding in the bay region which blocks association of the monoxygenase with this bond. In bacterial mutagenicity assays,
in the presence of a rat postmitochondrial fraction, the 3,4-dihydrodiol was
about sixfold more active than DMBA itself. Similarly, in Chinese hamster
V79 cells the 3,4- and 8,9-dihydrodiols were more active in inducing
mutation than either DMBA or the 5,6- or 10,11-dihydrodiols. In the
induction of skin tumors in mice, the 3,4-dihydrodiol was again more active
than the parent hydrocarbon (Slaga *et al.*, 1979). Substitution of methyl
groups in the 2- or 3-positions and fluorine in the 1- or 2-positions of DMBA
led to a loss of biological activity (Harvey & Dunne, 1978). These results are
consistent with either, or both, the *anti* or *syn* bay region diol epoxide
metabolite being the ultimate carcinogenic form of DMBA. On the other
hand, substitution of methyl into the 4-position of DMBA failed to abolish
activity, and 1,2,3,4-tetrahydro-DMBA exhibited relatively high tumorigenic
activity (DiGiovanni *et al.*, 1982), suggesting that additional active
metabolites, other than the bay region diol epoxide, may be partially
responsible for the carcinogenic activity of DMBA.

Chrysene can form only three dihydrodiols because of its symmetry, and
the 1,2-, 3,4-, and 5,6-dihydrodiols have all been detected as metabolic
products. When chrysene was incubated with hepatic microsomal fractions
from 3-MC-treated rats, the 3,4-dihydrodiol was the principal isomer formed,
and the 5,6-dihydrodiol was only a minor metabolite. In bacterial assays in
the presence of activating enzymes the 1,2-dihydrodiol, which could be
converted to the bay region diol epoxide on further metabolism, showed 20-
fold greater activity than chrysene or the isomeric dihydrodiols (Wood *et al.*,
1979). The synthetic *anti*-diol epoxide was more active than the *syn*-isomer
in either *S. typhimurium* strains or Chinese hamster V79 cells. Chrysene
resembles BA in that both hydrocarbons are only weak tumor initiators, but
the dihydrodiols which give rise to the bay region diol epoxides are highly
active.

5-Methylchrysene is interesting in that it has two bay regions that can give
rise to diol epoxides one of which has a methyl group in a nonbenzo bay
region site. The major dihydrodiol metabolites of 5-methylchrysene were
shown by Hecht *et al.* (1978) to be the 1,2- and 7,8-dihydrodiols
accompanied by small amounts of the 9,10-dihydrodiol. 5-
Hydroxymethylchrysene and a number of phenolic metabolites were also
formed. In bacterial mutagenicity assays in the presence of a rat liver
homogenate, the 1,2-dihydrodiol was more active than the 7,8-dihydrodiol,
which was more active than the other metabolites tested. In Chinese hamster
V79 cells the *anti*-1,2-diol-3,4-epoxide isomer was the most mutagenic diol
epoxide isomer (Brookes *et al.*, 1986). The 1,2-dihydrodiol exhibited higher

activity than the parent hydrocarbon or the isomeric dihydrodiols in the induction of skin tumors in mice, and the corresponding *anti*-diol epoxide was the most active diol epoxide isomer (Hecht *et al.*, 1985). These findings support the idea that the *anti*-1,2-diol-3,4-epoxide is the ultimate carcinogenic form of 5-MC. The low tumorigenicity of the 1-, 3-, and 12-fluoro derivatives of 5-MC provide further support, since substitution in these sites significantly reduces the amount of the 1,2-dihydrodiol formed as a metabolite.

The enzymatic formation of PAH oxidized metabolites generally proceeds with high stereoselectivity. The enantiomeric composition of the epoxides and *trans*-dihydrodiols formed in the metabolism of several representative PAHs is summarized in Table 4.1. The percentage of the S,R-enantiomers formed in the metabolism of the K-regions of several PAHs by liver microsomes from 3-MC-treated rats are 95–99% for BA, chrysene, and DMBA. The phenobarbitol-inducible cytochrome P-450 isozyme (P-450b) showed a lower preference for the S,R-enantiomer, resembling more closely that of the cytochrome P-450 isozymes from untreated rats.

Epoxide hydrase frequently has a higher affinity toward one of the two arene oxide enantiomers formed by metabolism, resulting in differential rates of metabolism. Consequently, EH tends to exert an enantioselective effect on the ratio of dihydrodiol isomers formed. Hydration of the K-oxides of the planar polyarenes BA and chrysene, like that of BaP 4,5-oxide, proceeds via preferential attack at the S-center to afford predominantly the R,R-dihydrodiol enantiomers. In contrast, hydration of the K-oxides of the nonplanar polyarenes benzo[c]phenanthrene and DMBA involves reaction by EH predominantly at the R-center to form the dihydrodiols enriched in the S,S-enantiomers. Further studies on the mechanism of hydration of the K-oxides of additional planar and nonplanar PAHs are needed before it can be established whether or not this is a general rule.

A stereochemical model to predict the stereochemistry of epoxidation of polyarenes by the cytochrome P-450 isozyme was proposed by Jerina *et al.* (1982). This model was developed for cytochrome P-450c and it is not necessarily applicable to other cytochromes P-450. The cytochromes P-450 contained in liver microsomes from untreated and PB-treated rats generally exhibit lower stereoselectivity than cytochrome P-450c. According to the proposed model, the minimum boundary for the catalytic binding site is represented by the structure in Fig. 4.7. Oxygenation is assumed to take place from the underside of the polyarene in the molecular region indicated. For example, in the oxygenation of BaP in the K-region the allowed binding mode yields the 4S,5R-oxide which is obtained as the major product. Formation of the enantiomeric 4R,5S-oxide requires orientation of the hydrocarbon in an unfavorable binding mode with the benzo ring in the 'restricted area'. While this is a useful empirical model which correctly predicts the stereochemistry of PAH oxygenation in many of the cases examined, its general applicability has not been established. Yang (1988) has noted a number of exceptions and has stated that 'at this time, it is not possible to define the exact size [and dimensions] of the catalytic binding site in order to account for the observed results in the metabolism studies of PAHs'. It may be that the binding site possesses some degree of flexibility, allowing it to partially adjust its shape to fit the substrate.

4.5   Other metabolic pathways

Although the metabolic pathway leading to reactive diol epoxide metabolites has received major attention, there is evidence for several additional modes of metabolic activation of polyarenes. These include formation of radical-cations, hydroperoxide-dependent oxidation, dihydrodiol dehydrogenase-catalyzed oxidation of dihydrodiols to quinones, and, biomethylation by S-adenosyl-L-methionine.

One-electron oxidation of polyarenes by chemical oxidants, such as iodine in pyridine or $Mn(OAc)_3$ in acetic acid can afford products arising from trapping of radical-cation intermediates with nucleophiles (Cavalieri & Rogan, 1985). For unsubstituted PAHs, such as BaP, oxidation with these reagents yields pyridinium or acetoxy derivatives formed by direct attack of pyridine or acetate ion, respectively, on the radical-cation at C-6, the position of maximum charge density (Fig. 4.8). Reaction of the BaP radical-cation with the weak nucleophile H_2O affords a mixture of the BaP 1,6-, 3,6-, and 6,12-diones arising from secondary oxidation of the primary product 6-hydroxy-BaP. Analogous reaction of a methyl-substituted hydrocarbon, such as 6-methyl-BaP, which has a methyl group at the position of maximum charge density has the additional possibility of loss of a proton from the

Fig. 4.7. (A) The minimum boundary for the catalytic binding site and the site of oxygenation of cytochrome P-450c proposed by Jerina et al. (1982). (B) The allowed binding mode which yields the 4S,5R-oxide. (C) The unfavorable binding mode that leads to the 4R,5S-oxide of BaP contains a ring in the 'restricted ' area.

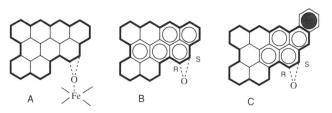

methyl group to form a benzylic radical followed by a second oxidation to generate a benzylic cation which, in turn, undergoes trapping by a nucleophile (Fig. 4.8).

Assuming that radical–cation intermediates can be generated *in vivo*, they may react with water to form phenolic and quinone metabolites or with other cellular nucleophiles, such as DNA, to form adducts. The ability of PAH radical–cations to bind covalently to cellular macromolecules is expected to depend upon their ease of formation as measured by PAH ionization potential and the degree of localization of the charge at a particular site in the molecule. According to Cavalieri & Rogan (1985), only PAHs with a relatively low ionization potential (< 7.35 eV) can be biologically activated by one-electron oxidation. Thus, in the binding of PAHs to DNA using horseradish peroxidase/H_2O_2, a system which catalyzes one-electron oxidation, only PAHs with IP < 7.35 eV are significantly bound. The ionization potentials (IPs) of a series of representative PAHs are presented in Table 4.2.

The carcinogenicity of the PAHs in Table 4.2 correlates approximately with their ionization potentials. However, a number of exceptions are also evident. Thus, 5-methylchrysene which is equipotent as a carcinogen with BaP on mouse skin and 7-methyl-BA which is also a relatively potent carcinogen have IPs above the range for activity, while perylene which is noncarcinogenic has a low IP. Cavalieri & Rogan (1985) have suggested that the carcinogenic activity of PAHs with relatively high IPs, such as 5-

Fig. 4.8. One-electron oxidation of BaP and 6-methyl-BaP and trapping of the intermediates with a nucleophile (Nu).

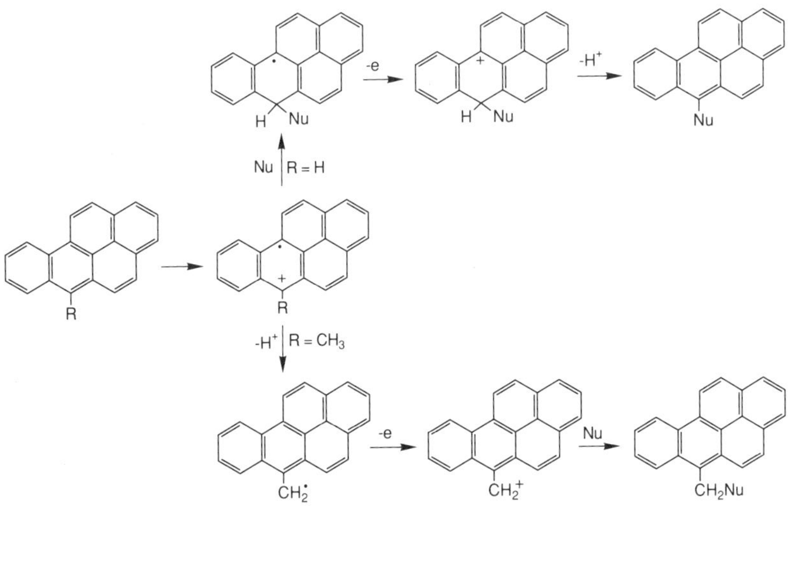

Table 4.2. *Ionization potentials of PAHs in relation to carcinogenicity*[a]

Hydrocarbon	Ionization potential (eV)	Carcinogenicity
phenanthrene	8.19	0
benzo[c]phenanthrene	7.93	+
chrysene	7.8	±
5-methylchrysene	7.7	+++
benzo[e]pyrene	7.62	±
dibenz[a,h]anthracene	7.57	++
benz[a]anthracene	7.54	±
pyrene	7.50	0
anthracene	7.43	0
7-methylbenz[a]anthracene	7.37	+++
dibenzo[a,e]pyrene	7.35	+++
dibenzo[a,l]pyrene	7.26	+++
dibenzo[a,i]pyrene	7.25	++++
BaP	7.23	+++
DMBA	7.22	+++++
3-MC	7.12	++++
6-methyl-BaP	7.08	++
perylene	7.06	0
dibenzo[a,h]pyrene	6.97	++++
anthanthrene	6.96	±

[a]Ionization potential data are from Cavalieri & Rogan, 1985.

methylchrysene, may involve diol epoxide intermediates, while the activity of PAHs having IPs < 7.35 eV may involve, at least partially, radical–cation intermediates. There is, however, little direct evidence in support of this hypothesis. DNA binding experiments of PAH carcinogens in mouse skin and other animal tissues indicate that the major DNA-bound metabolites are formed from diol epoxide intermediates. If PAH–DNA adducts arising from radical–cations are present, they must be formed in relatively small amounts. This, of course, does not prove that they might not be more important for tumor induction. In the case of 6-methyl-BaP, Rogan *et al.* (1983) have identified a DNA adduct in mouse skin in which the methyl group is covalently bound to the 2-amino group of deoxyguanosine. While this was taken as evidence for a radical–cation intermediate, it is also conceivable that it may have arisen via an ionic mechanism involving the sulfate ester of 6-hydroxy-BaP.

In related studies, Marnett (1985) has shown that fatty acid hydroperoxides in the presence of heme complexes and heme proteins oxidize BaP and its 7,8-dihydrodiol to quinones and diol epoxides, respectively. The active oxidant is a peroxyl radical derived from the fatty acid hydroperoxides. The latter are the products of prostaglandin H synthase (PGH) and lipoxygenase oxidation of unsaturated fatty acids, such as arachidonic acid. Incubation of BaP with arachidonic acid and ram seminal vesicle microsomes, a rich source of PGH synthase, produces the 1,6-, 3,6-, and 6,12-quinones of BaP as the exclusive products. This oxidation is inhibited by antioxidants, suggesting that it entails a free radical mechanism. Analogous oxidation conducted in the presence of DNA or RNA results in substantial nucleic acid binding. However the structures of the nucleic acid adducts have not been determined, so the identity of the reactive intermediate is unknown. Despite the high level of nucleic acid binding, no mutagenic species could be detected when oxidation of BaP was conducted in the presence of *S. typhimurium* strains. It may be that the intermediate responsible for the nucleic acid binding is too unstable to survive transit across the bacterial cell wall.

Similar oxygenation of racemic BaP 7,8-dihydrodiol with PGH synthase and arachidonic acid hydroperoxide results in stereospecific formation of the corresponding *anti*-diol epoxide; the *syn*-diol epoxide isomer is not detected. In contrast to epoxidation by cytochrome P-450, both enantiomers are epoxidized at equal rates to the corresponding *anti*-diol epoxide enantiomers. Marnett (1985) has proposed a mechanism for the epoxidation of BaP 7,8-dihydrodiol that involves hematin-catalyzed generation of peroxyl radicals from fatty acid hydroperoxides (Fig. 4.9). According to this proposal, hematin reduces the hydroperoxide to an alkoxyl radical that cyclizes to the adjacent double bond. This incipient carbon-centered radical couples with O_2 to form a peroxyl radical that serves to epoxidize BaP 7,8-dihydrodiol. PGH synthase has also been shown to catalyze the activation of benz[a]anthracene 3,4-dihydrodiol and chrysene 1,2-dihydrodiol to bay region diol epoxides (Guthrie *et al.*, 1982). In the benz[a]anthracene case, the *anti*-diol epoxides predominate over the *syn*-diol epoxides by a ratio of 2:1 (Dix *et al.*, 1986). The relative importance of this mode of oxidation in the mechanism of PAH carcinogenesis is presently uncertain. Pretreatment of mice with aspirin or

Fig. 4.9. Mechanism proposed by Marnett (1985) for the generation of peroxyl radicals that epoxidize PAH dihydrodiols.

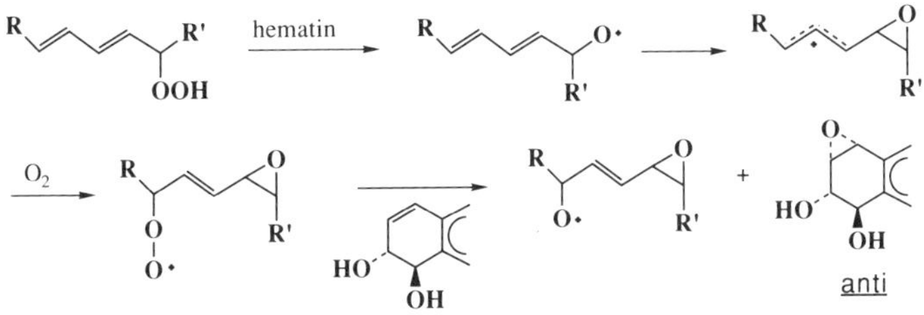

indomethacin, inhibitors of PGH synthase activity, does not lower the levels of DNA adducts formed from BaP in lung, nor does it reduce the incidence of lung neoplasms induced by BaP (Adriaenssens *et al.*, 1983). This suggests that PGH synthase-dependent oxidation does not play an important role in lung tumorigenesis by BaP in this system.

DNA damage may also be induced indirectly by reactive oxygen radical species produced as a consequence of metabolism of benzo[a]pyrene. A redox cycle (Fig. 4.10), involving the isomeric quinones of BaP and the corresponding hydroquinones on the one hand and molecular O_2 and NADPH on the other, leading to the formation of superoxide radicals has been demonstrated by Lorenzten & Ts'o (1977). Decomposition of the superoxide radicals gives rise to H_2O_2 and hydroxyl radicals. Cerutti (1974) has shown that hydroxyl radicals are the major active species responsible for DNA base damage induced by ionizing radiation in mammalian cells. Similar damage may also occur as a consequence of BaP metabolism in BHK cells in culture (Cerutti *et al.*, 1978).

Another metabolic pathway involves dihydrodiol dehydrogenase-catalyzed oxidation of PAH dihydrodiols to *ortho*-quinones (Smithgall *et al.*, 1986, 1988). The dihydrodiol dehydrogenase enzyme readily oxidizes the non-K-region *trans*-dihydrodiols of benzene, naphthalene, phenanthrene, chrysene, 5-methylchrysene, and BaP under physiological conditions, but fails to oxidize the K-region *trans*-dihydrodiols of phenanthrene and BaP. The mechanism of this NADP-dependent transformation is believed to involve initial formation of catechols by the action of dihydrodiol dehydrogenase, followed by autoxidation of the catechols to quinones (Smithgall et al., 1988a). These quinones exhibited exceptional reactivity towards the cellular thiols glutathione and cysteine, leading to formation of water soluble oxidized adducts. These findings suggest that the dihydrodiol dehydrogenase-catalyzed oxidation of proximate carcinogenic metabolites, such as the *trans-*

Fig. 4.10. Involvement of BaP quinone–hydroquinone redox couples in the production of reactive oxygen species at the expense of cellular reducing power.

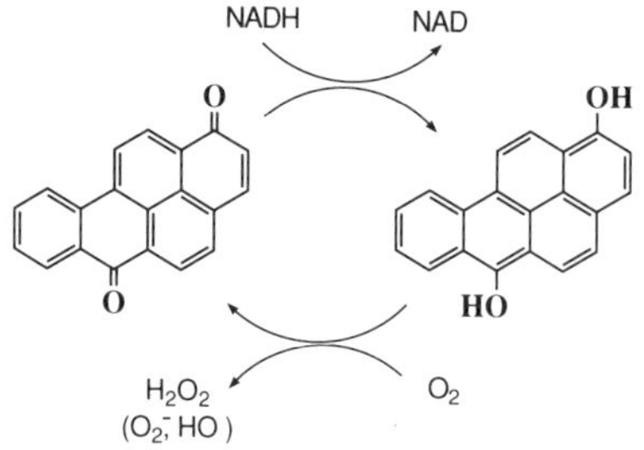

7,8-dihydrodiol of BaP, may be an important pathway for their detoxification.

In related studies, Jarabak and coworkers (Chung *et al.*, 1987) have shown that both K-region and non-K-region *o*-quinones of PAHs are excellent substrates for the human placental NADP-linked 15-hydroxyprostaglandin dehydrogenase enzyme. This, therefore, represents another potential pathway for the detoxification of PAH quinones.

Another potential mode of metabolic activation involves biomethylation of polyarenes in *meso*-anthracenic positions by S-adenosyl-L-methionine. Myers *et al.* (1988) have shown that incubation of anthracene in rat liver cytosol preparations fortified with S-adenosyl-L-methionine leads to formation of the weakly carcinogenic 9-methyl- and 9,10-dimethylanthracene. Further oxidation leads to formation of the corresponding hydroxymethyl and formyl derivatives. Flesher *et al.* (1986) have proposed that this pathway of metabolic activation may be general for unsubstituted polyarenes. However, the very weak tumorigenicity of BA and other PAHs which possess a reactive *meso*-region suggests that this mode of activation may be of only minor importance.

Therefore, although the adducts formed by the BaP diol epoxide metabolites with DNA represent the predominant covalent adducts produced in intact mammalian cells, there is evidence for minor adducts arising from the alternative metabolic pathways outlined herein as well as for indirect DNA damage caused by reactive oxygen radical species produced in redox cycles involving the quinone metabolites. The relative importance of these various pathways remains to be established.

4.6 Binding of metabolites to cellular macromolecules

The early studies which led to identification of the ultimate carcinogenic diol epoxide metabolites were based on the assumption that DNA binding was a critical step in the mechanism of PAH carcinogenesis. Following the demonstration of a correlation between carcinogenic potency and extent of binding to DNA in mouse skin for a series of polyarenes (Brookes & Lawley, 1964), Brookes and coworkers utilized rodent embryo cells in culture to obtain DNA modified by PAH metabolites, and they developed procedures for the enzymic degradation of the modified DNA and for the chromatographic analysis of the resulting PAH-nucleoside adducts (Brookes & Heidelberger, 1969; Duncan *et al.*, 1969; Baird & Brookes, 1973). Using these methodologies, Baird *et al.* (1973, 1975) demonstrated that the metabolites of 7-methyl-BA and BaP that were bound covalently to DNA in mammalian cells were not the K-region oxides. This finding shifted attention away from the K-region, where it so long resided, to other molecular regions.

A vital clue in the identification of the active species was the observation by Borgen *et al.* (1973) that a metabolite of BaP tentatively identified as the 7,8-dihydrodiol was metabolized by rat liver microsomes to an intermediate which bound to a greater extent to DNA than other BaP metabolites. Sims *et al.* (1974) proposed a diol epoxide structure of unspecified stereochemistry and showed that a crude preparation of the BaP diol epoxide, prepared from oxidation of the radioactive 7,8-dihydrodiol metabolite with *m*-chloroper-benzoic acid, reacted with DNA *in vitro* to yield products similar to those formed when rodent embryo cells were exposed to BaP. Proof for this hypothesis came from the chemical synthesis of the pure *anti-* and *syn*-BaP diol epoxides (*anti-* and *syn*-BPDE) in Harvey's and Jerina's laboratories (Beland & Harvey, 1976; Yagi *et al.*, 1975) and reaction of these authentic compounds with DNA.

The major product from reaction of *anti*-BPDE with DNA *in vitro* was found following degradation to the nucleoside level to be identical with the major adduct formed in metabolism and binding of BaP to DNA and RNA in rodent, bovine, and human cells (King *et al.*, 1976; Weinstein *et al.*, 1976; Jeffrey *et al.*, 1977). This adduct was shown by NMR and mass spectral analysis to be a guanosine derivative of (+)-*anti*-BPDE with the structure shown in Fig. 4.11 (Jeffrey *et al.*, 1977a; Nakanishi *et al.*, 1977). Minor nucleic acid-bound products arising from reaction of (+)-*anti*-BPDE on the

Fig. 4.11. Structures of the nucleoside adducts formed in the covalent binding of *anti*-BPDE with DNA.

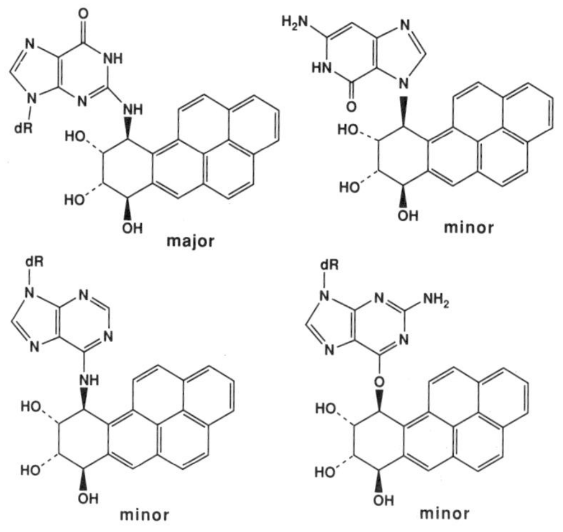

[7]N- and [6]O-positions of dG and the [6]N-position of dA and adducts of (–)-*anti*-BPDE and *syn*-BPDE were also subsequently identified (reviews on PAH–DNA binding: Harvey, 1981; Singer & Grunberger, 1983; Dipple *et al.*, 1984; Harvey & Geacintov, 1988).

Mutagenicity and tumorigenicity assays support the hypothesis that the diol epoxide metabolites are the ultimate carcinogenic forms of BaP (review: Sims & Grover, 1981). While *anti*- and *syn*-BPDE are both strongly mutagenic in bacterial and mammalian cells, *anti*-BPDE shows a higher level of activity in most assays (Newbold & Brookes, 1976; Huberman *et al.*, 1976). *Anti*-BPDE also exhibits higher activity in the inhibition of replication of bacterial viruses, in the induction of malignant transformation of mouse fibroblasts, and as a carcinogen on mouse skin and in newborn mouse lung.

Information on the structures of the covalent adducts formed by *anti*-BPDE with DNA has been obtained mainly from spectroscopic studies (Geacintov, 1985; Harvey & Geacintov, 1988). Two types of adducts, designated 'site I' and 'site II', have been detected. The site I adducts, which are relatively minor products, are characterized by a negative linear dichroism (LD) spectrum and a 10nm red shift in the ultraviolet absorption spectrum. The site II adducts exhibit a positive LD spectrum and a smaller 2–3nm red shift in the UV region. Geacintov proposed an intercalated structure for the site I adduct and an externally bound conformation for the site II adduct with the hydrocarbon moiety in the minor groove and its long axis inclined at an angle ≈35° to the DNA helix. These structural assignments are consistent with the findings of subsequent studies using the optical detection of magnetic resonance, flow dichroism, and electric field pulse-induced fluorescence polarization techniques.

On the basis of fluorescence quenching experiments Hogan *et al.* (1981) proposed an alternative structure for the major adduct in which the hydrocarbon is intercalated in a bent region of the DNA double helix forming a wedge-shaped structure. However, recent reinvestigation of the fluorescence properties of the *anti*-BPDE–DNA adducts has shown the presence of three different fluorescence decay components (Geacintov *et al.*, 1987; Zinger *et al.*, 1987). The first two of these are most satisfactorily interpreted in terms of the site I and site II adducts originally proposed. The third unusually long-lived fluorescence decay component was identified as tetraol formed by UV-induced hydrolysis of the covalent adducts. This previously unrecognized photodecomposition accounts for most of the discrepancies in the prior literature. Thus, the site II externally bound structure appears to be most consistent with the spectroscopic properties of the major *anti*-BPDE adduct.

DNA binding studies with the *syn* diastereomer of BPDE (Shahbaz *et al.*,

1986) indicate that the conformation of the major bound adduct contains the hydrocarbon molecule intercalated within the DNA helix. The structural difference between the *syn-* and *anti*-BPDE adducts may be of great importance in the recognition, repair, and fidelity of replication of these lesions by the appropriate enzymes. The possible relation between adduct conformation and differences in the mutagenic and tumorigenic activities of *anti*- and *syn*-BPDE has been discussed by Shahbaz *et al.* (1986).

Kinetic studies of the mechanism of interaction of *anti*-BPDE with calf thymus DNA (Harvey & Geacintov, 1988) are consistent with a mechanism involving initial rapid intercalation (complete in <5 ms) of the diol epoxide between the base pairs of DNA (Fig. 4.12). This complex is detectable by a red shift in its UV absorption maximum and by its linear dichroism spectrum, both of which are consistent with an intercalated structure. It undergoes rate-determining protonation to yield an intercalated triol carbonium ion intermediate which decomposes to products via two pathways. The major path (A) which accounts for >90 % of BPDE, is hydrolysis to yield tetraols which also physically associate with DNA. DNA catalyzes the rate of hydrolysis of BPDE, increasing the rate by a factor of 80. The minor, more biologically important, path (B) is covalent binding to DNA. The overall rate of BPDE–DNA interaction is dependent upon pH, temperature, ionic strength, solvent, and other factors, but the ratio of A/B is independent of these variables. This mechanism is also consistent with the findings of theoretical molecular modeling studies.

Subsequent studies of the metabolism and DNA binding of other alternant polyarenes support the hypothesis that diol epoxide metabolites are also their ultimate carcinogenic forms (reviews: Sims & Grover, 1981; Conney, 1982; Harvey & Geacintov, 1988). In most cases the evidence rests mainly on

Fig. 4.12. Mechanism of binding of *anti*-BPDE to DNA.

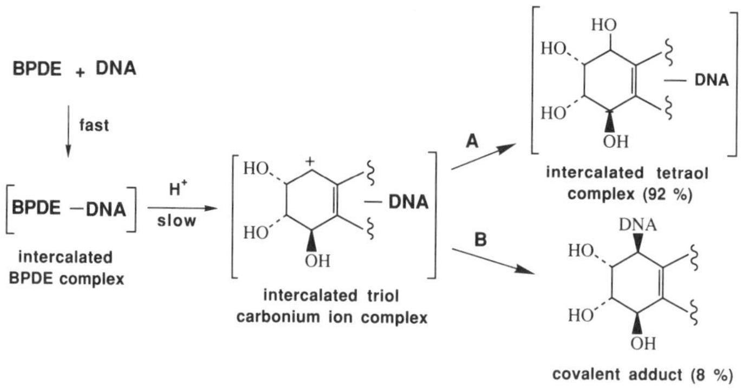

metabolism studies and comparison of the mutagenicities of the possible dihydrodiol and diol epoxide metabolites obtained synthetically. In only relatively few cases have DNA binding studies and characterization of the PAH–nucleoside adducts been carried out. On the basis of the findings to date it may be generalized that the active carcinogenic forms of all alternant PAHs are the bay region diol epoxide metabolites analogous to *anti-* and/or *syn*-BPDE in which the epoxide ring is located in a bay molecular region. However, there is evidence which indicates that in specific cases adducts arising from non-bay region diol epoxide and triol epoxide intermediates are also formed and may play an important role.

Benz[a]anthracene is a case in point. While the tumor-initiating activities of the BA 3,4-dihydrodiol and its diol epoxide derivative are consistent with the bay region diol epoxide generalization, DNA binding studies in mouse skin or hamster embryo cells show that the BA 8,9-dihydrodiol 11,12-oxide also binds to DNA to significant extent (Cooper *et al.*, 1980). The major products formed in the reactions of the BA 1,2,3,4- or 8,9,10,11-diol epoxides with DNA are the ^{2}N-dG adducts, but lesser amounts of the ^{6}N-dA adducts are also detected (Cooper *et al.*, 1980a; Hemminki *et al.*, 1980). Spectroscopic studies of the reactions of the stereoisomeric bay region diol epoxides of BA (*anti-* and *syn*-BADE) with DNA show that both diastereomers form noncovalent complexes with DNA, but the association constant for *syn*-BADE is six to seven times smaller (Carberry *et al.*, 1988a). The covalent DNA adduct of *anti*-BADE exists predominantly in a site II conformation, although a small fraction remains quasi-intercalated. In contrast, the covalent adduct of the less tumorigenic *syn*-BADE retains the site I conformation of the noncovalent complex.

Similar spectroscopic studies of the stereoisomeric *anti-* and *syn*-BA 8,9,10,11-diol epoxides (*anti-* and *syn*-BADE-II) indicate that both diastereomers form noncovalent intercalative complexes with double-stranded DNA prior to covalent binding (Carberry *et al.*, 1988). The association constant for the *anti*-BADE-II complex is twice that of the *syn*-BADE-II complex, qualitatively paralleling the relationship previously established for the bay region diol epoxide isomers of BaP and BA. However, the levels of covalent binding to DNA are about half those for *anti-* and *syn*-BADE. The conformations of the adducts resemble those derived from the *anti-* and *syn-* diastereomers of BaP and BA, providing an additional example of the correlation between adduct structure and relative biological activity.

The nature of the products obtained when 3-methylcholanthrene binds to DNA in cells in culture or in mouse tissue are less certain (Sims & Grover, 1981). Osborne *et al.*, 1986 have shown that the DNA derived from mouse embryo cells exposed to 3-MC yields a series of nucleoside adducts, only a minority of which are derived from the bay region diol epoxide, *anti*-3-MCDE. Two of the major DNA-bound products were tentatively identified as triol epoxide derivatives, probably the bay region *anti*- and *syn*-diol epoxide metabolites of 3-hydroxymethylcholanthrene. However, since the only diol epoxide derivative of 3-MC available through synthesis was *anti*-3-MCDE (Jacobs *et al.*, 1983), more precise characterization awaits the synthesis of a more complete set of metabolite standards. The reaction of *anti*-3-MCDE with DNA *in vitro* gave principally the ^{2}N-dG adduct, but minor products containing guanine, adenine, and cytosine were also obtained (Osborne *et al.*, 1986). Like *anti*-BPDE, *anti*-3-MCDE was an efficient mutagen in hamster V79 cells, even at low doses which caused no cytotoxicity. Spectroscopic studies of the reaction of *anti*-3-MCDE with DNA indicate that a physical noncovalent complex is formed which is not intercalated in the classical sense (Carberry *et al.*, 1988a). Nevertheless, covalent binding of *anti*-3-MCDE to DNA takes place at the same level as *anti*-BADE, indicating that intercalation is not a prerequisite to such binding. The conformations of the adducts formed by *anti*-3-MCDE with DNA closely resemble those of *anti*-BADE, i.e. a major externally bound site II adduct and a minor quasi-intercalated site I adduct.

The structure of the DNA adduct formed by metabolism of 7-methyl-BA, though based on more limited evidence, is again consistent with a bay region diol epoxide metabolite (Sims & Grover, 1981). Thus, fluorescence measurements of the adducts formed by metabolism of 7-MBA in cellular systems confirm the presence of an anthracene fluorophore. Also, both the 1,2- and 3,4-dihydrodiols, but not the 8,9-dihydrodiol, bind to the DNA of mouse skin *in vivo*, and the chromatographic properties of the *in vivo* adduct match those of the adduct obtained by treatment of DNA with the bay region diol epoxide of 7-MBA. However, the adducts have not been chemically characterized, and information is lacking concerning the three-dimensional structures of the DNA adducts.

The nucleic acid binding properties of DMBA are of particular interest because of the exceptional carcinogenic potency of this hydrocarbon. As with other PAHs, the weight of the evidence implicates a bay region diol epoxide metabolite as the principal species which binds to DNA in cellular systems. However, in contrast to other PAHs, there is substantial evidence that both *syn*- and *anti*-diol epoxides mediate the binding of this carcinogen to DNA, and that substantial amounts of dA as well as dG adducts are formed (Sawicki *et al.*, 1983). Three of the DNA adducts produced by metabolism of DMBA in cells were shown to be derived from reaction of the *syn*-diol epoxide with dA, while a fourth adduct was derived from its reaction with dG

(Cheng *et al.*, 1988, 1988a). The successful synthesis of the highly reactive *anti*- and *syn*-DMBA diol epoxides (Lee & Harvey, 1986) made it possible to prepare larger amounts of these adducts and determine their structures. The principal adducts were shown to be *cis* and *trans* addition products of ^{6}N-dA to the epoxide ring of the enantiomeric *syn*-DMBA diol epoxide. Reaction of the *anti*-DMBA diol epoxide to DNA was shown to afford an adenine and a guanine product in roughly equal amounts. The exceptionally high reactivity of the DMBA diol epoxides with dA residues in DNA has led to the suggestion that PAH-dA adducts may have greater potential for tumor initiation than the adducts with dG (Bigger *et al.*, 1983).

The metabolic activation and DNA binding of chrysene was examined in mouse, rat, and human skin using short term organ culture techniques (Weston *et al.*, 1985; Phillips *et al.*, 1987). Mouse skin exhibited greater propensity for metabolic activation, consistent with its greater sensitivity to PAH carcinogens. The major chrysene–deoxyribonucleoside adduct in all three tissues was the bay region *anti*-1,2-diol 3,4-oxide adduct with dG. A lesser amount of a dA adduct was also detected. In rodent, but not in human skin, a small quantity of a third adduct, determined to arise from the 9-hydroxychrysene *anti*-1,2-diol 3,4-oxide metabolite, was also characterized. Mutagenicity studies show that the *syn* and *anti* diastereomers of the latter are potent direct-acting mutagens. Evidence has been obtained that 9-hydroxychrysene *anti*-1,2-diol 3,4-oxide can be formed metabolically from the related chrysene diol epoxide (Hall *et al.*, 1988). The extent to which the triol epoxide contributes to tumorigenesis is unknown.

The comparative binding properties of chrysene and 5-methylchrysene are of interest in view of the striking differences in their carcinogenic properties. However, the situation is complicated by the asymmetry of 5-methylchrysene which contains two bay regions that can give rise to nonidentical bay region diol epoxides designated DE-I and DE-II (Fig. 4.13). The former exhibits a greater extent of binding to DNA *in vivo* and *in vitro* than the latter (Melikian *et al.*, 1982, 1988). This is somewhat surprising in view of the steric interference to binding anticipated to be imposed by the bay region methyl

Fig. 4.13. Structures of the *anti*- and *syn*-diol epoxide isomers of 5-methylchrysene in both bay regions.

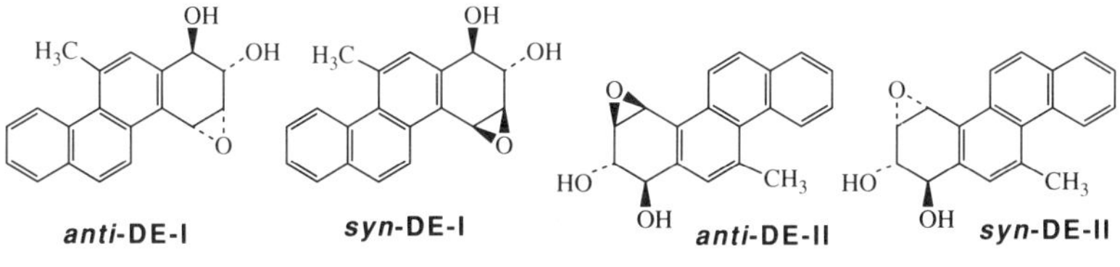

anti-DE-I   *syn*-DE-I   *anti*-DE-II   *syn*-DE-II

group of DE-I. The structures of the principal deoxyribonucleoside adducts formed in the metabolism and covalent binding of 5-methylchrysene to DNA are the *anti*-DE-I and DE-II derivatives attached to ^{2}N-dG. Minor adducts arising from *cis* and *trans* addition of both stereoisomeric *anti*- and *syn*-diol epoxides to dG and dA have also been characterized (Reardon *et al.*, 1987; Melikian *et al.*, 1988). A marked stereoselectivity in the formation of these products was observed. The extent of the reactions of the R,S,S,R-enantiomers of *anti*-DE-I and DE-II with dG exceeded those of the corresponding S,R,R,S-enantiomers by sixfold. The formation of dA adducts exhibited lower stereoselectivity, with the ratio of R,S,S,R/S,R,R,S adducts being approximately two. The higher reactivity of the R,S,S,R-enantiomers with DNA and the greater stereoselectivity of their binding to dG in comparison with the S,R,R,S-enantiomers parallel the results obtained with the enantiomers of BPDE. Spectroscopic studies indicate that the mechanism of interaction of *anti*-DE-I and DE-II with DNA also parallels that of *anti*-BPDE and involves initial formation of an intercalated complex followed by covalent bond formation and rearrangement to yield predominantly site II adducts (Kim *et al.*, 1985; Harvey & Geacintov, 1988).

Another carcinogen with a methyl group in a bay region is 16,17-dihydro-11-methyl-15H-cyclopenta[a]phenanthren-17-one (Fig. 4.14). Like 5-methylchrysene and DMBA, this compound is an example of the 'bay region methyl effect', i.e. enhancement of carcinogenicity by introduction of a methyl group into a nonbenzo bay region site (DiGiovanni *et al.*, 1983). Evidence has been obtained that the major hydrocarbon–deoxyribonucleoside adduct formed from the cyclopenta[a]phenanthrene compound arises from reaction of the bay region diol epoxide (Fig. 4.14) on the amino groups of dG residues in DNA (Coombs & Bhatt, 1987). More thorough characterization awaits studies with the authentic diol epoxides whose synthesis has recently been accomplished in the author's laboratory (Lee & Harvey, 1988; Young & Harvey, unpublished studies).

Although benzo[c]phenanthrene (BcP) is only very weakly carcinogenic, its fjord region diol epoxide is stated to be the most tumorigenic diol epoxide

Fig. 4.14. 16,17-Dihydro-11-methyl-15*H*-cyclopenta[a]phenanthren-17-one and its bay region *anti*- and *syn*-diol epoxides.

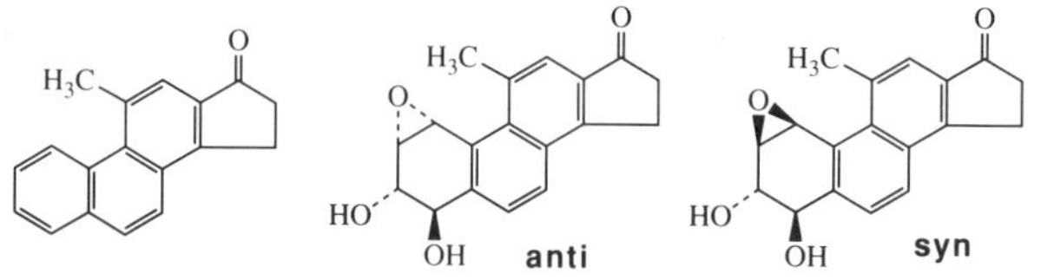

derivative tested to date (Levin *et al.*, 1980). The primary oxidative metabolites formed from BcP are the 3,4- and 5,6-oxides. They constitute 3–17% and 77–97%, respectively, of the total metabolites as determined by trapping with *N*-acetyl-L-cysteine. The stereochemistry of metabolic activation and DNA-binding of BcP have recently been studied in detail (leading references: Pruess-Schwartz *et al.*, 1987). Incubation of 5-^{3}H-BcP with rodent embryo cells in culture afforded dA and dG adducts of BcP in a ratio of 3:1. These were shown to be formed principally from reaction of the (-)-*anti* bay region diol epoxide. This isomer has the R,S,S,R absolute configuration shown previously to be associated with maximum carcinogenic activity of other PAHs. The fact that a high proportion of adducts are dA adducts, as observed earlier for DMBA, accords with Dipple's suggestion that binding to adenosine may be more important for carcinogenic activity than binding to guanine. It is probably also significant that BcP and DMBA are both distorted from planarity.

While the DNA-binding properties of additional alternant PAH metabolites have been reported, the evidence is minimal so far concerning the structures of the adducts formed. Nevertheless, the data appear consistent with the generalization that bay region diol epoxide metabolites are the principal active intermediates that bind to DNA leading ultimately to tumor induction.

4.7   Nonalternant polyarenes

Although nonalternant PAHs are common environmental pollutants, very little is known concerning their carcinogenic properties or their mechanisms of tumor induction. This is partly due to the historical fact that the carcinogenic properties of the alternant polyarenes were the first to be discovered. Also contributing to the relative neglect of this class of hydrocarbons is the less developed state of their chemistry, the unavailability for biological studies of all but a few simple nonalternant PAHs, and the weak carcinogenicity of the nonalternant PAHs investigated in early studies. There is also an assumption by many investigators that the mechanisms of carcinogenesis of nonalternant PAHs are likely to parallel those of the more intensively investigated alternant polyarenes. However, this assumption is not supported by any convincing scientific evidence.

While it is true that the nonalternant PAHs tested to date tend to exhibit weak activity, the effects of substitution by methyl and other groups on activity are relatively unexplored, and it is likely that more potent substituted nonalternant polyarenes will be discovered. More importantly, many of the highly tumorigenic alternant PAHs, such as DMBA and 3-MC, are not environmental contaminants, while some of the weakly active nonalternant

Table 4.3. *Names and numbering of representative nonalternant polycyclic aromatic hydrocarbons*

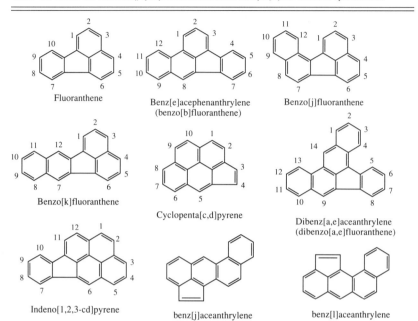

Fluoranthene

Benz[e]acephenanthrylene
(benzo[b]fluoranthene)

Benzo[j]fluoranthene

Benzo[k]fluoranthene

Cyclopenta[c,d]pyrene

Dibenz[a,e]aceanthrylene
(dibenzo[a,e]fluoranthene)

Indeno[1,2,3-cd]pyrene

benz[j]aceanthrylene

benz[l]aceanthrylene

*Nomenclature is in accord with Chemical Abstracts; common names are given in parentheses.

compounds, such as fluoranthene and cyclopenta[c,d]pyrene, constitute a significant percentage of the environmental hazards to which human populations are commonly exposed. Moreover, the assumption that the mechanisms of carcinogenesis of nonalternant polyarenes are likely to parallel those of alternant polyarenes appears unjustified; recent studies that show that some nonalternant PAHs which are structurally incapable of forming a bay region diol epoxide, nevertheless exhibit tumorigenic properties.

The most studied nonalternant PAHs are fluoranthene, benz[e]acephenanthrylene (benzo[b]fluoranthene), benzo[j]fluoranthene, benzo[k]fluoranthene, indeno[1,2,3-cd]pyrene, cyclopenta[c,d]pyrene, benz[j]aceanthrylene, benz[l]aceanthrylene, and dibenz[a,e]aceanthrylene (dibenzo[a,e]fluoranthene) (Table 4.3). The state of current knowledge concerning each of these compounds will be reviewed briefly.

Fluoranthene is a widespread environmental contaminant present in urban air, common foods, tobacco smoke, and industrial emissions. Although fluoranthene was once considered to be noncarcinogenic because it failed to induce tumors in mice with several bioassay systems, it has recently been shown to be tumorigenic in a newborn mouse lung adenoma assay (Busby Jr *et al.*, 1984). The major mutagenic metabolite of fluoranthene in the Ames assay has been identified as the 2,3-dihydrodiol (LaVoie *et al.*, 1982). Therefore, the ultimate mutagenic metabolite is presumably the corresponding 2,3-diol 1,10b-oxide in which the epoxide ring is attached to a fused ring position. This assignment is supported by DNA binding studies with microsomally activated fluoranthene which indicate that the major DNA-bound product is a ^{2}N-dG adduct of *trans*-2,3-dihydroxy-*anti*-1,10b-epoxy-1,2,3-trihydrofluoranthene (Babson *et al.*, 1986). While it is not yet established that this diol epoxide is also the ultimate carcinogenic metabolite that binds to DNA in animal tissues, this seems likely. If so, it is the first example of an active diol epoxide that is not a bay region diol epoxide.

Benz[e]acephenanthrylene (commonly known as benzo[b]fluoranthene) (BbF) is also widely distributed in the environment. Its tumor-initiating activity on mouse skin is about equivalent to that of dibenz[a,h]anthracene. The major dihydrodiol metabolites of BbF formed by rat liver microsomes or in mouse epidermis were the 1,2- and 11,12-dihydrodiols; for leading references on the properties of BbF and its metabolites see Geddie *et al.*, 1987. Both of these dihydrodiols exhibited mutagenic activity lower than that of the parent hydrocarbon in the Ames assay. This result is not surprising, since they are both bay region dihydrodiols. In contrast, the 9,10-dihydrodiol, which could not be detected as a metabolite of BbF but which is capable of forming a bay region diol epoxide, was equipotent with BbF as a mutagen and as a tumor initiator on mouse skin. The identity of the principal carcinogenic metabolite(s) of BbF is unknown. DNA binding studies, which are likely to provide the greatest insight, have apparently not been carried out.

Benzo[j]fluoranthene (BjF) and *benzo[k]fluoranthene* (BkF) are both commonly detected in urban air, automobile exhaust, cigarette smoke, and various foods. The levels of these hydrocarbons in the environment are comparable to those of BaP. BjF is a complete carcinogen on mouse skin with activity less than that of BbF, whereas BkF is inactive at the same dose. However, BkF is active as a tumor initiator on mouse skin and induces fibrosarcomas when administered by subcut. injection to mice. For leading references on the properties of BjF, BkF, and their metabolites see Rice *et al.*, 1987. Metabolism of BjF with microsomal enzymes or in mouse skin afforded two dihydrodiols identified as the 4,5- and 9,10-dihydrodiols, 4- and 10-hydroxy-BjF, and BjF 4,5-dione. The tumor initiating activity of the 4,5-dihydrodiol on mouse skin exceeded that of BjF, while the BjF 9,10-dihydrodiol exhibited lower activity; BjF 2,3-dihydrodiol was inactive as a tumor initiator. These findings suggest that BjF 4,5-dihydrodiol is a proximate tumorigenic metabolite of BjF that undergoes further metabolic activation to the corresponding 4,5-diol 6,6a-oxide. The latter is structurally analogous to the 2,3-diol 1,10-oxide of fluoranthene implicated as its ultimate carcinogenic metabolite. The BjF 9,10-dihydrodiol may also contribute to the overall tumorigenic activity of BjF. BkF 8,9-dihydrodiol, which was identified as the major mutagenic metabolite of BkF, was inactive as a tumor initiator on mouse skin. DNA binding studies have not been conducted with these hydrocarbons, and the identity of their principal ultimate carcinogenic metabolites have not been definitively established.

Indeno[1,2,3-cd]pyrene (IP) is listed as a priority pollutant by the Environmental Protection Agency. For leading references on the occurrence and properties of IP see Rice *et al.*, 1986. IP is active as a tumor initiator and a complete carcinogen on mouse skin and is also active as a carcinogen in rat lung. The major metabolites of IP formed *in vivo* in mouse skin are the K-region 1,2-dihydrodiol and 8- and 9-hydroxy-IP. Detected as minor metabolites were the 1,2-dihydrodiols of 8- and 9-hydroxy-IP, 10-hydroxy-IP, and IP-1,2-dione. While the 1,2-dihydrodiol is inactive as a mutagen *Salmonella typhimurium* TA 100, its precursor the 1,2-oxide is a potent direct-acting mutagen in this assay. The 1,2-dihydrodiol and the 1,2-oxide of IP exhibited equal potency as tumor initiators on mouse skin. However, this activity was less than that of the parent hydrocarbon. DNA binding studies have not yet been conducted with IP, and the identity of its principal active metabolite(s) is not established.

Cyclopenta[c,d]pyrene (CPP) occurs ubiquitously in products of incomplete combustion. It is especially prevalent in gasoline engine emissions, where it occurs at levels considerably higher than BaP, and in carbon black. For leading references on the occurrence and biological properties of CPP see Busby, Jr *et al.*, 1988. Although CPP is several-fold more mutagenic than BaP in bacterial assays with microsomal activation, it is less potent than BaP as a tumor initiator or as a complete carcinogen on mouse skin. However, CPP is a potent tumorigen in the newborn mouse lung adenoma assay. Metabolism of CPP in the presence of a microsomal activation system gives principally the 3,4-dihydrodiol. The 3,4-oxide, which is the putative metabolic precursor of the latter, is a potent direct-acting mutagen in the Ames assay (Gold & Eisenstadt, 1980). It is presumably the ultimate mutagenic metabolite of CPP. The relatively weak carcinogenicity of CPP may be due to the ease of enzymatic hydrolysis of the relatively reactive epoxide ring. Theoretical calculations predict the latter to be more reactive than a typical arene oxide, and it is sterically uncrowded, in contrast to bay region epoxides. DNA binding studies have not yet been conducted with CPP.

Benz[j]aceanthrylene (cholanthrylene) (BjA) and *benz[l]aceanthrylene* (BlA) are additional examples of cyclopenta-fused PAHs that have been obtained synthetically. For leading references on BjA and BlA see Nesnow *et al.*, 1988. While their environmental occurrence is unknown, BjA and BlA are both potent mutagens in bacterial and mammalian cell systems. Although BjA has not been examined for its tumorigenic effects, BlA is a potent mouse skin tumor initiator. The major metabolite of BjA produced by incubation with S9 rat liver proteins was the 1,2-dihydrodiol; the 9,10- and 11,12-dihydrodiols and 10-hydroxy-BjA were detected as minor metabolites. Oxidation of BlA takes place principally in the K-region to yield the 7,8-dihydrodiol; the 1,2- and 4,5-dihydrodiols are minor metabolites. Oxidation of the cyclopenta ring is approximately 50% of that observed for oxidation of the K-region. DNA binding studies have not yet been conducted with these hydrocarbons, and the identity of their principal active metabolites have not been established.

Dibenz[a,e]aceanthrylene (dibenzo[a,e]fluoranthene) (DBaeA) is a minor component of the PAHs present in the environment. Human exposure to DBaeA occurs primarily through tobacco smoke. In the earlier literature DBaeA was mistaken for its isomer dibenzo[a,l]pyrene, leading to some confusion. DBaeA exhibits moderate activity as a tumor initiator on mouse skin. Its metabolic activation and DNA binding has been extensively explored by French investigators; for leading references see Perin-Roussel *et al.*, 1988. Incubation of DBaeA with rat and mouse liver microsomes affords a complex pattern of metabolites, 19 of which have been identified. Oxidative attack occurs on all three peripheral rings. Primary metabolic transformation leads principally to the 3,4- and 12,13-dihydrodiols on ring A and D, respectively, and the 3-, 4-, and 7-phenols on rings A and E. Incubation of DBaeA or its major metabolites with calf thymus DNA in the presence of microsomes leads to a complex spectrum of adducts. The most abundant of these were characterized as the products of covalent reaction of the bay region (DE-I) and pseudo bay region (DE-II) diol epoxides derived from the 3,4- and 12,13-dihydrodiols, respectively, with guanosine. It is tentatively assumed by analogy with BPDE that these are ^{2}N-dG adducts, but it is not known whether they are derived from the *anti-* or *syn-*isomers. Comparison of the *in vivo* binding of DBaeA to mouse embryo fibroblast DNA with that observed *in vitro* with microsomal activation reveals some significant differences. The most notable is a reversal in the reactivities of the 3,4- and 12,13-dihydrodiols. *In vitro* the pseudo bay region dihydrodiol affords twice the level of adducts as the bay region dihydrodiol. *In vivo*, the opposite extents of reaction are observed, and the major adduct derives from DE-I rather than DE-II. Minor adducts arising from 3-hydroxy-DE-II and 7-

hydroxy-DE-I are also detected. These findings indicate that the principal ultimate carcinogenic metabolite of DBaeA is DE-I, but that DE-II and other minor diol epoxide metabolites very likely also contribute to overall tumorigenic activity.

The three-dimensional distribution of nuclear DNA damage induced by DBaeF in supercoiled nuclear DNA from nucleoids of mouse fibroblasts was examined (Perin-Roussel *et al.*, 1988). Preferential binding was observed to take place to the DNA of the extremities of loops which are rich in regulatory sequences.

4.8   Generalizations

On the basis of the foregoing experimental evidence, some tentative generalizations are possible. For most alternant PAHs it appears that the principal ultimate carcinogenic metabolites are the bay region diol epoxides. These metabolites are chemically reactive electrophiles that undergo relatively facile hydrolysis and react readily with nucleic acids, proteins, and other cellular molecules.

The evidence supporting diol epoxides as ultimate carcinogenic metabolite derives mainly from DNA binding studies and from mutagenesis and carcinogenesis experiments. It was first shown for BaP that the *anti*-diol epoxide metabolite gives rise to the principal DNA-bound adduct detected in mammalian cells, and similar adducts are formed in the cells of humans as well as in experimental animals. Similar DNA-bound adducts have been shown subsequently to be formed from the *in vivo* metabolism of several other PAHs. However, in only relatively few cases have the adducts been fully characterized chemically. Although attention has tended to focus on the principal nucleoside adducts derived from covalent binding of the *anti*-diol epoxide isomers to the amino function of dG, numerous minor adducts arising from binding of the (+) and (−)-*anti*- and *syn*-diol epoxide isomers at other sites are also formed, and there is no inherent reason to assume that the major adducts are more important than the minor adducts for carcinogenesis. Indeed, Dipple and coworkers (Bigger *et al.*, 1983; Cheng *et al.*, 1988) have shown that the potent tumorigen DMBA affords relatively high levels of dA adducts, leading them to suggest that dA adducts may be more relevant for tumorigenesis than dG adducts. Consistent with this hypothesis, the benzo[c]phenanthrene *anti*- and *syn*-3,4-diol-1,2-epoxides, stated to be the most active diol epoxide tumor initiators tested to date, also exhibit a high level of binding to adenines in DNA (Agarwal *et al.*, 1987). It will be interesting to see how closely the reactivity of other PAH compounds with adenine residues correlates with their carcinogenic potencies.

The reasons why bay region diol epoxides play a more important role in carcinogenesis than other reactive PAH metabolites are not established with certainty. According to the 'bay region theory' proposed by Jerina, Lehr and their associates, bay region diol epoxides are distinguished by their exceptional chemical reactivity as predicted by molecular orbital theoretical calculations (Lehr *et al.*, 1985). However, reactivity alone cannot account for their unique character, since K-region oxides and other types of diol epoxides readily enter into reaction with nucleic acids to yield covalent adducts. For example, BaP 4,5-oxide (Jennette *et al.*, 1977) and DMBA 5,6-oxide (Blobstein *et al.*, 1975) react with nucleic acids to afford principally 2-amino–guanosine adducts. This is the same site preferentially attacked by *anti*-BPDE. While the data is not adequate to permit direct comparison of the extent of binding of K-region oxides and bay region diol epoxides under the same experimental conditions, the level of binding of both to nucleic acids *in vitro* is of the same general order of magnitude. The primary reasons that K-region oxides are not important in tumorigenesis are most probably that K-region metabolism is generally not an important metabolic pathway for most hydrocarbons and K-region oxides are highly susceptible to enzymatic detoxification, principally by epoxide hydrolase. Consequently, relatively low levels of K-oxides are formed metabolically, and these are converted rapidly to water soluble conjugates which are excreted in the urine.

If reactivity were the principal determinant of biological activity, the esters of the hydroxymethyl metabolites of DMBA and other methyl-substituted carcinogenic PAHs might be expected to be among their principal active forms. Meso region hydroxymethyl esters of BA and BaP bearing a good leaving group (e.g. sulfate, phosphate, or acetate) can generate highly electrophilic benzylic carbonium ions that are predicted theoretically to be as reactive or more reactive than bay region diol epoxides (Fu *et al.*, 1978). The formation of reactive sulfuric acid esters of several hydroxymethyl derivatives of BA in the presence of rat liver cytosols and 3'-phosphoadeno-sine-5'-phosphosulfate (PAPS) was demonstrated by Watabe and coworkers (Watabe *et al.*, 1982; Watabe *et al.*, 1987 and earlier papers cited therein). It was also demonstrated that sulfate esters of this type can react with calf thymus DNA to yield adducts covalently attached to the amino groups of deoxyguanosine and deoxyadenosine. These findings have been confirmed by Miller and coworkers (Surh *et al.*, 1987; Surh *et al.*, 1989) who have shown that sulfotransferase mediates the formation of sulfate esters of 7-hydroxymethyl-12-methyl-BA and 6-hydroxymethyl-BaP in rat liver cytosols and these reactive intermediates bind covalently to DNA *in vivo* in rat liver to form adducts principally to deoxyguanosine. On the other hand, liver is poorly susceptible to the action of PAH carcinogens, and benzylic adducts arising from hydroxymethyl esters are generally not detected among the carcinogenic PAH–DNA adducts found in the usual target tissues. The apparent relative unimportance of hydroxymethyl sulfate esters as active metabolites may be a consequence of their exceptional chemical reactivity that is responsible for their relatively rapid intracellular destruction by indiscriminate reaction with proteins and other cellular nucleophiles.

If reactivity is the principal determinant of carcinogenic activity, it is also difficult to explain why the benzo[c]phenanthrene diol epoxides, reported to be exceptionally mutagenic and the most tumorigenic diol epoxides tested on mouse skin (Levin *et al.*, 1980), are found to be 'the most chemically unreactive bay region diol epoxides studied to date' in both SN_2 and solvolysis reactions (Sayer *et al.*, 1981).

An attractive hypothesis to explain the uniqueness of the bay region diol epoxides in comparison with other reactive PAH metabolites is that they are distinguished not by their special reactivity, but by their *resistance to enzymatic detoxification*. According to this concept, the bay region provides a pocket of protection that sterically interferes with the approach and proper orientation of epoxide hydrolase and other detoxifying enzymes (Harvey, 1981). Since the rates of nonenzymatic destruction, e.g. by hydrolysis, are considerably slower, these chemically reactive intermediates are able to survive sufficiently long to reach the critical target sites in the nucleic acids. Other reactive electrophilic metabolites, such as K-region oxides, nonbay region diol epoxides, and hydroxymethyl esters are often sufficiently reactive to attack DNA with formation of covalent bonds, but they are rapidly destroyed by the action of the microsomal enzymes before they are able to effect damage. Thus, the bay region diol epoxide metabolites of BaP and BA have been shown to be poorer substrates for epoxide hydrolase than the corresponding K-region oxides (Oesch, 1980; Gozukara *et al.*, 1980; Wood *et al.*, 1976). Although extensive kinetic data is lacking, the presence of high levels of epoxide hydrolase generally has little influence on the mutagenicity of diol epoxides, indicating that the presence of this enzyme does not significantly increase their rate of conversion to nonmutagenic products (Guenthner & Oesch, 1981). On the other hand, there is evidence that *anti*-BPDE is a moderately good substrate for glutathione-S-transferase (Jernstrom *et al.*, 1985), and it has been shown that the purified soluble GST inhibits the binding of the diol epoxide to DNA (Hesse *et al.*, 1982). GST is high in rat liver and low in mouse skin and rat mammary gland. Correspondingly, the amount of BaP bound to hepatic DNA after a single intraperitoneal injection is 35 times lower than the amount bound to skin DNA by an equimolar dose of the carcinogen (Lutz *et al.*, 1978). Presumably, this is the principal reason why BaP is a skin carcinogen, but not a liver carcinogen, in the mouse.

It is likely that the activity of the reactive electrophilic metabolites of BaP and other alternant polyarenes is also influenced by their ability to intercalate into DNA with the proper orientation to form adducts (Harvey & Geacintov, 1988), the conformations and relative stabilities of the adducts formed, and their susceptibility to DNA repair mechanisms (Feldman *et al.*, 1980; Rojas & Alexandrov, 1986). However, these latter factors are likely to be relatively less important for metabolites that are rapidly destroyed by enzymatic detoxification.

In summary, although the 'bay region theory' has been accepted uncritically by many investigators because it predicts correctly that bay region diol epoxides should be the ultimate carcinogenic forms of most alternant polyarenes, there is substantial reason to suspect that this relation may be only fortuitous. The bay region diol epoxides predicted theoretically to be the most reactive metabolic intermediates are also the metabolites most resistant to enzymatic detoxification by epoxide hydrolase. It is proposed that this property is the principal reason that bay region diol epoxides are the major carcinogenic forms of alternant polyarenes. Further investigations will be required to determine the validity of this hypothesis.

4.9   References

Adriaenssens, P. I., Sivarajah, K., Boorman, G. A., Eling, T. E. & Anderson, M. W. (1983). Effect of aspirin and indomethacin on the formation of benzo[a]pyrene-induced pulmonary adenomas and DNA adducts in A/Hej mice. *Cancer Res.* **43**, 4762–7.

Agarwal, S. K., Sayer, J. M., Yeh, H. J. C., Pannell, L. K., Hilton, B. D., Pigott, M. A., Dipple, A., Yagi, H. & Jerina, D. M. (1987). Chemical characterization of DNA adducts derived from the configurationally isomeric benzo[c]phenanthrene-3,4-diol 1,2-epoxides. *J. Am. Chem. Soc.* **109**, 2497–504.

Babson, J. R., Russo-Rodriguez, S. E., Rastetter, W. H. & Wogan, G. N. (1986). In vitro DNA-binding of microsomally-activated fluoranthene: Evidence that the major product is a fluoranthene N2-deoxyguanosine adduct. *Carcinogenesis*, **7**, 859–65.

Baird, W. M. & Brookes, P. (1973). Isolation of hydrocarbon–deoxyribonucleoside products from the DNA of mouse embryo cells treated in culture with 7-methylbenz[a]anthracene-[3]H. *Cancer Res.* **33**, 2378–85.

Baird, W. M., Dipple, A., Grover, P. L., Sims, P. & Brookes, P. (1973). Studies on the formation of hydrocarbon-deoxyribonucleoside products by the binding of derivatives of 7-methylbenz[a]anthracene to DNA in aqueous solutions and in mouse embryo cells in culture. *Cancer Res.* **33**, 2386–92.

Baird, W. M., Harvey, R. G. & Brookes, P. (1975). Comparison of the cellular DNA-bound products of benzo[a]pyrene with the products formed by reaction of benzo[a]pyrene 4,5-oxide with DNA. *Cancer Res.* **35**, 54–7.

Beland, F. A. & Harvey, R. G. (1976). The isomeric 9,10-oxides of trans-7,8-dihydroxy-7,8-dihydrobenzo[a]pyrene. *J. Chem. Soc. Chem. Commun.* 84–5.

Bigger, C. A. H., Sawicki, J. T., Blake, D. M., Raymond, L. G. & Dipple, A. (1983). Products of binding of 7,12-dimethylbenz[a]anthracene to DNA in mouse skin. *Cancer Res.* **43**, 5647–51.

Blobstein, S. H., Weinstein, I. B., Grunberger, D., Weisgras, J. & Harvey, R. G. (1975). Products obtained after *in vitro* reaction of 7,12-dimethylbenz[a]anthracene-5,6-oxide with nucleic acids. *Biochemistry*, **14**, 3451–8.

88   *Mechanisms of carcinogenesis*

Borgen, A., Darvey, H., Castagnoli, N., Crocker, T., Rasmussen, R. & Wang, I. (1973). Metabolic conversion of benzo[a]pyrene by Syrian hamster liver microsomes and binding of metabolites to DNA. *J. Med. Chem.* **16**, 502–6.

Brookes, P., Ellis, M. E., Pataki, J. & Harvey, R. G. (1986). Mutation in mammalian cells by isomers of 5-methylchrysene diol epoxide. *Carcinogenesis*, **7**, 463–6.

Brookes, P. & Heidelberger, C. (1969). Isolation and degradation of DNA from cells treated with tritium-labeled 7,12-dimethylbenz[a]anthracene: Studies on the nature of the binding of this carcinogen to DNA. *Cancer Res.* **29**, 157–65.

Brookes, P. & Lawley, P. D. (1964). Evidence for the binding of polynuclear aromatic hydrocarbons to the nucleic acids of mouse skin: Relation between carcinogenic power of hydrocarbons and their binding to deoxyribonucleic acid. *Nature (Lond.)*, **202**, 781–4.

Busby, W. F. J., Goldman, M. E., Newberne, P. M. & Wogan, G. N. (1984). Tumorigenicity of fluoranthene in a newborn mouse lung adenoma bioassay. *Carcinogenesis*, **5**, 1311–16.

Busby, W. F. J., Stevens, E., Kellenbach, E. R., Cornelisse, J. & Lugtenburg, J. (1988). Dose-response relationships of the tumorigenicity of cyclopenta[cd]pyrene, benzo[a]pyrene, and 6-nitrochrysene in a mouse lung adenoma assay. *Carcinogenesis*, **9**, 741–6.

Carberry, S. E., Geacintov, N. E. & Harvey, R. G. (1989). Reactions of stereoisomeric non-bay region benz[a]anthracene diol epoxides with DNA and conformations of non-covalent complexes and covalent adducts. *Carcinogenesis*, **10**, 97–103.

Carberry, S. E., Shahbaz, M., Geacintov, N. E. & Harvey, R. G. (1988). Reactions of stereoisomeric and structurally related bay region diol epoxide derivatives of benz-[a]anthracene with DNA. Conformations of non-covalent complexes and covalent carcinogen-DNA adducts. *Chem.–Biol. Interact.* **66**, 121–45.

Cavalieri, E. L. & Rogan, E. G. (1985). One-electron oxidation in aromatic hydrocarbon carcinogenesis. *Polycyclic Hydrocarbons and Carcinogenesis*. Am. Chem. Soc. Monogr. 283, ed. R. G. Harvey, 289–305, Washington, DC: American Chemical Society.

Cerutti, P. (1974). Effects of ionizing radiation on mammalian cells. *Naturwissenschaften*, **61**, 51–9.

Cerutti, P., Shinohara, K., Ide, M.-L. & Remsen, J. (1978). Formation and repair of benzo[a]pyrene-induced DNA damage in mammalian cells. *Polycyclic Hydrocarbons and Cancer*, 2, eds H. V. Gelboin & P O. P. Ts'o pp. 203–12, New York: Academic Press.

Cheng, S. C., Prakash, A. S., Pigott, M. A., Hilton, B. D., Lee, H., Harvey, R. G. & Dipple, A. (1988). A metabolite of the carcinogen 7,12-dimethylbenz[a]anthracene that reacts with adenine residues in DNA. *Carcinogenesis*, **9**, 1721–3.

Cheng, S. C., Prakash, A. S., Pigott, M. A., Hilton, B. D., Roman, J. M., Lee, H., Harvey, R. G. & Dipple, A. (1988a). Characterization of 7,12-dimethylbenz[a]anthracene–adenine nucleoside adducts. *Chem. Res. Tox.* **1**, 216–21.

Chung, H., Harvey, R. G., Armstrong, R. N. & Jarabak, J. (1987). Polycyclic aromatic hydrocarbon quinones and glutathione thioethers as substrates and inhibitors of the human placental NADP-linked 15-hydroxyprostaglandin dehydrogenase. *J. Biol. Chem.* **262**, 12448–51.

Conney, A. (1982). Induction of microsomal enzymes by foreign chemicals and carcinogenesis by polycyclic aromatic hydrocarbons. *Cancer Res.* **42**, 4875–17.

Coombs, M. M. & Bhatt, T. S. (1987). *Cyclopenta[a]phenanthrenes*, Cambridge: Cambridge University Press.

Cooper, C. S., Ribeiro, O., Farmer, P. B., Hewer, A., Walsh, C., Pal, K., Grover, P. L. & Sims, P. (1980a). The metabolic activation of benz[a]anthracene in hamster embryo cells: Evidence that diol epoxides react with guanosine, deoxyguanosine, and adenosine in nucleic acids. *Chem.–Biol. Interact.* **32**, 209–31.

Cooper, C. S., Ribeiro, O., Hewer, A., Walsh, C., Pal, K., Grover, P. L. & Sims, P. (1980). The involvement of a 'bay-region' and non-'bay-region' diol-epoxide in the metabolic activation of benz[a]anthracene in mouse skin and in hamster embryo cells. *Carcinogenesis*, **1**, 223–43.

Coulson, C. A. (1953). Electronic configuration and carcinogenesis. *Adv. Cancer Res.* **1**, 1–56.

Dannenberg, H. (1957). Stearanthene, a link between steroids and carcinogenic hydrocarbons. *Z. Krebsforsch.* **62**, 217–29.

Dannenberg, H. (1959). The relation between steroids and carcinogenic hydrocarbons. *Z. Krebsforsch.* **63**, 523–31.

DeSombre, E. R. & Arbogast, L. V. (1974). Effect of antiandrogen C1628 on the growth of rat mammary tumors. *Cancer Res.* **34**, 1971–6.

Deutsch, J., Vatsis, K. P., Coon, M. J., Leutz, J. C. & Gelboin, H. V. (1979). Catalytic activity and stereoselectivity of purified forms of rabbit liver microsomal cytochrome P-450 in the oxygenation of the (+) and (–) enantiomers of trans-7,8-dihydroxy-7,8-dihydrobenzo-[a]pyrene. *Mol. Pharmacol.* **16**, 1011–18.

Dewar, M. J. S. & Dougherty, R. C. (1975). *The PMO Theory of Organic Chemistry*, New York: Plenum Press.

DiGiovanni, J., Diamond, L., Harvey, R. G. & Slaga, T. J. (1983). Enhancement of the skin tumor-initiating activity of polycyclic aromatic hydrocarbons by methyl substitution of nonbenzo 'bay-region' positions. *Carcinogenesis*, **4**, 403–7.

DiGiovanni, J., Diamond, L., Singer, J. M., Daniel, F. B., Witiak, D. & Slaga, T. J. (1982). Tumor-initiating activity of 4-fluoro-7,12-dimethylbenz[a]anthracene and 1,2,3,4-tetrahydro-7,12-dimethylbenz[a]anthracene in female SENCAR mice. *Carcinogenesis*, **3**, 651–5.

Dipple, A., Moschel, R. C. & Bigger, C. A. H. (1984). Polynuclear aromatic carcinogens. *Chemical Carcinogens.* 1, ed. C. E. Searle, 41–163, Washington, DC: American Chemical Society.

Dix, T. A., Buck, J. R. & Marnett, L. J. (1986). Hydroperoxide-dependent epoxidation of 3,4-dihydroxy-3,4-dihydrobenzo[a]anthracene by ram seminal vesicle microsomes and by hematin. *Biochem. Biophys. Res. Commun.* **140**, 181–7.

Duncan, M. E., Brookes, P. & Dipple, A. (1969). Metabolism and binding to cellular macromolecules of a series of hydrocarbons by mouse embryo cells in culture. *Int. J. Cancer*, **4**, 813–19.

Feldman, G., Remsen, J., Wang, T. V. & Cerutti, P. (1980). Formation and excision of covalent deoxyribonucleic acid adducts of benzo[a]pyrene 4,5-epoxide and benzo[a]pyrene epoxide I in human lung cells A549. *Biochemistry*, **19**, 1095–101.

Flesher, J., Myers, S. R. & Blake, J. W. (1986). Bioalkylation of polynuclear aromatic hydrocarbons: A predictor of carcinogenic activity. *Polynuclear Aromatic Hydrocarbons*, eds M. Cooke & A. J. Dennis, 271–84, Columbus, OH: Battelle Press.

Fu, P. P., Harvey, R. G. & Beland, F. A. (1978). Molecular orbital theoretical prediction of the isomeric products formed from reactions of arene oxides and related metabolites of polycyclic aromatic hydrocarbons. *Tetrahedron*, **34**, 857–66.

Geacintov, N. E. (1985). Mechanisms of interaction of polycyclic aromatic diol epoxides with DNA and structures of the adducts. *Polycyclic Hydrocarbons and Carcinogenesis*, Amer. Chem. Soc. Monogr. 283, ed. R. G. Harvey, 107–24, Washington, DC: American Chemical Society.

Geacintov, N. E., Zinger, D., Ibanez, V., Santella, R., Grunberger, D. & Harvey, R. G. (1987). Properties of covalent benzo[a]pyrene diol epoxide–DNA adducts investigated by fluorescence techniques. *Carcinogenesis*, **8**, 925–35.

Geddie, J. E., Amin, S., Huie, K. & Hecht, S. S. (1987). Formation and tumorigenicity of benzo[b]fluoranthene metabolites in mouse epidermis. *Carcinogenesis*, **8**, 1579–84.

Gold, A. & Eisenstadt, E. (1980). Metabolic activation of cyclopenta(c,d)pyrene to 3,4-epoxycyclopenta(c,d)pyrene by rat liver microsomes. *Cancer Res.* **40**, 3940–4.

Goshman, L. M. & Heidelberger, C. (1967). Binding of tritium-labeled polycyclic hydrocarbons to DNA of mouse skin. *Cancer Res.* **27**, 1678–88.

Gozukara, E. H., Belvedere, G., Robinson, R. C., Deutsch, J., Guengerich, F. P. & Gelboin, H. V. (1981). The effect of epoxide hydratase on benzo(a)pyrene diol epoxide hydrolysis and binding to DNA and mixed function oxidase proteins. *Mol. Pharmacol.* **19**, 153–61.

Grover, P. L. & Sims, P. (1968). Enzyme-catalyzed reactions of polycyclic hydrocarbons with deoxyribonucleic acid and protein *in vitro. Biochem. J.* **110**, 159–60.

Guenthner, T. M. & Oesch, F. (1981). Microsomal epoxide hydrolase and its role in polycyclic aromatic hydrocarbon biotransformation. *Polycyclic Hydrocarbons and Cancer*, 3, eds H. V. Gelboin & P. O. P. Ts'o, 183–212, New York: Academic Press.

Guthrie, J., Robertson, I. G. C., Zeiger, E., Boyd, J. A. & Eling, T. E. (1982). Selective activation of some dihydrodiols of several polycyclic aromatic hydrocarbons to mutagenic products by prostaglandin synthetase. *Cancer Res.* **42**, 1620–3.

Hall, M., Parker, D. K., Hewer, A. J., Philips, D. H. & Grover, P. L. (1988). Further metabolism of diol-epoxides of chrysene and dibenz[a,c]anthracene to DNA binding species as evidenced by ^{32}P-postlabelling analysis. *Carcinogenesis*, **9**, 865–8.

Harvey, R. G. (1981). Activated metabolites of carcinogenic hydrocarbons. *Acc. Chem. Res.* **14**, 218–26.

Harvey, R. G. (1985). Synthesis of the dihydrodiol and diol epoxide metabolites of carcinogenic polycyclic hydrocarbons. *Polycyclic Hydrocarbons and Carcinogenesis*. Am. Chem. Soc. Monogr. 283, ed. R. G. Harvey, 35–62, Washington, DC: American Chemical Society.

Harvey, R. G. (1986). Synthesis of oxidized metabolites of carcinogenic hydrocarbons. *Synthesis*, 605–19.

Harvey, R. G. & Dunne, F. B. (1978). Multiple regions of metabolic activation of carcinogenic hydrocarbons. *Nature (Lond.)*, **273**, 566–8.

Harvey, R. G. & Fu, P. P. (1978). Synthesis and reactions of diol epoxides and related metabolites of carcinogenic hydrocarbons. *Polycyclic Hydrocarbons and Cancer*, 1, eds H. V. Gelboin & P. O. P. Ts'o, 133–65, New York: Academic Press.

Harvey, R. G. & Geacintov, N. E. (1988). Interaction and binding of carcinogenic hydrocarbon metabolites to nucleic acids. *Acc. Chem. Res.* **21**, 66–73.

Hecht, S. S., LaVoie, E., Mazzarese, E., Amin, S., Bedenko, V. & Hoffmann, D. (1978). 1,2-Dihydro-1,2-dihydroxy-5-methylchrysene, a major activated metabolite of the environmental carcinogen 5-methylchrysene. *Cancer Res.* **38**, 2191–4.

Hecht, S. S., Radock, R., Amin, S., Huie, K., Melikan, A. A., Hoffmann, D., Pataki, J. & Harvey, R. G. (1985). Tumorigenicity of 5-methylchrysene dihydrodiols and dihydrodiol epoxides in newborn mice and on mouse skin. *Cancer Res.* **45**, 1449–52.

Hemminki, K., Cooper, C. S., Ribeiro, O., Grover, P. L. & Sims, P. (1980). Reactions of 'bay-region' and non-'bay-region' diol epoxides of benz[a]anthracene with DNA: Evidence indicating that the major products are hydrocarbon–N2–guanosine adducts. *Carcinogenesis*, **1**, 277–86.

Herndon, W. C. (1974). Theory of carcinogenic activity of aromatic hydrocarbons. *Trans. NY Acad. Sci.* **36**, 200–17.

Herndon, W. C. (1981). Model calculations for reactivities of polycyclic aromatic hydrocarbon metabolites. *Tetrahedron Lett.* **22**, 983–6.

Hesse, S., Jernstrom, B., Martinez, M., Moldeus, P., Christodoulides, L. & Ketterer, B. (1982). Inactivation of DNA binding metabolites of benzo[a]pyrene and benzo[a]pyrene-7,8-dihydrodiol by glutathione and glutathione S-transferases. *Carcinogenesis*, **3**, 757–60.

Hoffman, F. (1960). LCAO-MO-SCF indices of chemical reactivity and carcinogenic activity of polycyclic hydrocarbons. *Theor. Chim. Acta.* **15**, 393–412.

Hogan, M. E., Dattagupta, N. & Whitlock, J. P. Jr (1981). Carcinogen-induced alteration of DNA structure. *J. Biol. Chem.* **256**, 4504–13.

Huberman, E., Sachs, L., Yang, S. K. & Gelboin, H. V. (1976). Identification of mutagenic metabolites of benzo[a]pyrene in mammalian cells. *Proc. Natl. Acad. Sci. USA*, **73**, 607–11.

Huggins, C. B. (1979). *Experimental Leukemia and Mammary Cancer*, Chicago: University of Chicago Press.

Huggins, C. B. & Yang, N. C. (1962). Induction and extinction of mammary cancer. *Science*, **137**, 257–62.

Ioannides, C. & Parke, D. V. (1987). The cytochromes P-448 – a unique family of enzymes involved in chemical toxicity and carcinogenesis. *Biochem. Pharmacol.* **36**, 4197–207.

Jacobs, S. A., Cortez, C. & Harvey, R. G. (1983). Synthesis of potential proximate and ultimate carcinogenic metabolites of 3-methylcholanthrene. *Carcinogenesis*, **4**, 519–22.

Jeffrey, A. M., Jennette, K., Blobstein, S. H., Weinstein, I. B., Beland, F. A., Harvey, R. G., Kasai, H., Miura, I. & Nakanishi, K. (1976). Benzo[a]pyrene–nucleic acid derivatives found *in vivo*: Structure of a benzo[a]pyrenetetrahydrodiol epoxide guanosine adduct. *J. Amer. Chem. Soc.* **98**, 5714–16.

Jeffrey, A. M., Weinstein, I. B., Jennette, K., Grzeskowiak, K., Nakanishi, K., Harvey, R. G., Autrup, H. & Harris, C. (1977). Structures of benzo[a]pyrene–nucleic acid adducts formed in human and bovine bronchial explants. *Nature (Lond.)*, **269**, 348–50.

Jennette, K. W., Jeffrey, A. M., Blobstein, S. H., Beland, F. A., Harvey, R. G. & Weinstein, I. B. (1977). Nucleoside adducts from the *in vitro* reaction of benzo[a]pyrene-7,8-dihydrodiol 9,10-oxide or benzo[a]pyrene 4,5-oxide with nucleic acids. *Biochemistry* **16**, 932–8.

Jerina, D. M., Michaud, D. P., Feldmann, R. J., Armstrong, R. N., Vyas, K. P., Thakker, D. R., Thomas, P. E., Ryan, D. E. & Levin, W. (1982). Stereochemical modeling of the catalytic site of cytochrome P-450c. *Microsomes, Drug Oxidations, and Drug Toxicity*, ed., 195–201, Tokyo: Japan Scientific Societies Press.

Jernstrom, B., Martinez, M., Meyer, D. J. & Ketterer, B. (1985). Glutathione conjugation of the carcinogenic and mutagenic electrophile (±)-7ß,8α-dihydroxy-9α,10α-oxy-7,8,9,10-tetrahydrobenzo[a]pyrene catalyzed by purified rat liver glutathione transferases. *Carcinogenesis*, **6**, 85–9.

Johnson, D. M. & Bruice, T. C. (1975). Nucleophilic catalysis of the aromatization of an arene oxide. The reaction of trimethylamine with 4-carbo-*tert*-butoxybenzene oxide. *J. Am. Chem. Soc.* **97**, 6901–3.

Jull, J. W. (1956). Hormones as promoting agents in mammary carcinogenesis. *Acta Union Internat. Cancer*, **12**, 653–60.

Kim, M.-H., Roche, C. J., Pope, N., Pataki, J. & Harvey, R. G. (1985). Conformations of complexes derived from the interactions of two stereoisomeric bay-region 5-methylchrysene diol epoxides with DNA. *J. Biomol. Struct. Dynam.* **3**, 949–65.

King, H. W. S., Osborne, M. R., Beland, F. A., Harvey, R. G. & Brookes, P. (1976). (±)-7α,8ß-dihydroxy-9ß,10ß-epoxy-7,8,9,10-tetrahydrobenzo[a]pyrene is an intermediate in the metabolism and binding to DNA of benzo[a]pyrene. *Proc. Natl. Acad. Sci. USA*, **73**, 2679–81.

Koutecky, J. & Zahradnick, R. (1961). On the problem of the connection between the electronic structure of polynuclear aromatic hydrocarbons and their carcinogenic effect. *Cancer Res.* **21**, 457–62.

Lacassagne, A., Buchta, E., Kiessling, D., Zajdela, F. & Buu-Hoi, N. P. (1963). Particular carcinogenic activity of F-norstearanthrene. *Nature (Lond.)*, **200**, 183–184.

LaVoie, E. J., Hecht, S. S., Bendenko, V. & Hoffmann, D. (1982). Identification of the mutagenic metabolites of fluoranthene, 2-methylfluoranthene, and 3-methylfluoranthene. *Carcinogenesis*, **3**, 841–6.

Lee, H. & Harvey, R. G. (1986). Synthesis of the active diol epoxide metabolites of the potent carcinogenic hydrocarbon 7,12-dimethylbenz[a]anthracene. *J. Org. Chem.* **51**, 3502–7.

Lee, H. & Harvey, R. G. (1988). New synthetic approaches to cyclopenta[a]phenanthrenes and their carcinogenic derivatives. *J. Org. Chem.* **53**, 4253–6.

Lehr, R., Kumar, S., Levin, W., Wood, A. W., Chang, R. L., Conney, A., Yagi, H., Sayer, J. M. & Jerina, D. M. (1985). The bay region theory of polycyclic aromatic hydrocarbon carcinogenesis. *Polycyclic Hydrocarbons and Carcinogenesis*, Am. Chem. Soc. Monogr. 283, ed. R. G. Harvey, 63–84, Washington, DC: American Chemical Society.

Levin, W., Wood, A. W., Chang, R. L., Ittah, Y., Croisy-Delcey, M., Yagi, H., Jerina, D. M. & Conney, A. H. (1980). Exceptionally high tumor-initiating activity of benzo(c)phenanthrene bay-region diol-epoxides in mouse skin. *Cancer Res.* **40**, 3910–14.

Lewis, D. F. V., Ioannides, C. & Parke, D. V. (1987). Structural requirements for substrates of cytochromes P-450 and P-448. *Chem.–Biol. Interact.* **64**, 39–60.

Lewis, D. F. V., Ioannides, C. & Parke, D. V. (1989). Molecular orbital studies of oxygen activation of cytochromes P-450 mediated oxidative metabolism of xenobiotics. *Chem.–Biol. Interact.* **70**, 263–80.

Lorentzen, R. J., Caspary, W. J., Lesko, S. A. & Ts'o, P. O. P. (1975). The autoxidation of 6-hydroxybenzo[a]pyrene and 6-oxobenzo[a]pyrene radical in rat liver homogenates from carcinogenic benzo[a]pyrene. *Biochemistry*, **14**, 3970–7.

Lowe, J. P. & Silverman, B. D. (1984). Predicting carcinogenicity of polycyclic aromatic hydrocarbons. *Acc. Chem. Res.* **17**, 332–8.

Lutz, W. K., Viviani, A. & Schlatter, C. (1978). Nonlinear dose–response relationship for the binding of the carcinogen benzo(a)pyrene to rat liver DNA *in vivo*. *Cancer Res.* **38**, 575–8.

Mainster, M. A. & Memory, J. D. (1967). Superdelocalizability indices and the Pullman theory of chemical carcinogenesis. *Biochim. Biophys. Acta*, **148**, 605–8.

Marnett, L. (1985). Hydroperoxide-dependent oxygenation of polycyclic aromatic hydrocarbons. *Polycyclic Hydrocarbons and Carcinogenesis*, ACS Symp. Monogr. 283, ed. R. G. Harvey, 307–26, Washington, DC: American Chemical Society.

McCaustland, D. J., Fischer, D. L., Kolwyck, K. C., Duncan, W. P., Wiley, J. C. Jr Engel, J. F., Selkirk, J. K. & Roller, P. P. (1976). Polycyclic aromatic hydrocarbon derivatives: Synthesis and physiochemical characterization. *Carcinogenesis*, 1, eds R. I. Freudenthal & P. W. Jones, 349–411, New York: Raven Press.

Melikian, A. A., Amin, S., Hecht, S. S., Hoffmann, D., Pataki, J. & Harvey, R. G. (1982). Identification of the major adducts formed by reaction of 5-methylchrysene *anti*-dihydrodiol-epoxides with DNA *in vitro*. *Cancer Res.* **44**, 2524–9.

Melikian, A. A., Amin, S., Huie, K., Hecht, S. S. & Harvey, R. G. (1988). Reactivity with DNA bases and mutagenicity toward Salmonella typhimurium of methylchrysene diol epoxide enantiomers. *Cancer Res.* **48**, 1781–7.

Melikian, A. A., LaVoie, E. J., Hecht, S. S. & Hoffmann, D. (1982a). Influence of a bay-region methyl group on formation of 5-methylchrysene dihydrodiol epoxide: DNA adducts in mouse skin. *Cancer Res.* **42**, 1239–42.

Miller, E. C. (1978). Some current perspectives on chemical carcinogenesis in humans and experimental animals: Presidential address. *Cancer Res.* **38**, 1479–96.

Myers, S. R., Blake, J. W. & Flesher, J. W. (1988). Bioalkylation and biooxidation of anthracene *in vitro* and *in vivo*. *Biochem. Biophys. Res. Commun.* **151**, 1441–5.

Nagata, C., Fukui, K., Yonezawa, T. & Tagashira, Y. (1955). Electronic structure and carcinogenic activity of aromatic compounds. I. Condensed aromatic hydrocarbons. *Cancer Res.* **15**, 233–9.

Nakanishi, K., Kasai, H., Cho, H., Harvey, R. G., Jeffrey, A. M., Jennette, K. W. & Weinstein, I. B. (1977). Absolute configuration of an RNA adduct formed *in vivo* by metabolism of benzo[a]pyrene. *J. Amer. Chem. Soc.* **99**, 258–60.

Nemoto, N. (1981). Glutathione, glucuronide, and sulfate transferase in polycyclic aromatic hydrocarbon metabolism. *Polycyclic Hydrocarbons and Cancer*, 3, eds H. V. Gelboin & P. O. P. Ts'o, 213–58, New York: Academic Press.

Nes, W. R. & Ford, D. L. (1962). The conversion of a steroid to 4',10-dimethyl-1,2-benzanthracene by a model of a biochemical route. *Tetrahedron Lett.* 209–12.

Nesnow, S., Easterling, R. E., Ellis, S., Watts, R. & Ross, J. (1988). Metabolism of benz[j]aceanthrylene by induced rat liver S9. *Cancer Lett.* **39**, 19–27.

Newbold, R. F. & Brookes, P. (1976). Exceptional mutagenicity of benzo{a}pyrene diol epoxide in cultured mammalian cells. *Nature(Lond.)*, **261**, 52–4.

Oesch, F. (1980). Microsomal epoxide hydrolase. *Enzymatic Basis of Detoxification*, II, ed. W. B. Jacoby, 277–90, New York: Academic Press.

Oesch, F., Timms, C. W., Walker, C. H., Guenther, T. M., Sparrow, A., Watabe, T. & Wolf, C. R. (1984). Existence of multiple forms of microsomal epoxide hydrolases with radically different substrate specificities. *Carcinogenesis*, **5**, 7–9.

Ortez de Montellano, P. R. (1986). *Cytochrome P-450, Structure, Mechanism and Biochemistry*, New York: Plenum.

Osborne, M., Brookes, P., Lee, H. & Harvey, R. G. (1986). The reaction of a 3-methylcholanthrene diol epoxide with DNA in relation to the binding of 3-methylcholanthrene to the DNA of mammalian cells. *Carcinogenesis*, **7**, 1345–50.

Perin-Roussel, O., Barat, N. & Zajdela, F. (1988). Non-random distribution of dibenzo-[a,e]fluoranthene-induced DNA adducts in DNA loops in mouse fibroblast nuclei. *Carcinogenesis*, **9**, 1383–8.

Phillips, D. H., Hewer, A. & Grover, P. L. (1987). Formation of DNA adducts in mouse skin treated with metabolites of chrysene. *Cancer Lett.* **35**, 207–14.

Pruess-Schwartz, D., Baird, W. M., Yagi, H., Jerina, D. M., Pigott, M. A. & Dipple, A. (1987). Stereochemical specificity in the metabolic activation of benzo(c)phenanthrene to metabolites that covalently bind to DNA in rodent embryo cell cultures. *Cancer Res.* **47**, 4032–7.

Pullman, A. (1947). Study of the electronic structure of organic molecules. Carcinogenic hydrocarbons. *Ann. Chim.* **Ser. 12, 2**, 5–71.

Pullman, A. & Pullman, B. (1955). Electronic structure and carcinogenic activity of aromatic molecules. *Adv. Cancer Res.* **3**, 117–69.

Pullman, B. (1965). Steroids, purine–pyrimidine pairs, and polycyclic aromatic carcinogens. *Adv. Chem. Phys.* **8**, 163–76.

Reardon, D. B., Prakash, A. S., Hilton, B. D., Roman, J. M., Pataki, J., Harvey, R. G. & Dipple, A. (1987). Characterization of 5-methylchrysene-1,2-dihydrodiol-3,4-epoxide–DNA adducts. *Carcinogenesis*. **8**, 1317–22.

Rice, J. E., Hosted T. J. Jr., DeFloria, M. C., LaVoie, E. J., Fischer, D. L. & Wiley, J. C., Jr (1986). Tumor-initiating activity of major *in vivo* metabolites of indeno[1,2,3-cd]pyrene on mouse skin. *Carcinogenesis*, **7**, 1761–4.

Rice, J. E., Weyand, E. H., Geddie, N., DeFloria, M. C. & LaVoie, E. J. (1987). Identification of tumorigenic metabolites of benzo[j]fluoranthene formed *in vivo* in mouse skin. *Cancer Res.* **47**, 6166–70.

Robertson, I. G. C., Guthenberg, C., Mannervik, B. & Jernstrom, B. (1986). Differences in stereoselectivity and catalytic efficiency of three human glutathione transferases in the conjugation of glutathione with 7ß, 8α-dihydroxy-9α,10α-oxy-7,8,9,10-tetrahydrobenzo(a)pyrene. *Cancer Res.* **46**, 2220–4.

Rogan, E. G., Hakam, A. & Cavalieri, E. L. (1983). Structure elucidation of a 6-methylbenzo[a]pyrene-DNA adduct formed by horseradish peroxidase *in vitro* and mouse skin *in vivo*. *Chem.–Biol. Interact.* **47**, 111–22.

Rojas, M. & Alexandrov, K. (1986). *In vivo* formation and persistence of DNA and protein adducts in mouse and rat skin exposed to (±)-benzo[a]pyrene-4,5-oxide. *Carcinogenesis*, **7**, 235–40.

Sawicki, J. T., Moschel, R. C. & Dipple, A. (1983). Involvement of both *syn-* and *anti-*dihydrodiol epoxides in the binding of 7,12-dimethylbenz[a]anthracene to DNA in mouse embryo cell cultures. *Cancer Res.* **43**, 3212–18.

Sayer, J., Yagi, H., Croisy-Delcey, M. & Jerina, D. M. (1981). Novel bay-region diol epoxides from benzo[c]phenanthrene. *J. Am. Chem. Soc.* **103**, 4970–2.

Schmidt, O. (1941). Charakterisierung und Mechanismus der Krebs erzeugneden Kohlenwasserstoffe. *Naturwissenschaften*, **29**, 146–50.

Scribner, J. D. (1975). Molecular orbital theory in carcinogenesis research. *J. Natl. Cancer Inst.* **55**, 1035–8.

Selkirk, J. K., Croy, R. G. & Gelboin, H. V. (1974). Benzo[a]pyrene metabolites: Efficient and rapid separation by high-pressure liquid chromatography. *Science*, **184**, 169–71.

Shahbaz, M., Geacintov, N. E. & Harvey, R. G. (1986). Noncovalent intercalative complex formation and kinetic flow linear dichroism of racemic *syn-* and *anti-*benzo[a]pyrenediol epoxide-DNA solutions. *Biochemistry*, **25**, 3290–6.

Sims, P. & Grover, P. L. (1981). Involvement of dihydrodiols and diol epoxides in the metabolic activation of polycyclic hydrocarbons other than benzo[a]pyrene. *Polycyclic Hydrocarbons and Cancer*, 3, eds H. V. Gelboin & P. O. P. Ts'o, 117–81, New York: Academic Press.

Sims, P., Grover, P. L., Swaisland, A., Pal, K. & Hewer, A. (1974). Metabolic activation of benzo[a]pyrene proceeds by a diol epoxide. *Nature (Lond.)*, **252**, 326–8.

Singer, B. & Grunberger, D. (1983). *Molecular Biology of Mutagens and Carcinogens*, New York: Plenum Press.

Slaga, T. J., Gleason, G. L., DiGiovanni, J., Sukumaran, K. B. & Harvey, R. G. (1979). Potent tumor-initiating activity of the 3,4-dihydrodiol of 7,12-dimethylbenz[a]anthracene in mouse skin. *Cancer Res.* **39**, 1934–6.

Slaga, T. J., Gleason, G. L., Mills, G., Ewald, L., Fu, P. P., Lee, H. M. & Harvey, R. G. (1980). Comparison of the skin tumor-initiating activities of dihydrodiols and diol-epoxides of various polycyclic aromatic hydrocarbons. *Cancer Res.* **40**, 1981–4.

Smith, I. A., Berger, G. D., Seybold, P. G. & Serve, M. P. (1978). Relationships between carcinogenicity and theoretical reactivity indices in polycyclic aromatic hydrocarbons. *Cancer Res.* **38**, 2968–77.

Smithgall, T. E., Harvey, R. G. & Penning, T. M. (1986). Regio- and stereospecificity of homogeneous 3α-hydroxysteroid-dihydrodiol dehydrogenase for *trans*-dihydrodiol metabolites of polycyclic aromatic hydrocarbons. *J. Biol. Chem.* **261**, 6184–6.

Smithgall, T. E., Harvey, R. G. & Penning, T. M. (1988). Oxidation of the *trans*-3,4-dihydrodiol metabolites of the potent carcinogen 7,12-dimethylbenz[a]anthracene and other benz[a]anthracene derivatives by 3α-hydroxysteroid-dihydrodiol dehydrogenase: Effects of methyl substitution on velocity and stereochemical course of *trans*-dihydrodiol oxidation. *Cancer Res.* **48**, 1227–32.

Smithgall, T. E., Harvey, R. G. & Penning, T. M. (1988a). Spectroscopic identification of *ortho*-quinones as the products of polycyclic aromatic *trans*-dihydrodiol oxidation catalyzed by dihydrodiol dehydrogenase. *J. Biol. Chem.* **263**, 1814–20.

Surh, Y., Lai, C.-C., Miller, E. C. & Miller, J. (1987). Hepatic DNA and RNA formation from the carcinogen 7-hydroxymethyl-12-methylbenz[a]anthracene and its electrophilic sulfuric acid ester metabolite in preweaning rats and mice. *Biochem. Biophys. Res. Commun.* **144**, 576–82.

Surh, Y., Liem, A., Miller, E. C. & Miller, J. (1989). Metabolic activation of the carcinogen 6-hydroxymethylbenzo[a]pyrene: formation of an electrophilic sulfuric acid ester and benzylic DNA adducts in rat liver *in vivo* and in reactions *in vitro*. *Carcinogenesis*, **10**, 1519–28.

Svartholm, N. V. (1942). Electronic distribution and chemical reactivity in condensed unsaturated hydrocarbons. *Arkiv. Kemi Minerol. Geol.* **A15**, 1–13.

Thakker, D. R., Yagi, H., Levin, W., Wood, A. W., Conney, A. H. & Jerina, D. M. (1985). Polycyclic aromatic hydrocarbons: Metabolic activation to ultimate carcinogens. *Bioactivation of Foreign Compounds*, ed. M. W. Anders, 177–242, New York: Academic Press.

Watabe, T., Hiratsuka, A. & Ogura, K. (1987). Sulfotransferase-mediated covalent binding of the carcinogen 7,12–dihydroxymethylbenz[a]anthracene to calf thymus DNA and its inhibition by glutathione transferase. *Carcinogenesis*, **8**, 445–53.

Watabe, T., Ishizuka, T., Isobe, M. & Ozawa, N. (1982). A 7-hydroxymethyl sulfate ester as an active metabolite of 7,12-dimethylbenz[a]anthracene. *Science*, **215**, 403–4.

Weinstein, I. B., Jeffrey, A. M., Jennette, K., Blobstein, S., Harvey, R. G., Harris, C., Autrup, H., Kasai, H. & Nakanishi, K. (1976). Benzo[a]pyrene diol epoxides as intermediates in nucleic acid binding *in vitro* and *in vivo*. *Science*, **193**, 592–5.

Weston, A., Hodgson, R. M., Hewer, A. J., Kuroda, R. & Grover, P. L. (1985). Comparative studies of the metabolic activation of chrysene in rodent and human cells. *Chem.–Biol. Interact.* **54**, 223–42.

Wheland, G. W. (1942). A quantum mechanical investigation of the orientation of substituents in aromatic molecules. *J. Am. Chem. Soc.* **64**, 900–8.

Wieland, H. & Dane, E. (1933). The constitution of the bile acids. III. The site of attachment of the side chain. *Z. Physiol. Chem.* **219**, 240–4.

Wood, A. W., Levin, W., Lu, A. Y. H., Yagi, H., Hernandez, O., Jerina, D. M. & Conney, A. H. (1976). Metabolism of benzo[a]pyrene and benzo[a]pyrene derivatives to mutagenic products by highly purified hepatic microsomal enzymes. *J. Biol. Chem.* **251**, 4882–90.

Wood, A. W., Chang, R. L., Levin, W., Ryan, D. E., Thomas, P. E., Mah, H. D., Karle, J. M., Yagi, H., Jerina, D. M. & Conney, A. H. (1979). Mutagenicity and tumorigenicity of phenanthrene and chrysene epoxides and diol epoxides. *Cancer Res.*, **39**, 4069–77.

Yagi, H., Hernandez, O. & Jerina, D. M. (1975). Synthesis of (±)-7ß,8α-dihydroxy-9ß,10ß-epoxy-7,8,9,10-tetrahydrobenzo[a]pyrene, a potential metabolite of the carcinogen benzo[a]pyrene with stereochemistry related to the antileukemic triptolides. *J. Am. Chem. Soc.* **97**, 6881–3.

Yang, S. K. (1988). Stereoselectivity of cytochrome P-450 isozymes and epoxide hydrolase in the metabolism of polycyclic aromatic hydrocarbons. *Biochem. Pharmacol.*, **37**, 61–70.

Yang, S. K., Mustaq, M. & Chiu, P. L. (1985). Stereoselective metabolism and activations of polycyclic aromatic hydrocarbons. *Polycyclic Hydrocarbons and Carcinogenesis*, Amer. Chem. Soc. Monogr. 283, ed. R. G. Harvey, 19–34, Washington, DC: American Chemical Society.

Yang, S. K., Roller, P. P., Fu, P. P., Harvey, R. G. & Gelboin, H. V. (1977). Evidence for a 2,3-epoxide as the intermediate in the microsomal metabolism of benzo[a]pyrene to 3-hydroxybenzo[a]pyrene. *Biochem. Biophys. Res. Commun.* **77**, 1176–82.

Zinger, D., Geacintov, N. E. & Harvey, R. G. (1987). Conformations and selective photodissociation of heterogeneous benzo[a]pyrene diol epoxide enantiomer–DNA adducts. *Biophys. Chem.* **27**, 131–8.

5

Molecular properties of polyarenes

The essential features of the chemistry of polyarenes are surveyed in this and the next chapter. A comprehensive account of the chemistry of the polyarenes may be found in Clar's classic two volume work *Polycyclic Hydrocarbons* (Clar, 1964). However, the majority of the references in this work are to the older literature, and the emphasis is on classical hydrocarbon chemistry. More modern sources include the other volumes of the *Cambridge Monographs on Cancer Research*, the *IARC monographs* (1973, 1983), the reviews by Campbell & Andrew (1979) and Zander (1983), and the books by Badger (1954, 1969) and Dias (1987).

5.1   Aromaticity

The nature of aromaticity has long intrigued chemists. In the last century it was recognized that compounds, such as benzene and naphthalene, that contain completely unsaturated six-membered carbocyclic rings are characterized by a special stability and a tendency to undergo substitution rather than addition reactions. The conventional Kekulé structural formulae with their alternate double and single bonds fail to adequately represent these special properties of aromatic ring systems.

Benzene has hexagonal symmetry and the length of each carbon–carbon bond is 1.39 Å in the ground state, intermediate between the values anticipated for alternating single (1.54 Å) and double (1.33 Å) bonds. The bond lengths of higher polycyclic aromatic compounds have been determined by X-ray diffraction analysis of the crystal structures and found to be generally unequal and between the limiting values for pure single or double bonds (Glusker, 1985). The bonding electrons of aromatic ring systems are said to be delocalized.

In the *valence-bond method* of solving the wave equation for aromatic molecules the structure of the molecule is represented by the sum of the structural forms, called *canonical forms*, that can be drawn (Wheland, 1955). The energy of the molecule is calculated as a weighted average of the combinations: $\Psi = C_A \Psi_A + C_B \Psi_A + \cdots\cdots$ For benzene, the principal canonical forms are the two Kekulé structures **1** and **2** and the three Dewar structures **3**, **4**, and **5** (Fig. 5.1). These forms are said to be in resonance, indicated by double-headed arrows. Solution of the wave equation shows that **1** and **2** each contribute 39% to the actual molecule, and structures **3–5** each contribute 7.3%. The *bond order* is the weighted sum of those canonical forms in which the bond is double. For benzene, the carbon–carbon bond order is 0.463; it would be 0.5 if only **1** and **2** contributed. Bond order provides a measure of the double bond character of the linkage between the atoms concerned.

For polycyclic ring systems the difficulty of the theoretical calculations expands as the number of fused rings increases, due to the rapid increase in the number of contributing structures (Herndon, 1974). However, it is found that a simplified theoretical treatment that uses only the Kekulé structures gives virtually as good results as more refined valence-bond or molecular orbital methods (Herndon, 1974a). There is relatively good agreement between calculated and experimental bond lengths (Table 5.1). The K-region bonds of phenanthrene and pyrene show exceptionally high bond order, indicative of their strong olefinic character. In contrast, the central bonds of triphenylene that link the outer benzenoid rings, and the central bonds of perylene that join the outer naphthalene ring systems, exhibit very low or zero bond order, indicating that the central rings in these systems are essentially nonaromatic.

Molecular orbital methods are also often employed to describe the structures of polyarenes. In benzene, each carbon atom is connected to three other atoms using $sp2$ orbitals to form σ bonds, so that all 12 atoms are in one plane. Each carbon atom has a p orbital remaining that contains one electron and overlaps with the two adjacent p orbitals to produce six new orbitals. These six electrons are commonly referred to as the *aromatic sextet*. Three of the orbitals formed, called π orbitals, are bonding and occupy approximately the same space. They each have the plane of the ring as the node and are split into two parts, one above and one below the plane. Two of the orbitals are of high energy and have another node.

Fig. 5.1. Valence bond representation of the structure of benzene.

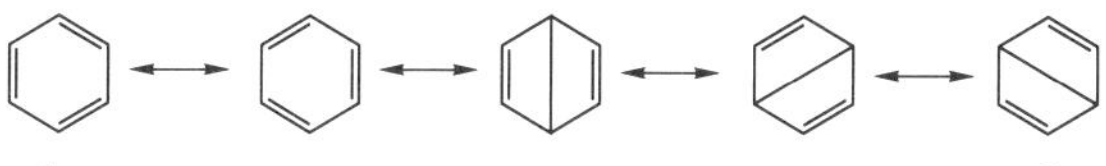

1   2   3   4   5

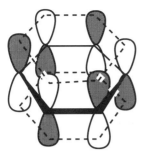

Various modifications of the molecular orbital approach are available that differ in their assumptions and levels of complexity. The oldest and simplest of these is the Huckel molecular orbital (HMO) theory which assumes that the σ orbitals can be treated as localized bonds and considers only the π electrons (Streitweiser, 1961). An alternative theoretical approach that takes into account electron–electron repulsions is the self-consistent field (SCF) method. Perhaps the most useful methods for carcinogenic polyarenes is Dewar's perturbational molecular orbital (PMO) theory (Dewar & Dougherty, 1975) which allows calculations of the π-electron densities of alternant PAHs by 'pencil and paper' methods.

Aromatic molecules exhibit greater stability, i.e. lower energy, than would be expected for the individual Kekulé structures. In valence-bond theory the difference between the energy of the actual compound and that represented by the most stable canonical structure is defined as the *resonance energy*. The latter is a theoretical concept that provides a useful index of the stabilities of the actual molecules in relation to those expected for the structural formulae usually written. In the case of benzene, if we add the energies of all the bonds for the structures **1** or **2**, taking the energies for the carbon–carbon double and single bonds from cyclohexene and cyclohexane (148.8 and 81.8 kcal, respectively) and for the carbon–hydrogen bonds from methane (99.5 kcal), we get a total of 1289 kcal/mol. The actual heat of atomization of benzene is 1323 kcal/mol. Therefore, the resonance energy of

Fig. 5.2. Resonance energy of benzene (kcal/mol).

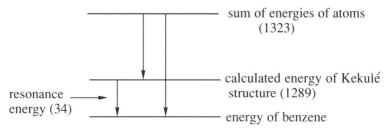

Table 5.1. *Pauling bond orders and bond lengths in typical polyarenes* $(\mathring{A})^a$

hydrocarbon	bond	bond order	bond length exptl	calcd
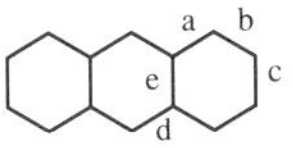 anthracene	a	0.250	1.444	1.433
	b	0.750	1.375	1.370
	c	0.250	1.418	1.433
	d	0.500	1.408	1.405
	e	0.250	1.433	1.433
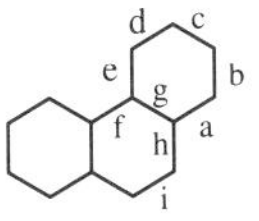 phenanthrene	a	0.400	1.432	1.414
	b	0.600	1.386	1.389
	c	0.400	1.394	1.414
	d	0.600	1.401	1.389
	e	0.400	1.409	1.414
	f	0.200	1.465	1.439
	g	0.400	1.420	1.414
	h	0.200	1.453	1.439
	i	0.800	1.350	1.364
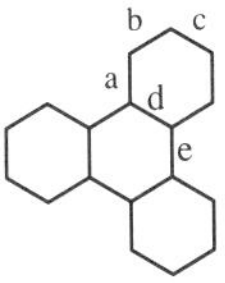 triphenylene	a	0.444	1.410	1.409
	b	0.556	1.381	1.395
	c	0.444	1.347	1.409
	d	0.444	1.413	1.409
	e	0.111	1.458	1.450
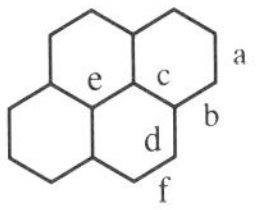 pyrene	a	0.500	1.395	1.401
	b	0.500	1.406	1.401
	c	0.333	1.425	1.422
	d	0.167	1.438	1.433
	e	0.333	1.430	1.422
	f	0.833	1.367	1.360
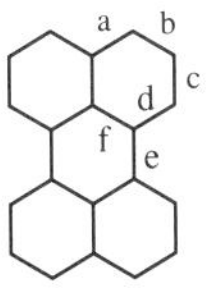 perylene	a	0.333	1.400	1.422
	b	0.667	1.370	1.381
	c	0.333	1.418	1.422
	d	0.667	1.397	1.381
	e	0.000	1.471	1.464
	f	0.333	1.425	1.422
	g	0.333	1.424	1.422

[a]Data are from Herndon, 1974

benzene is 34 kcal/mol (Fig. 5.2). Resonance energies may be computed from experimental values for heats of combustion or heats of hydrogenation, or calculated by theoretical quantum mechanical methods (Herndon, 1974). The resonance energies of fused ring systems increase as the number of aromatic rings and the number of principal canonical forms increases. Thus, for benzene, naphthalene, anthracene, and phenanthrene for which we can draw two, three, four, and five principal canonical forms, respectively, the resonance energies are 36, 61, 84, and 92 kcal/mol, respectively, calculated from heats of combustion data.

The energies of PAH ring systems are dependent upon both *size* (i.e. number of rings) and *topology* (i.e. spatial arrangement of the rings), particularly whether they are fused linearly or angularly. The importance of topology can be illustrated by plotting the resonance energies of the isomeric isoelectronic four-ring PAH systems (tetracene, benz[a]anthracene, chrysene, benzo[c]phenanthrene, triphenylene) against their angularity (equivalent to the number of bay molecular regions). The relation is essentially linear (Fig. 5.3).

According to Clar (1972), the effect of annelation on the chemical and physical properties of a PAH system is dependent upon the number of aromatic sextets that can be formed. In simple terms, he proposed to assign the π-electrons which can participate in aromatic sextets to particular rings. This is accomplished in such a way that the structure with the maximum number of aromatic sextets, considered a favored structure, is drawn. Any π-electrons that remain but do not participate in aromatic sextets are depicted as double bonds (Fig. 5.4). In the case of phenanthrene, the only favorable structure that can be written contains aromatic sextets in both outer rings. The alternative structure having a single aromatic sextet in the central ring is clearly less energetically favorable. Clar's π-formulae for phenanthrene, pyrene, and other angular PAHs are consistent with the olefinic character and unique chemical reactivities of the K-region bonds in these molecules.

Fig. 5.3. Correlation between resonance energy (RE) and angularity of isoelectronic polyarenes: (0) tetracene, (1) BA, (2) chrysene and benzo[c]phenanthrene, and (3) triphenylene. Based on Zander, 1983.

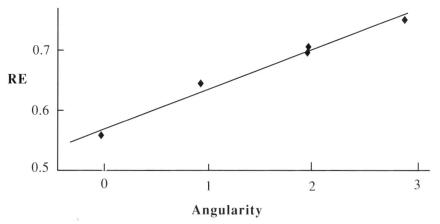

Other chemical and physical evidence suggests that Clar's model, with its emphasis on π-electron sextets, is relevant to chemical properties. For example, Diels–Alder addition of maleic anhydride to PAHs is generally regioselective, and the preferred site of addition is that which affords the adduct with the largest number of aromatic sextets (Biermann & Schmidt, 1980; Zander, 1983). Moreover, for the Diels–Alder addition to take place, it is necessary for at least one aromatic sextet to be gained, i.e. the number of sextets in the product must be at least one greater than in the PAH undergoing reaction. Thus, the adduct between maleic anhydride and benzo[a]tetracene has the structure **A** formed by addition at the 8,13-positions, rather than the alternative structure **B** formed by addition at the 7,14-positions (Fig. 5.5).

Comparison of the properties of PAHs of different sizes, but with the same number of aromatic sextets ('sextet isomers') is also instructive. The parameter $(n - 2)/n^2$, where n is the total number of π-electrons, may be employed as a measure of the size of the PAH ring system. Plots of $(n - 2)/n^2$ against the resonance energy per π-electron (REPE) for the acene, benz[a]acene, and dibenz[a,c]acene series of annellated hydrocarbons yield linear correlations in each case (Zander, 1983). These differences are also reflected in the electronic spectra of the sextet isomers. The effect of annelation in any series is to cause a bathochromic shift to higher wavelengths.

Nuclear magnetic resonance (NMR) spectroscopy provides a convenient

Fig. 5.4. Representation of PAHs by Clar's π-aromatic sextet formulae.

Fig. 5.5. The structure A is formed preferentially in the Diels–Alder reaction.

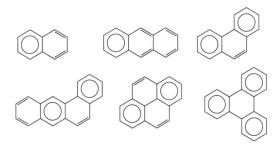

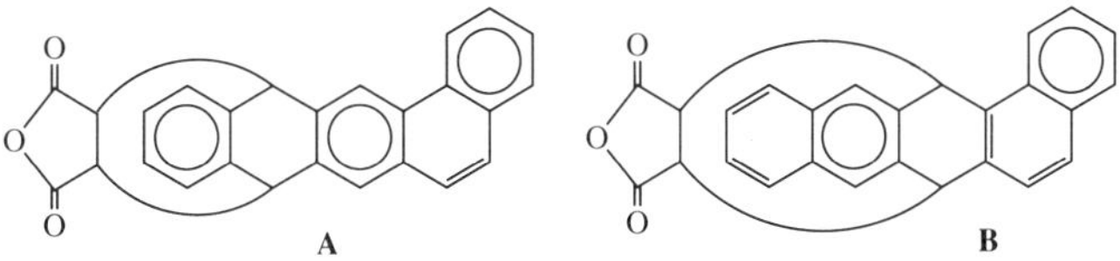

direct experimental measure of aromaticity. Indeed, a modern definition of aromaticity is *the ability to sustain an induced ring current*. When an external magnetic field is imposed upon an aromatic ring, the π-electrons circulate in a diamagnetic ring current (Fig. 5.6). The latter induces a magnetic field of its own which parallels and reinforces the external field in the vicinity of the aromatic protons. Consequently, the aromatic proton signals are shifted downfield from where they would be found in the absence of the diamagnetic ring current. Thus, while ordinary olefinic protons appear at δ 7–8 ppm, the benzenoid proton signals appear in the range of δ 7–8.5 ppm. Moreover, the greater the number of fused aromatic rings in the vicinity of a proton, the greater the shift. Thus, the chemical shift of the benzene protons is δ 7.27 ppm, whereas the proton resonances of anthracene appear at δ 7.39 to 8.36 ppm.

The chemical shifts of aromatic protons are also influenced by local contributions from other atoms as well as by steric and other structural effects. Consequently, the chemical shift and coupling constant patterns of PAH molecules vary widely, providing a wealth of information on PAH molecular structure. Theoretical analysis of the NMR spectra of polyarenes has met with considerable success, and there is generally reasonably good agreement between calculated and observed spectral properties. A review of this topic is available (Memory & Wilson, 1982). Application of NMR spectroscopic techniques to analysis of the structures of PAHs and PAH metabolites is discussed later in this chapter.

5.2   Planarity and intramolecular crowding

Fully aromatic polyarenes are generally planar with a molecular thickness of ≈ 3.7 Å. However, intramolecular crowding may lead to distortion of normal molecular geometry. X-ray crystallographic analysis of DMBA which contains a crowded methyl in the bay region, indicates that the

Fig. 5.6. Ring current induced in a benzoid ring by an external magnetic field.

induced field

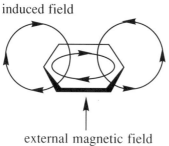

external magnetic field

benzo ring is bent out of the general plane by about 20° (Klein *et al.*,1987; Glusker, 1985). 5-Methylchrysene, which also contains a bay region methyl group, exhibits less distortion from planarity, but relieves the strain by in-plane expansion of the bay region angle (Kashino *et al.*, 1984; Zacharias *et al.*, 1984). 1-Methylbenzo[c]phenanthrene, which contains a methyl group in a more severely crowded 'fjord' region is also nonplanar (Hirschfeld *et al.*, 1963). Molecules which are sufficiently distorted from planarity may potentially exist as pairs of enantiomers.

Another important consequence of nonplanarity is loss of resonance energy resulting in increased olefinic character of the aromatic bonds. In extreme cases, aromaticity may be lost. For example, 9-isopropyl-10-isopropylidene-9,10-dihydroanthracene is found to be stable with respect to its fully aromatic tautomer 9,10-diisopropylanthracene (Fig. 5.7) (Cho *et al.*, 1975). The loss in delocalization energy is apparently more than compensated for by the relief in steric compression.

It is interesting to consider the relation between carcinogenicity and nonplanarity. X-ray analyses of the hydrocarbons chrysene, BA, DBA, BaP, and 3-MC indicate that all are essentially planar (Glusker, 1985). While these PAHs exhibit a range of tumorigenic activity from inactive to relatively potent, introduction of a methyl group into the nonbenzo bay region of each of these molecules results in a marked enhancement of potency (Harvey *et al.*, 1987; Hecht *et al.*, 1985; DiGiovanni *et al.*, 1983). Consideration of molecular models indicates that a methyl group in a bay region position is too bulky to fit the available space and still allow the molecule to remain planar. In support of this, X-ray analyses of two bay region methyl-substituted hydrocarbons, 5-methylchrysene and DMBA, show both to be buckled. Distortion from planarity may be expected to decrease aromaticity in the benzo ring, thereby increasing the olefinic character of the ring bonds making them more susceptible to metabolic activation. However, current evidence suggests that this effect may be of only minor importance. Thus, while metabolism of DMBA affords somewhat higher levels of the proximate 3,4-dihydrodiol metabolite than does BA (Sims & Grover, 1981), metabolism of 5-methylchrysene affords approximately equal amounts of the

Fig. 5.7. Steric crowding results in a loss of aromaticity.

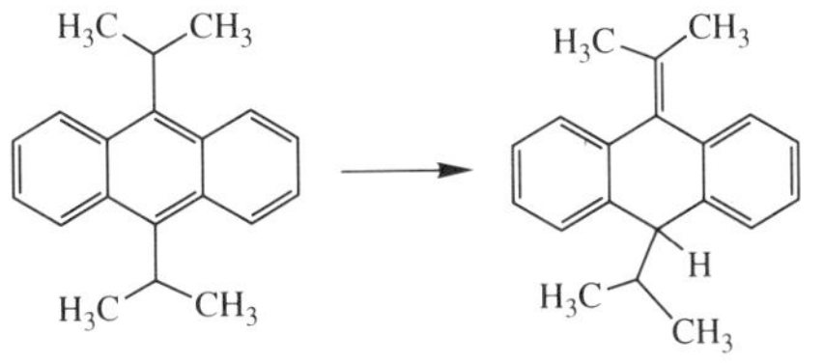

1,2- and 7,8-dihydrodiol metabolites in both bay regions (Melikian *et al.*, 1983). Since carcinogenesis is a multistage process, the bay region methyl effect may conceivably operate at other stages, e.g. by selectively blocking enzymatic detoxification of the active metabolite or by enhancing its reactivity with DNA. In the case of 5-methylchrysene, the latter effect appears to be important. Thus, comparison of the reactions with DNA of the pairs of enantiomers of the 1,2-diol-3,4-epoxide and 7,8-diol-9,10-epoxides of 5-MC reveal that the R,S,S,R enantiomer with the methyl group and epoxide ring in the same bay region is the most tumorigenic as well as the most reactive isomer with DNA (Melikian *et al.*, 1988). However, comparable studies have not been conducted with other methyl-substituted PAHs, and evidence concerning the possible importance of other factors is still limited.

5.3   Diamagnetic susceptibility

Polycyclic hydrocarbons are generally diamagnetic, i.e. they are repelled in a magnetic field. The molecular diamagnetic susceptibilities may be measured with a magnetic balance or calculated from the relation: $\chi_{mol} = \Sigma\chi_p + \Sigma \lambda$. The atomic increments (χ_p) are -2.93×10^{-6} for hydrogen and -6.0×10^{-6} for carbon and the structural increments (λ) are $+5.45 \times 10^{-6}$ for a double bond and -1.44×10^{-6} for a benzene ring. Due to the anisotropy of aromatic ring systems, the diamagnetic susceptibilities are different in each of the three dimensions of the molecule. K_1 and K_2 are designated as the susceptibilities in the molecular plane, while K_3 is perpendicular to the plane. These may be measured in a single crystal. Since this is not always feasible, the mean molecular susceptibility (χ_m) is often employed. If $\chi_m = 1/3(K_1 + K_2 + K_3)$ and one assumes $K_1 = K_2$ for the planar structure of the molecule, then the diamagnetic anisotropy of the molecule is $\Delta K = K_3 - K_1 = 3(\chi_m + K_1)$. ΔK is the anisotropic component of the susceptibility which derives from the circulation of the electrons in the molecular plane. K_1 and K_2 are isotropic components of the atomic susceptibility based on the spherical distribution of the electrons. The values of K_1 and K_2 may be calculated from the sum of the susceptibilities of the atoms concerned, where $\chi(C) = -3.36 \times 10^{-6}$ and $\chi(H) = -2.93 \times 10^{-6}$. In the acene series, ΔK increases proportionately to the number of rings (Akamatsu & Matsunaga, 1953) (Table 5.2).

5.4   Nuclear magnetic resonance spectroscopy

NMR spectroscopy, despite its potential for providing a wealth of information concerning PAH molecular structure, has not been utilized extensively in the synthetic and biological studies of these molecules until

Table 5.2. *Magnetic properties of acenes*

	Benzene	Naphthalene	Anthracene	Tetracene	Pentacene
$\chi_m \times 10^6 =$	55.6	92.2	130.3	168.0	205.4
$\Delta K \times 10^6 =$	54	106	162	217	272

quite recently. Partially this has been a consequence of historical developments. The early investigations in polyarene chemistry were conducted prior to the studies of the NMR spectra of polyarenes by Haigh & Mallion (1970) and others, and prior to the development of high field FT NMR instruments capable of resolving the complex patterns of the PAH proton resonances.

The most comprehensive source of information on the NMR spectroscopic properties of polyarenes is the book by Memory & Wilson (1982). This work provides extensive tables of chemical shift data for ^1H, ^{13}C, ^{19}F, and other nuclei. Another useful source of information is the review by Bartle & Jones (1972). A number of collections of reference NMR spectra are available. The most useful of these are the *Spectral Atlas of Polycyclic Aromatic Compounds* (Karcher *et al.*, 1985) and the serial collection of high resolution proton NMR spectra published by the Thermodynamics Research Center. The latter includes fully interpreted 500 MHz proton NMR spectra of many rare PAH compounds from the author's laboratory, including numerous carcinogenic PAHs and their oxidized metabolites. Other less extensive compilations of NMR spectral data are available from Aldrich (Pouchert & Campbell, 1983) and Sadtler.

The chemical shifts of aromatic protons are highly dependent upon their molecular environments. Methods for the calculation of chemical shift and coupling constants are discussed by Memory & Wilson (1982). In Table 5.3 is given a classification of the types of aromatic protons on the basis of their sites of attachment to polycyclic ring systems along with their chemical shifts. This classification is useful in the initial tentative assignments of the proton resonances in the NMR spectra of unknown PAH derivatives. While the absolute magnitudes of the chemical shifts of the aromatic protons may vary considerably with the number of fused aromatic rings and other structural factors, the relative chemical shifts of the different types of aromatic protons tend to be retained.

Substituents generally alter the chemical shifts of nearby protons, sometimes dramatically. Electron-donating groups tend to cause shifts to

Table 5.3. *Classification of Proton Types in Unsubstituted PAH* [a]

Proton Type (Chemical shift)	Designation	Proton Type (Chemical shift)	Designation
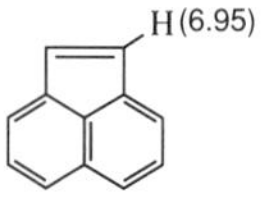 H (6.95)	Bridge	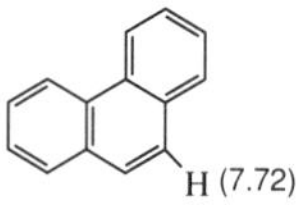 H (7.72)	K-region
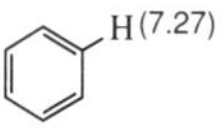 H (7.27)	Phenyl	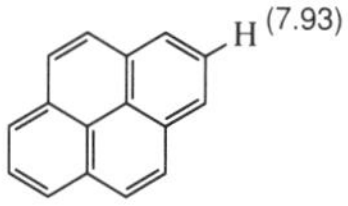 H (7.93)	β-pyrenyl
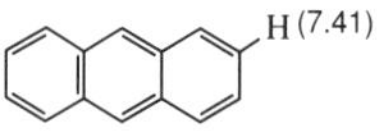 H (7.41)	Beta	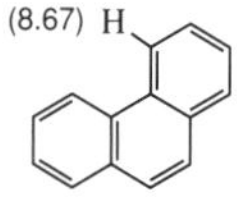 (8.67) H	Angular or bay
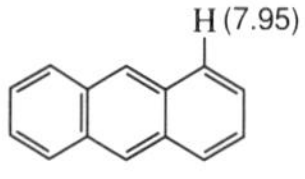 H (7.95)	Alpha	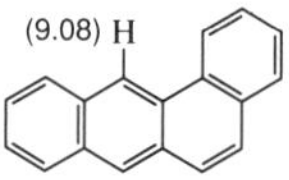 (9.08) H	Meso-bay
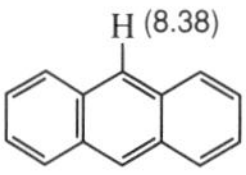 H (8.38)	Meso	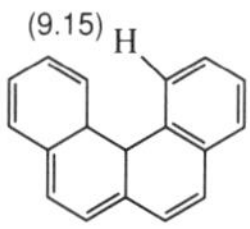 (9.15) H	Fjord

[a]Spectra are in CDCl₃ and chemical shifts are in ppm relative to tetramethylsilane

higher field, while electron-withdrawing groups have the opposite effect. In addition, there may be larger contributions from substituent magnetic anisotropies, local van der Waals interactions, and altered ring currents. In Table 5.4 are summarized the shielding or deshielding effects of various groups on the adjacent aromatic protons of benzene; data are from Ballantine & Pillinger (1967). Positive values correspond to a shift to higher field, and vice versa. Although these data are empirical, they are useful in providing an indication of the kind of effects to be expected. More extensive treatment of shielding effects may be found in other sources (Memory & Wilson, 1982; Bartle & Jones, 1972).

Nuclear spins within aromatic molecules interact through the bonds, and the energy of such interaction is proportional to the scalar product of the spin vectors of the nuclei affected. This coupling may be considered to arise from fixed increments in the total magnetic field produced at a given nucleus by the magnetic moments of neighboring nuclei. A proton coupled with a single

Table 5.4. *Shielding effects of substituents on benzene* [a,b]

Group	Ortho	Meta	Para
OH	0.45	0.10	0.40
OR	0.45	0.10	0.40
OCOR	0.20	–0.10	0.20
NH_2	0.55	0.15	0.55
CH_2R	0.10	0.10	0.10
CHR_2	0	0	0
CH=CHR	–0.10	0	–0.10
CHO	–0.65	–0.25	–0.10
C(=O)R	–0.70	–0.25	–0.10
CO_2R	–0.80	–0.25	–0.20
Cl	–0.10	0	0
Br	-0.10	0	0
NO_2	-0.85	-0.10	-0.55

[a] Data are from Ballantine & Pillinger (1967).
[b] ppm in $CDCl_3$.

neighboring proton will experience an effective magnetic field which has two possible values depending on the spin orientation of the second nucleus. Coupling constants for the aromatic protons of polyarenes are usually in the range: J_{ortho} = 6-10; J_{meta} = 1–3; and J_{para} = 0.1 Hz.

Carbon-13 NMR spectroscopy is an additional valuable source of information on the structures of polyarenes and their sites of substitution. A number of excellent books and review articles on ^{13}C NMR spectroscopy of PAH compounds are available (Memory & Wilson, 1982; Hansen, 1979; Levy & Nelson, 1972; Stothers, 1972). The chemical shifts of the ^{13}C nuclei of alternant hydrocarbons have a range of 10 ppm, while nonalternant hydrocarbons have a wider range of about 14–22 ppm, reflecting the less uniform distribution of electrons in the latter molecules. Introduction of substituents into aromatic molecules extends the range of shifts to about 50 ppm. The effects of substituents on the ^{13}C shieldings of aromatic polyarenes are approximately additive in the absence of steric interactions and other effects.

Complete ^1H and ^{13}C NMR assignment of benzo[a]pyrene, cyclopenta[cd]pyrene, benzo[b]fluoranthene, indeno[1,2,3-hi]chrysene, and indeno[1,2,3-cd]pyrene have recently been achieved by the application of two-dimensional NMR spectroscopic techniques (Bax *et al.*, 1985; Jans *et al.*, 1986; and Cho & Harvey, 1987). These new techniques provide a potentially powerful tool for the structural elucidation of complex polyarenes and their products of electrophilic substitution or metabolism.

The utilization of NMR spectroscopic methods for determination of the structures and conformations of polyarene metabolites will be discussed in later chapters.

5.5   Ultraviolet absorption and fluorescence spectroscopy

Polyarenes absorb strongly in the ultraviolet region to give distinctive spectral patterns. Ultraviolet spectroscopy is commonly employed for the analysis of PAH compounds in the environment and for the identification of PAH metabolites in animal tissues. UV spectra also find important application in the determination of the structures of the products formed in PAH reactions. For example, in reactions that lead to a decrease in the number of aromatic rings, such as hydrogenation or Diels–Alder addition, the possible isomeric products can often be distinguished by the UV spectrum of the remaining aromatic ring system. Thus, hydrogenation of BaP over palladium/C affords a single product identified as 4,5-dihydro-BaP by the presence of the chrysene chromophore in its UV spectrum (Lijinsky & Zechmeister, 1973). It is readily distinguished from 11,12-dihydrochrysene which contains the BA chromophore. Reference sources on the UV spectra of polyarenes include books by Friedel & Orchin (1951), Jaffe & Orchin (1962), Scott (1964), and Karcher *et al.* (1985), a review by Sawicki *et al.* (1960), and several compilations of standard spectra (Thermodynamics Research Center; Pouchert, 1981; Sadtler).

The ultraviolet absorption bands of PAHs have been classified and related to molecular structural features (Mason, 1961; Clar, 1964, 1972). Three classes of bands, designated as α, ß, and p in order of increasing wavelength are distinguishable in the absorption spectrum of benzene. As additional rings are fused angularly in the phene series, the α-, ß-, and p-bands retain their characteristic features and shift to longer wavelengths. In the linear acene series, the p-bands shift more to red with annellation than the α-, and ß-bands. The α-bands become obscured by the p-bands in anthracene and tetracene, then reappear faintly in the spectrum of pentacene. The theoretical basis of the electronic transitions that give rise to these bands is now relatively well understood (Dias,1987).

The p-bands have an intensity of approx. $\log \varepsilon = 4$ which changes minimally with annellation. The p-bands are shifted to the red with increasing temperature or change of solvent from hexane or alcohol to benzene. The shift of the p-bands to the red on linear annellation is constant for each additional ring. The p-bands have been correlated with localization of two electrons in meso ring positions, e.g. the 9,10-positions of anthracene. The red shift of the p-bands with annelation correlates with an observed increase in the chemical reactivity of the meso regions. The p-bands of acenes are also called L_α-bands (Platt, 1949; Moffit, 1954). This is based on the fact that the maximum absorption of light polarized in the molecular plane takes place in the direction of the long axis 'a' of the acenes. This means that the p-bands are polarized perpendicular to the long axis.

The intensities of the α-bands are usually in the range of log ε = 2–3, but can exhibit intensities as high as log ε = 4–5 in the fluorenes and fluoranthenes. The α-bands, also called L_b-bands, are polarized perpendicular to the short axis of the molecule. The ß-bands appear at shortest wavelength and are generally the most intense in the absorption spectra of PAHs. The intensities lie in the range log ε =4–6. the β-bands, which are also called $ß_b$-bands, are polarized perpendicular to the short axis of the molecule like the α-bands. Although both the α- and ß-bands are shifted toward the red upon linear annellation, because the ß-bands appear at longer wavelengths and are of greater intensity, they are never obscured by other absorption transitions.

Ultraviolet and ultraviolet fluorescence spectroscopic techniques have seen extensive use for the analysis and identification of the metabolites of carcinogenic hydrocarbons and their nucleic acid adducts formed in biological systems. The sensitivity of these techniques permits the detection of the tiny amounts of these products formed in animal cells without the necessity for labeling with radioisotopes. The introduction of HPLC methods for the efficient separation of PAH metabolites coupled with UV detection (Selkirk *et al.*, 1974) allowed the quantitative analysis of the patterns of PAH metabolites, contributing importantly to understanding of PAH metabolism. Ultraviolet absorption and fluorescence spectroscopy have also been utilized effectively in studies of the mechanism of interaction of PAH metabolites with nucleic acids and provide the most useful techniques for determination of the structures of the DNA adducts formed (Harvey & Geacintov, 1988).

5.6   Infrared spectroscopy

The infrared spectra of polyarenes exhibit three principal regions of absorption: C–H stretching frequencies range from 3090 to 3000 cm^{-1}; sharp medium intensity bands near 1600 and 1500 cm^{-1} arise from C–C stretching of the aromatic rings; and the C–H out-of-plane bending vibrations occur between 900 and 650 cm^{-1}. The latter absorption bands are particularly useful as structural diagnostic features. Their presence or absence allows one to distinguish molecular regions containing one (solo), two (duo), three (trio), and four (quartet) adjacent hydrogens (Fig. 5.8). The solo C–H bending vibrations require most energy and therefore occur in the highest frequency range of 900–860 cm^{-1}. Duo bending C–H vibrations are found between 860–800 cm^{-1}, trio bending C–H vibrations occur between 810–750 cm^{-1}, and quartet C–H bending frequencies require the least energy and are found between 770–735 cm^{-1}. Thus, naphthalene has a single strong absorption band in the quartet IR region, and phenanthrene with two duo and eight quartet C–H groupings gives rise to an IR spectrum containing a duo band and a quartet band. Pyrene with four duo and six trio C–H groups shows the two expected IR bands in the duo and trio regions. As molecular size and complexity increase, the complexity of these spectral patterns also increases, rendering analysis more difficult. However, even when interpretation is not obvious, IR spectral patterns often provide a characteristic fingerprint that allows one to distinguish one polycyclic aromatic system from another. Several compilations of standard IR spectra are available, most notably the Aldrich Library (Pouchert, 1981) and the Sadtler series.

5.7   Photoelectron spectroscopy

The photoelectron spectra of polyarenes contain more information than the UV and mass spectra, making them a valuable tool for the structural elucidation of unknown hydrocarbons (Clar *et al.*, 1981). On the other hand, the PE spectra are less useful for the characterization of PAH oxidized metabolites, because they are normally measured under conditions where the latter tend to decompose, namely in the gas phase at elevated temperatures.

In the alternant hydrocarbon series, the energies of the UV absorption bands correlate linearly with the ionization potentials (IPs) of the highest wavelength. In accord with theoretical prediction, the p- and ß'-band correlate linearly with IP$_1$ and IP$_2$, respectively, and the α- and ß-band energies both correlate with IP = 1/2(IP$_1$ and IP$_2$). From a study of a large number of cata-condensed and peri-condensed polyarenes Clar *et al.* (1981) have deduced the following semiempirical relationships:

$$E_\alpha = -3.750 + 0.5378IP_1 + 0.3862IP_2$$
$$E_p = -5.015 + 1.3947IP_1 - 0.2047IP_2$$
$$E_\beta = -6.232 + 0.6861IP_1 + 0.6999IP_2$$

These relationships are highly significant, having standard deviations of

Fig. 5.8. The C–H out-of-plane bending vibrations of aromatic molecules occur at characteristic frequencies.

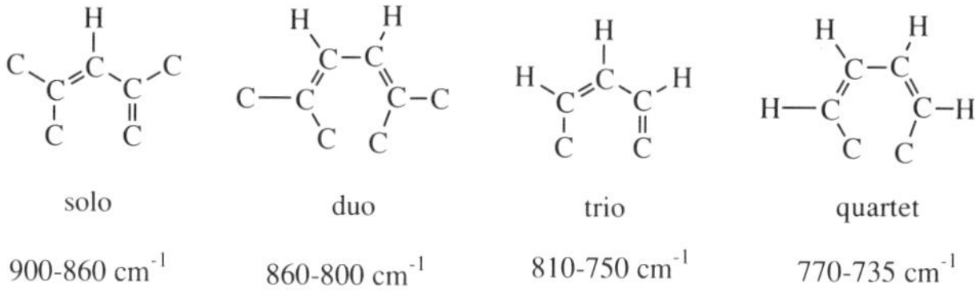

solo	duo	trio	quartet
900-860 cm^{-1}	860-800 cm^{-1}	810-750 cm^{-1}	770-735 cm^{-1}

0.047, 0.080, and 0.059 eV, respectively, and are valid for planar as well as nonplanar alternant hydrocarbons, irrespective of size, shape, and symmetry. On the other hand, in the nonalternant hydrocarbon series, there is no obvious relation between excitation energies and IPs.

The PE spectra of peri-condensed hydrocarbons, such as pyrene, contain additional bands originating from the orbitals of the insular structure (i.e. internal carbon atoms not part of the peripheral structure). For example, the spectra of most pyrene derivatives show a band at about 9.1 eV which derives from the insular ethene component. Moreover, the IPs of most larger PAHs are often simply related to those of the smaller basic components present (e.g. naphthalene, phenanthrene, pyrene, etc.). For example, the PE spectrum of hexaphene is essentially the superposition of the spectra of anthracene and tetracene, and the spectrum of heptacene resembles that of tetracene, with all the bands showing twice the normal integrated intensity. The bands in the PE spectra of the linearly annelated pyrenes and perylenes can be distinguished as pyrene, perylene, or acene type bands. Only the latter respond to annelation, and as a consequence are called 'moving bands'.

UV photoelectron spectroscopy has been employed to investigate the electronic structure of the mono-, di-, and trimethylbenz[a]anthracenes (Akiyama *et al.*, 1981). Trimethyl substitution reduced the IP_1 of BA more than dimethyl substitution, which in turn caused a larger perturbation than monomethyl substitution. The vertical IP of the carcinogenic DMBA is almost 0.4 eV lower than that of BA. Of the ten monomethyl-BAs studied, the two most carcinogenic isomers, 7- and 12-methyl-BA, have the lowest IPs. However, no simple correlation was found between the IPs of different methyl-BAs and their carcinogenicities. This finding is evidence against the radical cation theory of hydrocarbon carcinogenesis (Cavalieri & Rogan, 1985; see Chap. 4: **4.5**).

5.8   X-ray crystallography

X-ray diffraction analysis provides fundamental information concerning bond length, bond angles, planarity, conformation, and other features of the molecular structures of carcinogenic PAHs and their activated metabolites. This knowledge is useful in understanding the mechanisms of PAH activation and interaction of the active metabolites with nucleic acids. An excellent review of the application of X-ray analytical methods to PAH compounds is available (Glusker, 1985).

X-ray diffraction studies show that the carbon–carbon bonds of polycyclic aromatic molecules are not generally equivalent in length. Some localization of double bonds takes place. The experimentally measured bond lengths generally accord with those that would be expected from consideration of the various types of resonance hybrids present in the molecule. K-region bonds tend to be shorter than other aromatic bonds, i.e. closer to pure double bonds (1.34–1.35 Å), while most other ring bonds are in the range of 1.36–1.44 Å.

The structures of the K-region epoxide derivatives of several PAHs have been investigated by X-ray diffraction methods (Glusker, 1985). The epoxide ring of phenanthrene 9,10-oxide is approximately symmetrical and perpendicular to the plane of the aromatic ring system. However, K-region epoxidation of the nonplanar DMBA increases the angle between the outer rings from 24° to 35°, and the epoxide bond lengths are unequal (1.445 and 1.457 Å). It would be expected that the longer bond (to C6) would be cleaved more readily, and this is the case (Beland & Harvey, 1976).

Information on the conformational properties of the PAH dihydrodiol metabolites may also be obtained from X-ray diffraction analysis (Glusker, 1985; Harvey, 1989). Thus, the sterically hindered bay region *trans*-1,2-dihydrodiol of BA is shown by X-ray analysis to exist in the diaxial conformation, while the unhindered nonbay region *trans*-10,11-dihydrodiol isomer is found to adopt the diequatorial conformation (Fig. 5.9). NMR analysis indicates that the former is still 100% diaxial in solution, while the latter exists in solution as a mixture of the diequatorial (70%) and diaxial (30%) conformers in dynamic equilibrium (Zacharias *et al.*, 1979).

The structures of the *anti*- and *syn*-diol epoxides of BaP were determined by Neidle *et al.* (1980) and Neidle & Cutbush (1983), respectively, by X-ray diffraction analysis. The hydroxyl groups of the former are diequatorial in the crystal, as they are in solution as shown by NMR studies (Harvey, 1989), and the epoxide ring lies in a plane nearly perpendicular to the PAH ring system. In the *anti* isomer the saturated ring has a half-chair conformation with C8 as the atom most out of the plane. The *syn*-BPDE isomer was also found to exist

Fig. 5.9. Conformational equilibria between the diaxial and diequatorial forms of the dihydrodiols of benz[a]anthracene indicating the populations in solution and in the crystalline state.

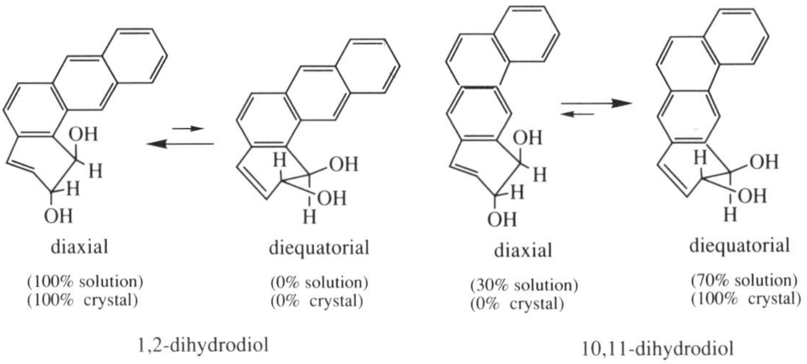

diaxial

(100% solution)
(100% crystal)

diequatorial

(0% solution)
(0% crystal)

diaxial

(30% solution)
(0% crystal)

diequatorial

(70% solution)
(100% crystal)

1,2-dihydrodiol   10,11-dihydrodiol

in the crystal lattice in a conformation in which the hydroxyl groups are oriented diequatorially. This finding is contrary to molecular orbital theoretical predictions (Hulbert, 1975; Yeh *et al.*, 1978; Klopman *et al.*, 1979) that the diaxial conformer should be stabilized by hydrogen bonding interaction between the benzylic hydroxylic group and the epoxide oxygen atom. In solution, *syn*-BPDE exists as a mixture of the diequatorial (major) and diaxial (minor) conformers in equilibrium; the ratio of conformers varies with solvent, temperature, and other factors.

5.9   References

Akamatsu, H. & Matsunaga, Y. (1953). The diamagnetic susceptibilities and anisotropies of polynuclear aromatic compounds. *Bull. Chem. Soc. Japan*, **26**, 364–72.

Akiyama, I., Harvey, R. G. & LeBreton, P. R. (1981). Ultraviolet photoelectron studies of methyl-substituted benz[a]anthracenes. *J. Am. Chem. Soc.* **103**, 6330–2.

Badger, G. M. (1954). *The Structures and Reactions of Aromatic Compounds*, London: Cambridge University Press.

Badger, G. M. (1969). *Aromatic Character and Aromaticity*, London: Cambridge University Press.

Ballantine, J. A. & Pillinger, C. T. (1967). An analysis of the chemical shift positions of the aromatic protons of phenolic compounds as a guide to orientation. *Tetrahedron*, **23**, 1691–6.

Bartle, K. E. & Jones, D. W. (1972). The application of proton magnetic resonance spectroscopy to structure identification in polycyclic aromatic molecules. *Adv. Org. Chem.* **8**, 317–423.

Bax, A., Ferretti, J. A., Nashed, N. & Jerina, D. M. (1985). Complete ^{1}H and ^{13}C NMR assignment of complex polycyclic aromatic hydrocarbons. *J. Org. Chem.* **50**, 3029–34.

Beland, F. & Harvey, R. G. (1976). Reactions of the K-region oxides of carcinogenic and related polycyclic hydrocarbons with nucleophiles: Stereochemistry and regioselectivity. *J. Am. Chem. Soc.* **98**, 4963–70.

Biermann, D. & Schmidt, W. (1980). Diels–Alder reactivity of polycyclic aromatic hydrocarbons. 1. Acenes and benzologs. *J. Am. Chem. Soc.* **102**, 3163–73.

Campbell, N. & Andrew, H. F. (1979). *Rodd's Chemistry of Carbon Compounds*, Amsterdam: Elsevier.

Cavalieri, E. & Rogan, E. G. (1985). One-electron oxidation in aromatic hydrocarbon carcinogenesis. *Polycyclic Hydrocarbons and Carcinogenesis*, Am. Chem. Soc. Monogr. 283, ed. R. G. Harvey, pp. 289–305, Washington, DC: American Chemical Society.

Cho, B. P. & Harvey, R. G. (1987). Complete ^{1}H and ^{13}C NMR assignment of polycyclic aromatic fluoranthenes by long-range optimized homo- and heteronuclear correlation spectroscopy. *J. Org. Chem.* **52**, 5679–84.

Cho, H., Harvey, R. G. & Rabideau, P. W. (1975). 9-Isopropylidene-9,10-dihydroanthracene. Synthesis, stereochemistry, and the effect of 10-alkyl group size on the equilibrium with 9-isopropyl-alkylanthracene. *J. Am. Chem. Soc.* **97**, 1140–5.

Clar, E. (1964). *Polycyclic Hydrocarbons*, New York: Academic Press.

Clar, E. (1972). *The Aromatic Sextet*, New York: Wiley.

Clar, E., Robertson, J. M., Schlogl, R. & Schmidt, W. (1981). Photoelectron spectra of polynuclear aromatics. 6. Applications to structural elucidation: 'Circumanthracene'. *J. Am. Chem. Soc.* **103**, 1320–8.

Dewar, M. J. S. & Dougherty, R. C. (1975). *The PMO Theory of Organic Chemistry*, New York: Plenum/Rosetta.

Dias, J. R. (1987). *Handbook of Polycyclic Hydrocarbons, Part A*, Amsterdam: Elsevier.

DiGiovanni, J., Diamond, L. & Harvey, R. G. (1983). Enhancement of the skin tumor initiating activity of polycyclic aromatic hydrocarbons by methyl substitution at non-benzo bay-region positions. *Carcinogenesis*, **4**, 403–7.

Friedel, R. A. & Orchin, M. (1951). *Ultraviolet Spectra of Aromatic Compounds*, New York: Wiley.

Glusker, J. P. (1985). X-Ray analysis of polycyclic hydrocarbon metabolite structures. *Polycyclic Hydrocarbons and Carcinogenesis*, Am. Chem. Soc. Monogr. 283, ed. R. G. Harvey, 125–85, Washington, DC: American Chemical Society.

Haigh, C. W. & Mallion, R. B. (1970). Proton magnetic resonance of planar condensed benzenoid hydrocarbons. II. Critical evaluation of the McWeeny 'ring-current' theory. *Mol. Phys.* **18**, 737–50.

Hansen, P. E. (1979). Carbon-13 NMR of polycyclic aromatic compounds. A review. *Org. Magn. Resonance*, **12**, 109–42.

Harvey, R. G. (1989). The conformational analysis of hydroaromatic metabolites of carcinogenic hydrocarbons and the relation of conformation to biological activity. *The Conformational Analysis of Cyclohexenes, Cyclohexadienes, and Related Hydroaromatics*, ed. P. W. Rabideau, 269–98, New York: VCH Publishers.

Harvey, R. G., Cortez, C., Sugiyama, T., Ito, Y., Sawyer, T. W. & DiGiovanni, J. (1987). Biologically active dihydrodiol metabolites of polycyclic aromatic hydrocarbons structurally related to the potent carcinogenic hydrocarbon 7,12-dimethylbenz[a]anthracene. *J. Med. Chem.* **31**, 154–9.

Harvey, R. G. & Geacintov, N. E. (1988). Intercalation and binding of carcinogenic hydrocarbon metabolites to nucleic acids. *Acc. Chem. Res.* **21**, 66–73.

Hecht, S. S., Amin, S., Melikian, A. A., LaVoie, E. J. & Hoffmann, D. (1985). Effects of methyl and fluorine substituents on the metabolic activation and tumorigenicity of polycyclic aromatic hydrocarbons. *Polycyclic Hydrocarbons and Carcinogenesis*, Am. Chem. Soc. Monogr. 283, ed. R. G. Harvey, 85–105, Washington, DC: American Chemical Society.

Herndon, W. C. (1974). Resonance theory. VI. Bond orders. *J. Am. Chem. Soc.* **96**, 7605–14.

Herndon, W. C. (1974a). Resonance theory and the enumeration of Kekulé structures. *J. Chem. Educ.* **51**, 10–15.

Hirshfeld, F. L., Sandler, S. & Schmidt, G. M. (1963). The structure of overcrowded aromatic compounds. Part VI. The crystal structure of benzo[c]phenanthrene. *J. Chem. Soc.* 2108–25.

Hulbert, P. B. (1975). Carbonium ion as ultimate carcinogen of polycyclic aromatic hydrocarbons. *Nature (Lond.)*, **256**, 146–8.

IARC. (1973). *IARC Monographs on the Evaluation of the Carcinogenic Risk of Chemicals to Humans: Polynuclear Aromatic Compounds*, Lyon, France: Internat. Agency Res. Cancer.

IARC. (1983). *IARC Monographs on the Evaluation of the Carcinogenic Risk of Chemicals to Humans: Polynuclear Aromatic Compounds, Part 1, Chemical, Environmental and Experimental Data*, Lyon, France: Internat. Agency Res. Cancer.

Jaffe, H. H. & Orchin, M. (1962). *Theory and Applications of Ultraviolet Spectroscopy*, New York: Wiley.

Jans, A. W. H., Tintel, C., Cornelisse, J. & Lughtenburg, J. (1986). Proton and carbon-13 assignment of cyclopenta[cd]pyrene by two-dimensional NMR spectroscopy. *Mag. Resonan. Chem.* **24**, 101–4.

Karcher, W., Fordham, R. J., Dubois, J. J., Glaude, P. G. & Lighthart, J. A. (1985). *Spectral Atlas of Polycyclic Aromatic Compounds*, Dordrecht, Holland: D. Reidel.

Kashino, S., Zacharias, D. E., Prout, C. K., Carrell, H. L., Glusker, J. P., Hecht, S. S. & Harvey, R. G. (1984). Structure of 5-methylchrysene, $C_{19}H_{14}$. *Acta Cryst C.* **C40**, 536–40.

Klein, C. L., Stevens, E. D., Zacharias, D. E. & Glusker, J. P. (1987). 7,12-Dimethyl-benz[a]anthracene: refined structure, electron density distribution and *endo*-peroxide structure. *Carcinogenesis*, **8**, 5–18.

Klopman, G., Grinberg, H. & Hopfinger, A. J. (1979). MINDO/3 calculations of the conformation and carcinogenicity of epoxy-metabolites of aromatic hydrocarbons; 7,8-dihydroxy-9,10-oxy-7,8,9,10-tetrahydrobenzo[a]pyrene. *J. Theor. Biol.* **79**, 355–66.

Levy, G. C. & Nelson, G. L. (1972). *Carbon-13 Nuclear Magnetic Resonance for Organic Chemists*, New York: Wiley-Interscience.

Lijinsky, W. & Zechmeister, L. (1973). On the catalytic hydrogenation of 3,4-benzpyrene. *J. Am. Chem. Soc.* **75**, 5495–7.

Mason, S. F. (1961). Molecular electronic absorption spectra. *Quart. Rev.* **15**, 287–371.

Melikian, A. A., Amin, S., Huie, K., Hecht, S. S. & Harvey, R. G. (1988). Reactivity with DNA bases and mutagenicity toward *Salmonella typhimurium* of methyl chrysene diol epoxide enantiomers. *Cancer Res.* **48**, 1781–7.

Melikian, A. A., LaVoie, E. J., Hecht, S. S. & Hoffmann, D. (1983). 5-Methylchrysene metabolism in mouse epidermis *in vivo*, diol epoxide–DNA adduct persistence, and diol epoxide reactivity with DNA as potential factors influencing the predominance of 5-methylchrysene-1,2-diol-3,4-epoxide–DNA adducts in mouse epidermis. *Carcinogenesis*, **4**, 843–49.

Memory, J. D. & Wilson, N. K. (1982). *NMR of Aromatic Compounds*, New York: Wiley.

Moffit, W. (1954). The electronic spectra of *cata*-condensed hydrocarbons. *J. Chem. Phys.* **22**, 320–33.

Neidle, S. & Cutbush, S. D. (1983). X-ray crystallographic analysis of (±)-7ß,8a-dihydroxy-9ß,10ß-epoxy-7,8,9,10-tetrahydrobenzo[a]pyrene: molecular structure of a '*syn*' diol epoxide. *Carcinogenesis*, **4**, 415–18.

Neidle, S., Subbiah, A., Cooper, C. S. & Ribeiro, O. (1980). Molecular structure of (±)-7α,8ß-dihydroxy-9ß, 10ß-epoxy-7,8,9,10-tetrahydrobenzo[a]pyrene; an X-ray crystallographic study. *Carcinogenesis*, **1**, 249–54.

Platt, J. R. (1949). Classification of spectra of cata-condensed hydrocarbons. *J. Chem. Phys.* **17**, 484–95.

Pouchert, C. E. (1981). *Aldrich Library of Infrared Spectra*, Milwaukee, Wisc.: Aldrich Chemical Co.

Pouchert, C. E. & Campbell, J. R. (1983). *Aldrich Library of NMR Spectra*, Milwaukee, Wisc.: Aldrich Chemical Co.

Pullman, B. & Pullman, A. (1958). Free valence in conjugated organic molecules. *Prog. Org. Chem.* **4**, 31–71.

Sadtler. (Serial publication). *The Sadtler Standard Spectra*, Philadelphia: Sadtler Research Laboratories.

Sawicki, E., Hauser, R. T. & Stanley, T. W. (1960). Ultraviolet, visible, and fluorescence spectral analysis of polynuclear hydrocarbons. *Int. J. Air Pollution*, **2**, 253–72.

Scott, A. I. (1964). *Interpretation of the Ultraviolet Spectra of Natural Products*, Oxford: Pergamon.

Selkirk, J. K., Croy, R. G. & Gelboin, H. V. (1974). Benzo[a]pyrene metabolites. Efficient and rapid separation by high-pressure liquid chromatography. *Science*, **184**, 169–71.

Sims, P. & Grover, P. L. (1981). Involvement of dihydrodiols and diol epoxides in the metabolic activation of polycyclic hydrocarbons other than benzo[a]pyrene. *Polycyclic Hydrocarbons and Cancer*, eds H. V. Gelboin & P. O. P. Ts'o, 117–81, New York: Acadmic Press.

Stothers, J. B. (1972). *Carbon-13 NMR Spectroscopy*, New York: Academic Press.

Streitweiser, A. (1961). *Molecular Orbital Theory for Organic Chemists*, New York: Wiley.

Thermodynamics Research Center. (Serial publication). *Selected ^{1}H Nuclear Magnetic Resonance Spectral Data*, College Station, TX: Thermodynamics Res. Center.

Thermodynamics Research Center. (Serial publication). *Selected Ultraviolet Spectral Data*, College Station, TX: Thermodynamics Res. Center.

Wheland, G. W. (1955). *Resonance in Organic Chemistry*, New York: Wiley.

Yeh, C. Y., Beland, F. A. & Harvey, R. G. (1978). Application of CNDO/2 theoretical calculations to interpretation of the chemical reactivity and biological activity of the *syn* and *anti* diol epoxides of benzo[a]pyrene. *Bioorg. Chem.* **7**, 497–506.

Zacharias, D. E., Glusker, J. P., Fu, P. P. & Harvey, R. G. (1979). Molecular structure of the dihydrodiols and diolepoxides of carcinogenic polycyclic hydrocarbons: X-ray crystallographic and NMR analysis. *J. Am. Chem. Soc.* **101**, 4043–51.

Zacharias, D. E., Kashino, S., Glusker, J. P., Harvey, R. G., Amin, S. & Hecht, S. S. (1984). The bay-region geometry of carcinogenic 5-methylchrysenes: Steric effects in 5,6- and 5,12-dimethylchrysenes. *Carcinogenesis*, **5**, 1421–30.

Zander, M. (1983). Physical and chemical properties of polycyclic aromatic hydrocarbons. *Handbook of Polycyclic Aromatic Hydrocarbons*, ed. A. Bjorseth, New York: Marcel Dekker.

6

Chemical reactivity

6.1 Electrophilic substitution

Electrophilic substitutions are the most common reactions of polyarenes. They proceed mainly via an SE_2 mechanism in which initial electrophilic attack by a positive electrophilic ion (E^+) gives rise to an *arenium ion* (also referred to as a σ-complex or a Wheland intermediate) (Fig. 6.1). This reactive intermediate stabilizes itself by loss of a proton to form a fully aromatic structure or by further reaction. Proton loss is nearly always faster than the addition step ($k_2 \gg k_1$), so that addition of the electrophile is rate-determining and the reaction is second order. The absence of a deuterium isotope effect in such reactions confirms that the C–H or C–D bond must be intact in the transition state. The ease with which polyarenes undergo electrophilic substitution is directly related to the degree of stabilization of the arenium ion intermediate by delocalization of the charge by the polycyclic aromatic ring system. This increases dramatically with the number of fused aromatic rings, as shown by the partial rate-factors for nitration of PAHs (Table 6.1). Generally only a small fraction of the peripheral ring positions of any polyarene undergo significant extent of substitution by electrophiles.

In strongly acidic media, polyarenes form protonated arenium ion complexes that are sufficiently stable to investigate by NMR, UV, and IR spectroscopic methods (Perkampus & Baumgarten, 1964). The protonated

Fig. 6.1. The SE_2 mechanism for electrophilic substitution of polyarenes.

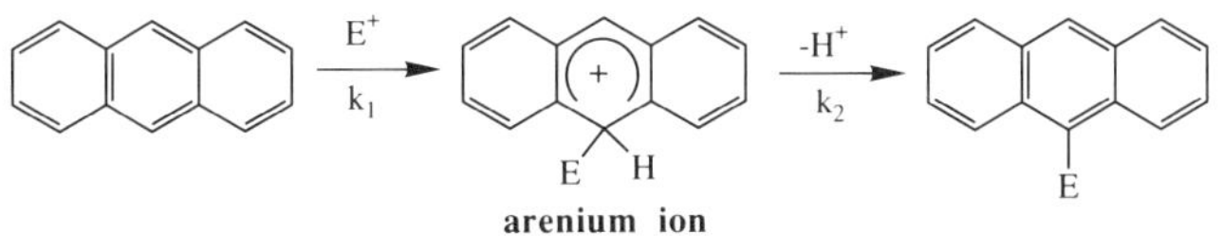

arenium ion

Table 6.1. *Nitration of polyarenes*[a]

Hydrocarbon	Site of attack	Partial-rate factor, PRF	Reactivity number, N_t
benzene		1	
naphthalene	2	50	2.12
	1	470	1.81
phenanthrene	4	79	1.96
	2	92	2.18
	3	300	2.04
	1	360	1.86
	9	490	1.80
triphenylene	1	600	2.00
	2	600	2.12
chrysene	6	3 500	1.67
pyrene	1	17 000	1.51
perylene	3	77 000	1.34
benzo[a]pyrene	6	108 000	1.15
anthanthrene	6	156 000	1.03

[a]Data are from Dewar *et al.*, 1956; Dewar, 1952.

complex formed by DMBA is shown by NMR spectroscopy to have the structure **1** in which proton addition has taken place exclusively in the 12-position (MacLean *et al.*, 1958). In the proton NMR spectrum of **1** the singlet assigned to the 12-methyl group of DMBA is replaced by a doublet and a new methine proton signal appears as a quartet, consistent with the assignment.

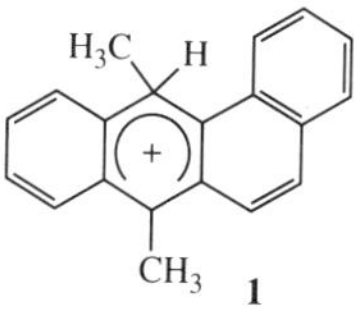

The sites of electrophilic substitution in alternant PAHs, as well as the relative rates of reaction, are predictable by the valence bond or molecular orbital theoretical methods. The perturbation molecular orbital (PMO) treatment of Dewar (1952) is particularly convenient, since it permits a semiquantitative estimation of the preferred sites of substitution using only simple arithmetical calculations. Since the intermediate undergoing substitution is an even alternant hydrocarbon, the arenium ion intermediate is odd. According to the pairing theorem, an odd alternant PAH has one unpaired MO which is neither bonding nor antibonding. The odd MO is, therefore, described as a nonbonding MO (NBMO). The NBMO is confined to alternate atoms and is zero at the remaining positions.

The π-energy of the reaction is given by the relation $\Delta E_\pi = 2\beta(a_{ox} + a_{oy})$ $= \beta N_t$ where a_{ox} and a_{oy} are the NBMO coefficients at the positions adjacent to the positions undergoing substitution in the arenium ion intermediate, and N_t is the corresponding reactivity number. The NBMO coefficients may be found by the procedure in Fig. 6.2. (a) First one stars the molecule, omitting the substituted atom and making sure the starred set is the more numerous one; from the pairing theorem, the NBMO is confined to starred atoms. (b) Assign the value 'a' to the coefficient of an arbitrary starred atom. (c) Consider one of the adjacent unstarred atoms indicated by a circle in (b); because the sum of the coefficients of atoms adjacent to the circled atom must be zero, the coefficient of the next adjacent atom must be '-a'. (d) Continue the process until (e) an unstarred atom is encountered with three neighbors, two of whose NBMO coefficients are unassigned. (f) One of the unknowns is designated as 'b', and the process is continued through (g) and (h) until all positions are assigned. The relation between 'a' and 'b' is derived from the requirement for the sum of the coefficients of the atoms adjacent to the circled atom in (h) to vanish. Therefore, $-2a + 2b = 0$. It follows that 'a' must equal 'b', giving (i) as the final assignment. Since the square of each NBMO coefficient is the fraction of the MO composed of the particular atomic orbital, the sum of the squares of the coefficients in (i) must add up to

Fig. 6.2. Calculation of NBMO coefficients for the 9-anthracenium ion.

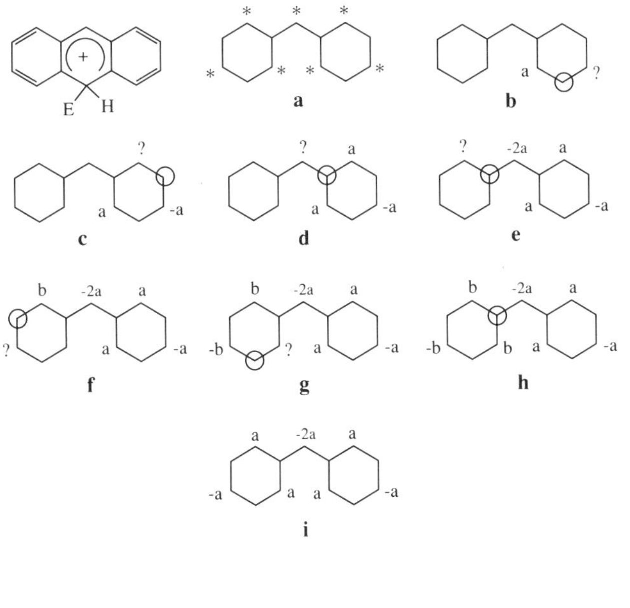

unity, so that:

$$a^2 + (-a)^2 + a^2 + (-2a)^2 + a^2 + (-a)^2 + a^2 = 1$$
$$10a^2 = 1$$
$$a = \sqrt{1/10} = 0.315$$

Utilizing this value for $a_{ox} = a_{oy}$ in the equation for ΔE_π, one obtains ΔE_π = 1.26ß, and N_t = 1.26 for substitution in the 9-position of anthracene. The calculated reactivity numbers for nitration reactions at various positions of other PAHs are given in Table 6.1.

The relative rates of electrophilic substitution in two different polyarenes can be estimated from the amounts of the products formed when a mixture of the two undergoes competitive substitution. The reactivities at two different positions in a single compound can be found from the proportions of the various isomers formed. The rate of reaction at a given position in a PAH relative to the rate of substitution in benzene under similar conditions is called the partial rate factor (PRF). The PRF for substitution at position 'i' in an alternant PAH is given by the relation, $PRF_i = \alpha ß(N_i - N_B)$, where N_i is the corresponding reactivity number, and N_B is the reactivity number for benzene. A plot of log (PRF_t) against N_t for nitration of a number of PAHs was shown by Dewar *et al.*, 1956 to give an approximately linear relationship.

The rates of reaction are also dependent upon the nature of the attacking electrophile. This is reflected in the values for 'α' in the equation for PRF_i. The nearer the transition state is to the arenium ion, the more endothermic and slower is the substitution reaction, and the larger will be the value of α. Therefore, the slope of the plot of log PRF against N_t should be greater, the slower the substitution reaction, i.e. the less active is the attacking electrophile. This is found to be the case.

A more thorough treatment of electrophilic substitution may be found in the volume by Dewar & Dougherty, 1975.

6.2   Addition reactions

The Diels–Alder reaction is the best known addition reaction of polyarenes. The 1,4-addition of dienophiles, such as maleic anhydride, to the *meso* regions of anthracene, BA, and other linear hydrocarbons has been extensively investigated (Wasserman, 1965; Zander, 1983; Biermann & Schmidt, 1980). In a series of classical papers, Clar showed that the Diels–Alder reactivity of polyarenes is increased by linear annelation, while angular annelation has the opposite effect (Clar, 1931, 1932, 1939, 1964). Anthracene slowly forms a Diels–Alder adduct with maleic anhydride in boiling xylene, while under the same conditions naphthacene reacts much more rapidly, and pentacene and hexacene react almost instantaneously.

Clar proposed that the preferred site of addition of a dienophile to a complex polyarene is that which affords the product with the maximum number of aromatic sextets. For reaction to occur, there must be a net gain in the number of aromatic sextets. More recently, the Diels–Alder reactivity of a large number of PAHs has been examined systematically by Biermann & Schmidt, 1980a. They observed second order rate constants that spanned a range of 10^7. The positional selectivity for the addition of maleic anhydride to acenes and their benzologs was correctly predicted by the six theoretical models tested (Clar's sextet theory, Brown's *para*-localization concept, Herndon's structure count method, the free valence indices, Fukui's frontier orbital theory, and complete second-order perturbational theory). However, these methods met with mixed success in predicting the relative rate constants. Herndon's treatment and second-order perturbational theory were the most successful, whereas frontier orbital theory failed completely. Alkyl substitution in the meso region generally enhances the Diels–Alder reactivity. 9,10-Dimethylanthracene and DMBA form meso region adducts much more rapidly than the corresponding unsubstituted parent PAHs (Bachmann & Chemerda, 1938).

Another important addition reaction of polyarenes is the 1,2-addition of osmium tetroxide to aromatic bonds. Addition is concerted and takes place regioselectively on the aromatic bond of highest order to afford a *cis*-dihydrodiol. The site of attack is generally predictable from the theoretically calculated *ortho*-localization energies (Dewar & Dougherty, 1975). Phenes are more susceptible to attack by OsO_4 than acenes, and reaction occurs preferentially in the electron-rich K-regions. If a K-region bond is lacking, reaction may take place on an alternative bond. Thus, anthracene forms an addition complex with OsO_4 which on hydrolysis affords the corresponding *cis*-1,2-dihydrodiol; reaction with additional OsO_4 yields the corresponding tetraol (Cook *et al.*, 1949). The addition of OsO_4 may also take place on alkyl-substituted ring positions. For example, reaction of 4,5-dihydropyrene with OsO_4 affords the products of addition to the 5a,6- and 11,12-bonds (**2** and **3**) in approximately equal ratio (Silverton *et al.*, 1976).

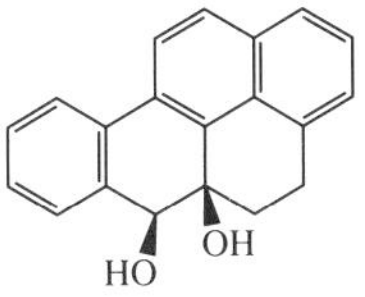

2 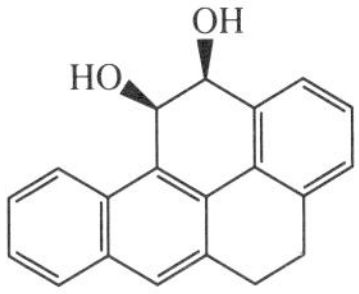   3

Photo-oxidation of many PAHs occurs on exposure to air and light (Rigaudy, 1968). One of the principal modes of reaction involves 1,4-addition of molecular oxygen in *meso* regions of acenes to yield epidioxides. The order of reactivity for the formation of epidioxides is the same as that for the Diels–Alder reactions, i.e. linear acenes are more reactive than angular PAHs, and reactivity increases with annelation. Carcinogenic benz[a]anthracene derivatives, such as DMBA and its 3,4-dihydrodiol, form epidioxides (**4** and **5**) with facility on exposure to light (Lee & Harvey, 1986), and great care must be exercised in their handling to prevent this mode of decomposition. The epidioxide of 9,10-diphenylanthracene (**6a**: R = C_6H_5) dissociates on heating to molecular oxygen and the parent hydrocarbon, while anthracene epidioxide (**6b**: R = H) is stable under these conditions.

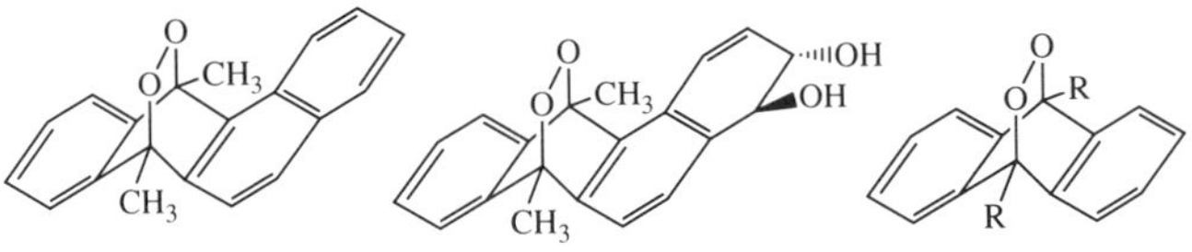

Addition of nucleophiles to polyarenes is less well studied than the corresponding addition reactions of electrophiles. Perhaps the best known such reaction is the addition of alkyllithium reagents to the meso regions of anthracene, BA, and other acenes (Harvey & Davis, 1969; Fu & Harvey, 1977) (Fig. 6.3). Association between the metal cation and the aromatic ring system may facilitate the initial step in these reactions. The intermediates produced on addition of a carbanion to an acene exhibit no tendency to spontaneously rearomatize with loss of hydride ion. Instead, the relatively

Fig. 6.3. Addition of nucleophiles (N^-), such as carbanions, to anthracene yields adducts that may be protonated or alkylated. Dehydrogenation gives mono- or dialkylated products.

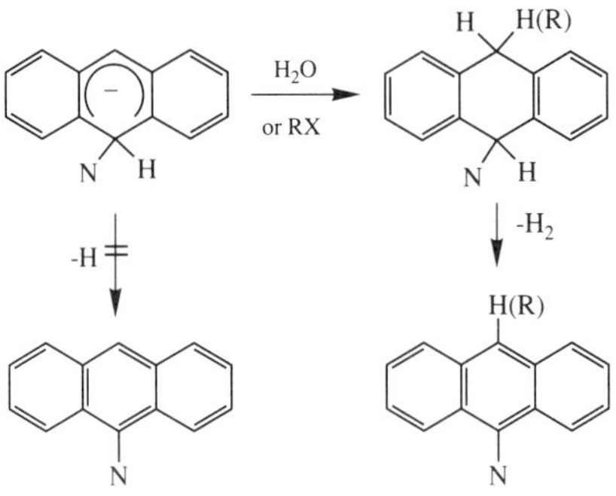

stable anionic intermediates can be protonated by water or dilute acid to yield monoalkyldihydroaromatics or alkylated to form dialkyldihydroaromatics. Since the latter products can be readily dehydrogenated catalytically or with reagents such as DDQ or the trityl cation (Fu & Harvey, 1978), this provides convenient synthetic route to alkyl-substituted polyarenes.

6.3   Hydrogenation

The addition of hydrogen to polyarenes is catalyzed by platinum group metal catalysts. For many years this was one of the least predictable and controllable reactions of PAHs, affording mixtures of products arising from hydrogen addition at various ring positions and varying degrees of hydrogenation. This situation changed with the discovery in the author's laboratory that hydrogenations of polycyclic hydrocarbons conducted under mild conditions of temperature and pressure could be controlled to afford hydroaromatic products arising from regiospecific hydrogen addition in different molecular regions, dependent upon the nature of the catalyst (Fu *et al.*, 1980). Hydrogenations over a palladium/charcoal catalyst occur regiospecifically in K-regions to afford dihydroarenes, while analogous reactions over platinum take place regioselectively on terminal rings to provide the corresponding tetrahydroarenes. For example, hydrogenation of BA in the presence of a Pd/C catalyst at 25 °C and 20 psig gives 5,6-dihydro-BA, while analogous reaction over a Pt catalyst furnishes the product of terminal ring hydrogenation, 8,9, 10,11-tetrahydro-BA (Fig. 6.4).

The mechanism of hydrogen addition with a palladium catalyst is proposed to involve essentially concerted addition of hydrogen from the catalyst surface to the PAH molecular region having minimum bond delocalization energy (Fu *et al.*, 1980). While the mechanism of hydrogen addition with platinum catalysts is not understood, the tetrahydroarenes formed are generally the most thermodynamically favored isomers. Thus, the BA 8,9,10,11-tetrahydro isomer, which retains the phenanthrene structural unit, is favored energetically by approximately 8 kcal over the other terminal ring isomer, 1,2,3,4-tetrahydro-BA, which contains the anthracene aromatic ring system.

Hydrogenation is frequently employed to control the site of substitution of

Fig. 6.4. Regiospecificity of hydrogen addition to polyarenes is dependent upon the catalyst.

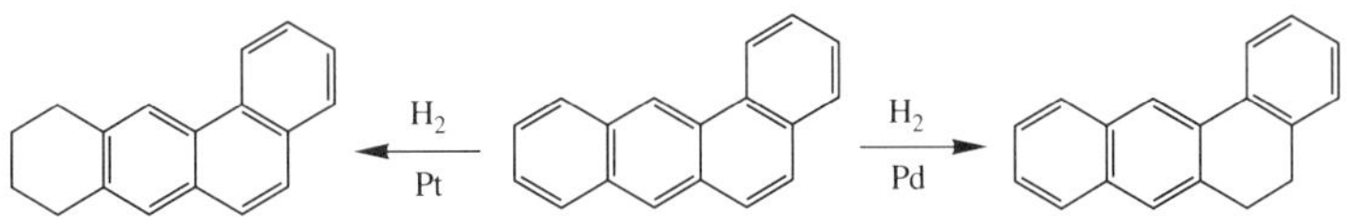

polyarenes and direct it to sites not normally favored for electrophilic attack. For example, bromination, acetylation, succinoylation, and other reactions of pyrene with electrophiles generally take place in the 1-position (Fig. 6.5). Consequently, the isomeric 2- and 4-substituted pyrene derivatives are not available via direct substitution. However, pyrene undergoes hydrogenation smoothly and essentially quantitatively over a palladium catalyst to 4,5,9,10-tetrahydropyrene which in turn reacts with electrophiles, such as bromine and acetyl chloride, in the 2-position (Harvey *et al.*, 1983; Harvey *et al.*, 1988). Dehydrogenation of these products yields the corresponding 2-substituted pyrenes. Conversely, reduction of pyrene with sodium and alcohol gives 1,2,3,6,7,8-hexahydropyrene which reacts with electrophiles in the 4-position. Dehydrogenation of these products yields the 4-substituted pyrenes.

6.4   Metal–ammonia reduction and reductive alkylation

Reduction of PAHs by alkali metals in liquid ammonia has also been shown to take place regiospecifically under appropriately controlled conditions (Harvey, 1970; Rabideau, 1989). The product structures are predictable by MO theory and are generally different than those obtained from either Pd or Pt catalyzed hydrogenation (Table 6.2). By appropriate choice of one of these methods it is possible to selectively hydrogenate virtually any ring of a polyarene. And by combination of these methods for regioselective ring reduction with electrophilic substitution one may effectively control to considerable degree the site of substitution of large polycyclic aromatic ring systems. Dehydrogenation of the substituted products is readily accomplished by chemical or catalytic methods (Fu & Harvey, 1978).

Metal–ammonia reductions of polyarenes involve addition of electrons to

Fig. 6.5. The site of substitution of polyarenes may be controlled by regioselective hydrogenation prior to reaction with electrophiles (E^+)

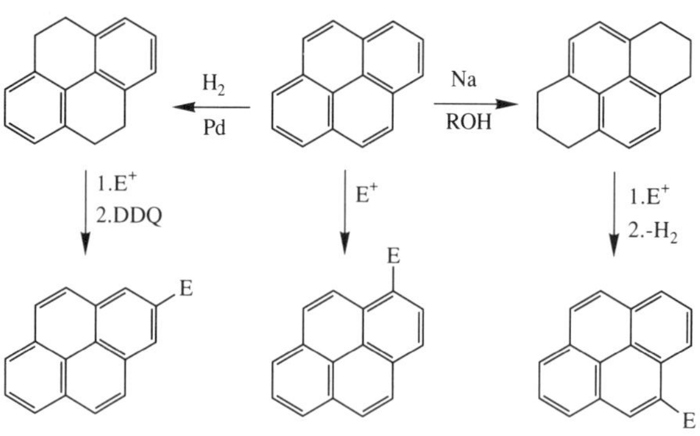

Table 6.2. *Comparison of the hydroaromatic products from hydrogenation*[a] *and lithium-ammonia reduction*[b] *of polyarenes*

polyarene	reduction, Li/NH$_3$	hydrogenation, Pd[c]	hydrogenation, Pt

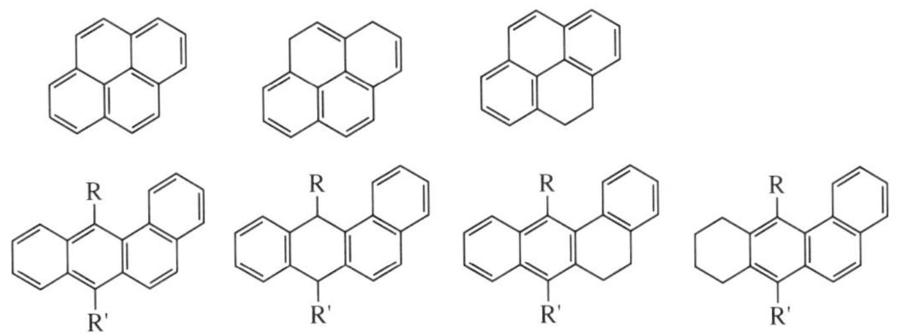

a: R = R' = H; **b**: R = H, R' = CH$_3$; **c**: R = R' = CH$_3$

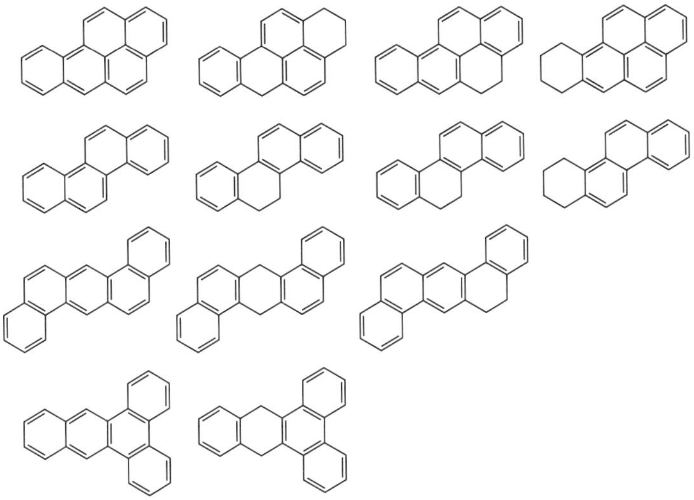

[a]Data are mainly from Fu et al., 1980; 7,12-dihydro-DMBA is a minor coproduct of hydrogenation of DMBA over a Pd catalyst. [b]Data are from Harvey, 1970, 1971; Harvey & Fu, 1980. [c]Further hydrogenation of dihydropyrene yields 4,5,9,10-tetrahydro-pyrene quantitatively (Harvey et al., 1983).

generate radical-anion (ArH$^-$) and dianion (ArH$^=$) intermediates (Fig. 6.6). Protonation occurs mainly at the latter stage to afford monoanionic intermediates (ArH$_2{}^-$) and dihydroaromatic products (ArH$_3$). In many cases, ammonia itself (pKa $\approx$ 34) serves as the proton source for the initial stage of proton addition. Protonation of the relatively stable AH$_2{}^-$ generally requires an external proton source; alcohol and ammonium chloride are most commonly employed for this purpose.

According to MO theory (Streitweiser, 1961), the incoming protons combine with the positions of highest electron density in the intermediate ion. This site is predicted by the coefficients of the lowest vacant MO; it is unimportant for alternant PAHs whether the orbital is singly or doubly occupied. Qualitative prediction may also be made on the basis of the expected relative stabilities of the various possible anions (secondary > tertiary and benzyl > allyl > primary). Product formation is generally controlled kinetically rather than thermodynamically, so that the less stable isomer frequently results. For example, reduction of naphthalene provides the unconjugated 1,4-dihydro- rather than the conjugated 1,2-dihydronaphthalene isomer.

Reduction beyond the initial stage can be prevented by the exclusion of alcohol or other external proton source during the reaction, taking advantage of the resistance of the stable anionic intermediates to addition of electrons. Reactions are quenched by the addition of a proton source. Although alcohol and water have frequently been employed in the older literature for this purpose, protonation by alcohol is relatively slow, resulting in isomerization and further reduction during quenching. For this reason, ammonium chloride is generally preferred. Overreduction may also be inhibited by conducting the reaction in the presence of small amounts of iron salts; the colloidal iron produced catalyzes the reaction of excess lithium metal with ammonia (Harvey, 1970). This method of carrying out metal–ammonia reduction, i.e. rapid quenching by the addition of the proton last, contrasts with the well known Birch reduction of benzenoid hydrocarbons which is conducted in the presence of alcohol (required to drive the equilibrium by trapping the benzene radical–anion). Stepwise reduction of polyarenes by this method affords a wide variety of hydroaromatic derivatives of polyarenes. For example, stepwise reduction of BA yields various di-, tetra-, and further hydroaromatic derivatives of BA (Fig. 6.7). The dihydroaromatic products of metal–ammonia reduction are useful starting compounds for the synthesis of dihydrodiols and other PAH oxidized metabolites (Harvey, 1985, 1986).

Alkylation of the anionic intermediates produced in metal–ammonia

Fig. 6.6. Mechanism of reduction of polyarenes by alkali metals in ammonia.

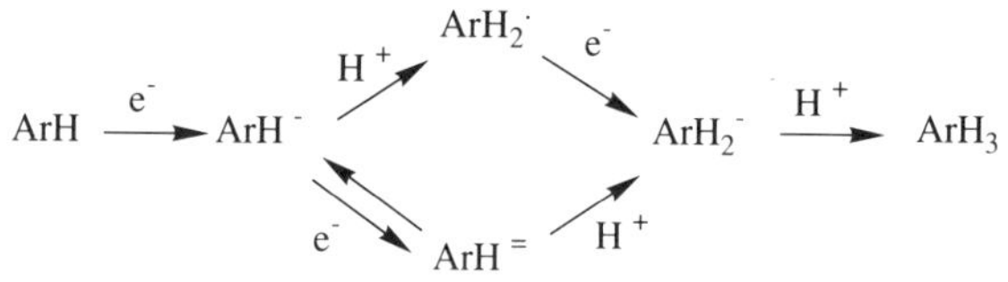

reactions with alkyl halides leads to formation of mono- and dialkylated hydroaromatic products. The dialkylated products were originally assumed to arise directly from reaction of the dianionic intermediates, however subsequent mechanistic studies (Lindow *et al.*, 1972; Rabideau & Burkholder, 1978) have shown that the dianionic species undergo relatively facile protonation by ammonia with formation of metal amide salts. The major pathway for formation of dialkylated products involves deprotonation of the initial monoalkylated product (ArH_2R) by reaction with amide anion followed by a second alkylation step (Fig. 6.8). Direct evidence for the formation of monanionic intermediates via back reaction with amide anion has been provided by ESR and NMR spectroscopic studies (Mullen *et al.*, 1985).

Relatively few examples of the analogous reduction and reductive alkylation of nonalternant PAHs have been investigated. The reduction of fluoranthene with lithium in ammonia and alkylation of the anionic intermediate proceed with high regiospecificity (Harvey *et al.*, 1972), whereas the analogous reactions of fluorene afford mixtures of isomeric products (Harvey *et al.*, 1976).

Fig. 6.7. Stepwise reduction of benz[a]anthracene with lithium and ammonia (Harvey & Urberg, 1968).

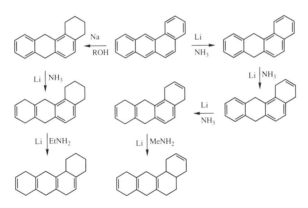

Fig. 6.8. Mechanism of reductive alkylation of polyarenes.

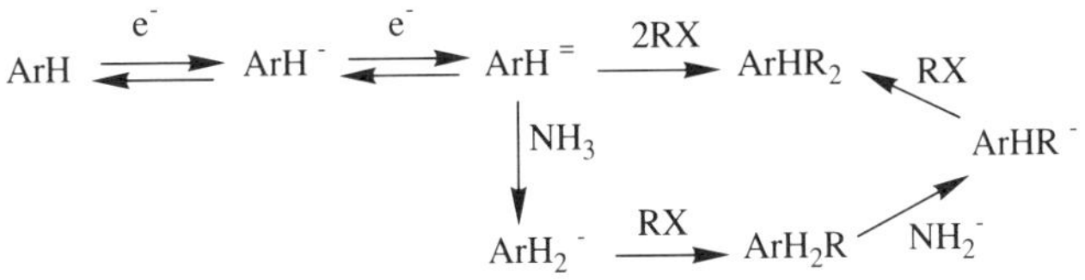

$$ArH \rightleftharpoons[e^-]{} ArH^{-} \rightleftharpoons[e^-]{} ArH^{=} \xrightarrow{2RX} ArHR_2 \xleftarrow{RX} ArHR^{-}$$

$$\downarrow NH_3$$

$$ArH_2^{-} \xrightarrow{RX} ArH_2R \xrightarrow{NH_2^-} $$

6.5   Oxidation

Oxidative transformations are of particular interest in view of the biological importance of oxidative metabolism by the P-450 microsomal enzymes (cf. Chap. 4). Oxidation by OsO_4 and photo-oxidation have been discussed along with other addition reactions in Section 6.2. Other reagents employed for the oxidation of the aromatic bonds and alkyl side chains of polycyclic aromatic rings include chromic acid, lead tetraacetate, DDQ, ozone, periodic acid, peracids, and hypochlorite.

Chromic acid is the most frequently employed reagent for the oxidation of polyarenes directly to the corresponding quinones. Where a *meso* region is present, as in anthracene and BA, oxidation occurs preferentially in this region to furnish the corresponding 1,4-quinones. In other cases, such as chrysene, oxidation tends to take place in the electron rich K-region. Alkyl substituents are readily oxidized by this reagent to carboxylic acids. On the other hand, neutral aqueous dichromate solutions oxidize aryl alkanes to the corresponding arylcarboxylic acids without attacking the aromatic ring system (Friedman *et al.*, 1965). Thus, oxidation of 2-methylanthracene with neutral dichromate occurs on the methyl group to afford anthracene 2-carboxylic acid, whereas reaction of the same hydrocarbon with chromic acid takes place in both the methyl group and the *meso* region to yield anthraquinone 2-carboxylic acid (Fig. 6.9). The utility of the neutral dichromate method is limited, however, by the high temperatures (250–275°C) and pressures required for these reactions. Chromyl chloride (CrO_2Cl_2) converts toluene derivatives to benzaldehydes and other alkyl-substituted aromatics to the corresponding ketones, but this reagent has seldom been employed for the oxidation of polyarenes.

Lead tetraacetate, $Pb(OAc)_4$, is one of the more versatile, and at the same time one of the more difficult to control, reagents employed for the oxidation of polyarenes (Criegee, 1965; Lee, 1969). Unsubstituted PAHs with a reactive *meso* region, or extended *meso* region, undergo preferential acetoxylation at this site with lead tetraacetate to yield the corresponding phenol acetates (Fieser & Hershberg, 1938, 1938a). Anthracene, BA, and BaP react with $Pb(OAc)_4$ to yield 9-acetoxyanthracene, 7-acetoxy-BA, and

Fig. 6.9. Neutral dichromate solutions oxidize arylalkanes selectively at benzylic sites.

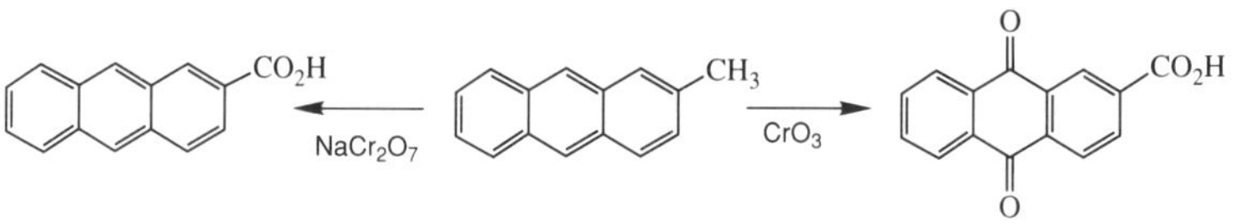

6-acetoxy-BaP, respectively. Alkyl-substituted PAHs undergo reaction with Pb(OAc)$_4$ in benzylic positions to yield benzyl acetates. This has been exploited as a synthetic approach to the hydroxymethyl metabolites of methyl-substituted carcinogenic PAHs, such as DMBA. Reaction of the latter with Pb(OAc)$_4$ affords a mixture of the two possible monoacetoxymethyl derivatives and the diacetoxymethyl derivative (Boyland & Sims, 1965).

2,3-Dichloro-5,6-dicyano-1,4-benzoquinone (DDQ), chloranil, and other quinone oxidants have long been employed as reagents for the dehydrogenation of hydroaromatic ring systems and for the introduction of double bonds into benzylic sites (Fu & Harvey, 1978). However, more recently it has been shown that DDQ in aqueous acetic acid efficiently oxidizes alkyl-substituted PAHs under mild conditions to provide good yields of arylketones and aldehydes (Lee & Harvey, 1988). Similar oxidations with DDQ/HOAc in the absence of water afford only the products of monoacetoxylation at benzylic positions (Lehr *et al.*, 1986). Oxidation with DDQ/HOAc/H$_2$O takes place regiospecifically at the site that affords the most stable carbocation intermediate predicted theoretically from the calculated ß-delocalization energies. For example, oxidation of 7,8,9,10-tetrahydrobenzo[a]pyrene with this reagent affords only the 10-keto derivative (ΔE_{deloc} = 0.794 ß), rather than the 7-keto derivative (ΔE_{deloc} = 0.488 ß), in agreement with theoretical prediction (Fig. 6.10). This reagent has recently been employed in the key step of a new synthetic approach to the carcinogenic cyclopenta[a]phenanthrenes (Lee & Harvey, 1988). Oxidation of 11-methyl-6,7,16,17-tetrahydro-15*H*-cyclopenta[a]phenanthrene with DDQ in aqueous acetic acid took place regiospecifically in the 17-position to furnish the 17-keto derivative (Fig. 6.10). Dehydrogenation of the latter gave 11-methyl-16,17-dihydro-15*H*-cyclopenta[a]phenanthren-17-one. Although there are five benzylic carbon atoms in the starting hydrocarbon, oxidative attack takes place exclusively in the 17-position in accord with theoretical

Fig. 6.10. Oxidation of benzylic positions with DDQ occurs regiospecifically in the theoretically predicted site of the most stable carbocation intermediate.

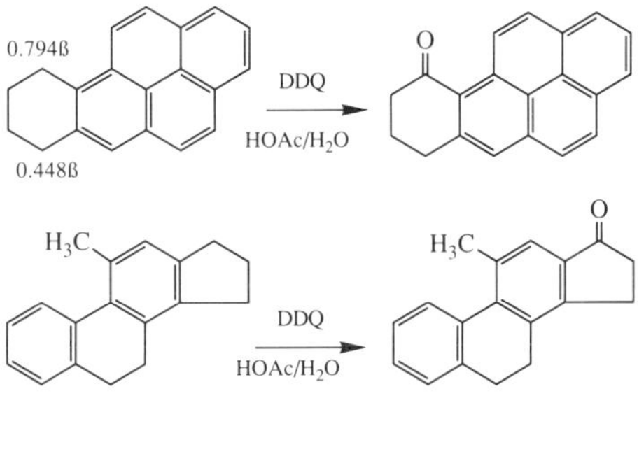

prediction. The DDQ/HOAc/H₂O reagent promises to be of considerable utility for the synthesis of PAH oxidized metabolites.

Ceric ammonium sulfate oxidations of phenanthrene, fluoranthene, BA, BaP, and chrysene afford principally quinone products (Fig. 6.11). However, the yields are low to moderate, and in some cases lactones and other products are also formed (Periasamy & Bhatt, 1977; Balanikas *et al.*, 1988). The method provides a useful synthetic route to fluoranthene-2,3-dione, but is of limited utility in other cases.

Ozone reacts readily with polyarenes to afford mainly products of oxidative ring cleavage. Ozonation of phenanthrene in methanol yields the

Fig. 6.11. Oxidation of polyarenes with ceric ammonium sulfate: [a]Periasamy & Bhatt, 1977; [b]Balanikas *et al.*, 1988.

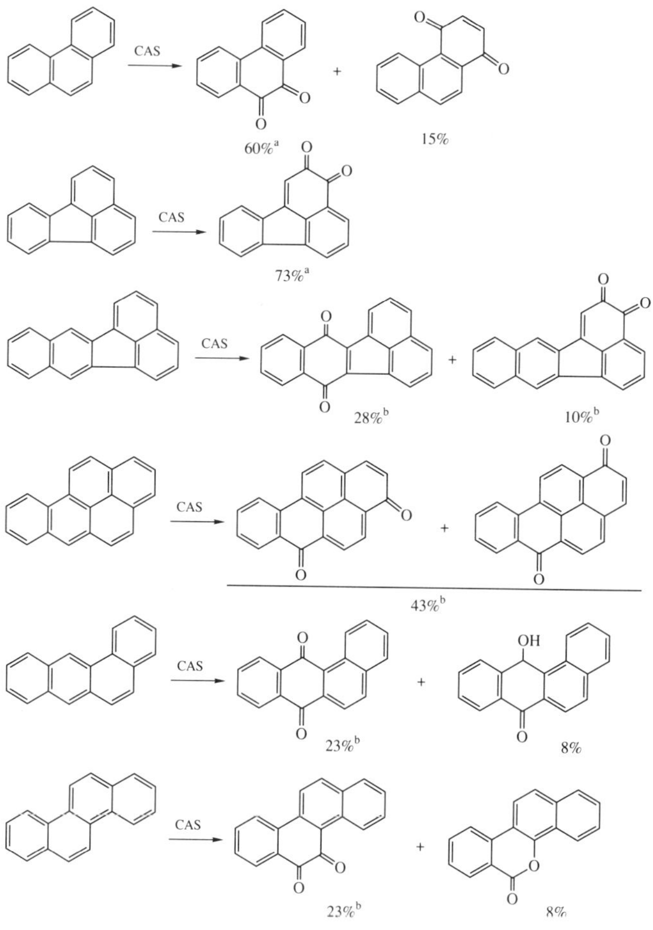

peroxidic ether **7** which undergoes reduction with NaI to yield 2,2'-diformylbiphenyl **8** (Bailey & Erickson, 1973). Reactions with ozone of PAHs having a meso region, such as anthracene and BA, takes place at this site to afford the corresponding 1,4-quinones along with other oxidized products (Moriconi *et al.*, 1959). Ozonation of BaP with ozone furnished a mixture of the 1,6- and 3,6-diones (1:3) and a trace of the 4,5-dione (Moriconi *et al.*, 1961). The reactions of polyarenes with ozone are difficult to control and tend to result in extensive degradation of the substrates.

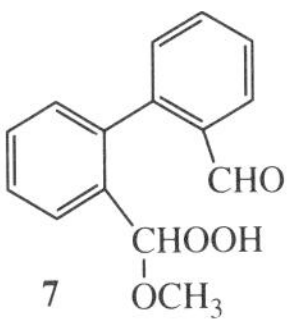

Periodic acid (H_5IO_6) has been used for the oxidation of PAHs with a *meso* region, e.g. naphthacene, pentacene, and BA, to the corresponding *meso*-region quinones (Fatiadi, 1974). Reaction of acenaphthylene and phenanthrene with this reagent gave acenaphthene 1,2-dione and phenanthrene 9,10-dione, respectively. However, triphenylene, perylene, and chrysene failed to react under similar conditions, and pyrene dimerized to yield 1,1'-bipyrene.

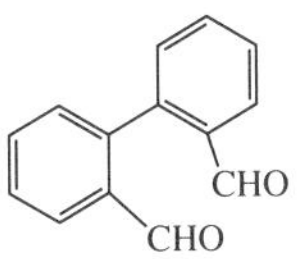

Other reagents that have been employed for the oxidation of polyarenes include *m*-chloroperbenzoic acid and other peracids, hypochlorite, *tert*-butylhydroperoxide, dimethyldioxirane, and manganese (VII) salts. While most of these have seen only limited application, several appear potentially useful. The peracids, hypochlorite, and dimethyldioxirane have been shown to convert polyarenes containing a K-region into the corresponding K-region oxides in variable yield (Ishikawa *et al.*, 1977; Krishnan *et al.*, 1977; Murray & Jeyaraman, 1985). However, the first two of these reagents are incompatible with the presence of a meso region in the molecule, limiting their utility. Rhodium catalyzed oxidation of anthracenes with *tert*-butylhydroperoxide furnishes the related anthraquinones in yields up to 90% (Muller & Bobillier, 1983). Recently, $KMnO_4$ in a biphasic medium in the presence of a phase-transfer catalyst has been shown to smoothly oxidize PAHs that contain a doubly benzylic carbon, such as fluorene, to the corresponding ketones (Gannon & Krause 1987).

6.6 Complexation

Polyarenes readily form colored donor–acceptor complexes with I_2, picric acid, trinitrobenzene, etc. Although these physical complexes are

Table 6.3. *Separation of partially saturated derivatives of polyarenes by 'charge-transfer chromatography' on TNF-silica gel*[a]

| | $R_f \times 100$ | | | $R_f \times 100$ | |
| | | Silica gel- | | | Silica gel- |
Hydrocarbon	Silica gel	5% TNF	Hydrocarbon	Silica gel	5% TNF
phenanthrene	48	14	anthracene	45	15
dihydro-	49	18	dihydro-	43	37
tetrahydro-	53	27	tetrahydro-	50	43
hexahydro-	54	44	hexahydro-	53	51
octahydro-	55	54			
chrysene	35	1			
dihydro-	36	16			
tetrahydro-	36	29			
hexahydro-	38	34			

[a]Data are from Harvey & Halonen, 1967; benzene–heptane (1:4)

commonly referred to as 'charge-transfer complexes', van der Waals forces, hydrogen bonding, and other intramolecular forces often contribute more to their stabilization than charge-transfer interaction (Foster, 1969). In the older literature before the development of modern chromatography methods, complexes of this type were frequently employed for the purification and characterization of PAHs in mixtures. They are still useful. For example, the modern technique of 'charge-transfer chromatography' (Harvey & Halonen, 1966) makes possible the separation of mixtures of PAH isomers and closely related PAH derivatives by chromatography on columns or thin layers of silica gel impregnated with a charge-transfer acceptor, such as 2,4,7-trinitrofluorenone. The effectiveness of the technique is illustrated by its ability to resolve the series of hydroaromatic compounds in Table 6.3.

6.7   References

Bailey, P. S. & Erickson, R. E. (1973). Diphenaldehyde. *Org. Syntheses,* **Col. Vol. 5**, 489–495.

Balanikas, G., Hussain, N., Amin, S. & Hecht, S. S. (1988). Oxidation of polynuclear aromatic hydrocarbons with ceric ammonium sulfate: Preparation of quinones and lactones. *J. Org. Chem.* **53**, 1007–10.

Biermann, D. & Schmidt, W. (1980). Diels–Alder reactivity of polycyclic aromatic hydrocarbons. 1. Acenes and benzologs. *J. Am. Chem. Soc.* **102**, 3163–73.

Boyland, E. & Sims, P. (1965). Metabolism of polycyclic compounds. The metabolism of 7,12-dimethylbenz[a]anthracene by rat liver homogenates. *Biochem. J.* **95**, 780–87.

Clar, E. (1931). Polynuclear aromatic hydrocarbons and their derivatives. XI. Constitution of anthracene. *Chem. Ber.* **64**, 2194–200.

Clar, E. (1932). Polynuclear aromatic hydrocarbons and their derivatives. XII. Distribution of the double bonds in condensed aromatic hydrocarbons. *Chem. Ber.* **65**, 503–19.

Clar, E. (1939). Aromatic hydrocarbons. XXIV. Hexacene. *Chem. Ber.* **72**, 1817–21.

Clar, E. (1964). *Polycyclic Hydrocarbons,* New York: Academic Press.

Clar, E. & Guzzi, A. (1932). Polynuclear aromatic hydrocarbons and their derivatives. 18. Synthesis of 1.9,5.10-di-[*peri*-naphthalen]-anthracene. *Chem. Ber.* **65**, 1521–5.

Clar, E. & Lombardi, L. (1932). Polynuclear aromatic hydrocarbons. XV. Constitution of phenanthrene and the polynuclear ring systems derived from it and a new method of separating aromatic hydrocarbons. *Chem. Ber.* **65**, 1411–20.

Cook, J. W., Hunter, L. & Schoental, R. (1949). Naphthalene-2:3-dialdehyde. *J. Chem. Soc.* S228.

Criegee, R. (1965). Oxidation with lead tetraacetate. *Oxidation in Organic Chemistry, Part A.* ed., 277–336, New York: Academic Press.

Dewar, M. J. S. (1952). A molecular theory of organic chemistry. VI. Aromatic substitution and addition. *J. Am. Chem. Soc.* **74**, 3357–63.

Dewar, M. J. S. & Dougherty, R. C. (1975). *The PMO Theory of Organic Chemistry*, New York: Plenum/Rosetta.

Dewar, M. J. S., Mole, T. & Warford, E. W. (1956). Electrophilic substitution. Part VI. The nitration of aromatic hydrocarbons; partial rate factors and their interpretation. *J. Chem. Soc.* 3581–86.

Fatiadi, A. (1974). New applications of periodic acid and periodates in organic and bioorganic chemistry. *Synthesis,* 229–72.

Fieser, L. & Hershberg, E. B. (1938). Substitution reactions and meso derivatives of 1,2-benzanthracene. *J. Am. Chem. Soc.* **60**, 1893–6.

Fieser, L. & Hershberg, E. B. (1938a). The oxidation of methylcholanthrene and 3,4-benzpyrene with lead tetraacetate; further derivatives of 3,4-benzpyrene. *J. Am. Chem. Soc.* **60**, 2542–8.

Foster, R. (1969). *Organic Charge-Transfer Complexes*, New York: Academic.

Friedman, L., Fishel, D. L. & Scheeter, H. (1965). Oxidation of alkylarenes with aqueous sodium dichromate. A useful method for preparing mono- and polyaromatic carboxylic acids. *J. Org. Chem.* **30**, 1453–7.

Fu, P. P. & Harvey, R. G. (1977). Synthesis and rearrangement of *tert*-butylanthracenes. *J. Org. Chem.* **42**, 2407–10.

Fu, P. P. & Harvey, R. G. (1978). Dehydrogenation of polycyclic hydroaromatic compounds. *Chem. Rev.* **78**, 317–61.

Fu, P. P., Lee, H. M. & Harvey, R. G. (1980). Regiospecific catalytic hydrogenation of polycyclic aromatic hydrocarbons under mild conditions. *J. Org. Chem.* **45**, 2797–803.

Gannon, S. & Krause, J. G. (1987). Phase-transfer permanganate oxidation of unfunctionalized benzylic positions. *Synthesis,* 915–17.

Harvey, R. G. (1970). Metal–ammonia reduction of aromatic molecules. *Synthesis,* 161–72.

Harvey, R. G. (1971). Metal–ammonia reduction. XI. Regiospecific and stereoselective reduction in the chrysene series. *J. Org. Chem.* **36**, 3306–11.

Harvey, R. G. (1985). Synthesis of the dihydrodiol and diol epoxide metabolites of carcinogenic polycyclic hydrocarbons. *Polycyclic Hydrocarbons and Carcinogenesis,* Am. Chem. Soc. Monogr. 283, ed. R. G. Harvey, 35–62, Washington, DC: American Chemical Society.

Harvey, R. G. (1986). Synthesis of oxidized metabolites of carcinogenic hydrocarbons. *Synthesis,* 605–19.

Harvey, R. G. & Davis, C. C. (1969). Metal–ammonia reduction. VI. Stereospecific alkylation of the 9-alkyl-9,10-dihydro-10-anthryl carbanion. *J. Org. Chem.* **34**, 3607–9.

Harvey, R. G. & Fu, P. P. (1980). Synthesis of oxidized metabolites of dibenz[a,c]anthracene. *J. Org. Chem.* **45**, 169–71.

Harvey, R. G., Fu, P. P. & Rabideau, P. W. (1976). Metal–ammonia reduction. XV. Regioselectivity of reduction and reductive methylation in the fluorene series. *J. Org. Chem.* **41**, 2706–10.

Harvey, R. G. & Halonen, M. (1966). Charge-transfer chromatography. *J. Chromatog.* **25**, 294–302.

Harvey, R. G., Konieczny, M. & Pataki, J. (1983). Synthesis of the isomeric *mono-* and *bis*-oxiranylpyrenes. *J. Org. Chem.* **48**, 2930–2.

Harvey, R. G., Lindow, D. F. & Rabideau, P. W. (1972). Metal–ammonia reduction. XVI. Fluoranthene: Correlation of primary product structure with MO theoretical prediction. *Tetrahedron,* **28**, 2909–19.

Harvey, R. G., Schmolka, S., Cortez, C. & Lee, H. (1988). Convenient syntheses of 2-bromopyrene and 2-hydroxypyrene. *Syn. Commun.* **18**, 2207–9.

Harvey, R. G. & Urberg, K. (1968). Metal–ammonia reduction. III. Stepwise transformation of polycyclic aromatic hydrocarbons. *J. Org. Chem.* **33**, 2206–11.

Ishikawa, K., Charles, H. C. & Griffin, G. W. (1977). Direct peracid oxidation of polynuclear hydrocarbons to arene oxides. *Tetrahedron Lett.* 427–30.

Krishnan, S., Kuhn, D. G. & Hamilton, G. W. (1977). Direct oxidation in high yield of some polycyclic aromatic compounds to arene oxides using hypochlorite and phase transfer catalysts. *J. Am. Chem. Soc.* **99**, 8121–3.

Lee, D. G. (1969). Hydrocarbon oxidation using transition metal compounds. *Oxidation,* ed. R. L. Augustine, pp. 1–51, New York: Marcel Dekker.

Lee, H. M. & Harvey, R. G. (1986). Synthesis of the active diol epoxide metabolites of the potent carcinogenic hydrocarbon 7,12-dimethylbenz[a]anthracene. *J. Org. Chem.* **51**, 3502–7.

Lee, H. M. & Harvey, R. G. (1988). 2,3-Dichloro-5,6-dicyano-1,4-benzoquinone (DDQ) in aqueous acetic acid, a convenient new reagent for the synthesis of aryl ketones and aldehydes via benzylic oxidation. *J. Org. Chem.* **53**, 4587–9.

Lehr, R. E., Kole, P. L. & Tschappat, D. (1986). Acetoxylation at benzylic positions of tetrahydrobenzo rings with DDQ in acetic acid. *Tetrahedron Lett.* **27**, 1649–52.

Lindow, D. F., Cortez, C. & Harvey, R. G. (1972). Metal–ammonia reduction. XI. Mechanism of reduction and reductive alkylation of aromatic hydrocarbons. *J. Am. Chem. Soc.* **94**, 5406–12.

MacLean, C., Waals, J. H. v. d. & Mackor, E. L. (1958). Proton magnetic resonance of aromatic carbonium ions. I. Structure of the conjugate acid. *Mol. Phys.* **1**, 247–56.

Moriconi, E. J., O'Connor, W. F. & Wallenberger, T. F. (1959). Ozonolysis of polycyclic aromatics. VI. Benz[a]anthracene and benz[a]anthracene-7,12-dione. Correlation of quinone-hydroquinone oxidation–reduction potentials with the positions of predominant ozone attack. *J. Am. Chem. Soc.* **81**, 6466–72.

Moriconi, E. J., Rakaczy, B. & O'Connor, W. F. (1961). Ozonolysis of polycyclic aromatics. VIII. Benzo[a]pyrene. *J. Am. Chem. Soc.* **83**, 4618–23.

Mullen, K., Huber, W., Neumann, G., Schneiders, C. & Unterberg, H. (1985). Alternative routes for reductive alkylation in liquid ammonia and their selection via spectroscopic evidence. *J. Am. Chem. Soc.* **107**, 801–7.

Muller, P. & Bobillier, C. (1983). Rh-catalyzed oxidation of anthracenes to anthraquinones using t-butylhydroperoxide. *Tetrahedron Lett.* **24**, 5499–500.

Murray, R. W. & Jeyaraman, R. (1985). Dioxiranes: Synthesis and reactions of methyldioxiranes. *J. Org. Chem.* **50**, 2847–53.

Periasamy, M. & Bhatt, V. (1977). A convenient method for the oxidation of polycyclic aromatic hydrocarbons to quinones. *Synthesis,* 330–2.

Perkampus, H. H. & Baumgarten, E. (1964). Proton-addition complexes of aromatic hydrocarbons. *Angew. Chem. Internat. Edit.* **3**, 776–83.

Rabideau, P. W. (1989). The metal–ammonia reduction of aromatic compounds. *Tetrahedron,* **45**, 1579–603.

Rigaudy, J. (1968). Photooxydation des derives aromatiques. *Pure Appl. Chem.* **16**, 169–86.

Silverton, J. V., Dansette, P. M. & Jerina, D. M. (1976). Oxidation of 4,5-dihydrobenzo[a]pyrene with osmium tetroxide. Stereochemistry of a substituted K-region diol. *Tetrahedron Lett.* 1557–60.

Streitwieser, A. Jr (1961). *Molecular Orbital Theory for Organic Chemists,* New York: Wiley.

Wasserman, A. (1965). *Diels–Alder Reactions,* New York: American Elsevier.

Zander, M. (1983). Physical and chemical properties of polycyclic aromatic hydrocarbons. *Handbook of Polycyclic Aromatic Hydrocarbons,* ed. A. Bjorseth, New York: Mercel Dekker.

7

General synthetic methods

The methods most frequently employed for the synthesis of polyarenes are surveyed in this chapter. Other procedures of less general utility may be found with application to the synthesis of specific polyarenes in Chapters 8–11. While many of the classical methods for building polycyclic ring systems, such as the Elbs reaction, involve relatively vigorous reaction conditions, the trend in recent years is toward the development of milder methods which proceed with greater regioselectivity and provide higher yields.

7.1 The Haworth synthesis

Cyclodehydration of ketonic or carboxylic acid intermediates is often a key step in the construction of PAH ring systems. One of the most powerful methods of synthesis involving cyclodehydration is the classical Haworth synthesis (Fig. 7.1) (Berliner, 1949). It entails initial Friedel–Crafts condensation of succinic anhydride with an appropriate polyarene, followed by reduction of the carbonyl group of the resulting keto acid, and acid-catalyzed cyclization to yield a cyclized ketone (Johnson, 1944). For

Fig. 7.1. Haworth synthesis of 1-keto-1,2,3,4-tetrahydrophenanthrene from naphthalene. Cyclization occurs preferentially in the more reactive α-position.

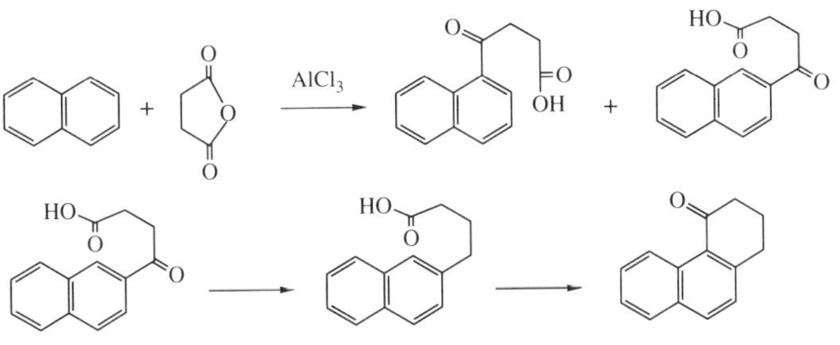

example, naphthalene undergoes AlCl$_3$-catalyzed condensation with succinic anhydride to give a mixture of the 4-keto-butyric acid derivatives of naphthalene in the 1- and 2-positions. These isomers can be individually transformed to the respective cyclic ketones via Clemmensen or Wolff–Kishner reduction followed by acidic cyclization. The cyclic ketone products are versatile intermediates that may, in turn be reduced and dehydrogenated to fully aromatic hydrocarbons or converted to various substituted PAH derivatives. For example, the 1- and 4-keto-tetrahydrophenanthrenes may be utilized for the synthesis of the corresponding phenols and methyl derivatives, or they may be employed as synthons for the construction of larger polycyclic ring systems.

The scope of the Haworth synthesis is limited by the regiospecificity of the initial Friedel–Crafts acylation which occurs preferentially in only a small number of the total PAH ring positions. Consequently, fusion of additional rings by this method can only take place on bonds in which at least one position is susceptible to electrophilic attack. This limitation can sometimes be circumvented by partial reduction of the PAH prior to acylation in order to alter the position of preferred electrophilic substitution. For example, while pyrene reacts with succinic anhydride preferentially in the 1-position, the 1,2,3,6,7,8-hexahydropyrene derivative undergoes analogous reaction in the 4-position (Fig. 6.5). The products of these reactions are convenient synthetic precursors of BaP and BeP, respectively.

Product structure in the Haworth synthesis is also determined by factors controlling the direction of cyclization. When the butyric acid side chain is in in a ß-position, subsequent cyclization tends to take place preferentially to the more reactive adjacent α-position with formation of an angular PAH (Fig. 7.1). However, steric hindrance may overcome this effect. For example, cyclization of 4-(3-phenanthryl)butyric acid takes place in the 2-position to provide a benz[a]anthracene derivative rather than in the more sterically crowded 4-position to furnish a benzo[c]phenanthrene derivative (Bachmann

Fig. 7.2. The direction of acid–catalyzed cyclization is determined by steric factors and by the nature of the acid catalyst.

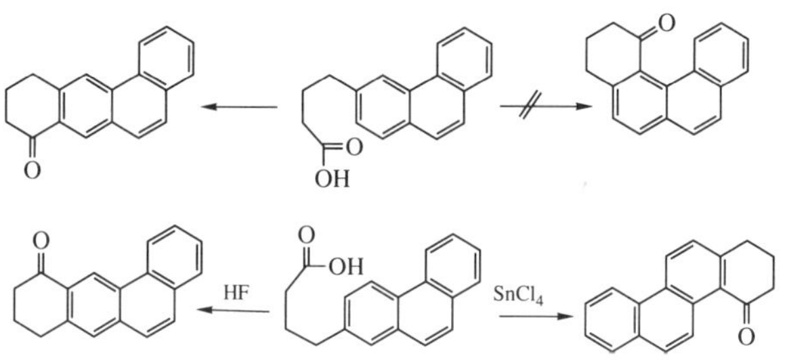

& Bradbury, 1937; Haworth & Marvin, 1933) (Fig. 7.2). The nature of the acidic catalyst employed may also influence the direction of ring closure. For example, SnCl$_4$-catalyzed cyclization of 4-(2-phenanthryl)butyric acid yields a chrysene derivative (Bachmann & Struve, 1939) (Fig. 7.2), whereas reaction of this same compound in liquid HF affords a benz[a]anthracene derivative (Fieser & Johnson, 1939).

A number of modifications of the Haworth synthesis are available for construction of larger polycyclic ring systems. Thus, phthalic anhydride may be employed in place of succinic anhydride for the fusion of two benzenoid rings to an existing aromatic system. This is illustrated by the reaction of naphthalene with phthalic anhydride in the presence of AlCl$_3$ to yield a keto acid that cyclizes directly to BA-7,12-dione in concentrated sulfuric acid (Fig. 7.3). This type of reaction has been modified and utilized extensively by Newman and others for the synthesis of substituted benz[a]anthracene derivatives for carcinogenesis studies (Newman *et al.*, 1988). Some of the common variations include: (i) reductive cyclization of the keto acid to the parent hydrocarbon with HI (Harvey *et al.*, 1978; Platt & Oesch, 1981); (ii) addition of a Grignard or alkyllithium reagent to the carbonyl function of the keto acid to generate a lactone intermediate that may be reduced to the carboxylic acid (e.g. with Zn/NaOH or Zn/HOAc) and cyclized to the corresponding phenol (Newman *et al.*, 1988); (iii) addition of an alkyllithium to the quinone product and reduction of the resulting diol to yield the dialkylated polyarene. The latter method provides the most convenient synthetic access to the potent carcinogen DMBA (Harvey & Cortez, 1986).

A practical alternative to the Friedel–Crafts acylation which avoids the problem of formation of multiple positional isomers involves reaction of the acid anhydride with an aryllithium or Grignard reagent. Thus reaction of phthalic anhydride with the Grignard reagent of 9-bromophenanthrene furnishes regiospecifically the keto acid arising from acylation in the 9-position of phenanthrene (Weizmann *et al.*, 1935) (Fig. 7.4). Reductive cyclization of this keto acid with hydriodic acid in acetic acid affords dibenz[a,c]anthracene in a single step (Harvey *et al.*, 1978).

Fig. 7.3. The keto acid from reaction of naphthalene with phthalic anhydride cyclizes in sulfuric acid to BA-7,12-dione.

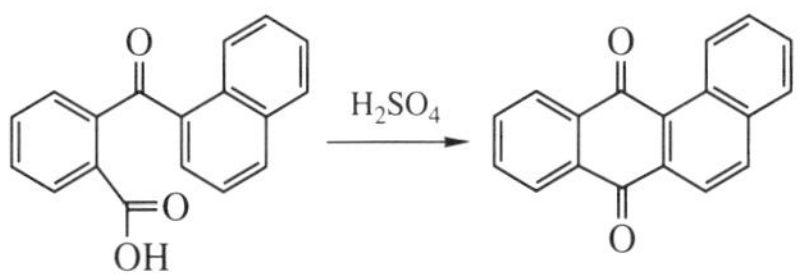

7.2   Alternative syntheses involving cyclodehydration

A number of alternative annelation methods which also involve cyclodehydration are available. The best known of these involve the *Reformatski reaction* of a cyclic benzylic ketone (e.g. the product of Haworth synthesis) (Fig. 7.5). Reformatski reaction of a nonbay region ketone with a bromocrotonate ester, followed by dehydration, dehydrogenation, and acid-catalyzed cyclization affords a new cyclic ketone with one additional ring (Cook & Schoental, 1945). An analogous reaction sequence with a bay region ketone using ethyl bromoacetate in the initial Reformatski reaction adds two carbon atoms to also form a hydrocarbon with an additional ring (Fieser & Heymann, 1941). A newer modification of this method that affords

Fig. 7.4. The reaction of acid anhydrides with aryllithium or Grignard reagents has the advantage of being regiospecific.

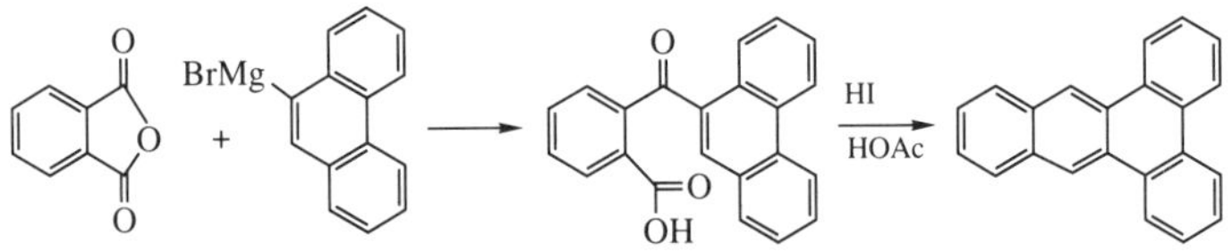

Fig. 7.5. Annelation of bay region and nonbay region ketones by Reformatski reaction with bromoacetate and bromocrotonate esters respectively

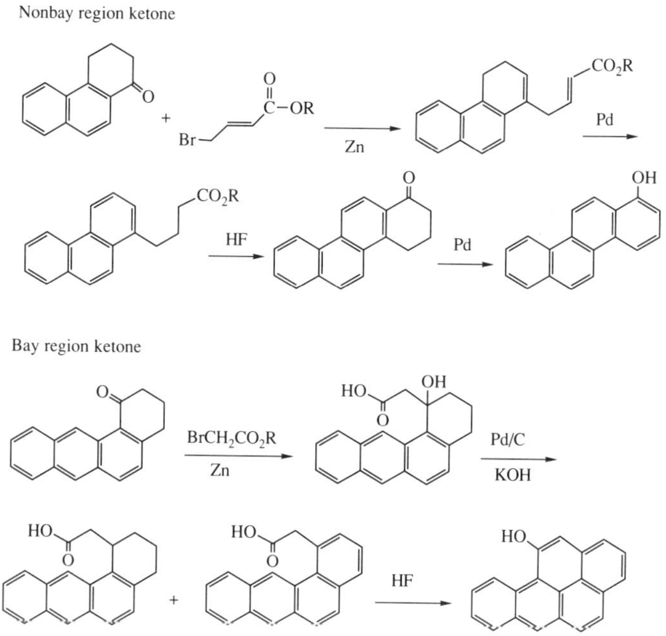

Nonbay region ketone

Bay region ketone

higher yields utilizes the α-lithio salt of ethyl acetate in place of the bromozinc derivative of ethyl acetate (Bodine *et al.*, 1978).

Although the foregoing examples all involve cyclodehydration of carboxylic acids, ketones and aldehydes also serve as useful intermediates for annelation to provide both alternant and nonalternant polyarenes. For example, cyclodehydration of 2-arylcyclohexanones provides synthetic access to polycyclic hydrocarbons derived from fluoranthene (Cho & Harvey, 1987) (Fig. 7.6). The requisite 2-arylcyclohexanones are obtainable from reaction of the appropriate aryllithiums with cyclohexene oxide, followed by oxidation of the resulting alcohol intermediate.

Recent advances in PAH carcinogenesis research have stimulated development of several new, milder and more efficient synthetic approaches to polyarenes that may be readily modified for the preparation of the oxidized metabolites of PAHs, including the biologically active diol epoxide derivatives.

One such method entails reaction of the ortho-lithio salt of an aryl *N,N*-dialkylamide (generated by metalation) with an arylketone or aldehyde (Harvey *et al.*, 1982) (Fig. 7.7). Reduction of the resulting lactone to the acid with zinc and alkali followed by cyclodehydration yields a phenol that may be readily reduced with HI or other appropriate reagent to the desired PAH,

Fig. 7.6. Cyclodehydration provides synthetic access to nonalternant as well as to alternant PAHs.

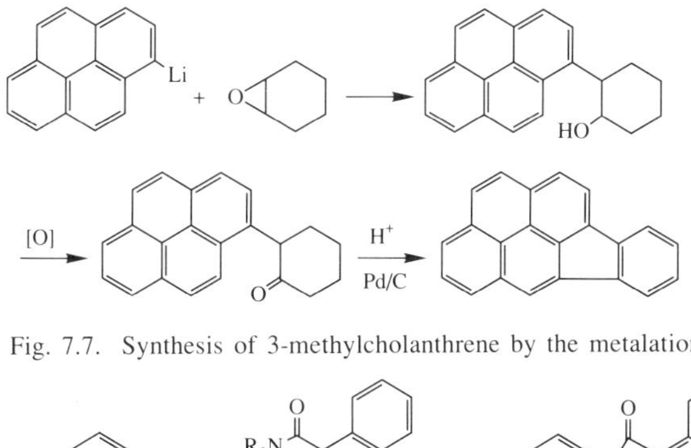

Fig. 7.7. Synthesis of 3-methylcholanthrene by the metalation route.

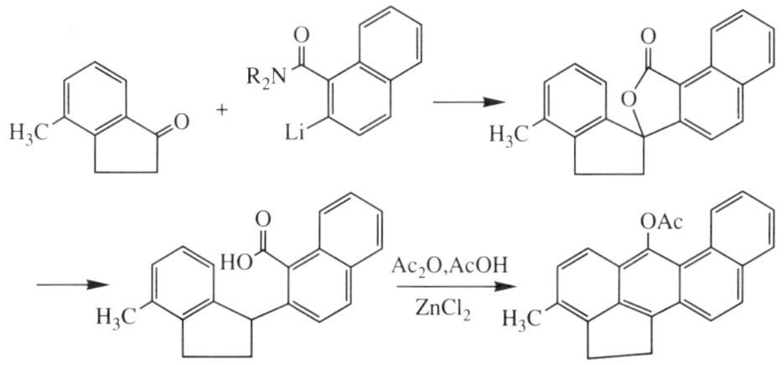

e.g. 3-methylcholanthrene (Jacobs & Harvey, 1981). Cyclodehydration is usually carried out with ZnCl$_2$ in acetic anhydride–acetic acid to yield the corresponding phenol acetate which is deoxygenated by treatment with hydroiodic acid. This method has been employed for the preparation of a number of polycyclic ring systems, including BA, BaP, dibenz[a,h]-anthracene, and dibenz[a,j]anthracene (Harvey *et al.*, 1982; Jacobs & Harvey, 1981; Pataki *et al.*, 1982; Harvey *et al.*, 1988, 1988a).

A second new method of potentially broad scope entails in the key step alkylation of the α-lithio salt of 1,3- or 1-4-dimethoxy-2,5-cyclohexadiene by a ß-arylethyl halide (Pataki *et al.*, 1983; Pataki & Harvey, 1982) (Fig. 7.8). The 1,3-cyclohexadiene derivative, which is readily available from Birch reduction of 1,3-dimethoxybenzene, is more satisfactory than the alkali metal salts of 1,3-cyclohexadione. The latter undergo alkylation predominantly on oxygen rather than carbon (Pataki & Harvey, 1982). Cyclodehydration of the diketone products takes place smoothly in polyphosphoric acid to provide the corresponding ketones containing two more rings than the starting PAH ring system. The ketonic products are convenient synthetic precursors of the corresponding phenols, quinones, dihydrodiols, and PAH derivatives. The choice between 1,3- or 1,4-dimethoxycyclohexadiene is dictated by the position it is desired to have the carbonyl function in the cyclized product. The use of the 1,4-isomer furnishes a ketonic product which on dehydrogenation yields a ß-type phenol, the preferred synthetic precursor of the corresponding diol epoxides. While this method was developed for the synthesis of derivatives of chrysene (Harvey *et al.*, 1986) and benzo[c]phen-anthrene (Pataki *et al.*, 1989), it may potentially be utilized for the preparation of any angular PAH ring system.

Additional new synthetic approaches to polyarenes involve alkylation of enol ethers or enamines (Fig. 7.9). One such method entails Ti(IV)-catalyzed aldol-type condensation between a 2-arylacetaldehyde and a silyl enol ether. In the presence of excess catalyst the primary condensation product undergoes cyclization and double dehydration to provide a partially saturated polyarene that may be readily dehydrogenated to a fully aromatic product, e.g. 5-methylchrysene (DiRaddo & Harvey, 1988). Alkylation of the bromo-magnesium salt of the enamine of cyclopentanone is the basis of a new

Fig. 7.8. Synthesis of angular PAHs by the method of Harvey *et al.*, 1986.

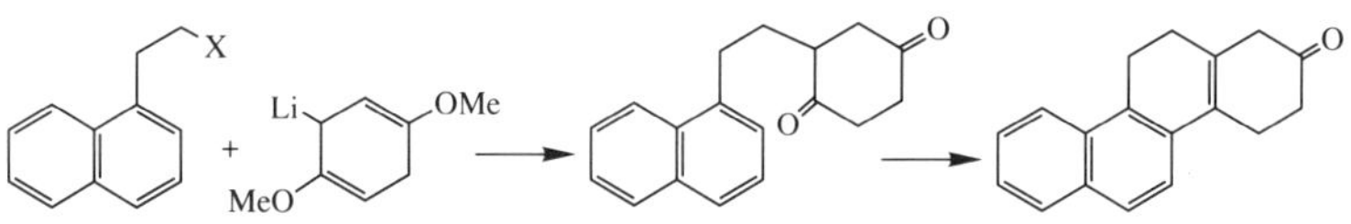

synthesis of the cyclopenta[a]phenanthrenes (Lee & Harvey, 1988) (Fig. 7.9). Acid-catalyzed cyclodehydration of the resulting alkylated cyclopentanone product, followed by dehydrogenation yields the desired cyclopenta[a]phenanthrene. The enamine derivatives of cyclohexanone and tetralone may be directly alkylated with bromomethylarenes to furnish alkylated ketones that may be cyclized in the presence of acidic catalysts and dehydrogenated to yield benzo- and dibenzofluorenes (Harvey *et al.*, 1991) (Fig. 7.9). The foregoing new methods all appear potentially broad in scope.

7.3   Diels–Alder cycloaddition

Diels–Alder reactions have been employed extensively for the construction of polycyclic aromatic ring systems. Maleic anhydride serves as a convenient dienophile for fusion of a ring with two additional carbon atoms onto a PAH. For example, perylene reacts with maleic anhydride in the presence of a dehydrogenating agent like nitrobenzene or chloranil to yield benzo[g,h,i]perylene dicarboxylic anhydride (Clar & Zander, 1957) (Fig. 7.10). Decarboxylation is accomplished by sublimation with soda-lime.

Fig. 7.9. New synthetic approaches to polyarenes are provided by alkylation of silyl enol ethers, bromomagnesium salts of enamines, and enamines.

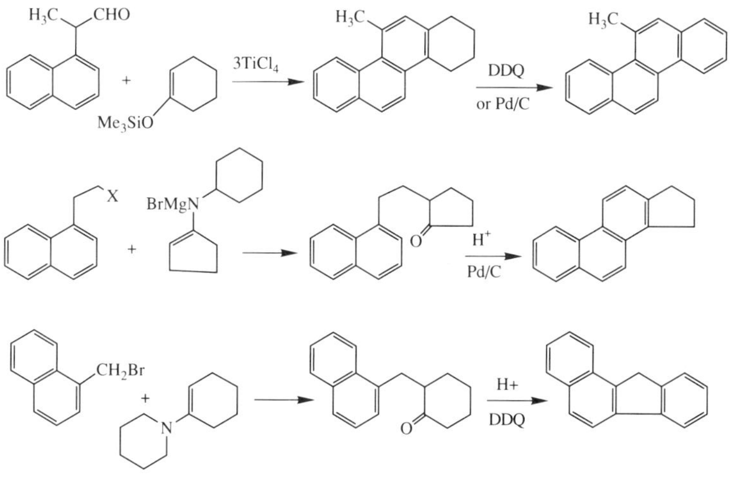

Fig. 7.10. Synthesis of polyarenes via Diels–Alder cycloaddition with maleic anhydride.

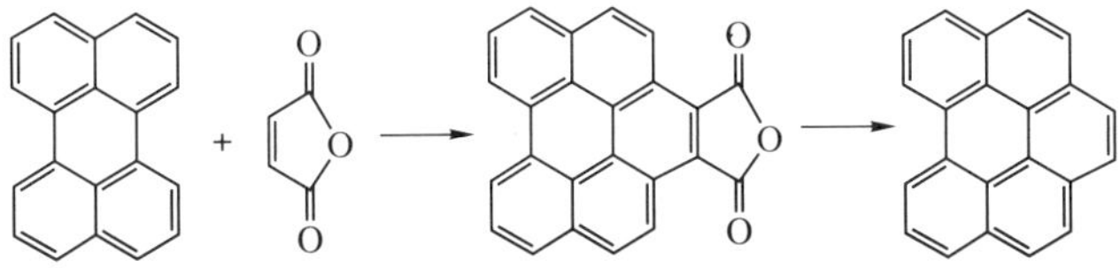

Quinones are frequently employed as dienophiles for the construction of PAH ring systems (Fig. 7.11). For example, substituted BA-7,12-diones are synthetically accessible by reaction of substituted styrenes with 1,4-naphthoquinone in the presence of chloranil or by reaction of substituted butadienes with phenanthrene-1,4-dione (Manning *et al.*, 1977; Rosen & Weber, 1977; Harvey *et al.*, 1977). Similar reaction of 1-vinylnaphthalene with *p*-benzoquinone furnishes chrysene-1,4-dione which undergoes reduction with LiAlH$_4$ to yield chrysene (Davies & Porter, 1957). Methoxy-substituted BA derivatives may be prepared via a Diels–Alder reaction between a methoxy-1,3-cyclohexadiene and 1,4-benzoquinone. On pyrolysis, ethylene is eliminated in a retro-Diels–Alder reaction to give the methoxy-substituted BA derivative (Wunderley & Weber, 1978).

Aryne intermediates may also serve as dienophiles for Diels–Alder cycloaddition reactions (Fig. 7.12). This is illustrated by the reaction of phenanthryne (generated *in situ* from 9-fluoro-10-lithiophenanthrene) with furan to produce 1,4-epoxytriphenylene (Wittig *et al.*, 1962). The latter undergoes rearrangement in acetic acid to 1-acetoxytriphenylene. Similar cycloaddition of 1,5-naphthodiyne to furan furnishes the bis adduct (LeHoullier & Gribble, 1983). The latter is converted to chrysene via hydrogenation and acidic dehydration.

Fig. 7.11. Diels–Alder synthetic routes to polyarenes.

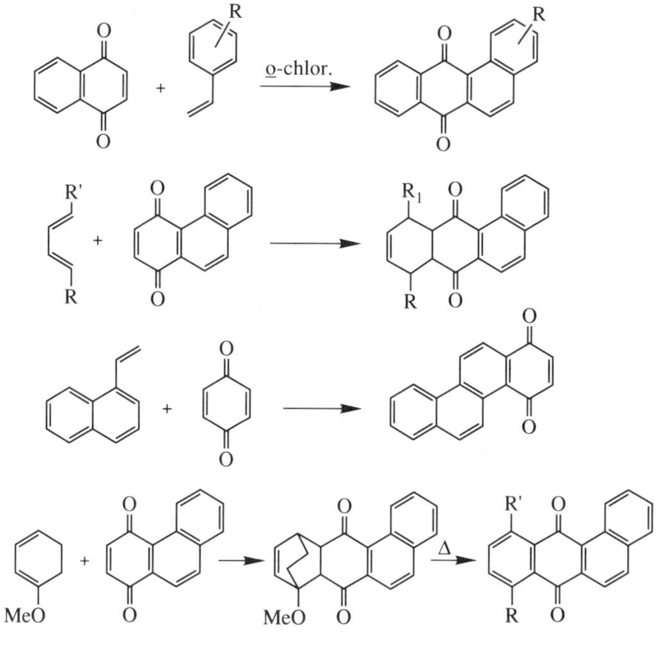

Nonalternant PAHs may also be prepared via 2 + 4 cycloaddition reactions (Fig. 7.13). For example, the addition of substituted butadienes to acenaphthylene and cyclopenta[c,d]pyrene provides synthetic access to fluoranthene (Kloetzel & Mertel, 1950) and indeno[1,2,3-cd] pyrene derivatives (Rice *et al.*, 1985).

7.4 Cyclodehydrogenation

Intramolecular cyclization accompanied by loss of hydrogen is frequently a key step in the synthesis of PAH. Cyclodehydrogenations are of the following types: (1) Lewis acid-catalyzed, (2) platinum or palladium catalyzed, (3) photochemical, and (4) potassium graphite.

Lewis acid-catalyzed cyclodehydrogenation, though frequently employed in the older literature, is seldom used today. In a typical example, 1,1'-binaphthyl on heating with $AlCl_3$ undergoes intramolecular loss of hydrogen to furnish perylene (Scholl & Weitzenbock, 1910) (Fig. 7.14). Ketones participate in similar cyclodehydrogenations, and tend to afford somewhat

Fig. 7.12. Diels–Alder reactions of aryne intermediates generated *in situ*.

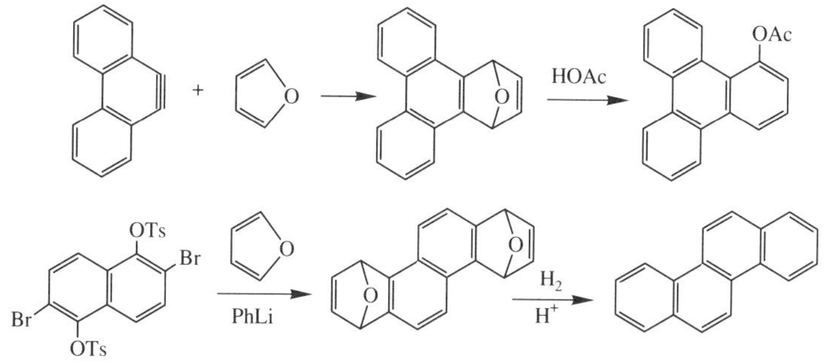

Fig. 7.13. Nonalternant PAHs are synthetically accessible via Diels–Alder reactions.

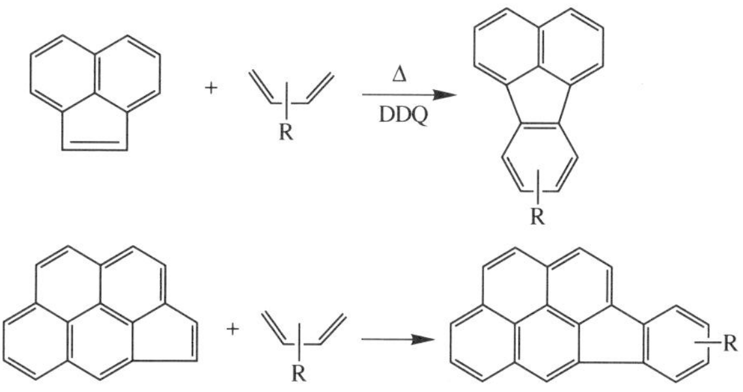

better yields of cyclized products. Thus, benzanthrone is conveniently synthesized from 1-benzoylnaphthalene via this route (Scholl & Seer, 1912). In view of the potential for rearrangement in reactions of this type, product structural assignments should be made with caution. Thus, the inital report that AlCl₃-catalyzed cyclodehydrogenation of 12-phenylbenz[a]anthracene gave dibenzo[a,l]pyrene (Clar & Stewart, 1951) (Fig. 7.15) was subsequently shown to be erroneous (Lavit-Lamy & Buu-Hoi, 1966; Vingiello *et al.*, 1966). The true product was identified as dibenzo[a,e]fluoranthene. The mechanism of this rearrangement is believed to involve migration of the phenyl group from the sterically crowded 12-position to the 7-position prior to cyclization.

Metal-catalyzed cyclodehydrogenation may be considered an electrocyclic reaction. Platinum and palladium metals are the most effective catalysts. Typical examples are the synthesis of triphenylene and benzo[g,h,i]perylene via this route (Copeland *et al.*, 1960; Altman & Ginsburg, 1959) (Fig. 7.16).

Photochemical cyclodehydrogenation has seen wide synthetic application for the preparation of fused aromatic systems. The conversion of stilbenes to

Fig. 7.14. Examples of Lewis acid-catalyzed cyclodehydrogenation

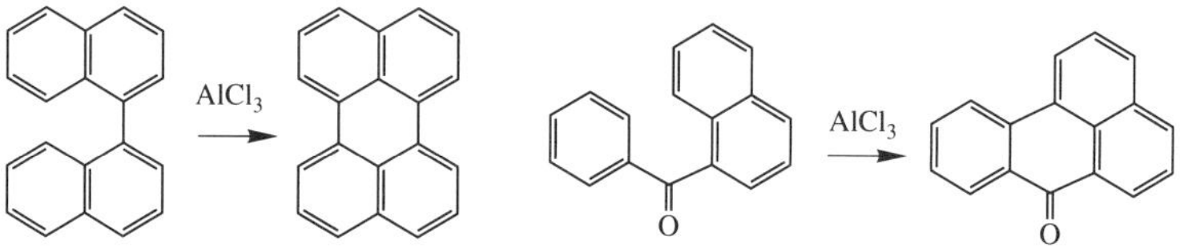

Fig. 7.15. AlCl₃-catalyzed reaction of 12-phenyl-BA involves rearrangement of the phenyl group prior to cyclodehydrogenation to yield dibenzo[a,e]fluoranthene.

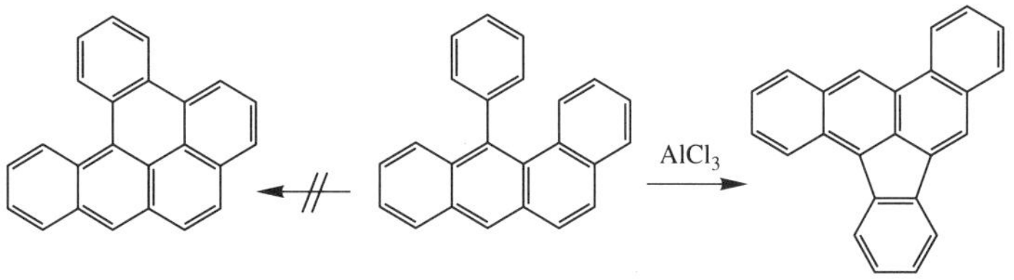

Fig. 7.16. Examples of metal-catalyzed cyclodehydrogenation.

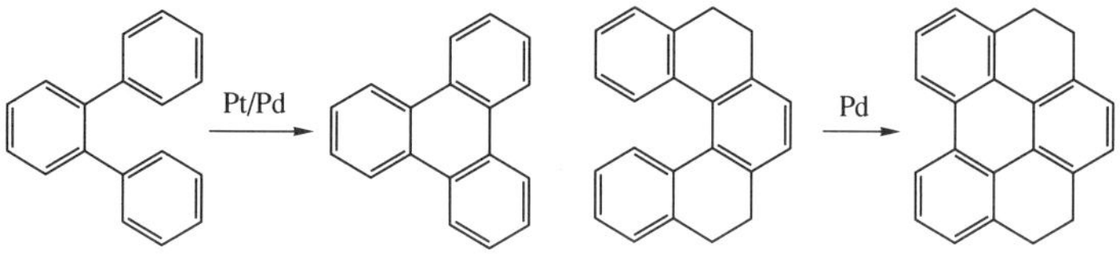

phenanthrenes by irradiation with UV light in the presence of an oxidant, such as I_2 or $FeCl_3$, has been most intensively investigated (Fig. 7.17), and several reviews are available (Mallory & Mallory, 1984; Laarhoven, 1983; Blackburn & Timmons, 1969). The reaction is a photochemically allowed conrotatory conversion of a 1,3,5-hexatriene to a cyclohexadiene with subsequent removal of the two hydrogen atoms by the oxidant. Although the reacting species must be a *cis*-stilbene, *trans*-stilbenes can be used because they are isomerized under the reaction conditions.

Studies conducted by Laarhoven, 1983 on a large number of photocyclizations have led to the following rules: (i) Photocyclization does not occur when ΣF_{rs} (the sum of the free valence numbers of the atoms r and s involved in the cyclization) is < 1.0; (ii) When two or more modes of ring closure are possible, only one product is formed if $\Delta (\Sigma F_{rs}) > 0.1$; (iii) When planar as well as nonplanar products are possible, the planar PAH is generally the main product. The introduction of substituents can also influence whether cyclization occurs. Thus, *p*-distyrylbenzene(**1** : R = H), for which $\Sigma F^* = 0.954$, fails to photocyclize (Laarhoven *et al.*, 1970), but its dimethyl derivative **1**: R = CH_3 ($\Sigma F^* = 1.077$) photocyclizes to yield 7,14-dimethyldibenz[a,h]anthracene (Blum & Zimmerman, 1972) (Fig. 7.18). Photocyclization is not limited to stilbenes, but occurs with all types of cyclohexatriene systems (Fig. 7.19). For example, the vinylogs of stilbene 1,4-diphenylbuta-1,3-diene (**2**) and 1,6-diphenylhexa-1,3,5-triene (**3**) undergo

Fig. 7.17. Photochemical cyclodehydrogenation of stilbene.

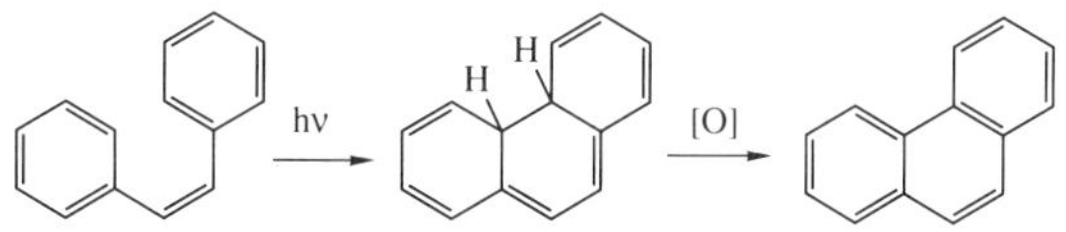

Fig. 7.18. Photocyclization of cyclohexatriene systems in the presence of an oxidant affords polycyclic aromatic hydrocarbons.

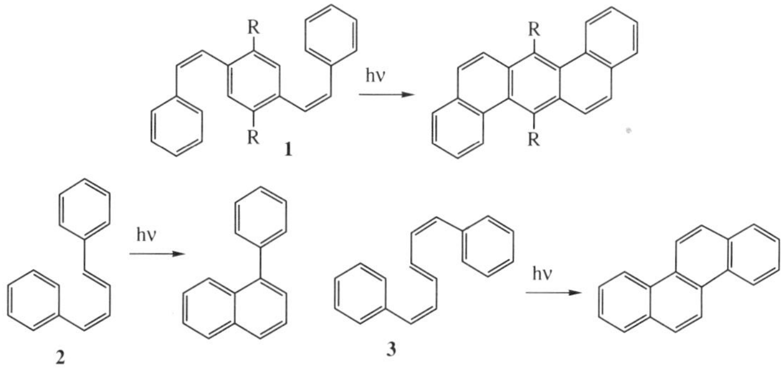

photocyclization to yield 1-phenylnaphthalene and chrysene, respectively (Fonken, 1962). Additional examples of hydrocarbons that undergo photocyclization (Fig. 7.19) are 1,2-divinylbenzene (**4**) (Pomerantz, 1967), *o*-terphenyl (**5**) (Karasch *et al.*, 1965), 4-phenylphenanthrene (**6**) (Hayward & Leznoff, 1971), 2-vinylbiphenyl (**7**) (Horgan *et al.*, 1973), and 4-vinylphenanthrene (**8**) (Horgan *et al.*, 1973); the products of their reactions are naphthalene, triphenylene, BeP, phenanthrene, and pyrene, respectively.

Finally, *cyclodehydrogenation with potassium graphite* (C_8K) of benzil is reported to afford phenanthrene quinone in 70% yield (Tamarkin *et al.*, 1984). The scope of this method has not been explored.

7.5   Jutz synthesis

One of the newest methods of polyarene synthesis is the method developed by Jutz and reviewed by him (Jutz, 1978). It involves base catalyzed condensation of a hydrocarbon containing an active methylene with a 'vinamidinium salt' such as **9** resulting in formation of a 1-dialkylaminohexatriene (Fig. 7.20). The latter on heating undergoes electrocyclic ring closure with elimination resulting in formation of a new aromatic ring. The broad scope of the method is illustrated by the examples in Fig. 7.21.

7.6   Cyclization of haloarenes

Polyarenes with a bromo or chloro substituent in a suitable ring position undergo ring closure with the elimination of hydrogen halide when heated in boiling quinoline with KOH. Typical examples are the cyclizations of the bromo compounds in Fig. 7.22 to yield the corresponding benzo[c]phenanthrene (Hewett, 1938) and benzo[b]fluoranthene (Amin *et al.*,

Fig. 7.19. Examples of hydrocarbons that undergo photocyclization.

4   5   6   7   8

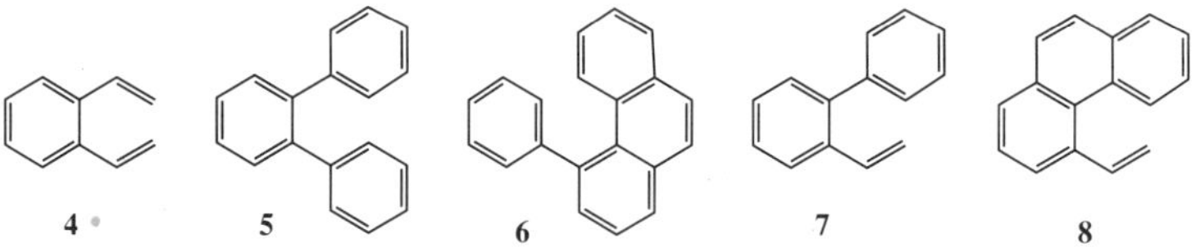

Fig. 7.20. The Jutz synthesis of polyarenes.

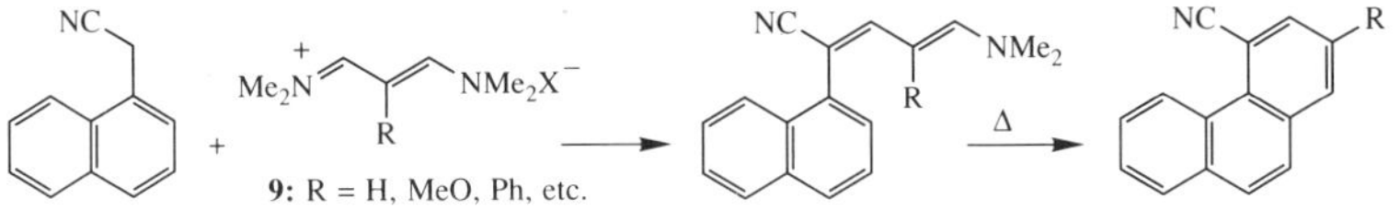

9: R = H, MeO, Ph, etc.

1985) derivatives. The method is limited mainly by the availability of the starting compounds and the susceptibility of substituent groups present to secondary reactions.

7.7   Elbs reaction

The Elbs reaction, which entails pyrolytic cyclization of *o*-alkyldiaryl-ketones at high temperature is one of the classical methods for the preparation of polyarenes (Fieser, 1942). The first practical synthesis of 3-methylcholanthrene was achieved by Elbs reaction (Fieser & Seligman, 1935, 1936) (Fig. 7.23). An example of the isomerization that may occur in the Elbs reaction is shown by the formation of dibenz[a,h]anthracene rather than the expected dibenz[a,j]anthracene in the pyrolysis of the ketone in Fig. 7.24 (Cook, 1931). It is likely that steric crowding is an important driving force in this rearrangement. The Elbs method has been utilized most

Fig. 7.21. Reactions of active methylene compounds with 'vinamidinium' salts followed by electrocyclic ring closure provides polyarenes.

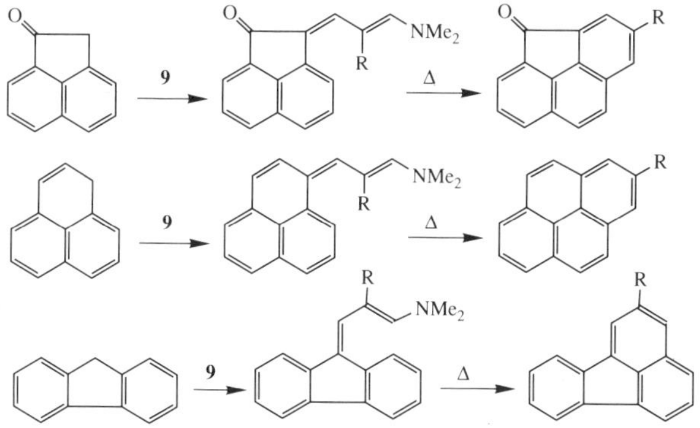

Fig. 7.22. Examples of cyclization of haloarenes under basic conditions.

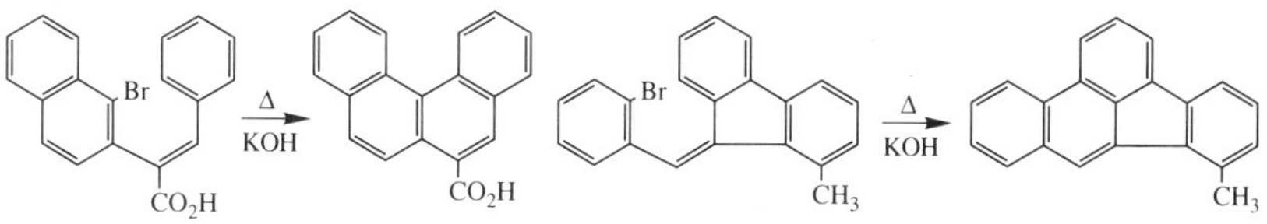

Fig. 7.23. Synthesis of 3-methylcholanthrene via the Elbs reaction.

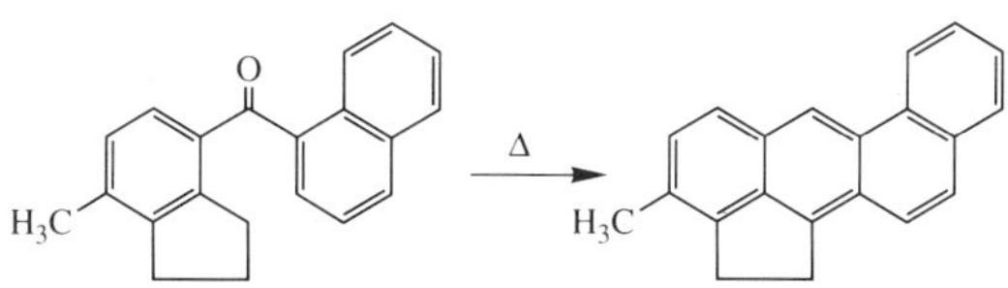

extensively for the synthesis of very large polyarenes (Clar, 1964). However, because the yields are often low and rearrangements may occur, this method is seldom now employed for synthesis of PAHs in the small or medium size range.

The mechanism of the Elbs cyclization may be rationalized as involving initial enolization, followed by sigmatropic rearrangement, isomerization into conjugation, and dehydration. This sequence is illustrated for conversion of 2-methylbenzophenone into anthracene (Fig. 7.25).

7.8   Pschorr synthesis

Another classic method of synthesis of PAH ring systems is the Pschorr synthesis involving cyclization of appropriately constituted diazonium salts (DeTar, 1957). These reactions are usually carried out in acidic solution in the presence of copper powder. There is evidence for both ionic and free radical mechanisms. Typical examples are the synthesis of fluorenone and phenanthrene 9-carboxylic acid from the corresponding diazonium salts (Fig. 7.26).

Several improvements in the Pschorr synthesis have been described in the more recent literature. Australian chemists have reported that both the rate

Fig. 7.24. Rearrangement may occur in the Elbs reaction.

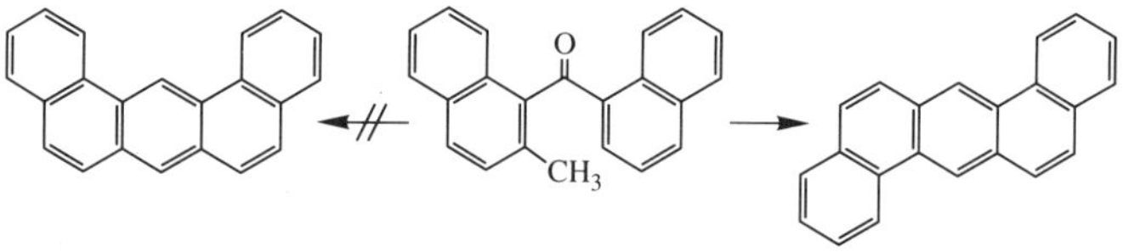

Fig. 7.25. Suggested mechanism for the Elbs reaction.

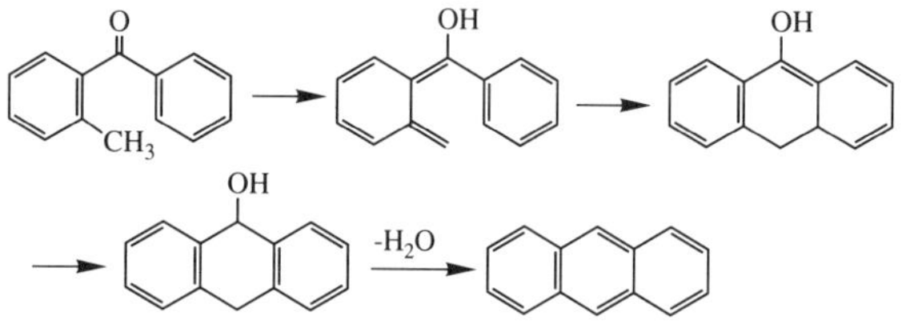

Fig. 7.26. Examples of the Pschorr synthesis.

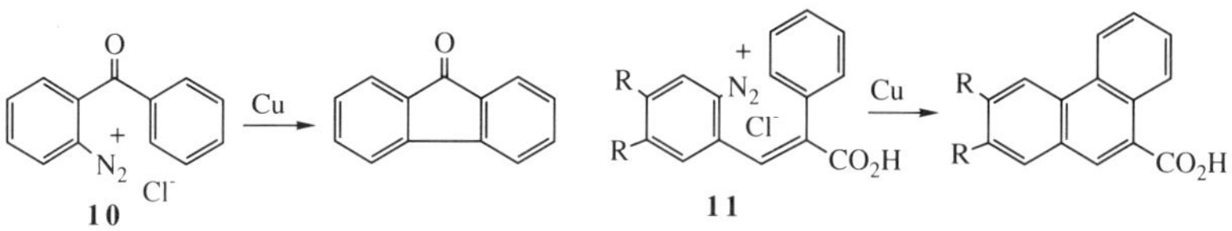

and the yield may be substantially enhanced by the use of sodium iodide in place of copper powder. Compound **11** (R = OMe) undergoes cyclization practically instantaneously in the presence of sodium iodide in acetone (72% yield), whereas similar reaction in the presence of copper powder gave a lower yield (55%) and required more than 10 hours (Chauncy & Gellert, 1969). More recently, ring closure reactions of diazonium ions have been found to occur under phase transfer conditions in the presence of a basic initiator (Beadle *et al.*, 1984). When **10** was stirred with KOAc and 18-crown-6 in Freon 113 at room temperature fluorenone was obtained in 73% yield. The copper powder/H_2SO_4 method afforded the same compound in 71% yield. Although oxygenated groups in the ring undergoing substitution tend to depress the yield in the Pschorr cyclization, it has been demonstrated that phenolic groups may be masked by conversion to the electron-withdrawing (phenylsulfonyl)oxy groups with significant enhancement in yield (Duclos *et al.*, 1984).

7.9   Annelation of quinones

An annelation method for the synthesis of polyarenes from *o*-quinones has recently been described (Sukumaran & Harvey, 1981). In a typical example, reaction of pyrene 4,5-dione with lithium acetylide followed by reduction of the resulting diacetylenic diol with $LiAlH_4$ furnished the corresponding *trans*-divinyldiol adduct (Fig. 7.27). The latter underwent concurrent cyclization and dehydration on treatment with HI or $POCl_3$ in pyridine to furnish benzo[e]pyrene. This method has also been employed to synthesize triphenylene, dibenz[a,c]anthracene, and benzo[g]chrysene in good overall yields.

7.10   Cyclization of bis-bromomethyl and diphosphonium derivatives

Examples of these methods are presented in Fig. 7.28. Treatment of 4,5-*bis*-(bromomethyl)phenanthrene with phenyllithium results in formation of 4,5-dihydropyrene (Marvel & Wilson, 1958). A closely related reaction is the synthesis of pentahelicene through treatment of the appropriate diphosphonium salt with sodium ethoxide (Bestmann *et al.*, 1969). The scope of these methods has not been explored.

Fig. 7.27. Annelation of quinones.

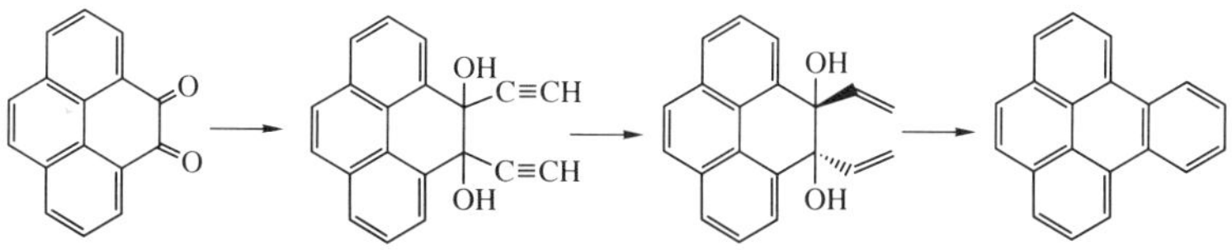

7.11   Dehydrogenation of hydroaromatic compounds

Dehydrogenation of partially saturated intermediates to fully aromatic products is frequently the final step in the synthesis of polyarenes. The scope and limitations of the various methods of catalytic and chemical dehydrogenation have been reviewed by Fu & Harvey, 1978. The traditional methods of aromatization using palladium or platinum metal catalysts or heating with sulfur or selenium have been augmented in recent years with a wide range of milder methods of chemical dehydrogenation. The most widely employed class of chemical oxidants is the high oxidation potential quinones, such as 2,3-dichloro-5,6-dichloro-5,6-dicyano-1,4-benzoquinone (DDQ) and chloranil. Other important classes of dehydrogenation reagents include trityl salts, alkyllithium-amine complexes, *N*-bromosuccinimide, and Lewis acids.

7.12   Reduction of quinones, catechols, and phenols

Quinones are often convenient starting materials for the preparation of polyarenes. Zinc and alkali is the reagent most commonly employed for the reduction of quinones in the older literature (Clar, 1964). Cyclohexanol and aluminum are also frequently employed for this purpose. This reagent is reported to efficiently reduce anthraquinone and other linear quinones, such as pentacene 6,13-dione, to the parent PAHs (Coffey & Boyd, 1954; Bruckner *et al.*, 1960).

Hydriodic acid, alone or in the presence of phosphorus or hypophosphorus acid, is one of the most convenient reagents for the reduction of polycyclic quinones, hydroquinones, and phenols to PAHs. A recent reinvestigation of HI reduction has shown that the more extensively reduced products reported

Fig. 7.28. Cyclization of bis-bromomethyl and diphosphonium derivatives.

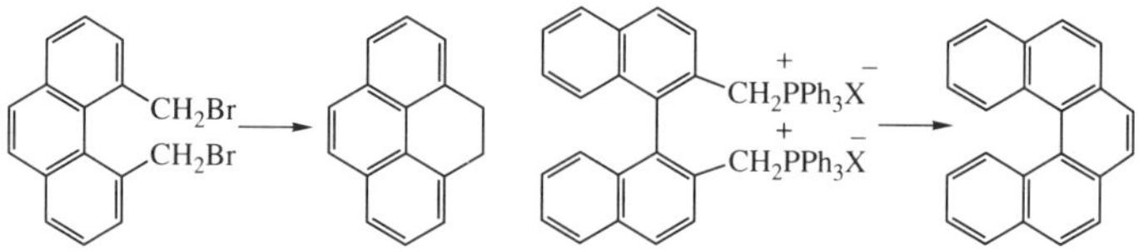

Fig. 7.29. Reductive methylation of quinones with methyllithium and HI.

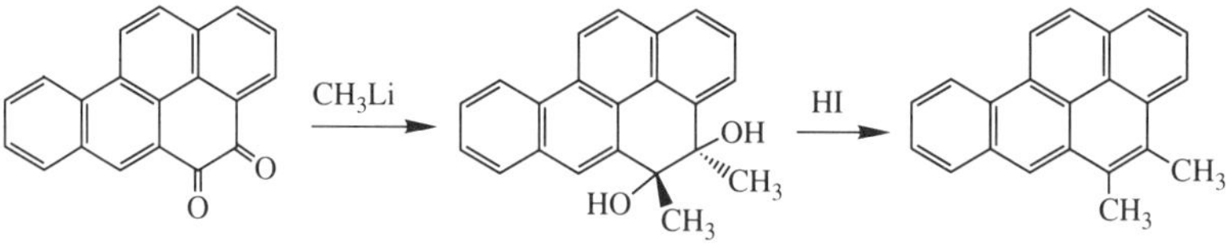

in the older literature are due to the relatively drastic conditions employed (Harvey *et al.*, 1978; Konieczny & Harvey, 1979, 1984, 1990). High yields of the fully aromatic polyarenes are readily obtainable from the reduction of quinones with HI under mild conditions.

A useful modification of the HI reduction method permits reductive methylation. For example, reaction of BaP-4,5-dione with methyllithium affords the dimethyl diol which is reduced with HI to the corresponding dimethylarene in good yield (Konieczny & Harvey, 1980) (Fig. 7.29).

7. 13   References

Altman, Y. & Ginsburg, D. (1959). Alicylic studies. Part XIV. An improved synthesis of 3:4-5:6-dibenzophenanthrene and 1:12-benzoperylene. *J. Chem. Soc.* 466–8.

Amin, S., Huie, K., Hussain, N., Balanikas, G. & Hecht, S. (1985). Synthesis of benzo-[b]fluoranthenes and benzo[k]fluoranthenes. *J. Org. Chem.* **50**, 1948–54.

Bachmann, W. E. & Bradbury, J. T. (1937). The synthesis of 5-phenyl-9,10-dialkyl-9,10-dihydroxy-9,10-dihydro-1,2-benzanthracenes and related compounds. *J. Org. Chem.* **2**, 175–82.

Bachmann, W. E. & Struve, W. S. (1939). The synthesis of derivatives of chrysene. *J. Org. Chem.* **4**, 456–63.

Beadle, J. R., Korzeniowski, S. H., Rosenberg, D. E., Garcia-Slanga, B. J. & Gokel, G. W. (1984). Phase-transfer-catalyzed Gomberg–Bachmann synthesis of unsymmetrical biarenes: A survey of catalysts and substrates. *J. Org. Chem.* **49**, 1594–603.

Berliner, E. (1949). The Friedel and Crafts reaction with aliphatic dibasic acid anhydrides. *Org. Reactions.* **5**, 229–89.

Bestmann, H. J., Armsen, R. & Wagner, H. (1969). Oxidation of phosphoalkenes with periodate. Synthesis of α,β-dicarbonyl compounds, olefins and polycyclic compounds. *Chem. Ber.* **102**, 2259–269.

Blackburn, E. V. & Timmons, T. J. (1969). The photocyclisation of stilbene analogues. *Quart. Rev. Chem. Soc.* **23**, 482–503.

Blum, J. H. & Zimmerman, M. (1972). Photocyclization of substituted 1,4-distyrylbenzenes to dibenz[a]anthracenes. *Tetrahedron,* **28**, 275–80.

Bodine, R. S., Hylarides, M., Daub, G. H. & VanderJagt, D. L. (1978). ^{13}C-Labelled benzo[a]pyrene and derivatives. 1. Efficient pathways to labeling the 4,5,11, and 12 positions. *J. Org. Chem.* **43**, 4025–8.

Bruckner, V., Karczag, A., Kormendy, K., Meszaros, M. & Tomasz, J. (1960). A simple synthesis of pentacene. *Tetrahedron Lett.* 5.

Chauncy, B. & Gellert, E. (1969). A new variation of the Pschorr synthesis. *Austr. J. Chem.* **22**, 993–5.

Cho, B. & Harvey, R. G. (1987). Polycyclic fluoranthene hydrocarbons. 2. A new general synthesis. *J. Org. Chem.* **52**, 5668–78.

Clar, E. (1964). *Polycyclic Hydrocarbons,* New York: Academic Press.

Clar, E. & Stewart, D. (1951). Aromatic hydrocarbons. Part LIX. 1:2-3:4-dibenzopyrene. *J. Chem. Soc.* 687–90.

Clar, E. & Zander, M. (1957). Synthesis of coronene and 1:2-7:8-dibenzocoronene. *J. Chem. Soc.* 4616–9.

Coffey, S. & Boyd, V. (1954). The reduction of anthraquinone and other polycyclic quinones with aluminum alkoxides (Meerwein-Pondorff reagent). *J. Chem. Soc.* 2468–70.

Cook, J. W. (1931). LXV. Polycyclic aromatic hydrocarbons. Part II. The non-existence of 1:2-7:8-dibenzanthracene. *J. Chem. Soc.* 487–9.

Cook, J. W. (1931a). LXVI. Polycyclic aromatic hydrocarbons. Part III. Derivatives of 1:2-5:6-dibenzanthracene. *J. Chem. Soc.* 489–99.

Cook, J. W. & Schoental, R. (1945). Polycyclic aromatic hydrocarbons. Part XXX. Synthesis of chrysenols. *J. Chem. Soc.* 288–92.

Copeland, P. G., Dean, R. E. & McNeil, D. (1960). The cyclodehydrogenation of o-terphenyl and 1,2'-biphenylyl-3,4-dihydronaphthalene. *J. Chem. Soc.* 1687–9.

Davies, W. & Porter, Q. N. (1957). The synthesis of polycyclic aromatic compounds. Part I. The reaction of quinones with vinylnaphthalenes and related dienes. *J. Chem. Soc.* 4967–70.

DeTar, D. F. (1957). The Pschorr synthesis and related diazonium ring closure reactions. *Org. Reactions*, **9**, 409–62.

DiRaddo, P. & Harvey, R. G. (1988). A new synthesis of polycyclic aromatic hydrocarbons via titanium(IV)-catalyzed aldol-type condensation of silyl enol ethers with 2-arylacetaldehydes. *Tetrahedron Lett.* **29**, 3885–6.

Duclos, R. I. J., Tung, J. S. & Rapoport, H. (1984). A high yield modification of the Pschorr synthesis. *J. Org. Chem.* **49**, 5243–6.

Fieser, L. F. (1942). The Elbs reaction. *Org. Reactions*, **1**, 129–54.

Fieser, L. F. & Heymann, H. (1941). Synthesis of 2-hydroxy-3,4-benzpyrene and 2-methyl-3,4-benzpyrene. *J. Am. Chem. Soc.* **63**, 2333–40.

Fieser, L. F. & Johnson, W. S. (1939). Synthesis in the 1,2-benzanthracene and chrysene series. *J. Am. Chem. Soc.* **61**, 1647–54.

Fieser, L. F. & Seligman, A. M. (1935). The synthesis of methylcholanthrene. *J. Am. Chem. Soc.* **57**, 942–6.

Fieser, L. F. & Seligman, A. M. (1936). An improved method for the preparation of methylcholanthrene. *J. Am. Chem. Soc.* **58**, 2482–7.

Fonken, G. J. (1962). Photochemical formation of polynuclear aromatic compounds from diaryl polyenes. *Chem. & Ind.* 1327.

Fu, P. P. & Harvey, R. G. (1978). Dehydrogenation of polycyclic hydroaromatic compounds. *Chem. Rev.* **78**, 317–61.

Harvey, R. G. & Cortez, C. (1986). Synthesis of 7,12-dimethylbenz[a]anthracene and its 1,2,3,4-tetrahydro derivative. *J. Org. Chem.* **51**, 5023–4.

Harvey, R. G., Cortez, C. & Jacobs, S. A. (1982). Synthesis of polycyclic hydrocarbons via a novel annelation method. *J. Org. Chem.* **47**, 2120–5.

Harvey, R. G., Cortez, C., Sawyer, T. W. & DiGiovanni, J. (1988). Synthesis of the tumorigenic 3,4-dihydrodiol metabolites of dibenz[a,j]anthracene and 7,14-dimethyldibenz[a]anthracene. *J. Medic. Chem.* **31**, 1308–12.

Harvey, R. G., Cortez, C., Sugiyama, T., Ito, Y., Sawyer, T. W. & DiGiovanni, J. (1988a). Biologically active dihydrodiol metabolites of polycyclic aromatic hydrocarbons structurally related to the potent carcinogenic hydrocarbon 7,12–dimethylbenz[a]anthracene. *J. Medic. Chem.* **31**, 154–9.

Harvey, R. G., Fu, P. P., Cortez, C. & Pataki, J. (1977). Synthesis of a biologically active D-ring diolepoxide of the potent carcinogen 7,12-dimethylbenz[a]anthracene. *Tetrahedron Lett.* 3533–6.

Harvey, R. G., Leyba, C., Fu, P. P., Konieczny, M. & Sukumaran, K. B. (1978). A novel and convenient synthesis of dibenz[a,c]anthracene. *J. Org. Chem.* **43**, 3423–5.

Harvey, R. G., Pataki, J., Cortez,C., DiRaddo, P. & Yang, C. (1991). A new general synthesis of polycyclic aromatic compounds based on enamine chemistry. *J. Org. Chem.* **56**, 1210–17.

Harvey, R. G., Pataki, J. & Lee, H. (1986). Synthesis of the dihydrodiol and diol epoxide metabolites of chrysene and 5-methylchrysene. *J. Org. Chem.* **51**, 1407–12.

Haworth, R. D. & Marvin, C. R. (1933). A new route to chrysene and 1:2-benzanthracene. *J. Chem. Soc.* 1012–6.

Hayward, R. J. & Leznoff, C. C. (1971). Photocyclization reactions of aryl polyarenes. II. The photocyclization of 1-aryl-4-phenyl-1,3-butadiene. *Tetrahedron*, **27**, 2085–90.

Hewett, C. L. (1938). Polycyclic aromatic hydrocarbons. Part XVIII. A general method for the synthesis of 3:4-benzphenanthrene derivatives. *J. Chem. Soc.* 1286–91.

Horgan, S. W., Morgan, D. D. & Orchin, M. (1973). The photochemistry of 2-vinylbiphenyl and 4-vinylphenanthrene. *J. Org. Chem.* **38**, 3801–3.

Jacobs, S. & Harvey, R. G. (1981). Synthesis of 3-methylcholanthrene. *Tetrahedron Lett.* **22**, 1093–6.

Johnson, W. S. (1944). The formation of cyclic ketones by intramolecular acylation. *Org. Reactions*, **2**, 114–77.

Jutz, J. C. (1978). Aromatic and heteroaromatic compounds by electrocyclic ring-closure with elimination. *Topics in Current Chem.* **73**, 127–230.

Karasch, N., Alston, T. G., Lewis, H. B. & Wolf, W. (1965). The photochemical conversion of *o*-terphenyl into triphenylene. *J. Chem. Soc. Chem. Commun.* 242–3.

Kloetzel, M. C. & Mertel, H. E. (1950). Fluoranthene derivatives. II. The reaction of acenaphthylene with butadiene derivatives. *J. Am. Chem. Soc.* **72**, 4786–91.

Konieczny, M. & Harvey, R. G. (1979). Efficient reduction of polycyclic quinones, hydroquinones, and phenols to polycyclic aromatic hydrocarbons with hydriodic acid. *J. Org. Chem.* **44**, 4813–6.

Konieczny, M. & Harvey, R. G. (1980). Reductive methylation of polycyclic aromatic quinones. *J. Org. Chem.* **45**, 1308–10.

Konieczny, M. & Harvey, R. G. (1984). Reduction of polycyclic quinones with hydriodic acid: Synthesis of benz[a]anthracene. *Org. Syn.* **62**, 165–9.

Konieczny, M. & Harvey, R. G. (1990). Reduction of quinones with hydriodic acid: Benz[a]anthracene. *Org. Syn.* Coll. Vol. VII, 18–22.

Laarhoven, W. H. (1983). Photochemical cyclization and intramolecular cycloadditions of conjugated arylolefins. Part I. Photocyclization with dehydrogenation. *Rec. Trav. Chim.* **102**, 185–204.

Laarhoven, W. H., Cuppen, T. J. & Nivard, R. J. (1970). Photodehydrocyclization in stilbene-like compounds. II. Photochemistry of distyrylbenzenes. *Tetrahedron*, **26**, 1069–83.

Lavit-Lamy, D. & Buu-Hoi, N. P. (1966). The true nature of 'dibenzo[a,l]pyrene' and its known derivatives. *J. Chem. Soc. Chem. Commun.* 92–4.

Lee, H. & Harvey, R. G. (1988). New synthetic approaches to cyclopenta[a]phenanthrenes and their carcinogenic derivatives. *J. Org. Chem.* **53**, 4253–6.

LeHoullier, C. S. & Gribble, G. W. (1983). Twin annulation of naphthalene via a 1,5-naphthodiyne synthon. New syntheses of chrysene and dibenzo[b,k]chrysene. *J. Org. Chem.* **48**, 1682–5.

Mallory, F. B. & Mallory, C. W. (1984). Photocyclization of stilbenes and related molecules. *Org. Reactions*, **30**, 1–456.

Manning, W. B., Tomaszewski, J. E., Muschik, G. M. & Sato, R. I. (1977). A general synthesis of 1-, 2-, 3-, and 4-substituted benz[a]anthracene-7-12-diones. *J. Org. Chem.* **42**, 3465–8.

Marvel, C. S. & Wilson, B. D. (1958). Synthetic studies in the dihydropyrene series. *J. Org. Chem.* **23**, 1483–8.

Newman, M. S., Tierney, B. & Veeraraghavan, S. (1988). *The Chemistry and Biology of Benz[a]anthracenes*, Cambridge: Cambridge University Press.

Pataki, J., DiRaddo, P. & Harvey, R. G. (1989). An efficient synthesis of the highly tumorigenic *anti*-diol epoxide derivative of benzo[c]phenanthrene. *J. Org. Chem.* **47**, 840–4.

Pataki, J. & Harvey, R. G. (1982). Benzo[c]phenanthrene and its oxidized metabolites. *J. Org. Chem.* **47**, 20–2.

Pataki, J., Lee, H. & Harvey, R. G. (1983). Carcinogenic metabolites of 5-methylchrysene. *Carcinogenesis*, **4**, 399–402.

Platt, K. L. & Oesch, F. (1981). Reductive cyclization of keto acids to polycyclic aromatic hydrocarbons by hydroiodic acid–red phosphorus. *J. Org. Chem.* **46**, 2601–3.

Pomerantz, M. (1967). Photochemical rearrangement of *o*-divinylbenzene. *J. Am. Chem. Soc.* **89**, 695–6.

Rice, J. E., Coleman, D. T., Hosted, T. J. Jr., LaVoie, E. J., McCaustland, D. J. & Wiley, J. C. Jr (1985). Identification of mutagenic metabolites of indeno[1,2,3-cd]pyrene formed *in vitro* with rat liver enzymes. *Cancer Res.* **45**, 5421–5.

Rosen, B. I. & Weber, W. P. (1977). Synthesis of 7,12-benz[a]anthraquinones via Diels–Alder reaction of 1,4-phenanthraquinones. *J. Org. Chem.* **42**, 3463–5.

Scholl, R. & Seer, C. (1912). Elimination of aromatically combined hydrogen and condensation of aromatic nuclei by means of aluminum chloride. *Liebigs Ann.* **394**, 111–77.

Scholl, R., Seer, C. & Weitzenbock, R. (1910). Perylene, a highly condensed aromatic hydrocarbon. *Chem. Ber.* **43**, 2202–9.

Sukumaran, K. B. & Harvey, R. G. (1981). Novel annelation reaction: Synthesis of polycyclic hydrocarbons from *o*-quinones. *J. Org. Chem.* **46**, 2740–5.

Tamarkin, D., Benny, D. & Rabinovitz, M. (1974). Formation of phenanthrenequinone from benzil: A novel reaction of graphite-potassium intercalates. *Angew. Chem. Int. Ed., Eng.* **23**, 642.

Vingiello, F. A., Yanez, J. & Greenwood, E. J. (1966). The synthesis of dibenzo[a,l]pyrene. *J. Chem. Soc. Chem. Commun.* 375.

Weizmann, C., Bergmann, E. & Bergmann, F. (1935). Grignard reactions with phthalic anhydrides. *J. Chem. Soc.* 1367–70.

Wittig, G., Uhlenbrock, W. & Weinhold, P. (1962). Formation and detection of 9,10-dehydrophenanthrene. *Chem. Ber.* **88**, 1692–702.

Wunderly, S. W. & Weber, W. P. (1978). Synthesis of 8-methoxy- and 11-methoxybenz-[a]anthraquinones via Diels–Alder reaction of 1,4-phenanthraquinone. *J. Org. Chem.* **43**, 2277–9.

8

Alternant tetracyclic polyarenes

The chemistry of the alternant polyarenes in the four to six ring range is summarized in this and the following two chapters. Information on the physical, chemical, and spectral properties, environmental occurrence, and carcinogenic properties of each hydrocarbon is provided along with a review of methods of synthesis and information on chemical reactivity. In the discussion of synthetic methodology, methods of broadest scope and utility are emphasized. Additional methods of less practical importance or of only historical interest are cited only briefly.

8.1 Triphenylene

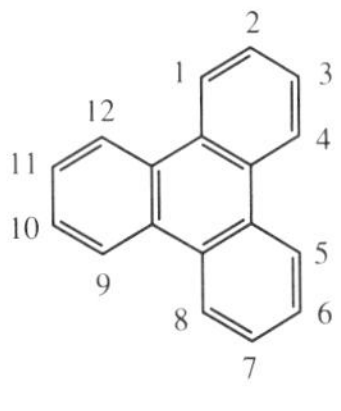

Other names: 9,10-benzophenanthrene, 1,2,3,4-dibenzonaph-thalene

Physical and spectral properties $C_{18}H_{12}$, mol. wt. 228.28, colorless needles (alcohol), mp 198 °C, sublimes. Soluble in benzene, chloroform, and alcohol; solutions exhibit blue fluorescence. Spectral data: UV (Karcher, 1988; TRC, 1982a; Clar, 1964; Friedel & Orchin, 1951; Jaffe & Orchin, 1962; Sadtler); UV fluorescence (Karcher, 1988; Berlman, 1971; Schoental & Scott, 1949); IR (Karcher, 1988; Sadtler; Pouchert, 1981); ^{1}H- and ^{13}C-NMR (Karcher, 1988; Memory & Wilson, 1982; Pouchert, 1983; TRC, 1982); mass spectrum (Karcher, 1988; Stenhagen *et al.*, 1974).

Occurrence and carcinogenicity Triphenylene occurs in coal tar and in fossil fuels. Low levels are found in atmospheric pollution and in cigarette smoke (Grimmer, 1979; Snook *et al.*, 1977). It has also been identified in gasoline engine exhaust and in exhaust tar (IARC, 1983). Triphenylene is generally considered to be noncarcinogenic. It also exhibits only borderline mutagenicity in the Ames assay with *Salmonella typhimurium* TA100 with microsomal activation (Wood *et al.*, 1980).

Synthesis The method most frequently employed for the preparation of triphenylene and its derivatives is a modified Haworth synthesis (Method 7.1). Reaction of succinic anhydride with 9-phenanthrylmagnesium bromide yields a ketoacid which undergoes Clemmensen reduction and cyclization with HF to provide a tricyclic ketone (Fig. 8.1) (Harvey *et al.*, 1979; Bergmann & Blum-Bergmann, 1937). The latter may be readily converted to triphenylene by reduction and dehydrogenation using standard methods, or it may be utilized to prepare substituted derivatives, such as 1- and 2-methyltriphenylene and 1-hydroxytriphenylene.

A newer synthetic approach involves reaction between phenanthrene-9,10-dione and lithium acetylide, followed by reduction of the resulting diacetylenic diol with LiAlH4, and cyclization with HI (Sukumaran & Harvey, 1981) (Method 7.9; Fig. 7.27).

Other syntheses include: self-condensation of cyclohexanone with sulfuric acid to yield dodecahydrotriphenylene followed by dehydrogenation over copper or selenium (Mannich, 1907; Diels & Karstens, 1927); reaction of *o*-diiodobenzene or *o*-bromoiodobenzene with lithium (via trimerization of benzyne) (Heaney & Millar, 1973); reaction of 1,2-dibromobenzene with activated nickel (Chao *et al.*, 1983); reaction between phenyllithium and 2,2'-dibromobiphenyl (Barton & McOmie, 1956); reaction between phenanthryne (generated from 9-fluorophenanthrene and butyllithium) and furan followed by treatment of the adduct with methanolic HCl and zinc dust distillation (Wittig & Pohmer, 1956; Wittig *et al.*, 1962); Diels–Alder cycloaddition of 1,3-naphthodiyne to furan followed by deoxygenation (Gribble *et al.*, 1985a); AlCl3-catalyzed condensation between octahydrophenanthrene and 1,4-

Fig. 8.1. Synthesis of the triphenylene ring system by a modified Haworth synthesis.

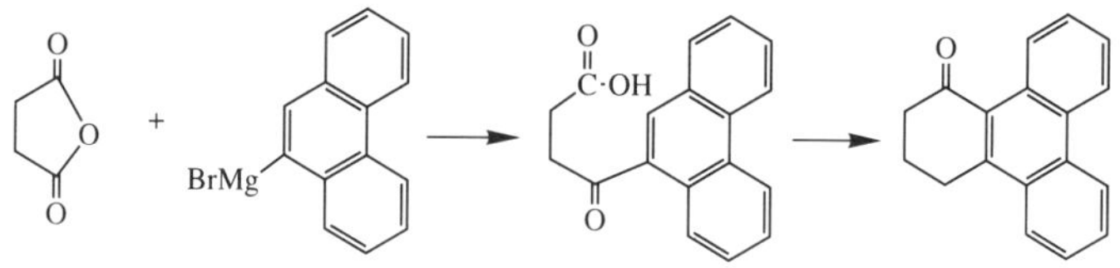

dichlorobutane followed by dehydrogenation (Reppe, 1955); and photochemical (Kharasch *et al.*, 1965) and Pd-catalyzed cyclization of *o*-terphenyl (Copeland *et al.*, 1960).

Reactions The most reactive site in triphenylene is predicted by MO theory to be the 1-position (Bolton *et al.*, 1969). However, electrophilic substitution is found to take place predominantly in the 2-position, probably due to steric resistance to attack in the hindered bay region. Thus, bromination yields 2-bromotriphenylene (Barker *et al.*, 1955), sulfonation with SO_3 in nitromethane gives the 2-sulfonic acid (Cerfontain *et al.*, 1982; Cook & Hewett, 1933), and reaction with oxalyl chloride and $AlCl_3$ furnishes the 2-carboxylic acid (Barker *et al.*, 1955). Analogous reactions of triphenylene with acetyl chloride, propionyl chloride, succinic anhydride, and phthalic anhydride and $AlCl_3$ provide the corresponding 2-substituted derivatives of triphenylene (Barker *et al.*, 1955; Buu-Hoi & Jacquignon, 1953; Clar, 1948). Nitration of triphenylene with N_2O_4 yields 2-nitrotriphenylene plus a lesser amount of the 1-nitro isomer (Radner, 1983), whereas nitration with HNO_3 in acetic anhydride gives a small excess of the latter isomer (Barker *et al.*, 1955). In contrast, chlorination (Bolton *et al.*, 1969) and deuteriation (Dallinga *et al.*, 1957) favor substitution in the 1-position of triphenylene.

Hydrogenation of triphenylene over platinum under mild conditions furnishes a mixture of 1,2,3,4-tetrahydro-, 1,2,3,4,5,6,7,8-octahydro-, and 1,2,3,4,5,6,7,8,9,10,11,12-dodecahydrotriphenylene in 7:4:3 ratio (Fu *et al.*, 1980). Hydrogenation over a Raney nickel catalyst under more vigorous conditions gives mainly dodecahydrotriphenylene (Ward *et al.*, 1945).

8.2   Benzo[c]phenanthrene

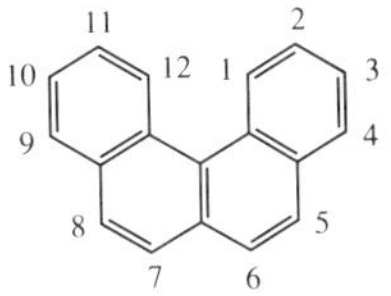

Other names: 3,4-benzophenanthrene (BcP)
Physical and spectral properties $C_{18}H_{12}$, mol. wt. 228.28, colorless needles, mp 68° C. Soluble in benzene, chloroform, and alcohol. X-ray analysis shows the molecule to be twisted out of planarity due to steric interaction in the 'fjord region' (Herbstein & Schmidt, 1954). Spectral data: UV (Karcher *et al.*, 1985; TRC, 1982a; Clar, 1964; Friedel & Orchin, 1951; Jaffe & Orchin, 1962), UV fluorescence (Berlman, 1971), IR (Sadtler), [1]H-

and ^{13}C-NMR (Bax *et al.*, 1985; TRC, 1982; Haigh & Mallion, 1971; Martin *et al.*, 1974); mass spectrum (Karcher *et al.*, 1985; Stenhagen *et al.*, 1974).

Occurrence and carcinogenicity Benzo[c]phenanthrene is a common component of coal tar, airborne pollutants, and cigarette smoke (Snook *et al.*, 1977; IARC,1983). It is generally considered inactive as a complete carcinogen and only a very weak initiator at best. However, its bay region diol epoxide derivative exhibits exceptionally high tumor-initiating activity (Levin *et al.*, 1980).

Synthesis One of the newest syntheses entails alkylation of the potassium salt of cyclohexan-1,3-dione with ß-(2-iodoethyl)naphthalene followed by acid-catalyzed cyclization of the alkylated diketone (**1**), reduction with NaBH$_4$, and dehydrogenation (Fig. 8.2) (Pataki & Harvey, 1982). The monoketone product (**2**), which may be readily converted to BcP, also serves as a precursor of its oxidized metabolites. Higher yields are obtainable by a modification of the method that involves similar alkylation of the lithium salt of 1,3- or 1,4-dimethoxycyclohexa-2,5-diene (Pataki *et al.*, 1989).

Additional syntheses include: Diels–Alder reaction of 2-vinylnaphthalene

Fig. 8.2. Synthetic approaches to benzo[c]phenanthrene.

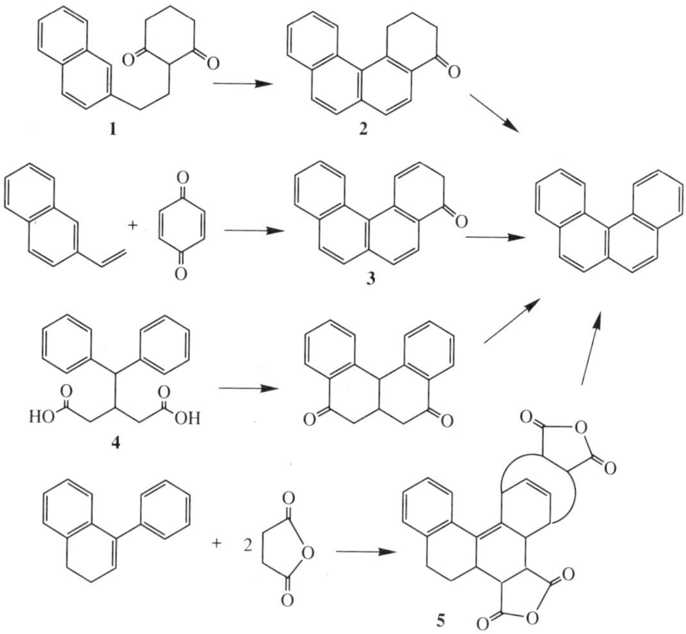

with excess benzoquinone followed by reduction of the quinone product (**3**) with LiAlH4 (Davies & Porter, 1957) (Fig. 8.2); acid-catalyzed cyclization of benzhydrylglutaric acid (**4**) followed by reduction of the carbonyl groups and catalytic dehydrogenation (Newman & Joshel, 1938); Diels–Alder reaction between 1-phenyl-3,4-dihydronaphthalene and two molecules of maleic anhydride, followed by catalytic dehydrogenation and decarboxylation of the adduct (**5**) (Smuszkovicz & Modest, 1948; Vickery & Eisenbraun, 1979); and photocyclization of 2-(ß-styryl)naphthalene (Carruthers, 1967; Scholtz *et al.*, 1967). Several syntheses of more limited application are cited by Clar, 1964.

Syntheses of all six monomethylbenzo[c]phenanthrenes (Nagel *et al.*, 1977; Newman & Wheatley, 1948; Newman *et al.*, 1953) and the 1-, 2-, 3-, 4-, and 6-fluorobenzo[c]phenanthrenes have been reported (Ittah & Jerina, 1980).

Reactions Electrophilic substitutions (bromination, nitration, and acetylation) take place regioselectively in the 5-position of BcP (Newman & Kosak, 1949), in accord with theoretical predictions. BcP reacts with N-bromoacetamide in acetic acid to furnish the K-region *trans*-5,6-bromohydrin acetate (van Bladeren & Jerina, 1983) which serves as a precursor for the BcP-5,6-oxide. Oxidation of BcP with sodium dichromate in glacial acid affords the K-region 5,6-dione (Cook, 1931).

Hydrogenation of BcP by a rhodium catalyst in a two phase system takes place selectively on the 5,6-bond to furnish 5,6-dihydro-BcP accompanied by lesser amounts of further hydrogenated products (Amer *et al.*, 1987). BcP on heating with a platinum catalyst at 400 °C undergoes cyclodehydrogenation to yield benzo[ghi]fluoranthene (Studt & Win, 1983).

8.3 Chrysene

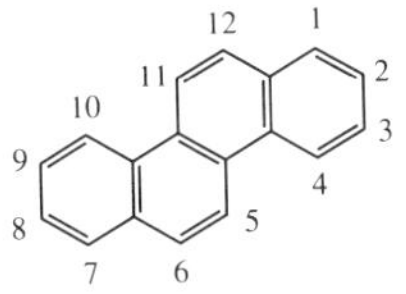

Physical and spectral properties $C_{18}H_{12}$, mol. wt. 228.28, color-less plates, mp 255–56 °C. Chrysene is only sparingly soluble in alcohol, acetic acid, and ether, but it is readily soluble in boiling toluene; solutions exhibit blue fluorescence. Spectral data: UV (Karcher et al., 1985; TRC, 1982a; Jaffe & Orchin, 1962; Friedel & Orchin, 1951); UV fluorescence (Berlman, 1971; Schoental & Scott, 1949); IR (Karcher et al., 1985;

Pouchert, 1981); NMR (Bax *et al.*, 1985; Karcher *et al.*, 1985; Memory & Wilson, 1982; TRC, 1982; Vysotskii & Mestechkin, 1975); mass spectrum (Karcher *et al.*, 1985; Stenhagen *et al.*, 1974).

Occurrence and carcinogenicity Chrysene is an important component of coal tar and a common atmospheric pollutant (Grimmer, 1979; Lao, 1973; IARC, 1983, 1973). It occurs at about the same level as BaP in products of incomplete combustion, and is a component of automobile exhaust and cigarette smoke (Grimmer, 1979; Snook *et al.*, 1977). It is also found in broiled and smoked meats, vegetables, and many common foods (IARC, 1983). Chrysene is inactive as a complete carcinogen on mouse skin, and exhibits only weak activity in initiation–promotion experiments (IARC, 1983).

Synthesis Numerous synthetic approaches to chrysene and its derivatives have been described. An efficient new synthesis involves $TiCl_4$-catalyzed condensation between 2-naphthylacetaldehyde and the silyl enol ether of cyclohexanone (Fig. 7.9) (DiRaddo & Harvey, 1988). In the presence of excess $TiCl_4$ the condensation product undergoes cyclization and dehydration to yield 1,2,3,4-tetrahydrochrysene in a single step. This is readily dehydrogenated to chrysene.

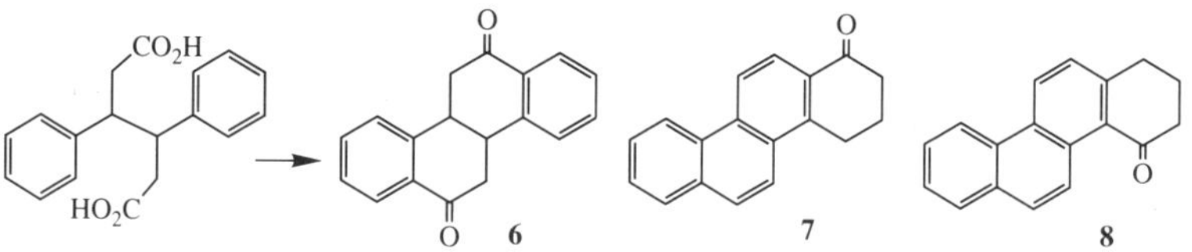

Cyclodehydration is a key step in several other syntheses. Thus, double cyclization of 3,4-diphenyladipic acid with sulfuric acid gives the diketone **6** which on reduction and dehydrogenation yields chrysene (Badger, 1948). Acidic cyclization of 4-(1-phenanthryl)butyric acid affords 1-oxo-1,2,3,4-tetrahydrochrysene (**7**), while analogous reaction of the 2-phenanthryl isomer provides either 4-oxo-1,2,3,4-tetrahydrochrysene (**8**) or 11-oxo-8,9,10,11-tetrahydro-BA, depending upon whether $SnCl_4$ or HF is employed as catalyst (Fig. 7.2) (Bachmann & Struve, 1939; Fieser & Johnson, 1939). The ketone **7** is more conveniently accessible via alkylation of the α-lithio derivative of 1,3- or 1,4-dimethoxy-2,5-cyclohexadiene by α-2-naphthylethyl iodide followed by acidic cyclization of the product (Fig. 7.8) (Harvey *et al.*, 1986). Another cyclodehydration route entails reaction of α-tetralone with the Grignard reagent from 2-phenylethylbromide followed by acidic dehydration, epoxidation, acidic rearrangement to the ketone, and acid-catalyzed cyclization to yield 5,6,11,12-tetrahydrochrysene (Lyle & Daub, 1979) (Fig. 8.3).

Fig. 8.3. Synthesis of tetrahydrochrysene.

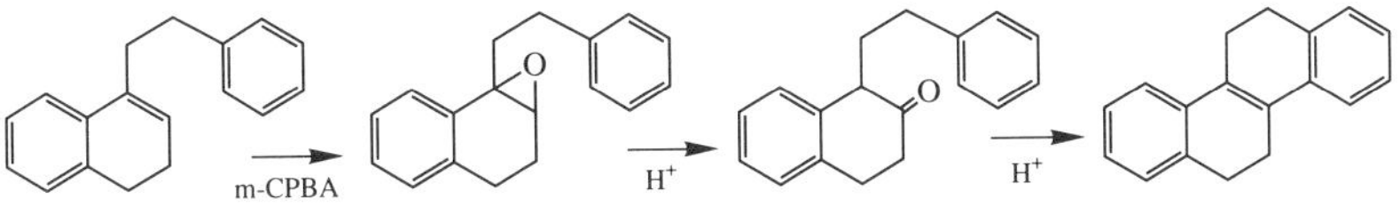

Several syntheses of chrysene involving Diels–Alder cycloaddition are also available. Reaction of 1-vinylnaphthalene with excess benzoquinone furnishes chrysene-1,4-dione which is reduced with $LiAlH_4$ to chrysene (Fig. 7.11) (Davies & Porter, 1957). Reaction of 1,5-naphthodiyne with furan provides a bis adduct which on hydrogenolysis and acidic dehydration yields chrysene (Fig. 7.12) (LeHoullier & Gribble, 1983). Intramolecular Diels–Alder reaction of the *o*-quinodimethane derivative **10a**, generated *in situ* from thermal elimination of SO_2 from **9**, gives hexahydrochrysene which on dehydrogenation furnishes chrysene (Fig. 8.4) (Levy & Sashikumar, 1985).

Chrysene is also synthetically accessible by photochemical cyclo-dehydrogenation of 1-styrylnaphthalene (Wood & Mallory, 1964) and 1,6-diphenylhexa-1,3,5-triene (Fonken, 1962) (Fig. 7.18). This method requires considerable dilution and is more suitable for small scale preparations. The Jutz synthesis involving base-catalyzed condensation of 1-phenanthrylaceto-nitrile with 1,3-bis(dimethylamino)trimethinium perchlorate followed by thermal electrocyclic ring closure and aromatization affords 4-cyanochrysene (Fig. 8.5) (Jutz, 1978). Although chrysene itself has not been prepared via this route, it is potentially obtainable through hydrolysis and decarboxylation of the 4-cyano compound. Another interesting new synthesis entails acid-catalyzed rearrangement of the cyclobutanone derivative **11** to afford **12** which is converted to chrysene via reduction with $LiAlH_4$, dehydration, and

Fig. 8.4. Synthesis of chrysene derivatives via intramolecular Diels–Alder intermediates.

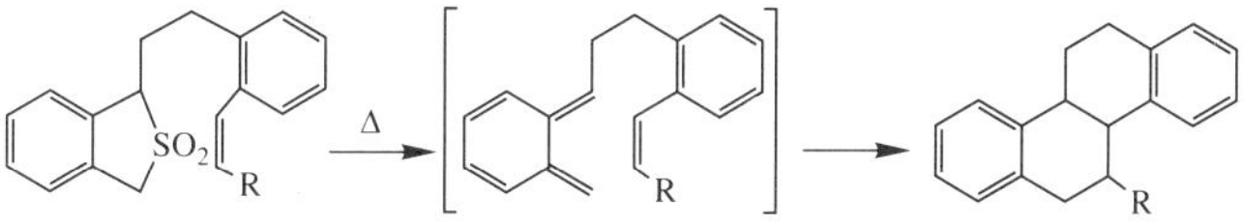

9   10a: R = H
         b: R = CH$_3$

dehydrogenation (Fig. 8.6) (Lee-Ruff *et al.*, 1981). Additional syntheses of less general utility are cited in Clar's book (Clar, 1964).

The six monomethyl isomers of chrysene are synthetically accessible by photocyclization of the appropriate naphthylstyrenes (Nagel *et al.*, 1977; Browne *et al.*, 1978). 5-Methylchrysene, the most carcinogenic isomer, is more conveniently prepared by reductive methylation of chrysene with lithium and methyl iodide (Harvey *et al.*, 1976) followed by dehydrogenation with trityl trifluoroacetate (Fu & Harvey, 1974). Other syntheses of 5-methylchrysene include: $TiCl_4$-catalyzed reaction between 2-(1-naphthyl)-propionaldehyde and 1-trimethylsiloxycyclohexene (Fig. 7.9) (DiRaddo & Harvey, 1988); and intramolecular Diels–Alder reaction of the quinodimethane derivative **10b** (Levy & Sashikumar, 1985).

Reactions Electrophilic attack on chrysene occurs selectively in the 6-position in agreement with theoretical prediction. Thus, the reactions of chrysene with sulfuryl chloride and bromine give 6-chloro- and 6-bromochrysene, respectively, and further halogenation affords the 6,12-dichloro and 6,12-dibromo derivatives (Clar, 1964). Halogenation of chrysene with $TiCl_4$ or $AlBr_3$ catalyzed by NO_2 also affords mainly the 6-halo derivatives (Sugiyama, 1982). Nitration with nitric acid in acetic anhydride (Dewar *et al.*, 1956) or dinitrogen tetroxide (Radner, 1983) give 6-nitrochrysene as the major product. Sulfonation of chrysene with chlorosulfonic acid affords chrysene-6-sulfonic acid (Clar, 1964). While acetylation with acetyl chloride and $AlCl_3$ in CH_2Cl_2 furnishes 6-acetylchrysene, similar reaction in nitrobenzene provides 2-, 3-, and 6-acetylchrysene in the ratio 3:2:1 (Carruthers, 1953). It is likely that the 6-acetyl

Fig. 8.5. Jutz synthesis of 4-cyanochrysene.

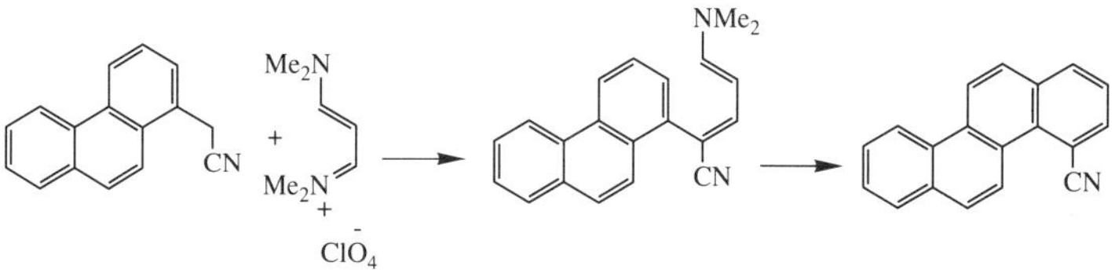

Fig. 8.6. Synthesis of chrysene via acid-catalyzed rearrangement of cyclobutanone derivatives.

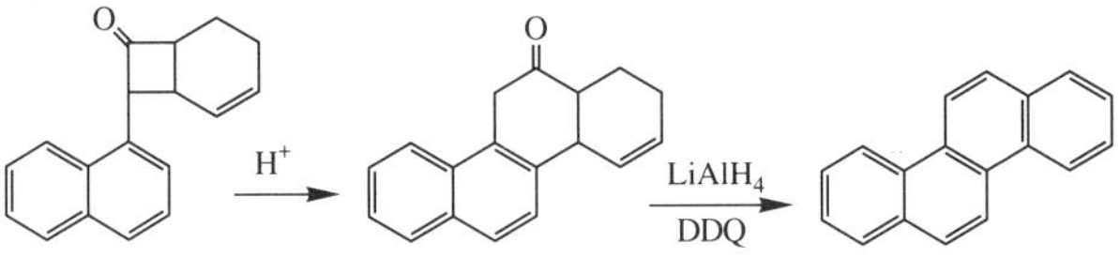

isomer is the *kinetic* product formed initially. It rearranges with greater facility in nitrobenzene to yield the *thermodynamic* product mixture. Analogous Friedel–Crafts reactions with benzoyl chloride (Mabille & Buu-Hoi, 1960), phthalic anhydride (Carruthers, 1953), and succinic anhydride (Beyer, 1938) also afford predominantly the 6-substituted derivatives. Reaction of oxalyl bromide and $AlCl_3$ with chrysene furnishes chrysene-6-carboxylic acid (Hauptmann & Hartig, 1963).

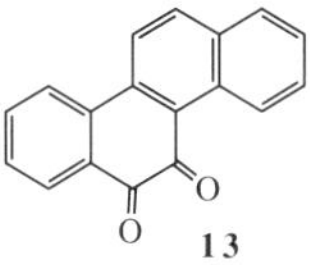

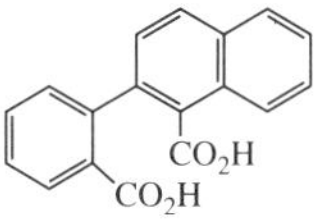

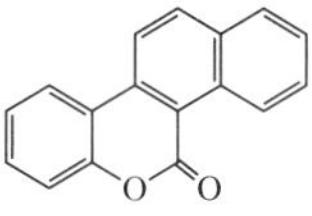

Oxidation of chrysene with sodium dichromate affords smoothly chrysene-5,6-dione **13** (Graebe & Honigsburger, 1900), and ozonolysis yields the dicarboxylic acid **14**. The latter is also obtained along with the lactone **15** on oxidation of chrysene with H_2O_2 in acetic acid (Copeland *et al.*, 1961). Reaction with OsO_4 also takes place in the K-region of chrysene to yield the *cis*-5,6-dihydrodiol **16** (Cook & Schoental, 1948). Chrysene reacts with *N*-bromoacetamide in acetic acid to provide the *trans*-bromohydrin acetate which on treatment with base is converted to chrysene-5,6-oxide (van Bladeren & Jerina, 1983).

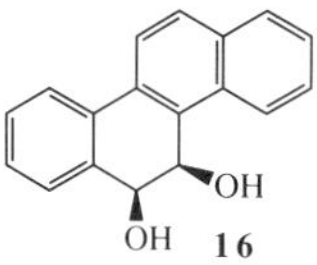

Reduction of chrysene with alkali metals in liquid ammonia can be carried out stepwise with addition of two hydrogens at each stage (Harvey, 1971). The initial product is 5,6-dihydrochrysene (**17**) which is also obtained by ethanolysis of the disodio adduct of chrysene in dimethoxyethane (Harvey *et al.*, 1976). Treatment of the disodio adduct with CO_2 affords the corresponding dicarboxylic acid (Hunt & Lindsey, 1958). Reduction of **17** with Li/NH_3 affords 4b,5,6,12-tetrahydrochrysene (**18**) which is isomerized by mild acid to the 5,6,11,12-isomer (**19**). Further reduction yields *cis*- and *trans*-4b,5,6,10b,11,12-hexahydrochrysene (**20**). Treatment of chrysene with sodium in decalin furnishes a mixture of 1,2,3,4,5,6-hexahydrochrysene (**21**) and **17** (Lang *et al.*, 1965).

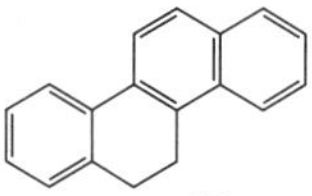

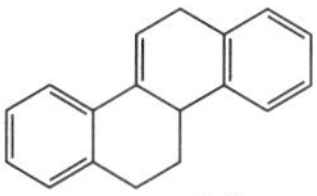

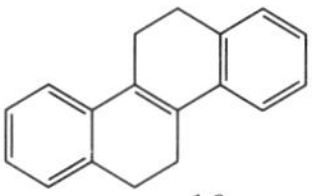

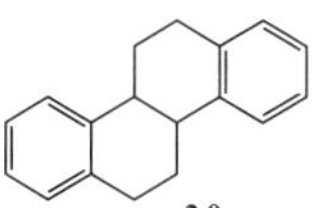

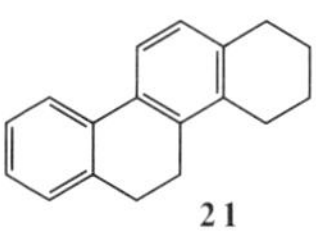

Hydrogenation of chrysene over a palladium catalyst at low pressure and ambient temperature affords regiospecifically the product of hydrogen addition to the K-region **17**, while similar reaction over a platinum catalyst furnishes 1,2,3,4-tetrahydrochrysene (Fu & Harvey, 1979). Hydrogenation over a mixed Pd/Pt catalyst under similar mild conditions yields **21**. With more vigorous conditions, more extensively hydrogenated products are obtained (Clar, 1964).

8.4   Benz[a]anthracene

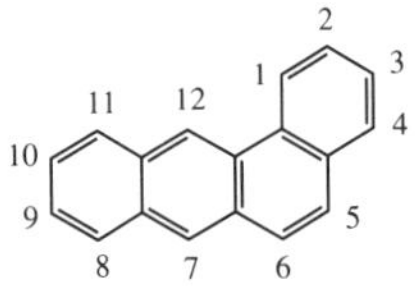

Other names: 1,2-benzanthracene, tetraphene (BA)
Physical and spectral properties $C_{18}H_{12}$, mol. wt. 228.28, colorless plates, mp 160.5-61 °C, sublimes. Dissolves in most common organic solvents, but is sparingly soluble in boiling alcohol; very soluble in benzene. Spectral data: UV (Karcher *et al.*, 1985; TRC, 1982a; Jaffe & Orchin, 1962; Friedel & Orchin, 1951), UV fluorescence (Karcher *et al.*, 1985; Schoental & Scott, 1949), PE (Clar & Schmidt, 1979a), IR (Karcher *et al.*, 1985; Pouchert, 1981; Sadtler), ^{1}H-NMR (Karcher *et al.*, 1985; Memory & Wilson, 1982; TRC, 1982), ^{13}C-NMR (Ozubuku *et al.*, 1974), mass spectrum (Karcher *et al.*, 1985; Stenhagen *et al.*, 1974).

Occurrence and carcinogenicity BA is a significant component of coal tar, atmospheric pollution (Grimmer, 1979; IARC, 1973,1983), automobile exhaust, and cigarette smoke (Snook *et al.*, 1977). It is only weakly carcinogenic in comparison with BaP in most test systems.

Synthesis BA and its derivatives are of central importance in PAH carcinogenesis research, and numerous syntheses of molecules of this class are recorded (Newman *et al.*, 1988; Clar, 1964). The classic method is the Haworth synthesis and its modifications. Reaction of phthalic anhydride with the Grignard reagent derived from 2-bromonaphthalene affords the corresponding ketoacid which undergoes acid-catalyzed cyclization to BA-7,12-dione (Badger & Cook, 1939) (Fig. 7.3). Reduction of BA-7,12-dione, which is commercially available, directly to BA is readily accomplished with HI in acetic acid (Konieczny & Harvey, 1979a, 1984, 1990). Cyclization of the ketoacid and subsequent reduction to BA may be compressed into a single step with the use of HI (Platt & Oesch, 1981). Other variations of the Haworth method include reaction of anthracene and phenanthrene with succinic anhydride and AlCl$_3$. γ-2-Anthranylbutyric acid obtained via this route undergoes SnCl$_4$-catalyzed cyclization to yield 1-oxo-1,2,3,4-tetrahydro-BA (Cook & Robinson, 1938). Similarly, acid-catalyzed cyclization of 4-(3-phenanthryl)butyric acid and 4-(2-phenanthryl)butyric acid yield 8-oxo-8,9,10,11-tetrahydro-BA and 11-oxo-8,9,10,11-tetrahydro-BA, respectively (Fig. 7.2).

One of the newest synthetic approaches to the BA ring system entails reaction of the *o*-lithio salt of *N,N*-diethyl-1-naphthamide (generated by metalation) with benzaldehyde, followed by reduction of the lactone product with zinc and alkali (or zinc and acetic acid), and cyclodehydration with ZnCl$_2$ and acetic anhydride to yield 12-acetoxy-BA (Harvey *et al.*, 1982) (Fig. 8.7). The latter is readily deoxygenated by treatment with HI.

Numerous syntheses of BA derivatives incorporating Diels–Alder cycloaddition have been reported (Fig. 8.8): reaction of 1,6-naphthodiyne (generated *in situ*) with furan affords a bis adduct which is converted to BA by hydrogenation and acidic dehydrogenation (Gribble *et al.*, 1985a); reaction of 1-naphthyne with lithium phthalide, followed by air oxidation of the hydroquinone product yields BA-7,12-dione (Sammes & Dodsworth, 1979); reaction between 1-naphthyne and isoindoles affords the corresponding BA-7,12-imine which on oxidative deamination gives BA (Gribble *et al.*, 1985); reaction between 1-naphthyne and 1,3-bis(trimethylsilyl)-isobenzofuran, both generated *in situ*, furnishes an adduct which may be converted to BA in two steps (Crump *et al.*, 1985); reaction of quinodimethane with 1,2-dihydronaphthalene yields hexahydro-BA which on treatment with DDQ provides BA (Levy & Pruitt, 1980); and reaction between 1,4-naphthoquinone and substituted styrenes furnishes substituted BA-7,12-diones (Muschik *et al.*, 1979).

Other syntheses include: Elbs reaction of α-naphthyl-*o*-tolyl ketone (analogous reaction of the isomeric ketone having the methyl group on the naphthalene ring affords a considerably lower yield) (Fieser, 1942); and Michael addition of methyl vinyl ketone to 2-formyl-1-oxo-1,2,3,4,5,6,7,8-octahydroanthracene, followed by acid-catalyzed cyclization, reduction of the

Fig. 8.7. Synthesis of BA derivatives from metalated arylamides.

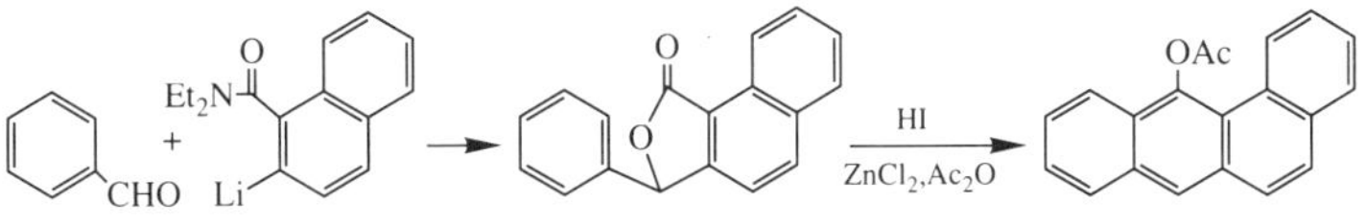

carbonyl, and dehydrogenation (Mukherji *et al.*, 1967; Buchta & Zollner, 1968).

Syntheses of all of the isomeric phenols of BA have also been reported (Fu *et al.*, 1979).

Reactions Electrophilic substitution takes place predominantly in the 7-position of BA in agreement with theoretical prediction. Reaction of BA with bromine in CS_2 (Badger & Cook, 1939,1940) or N-bromosuccinimide in CCl_4 (Lee & Harvey, 1979) furnishes 7-bromo-BA. Treatment of BA with PCl_5 yields 7-chloro-BA (Mikhailov & Kozminskaya, 1951), while chlorination with sulfuryl chloride furnishes both the 7-chloro- and 7,12-dichloro-BA derivatives (Muller & Hanke, 1949). 7-Fluoro-BA is synthetically accessible by pyrolysis of the 7-diazonium fluoroborate of BA (Newman & Lilje, 1979). Nitration of BA with nitrogen dioxide and $TiCl_4$ or with HNO_3 in CH_2Cl_2 yields 7-nitro-BA, apparently regiospecifically (Sugiyama, 1982; Newman & Lilje, 1979), while nitration with HNO_3 in

Fig. 8.8. Synthesis of benz[a]anthracene derivatives by various methods involving Diels–Alder cycloaddition.

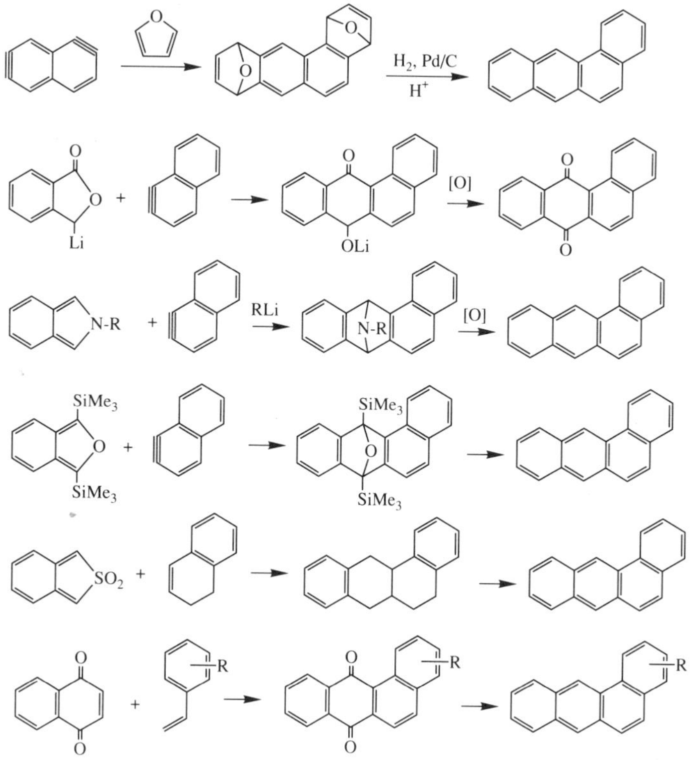

Ac$_2$O yields 7- and 12-nitro-BA and small amounts of four other isomers (Iversen *et al.*, 1985). Reaction of BA with oxalyl chloride and AlCl$_3$ yields BA-7-carboxylic acid along with the 1,2-dihydrobenz[e]aceanthrylene-1,2-dione and 1,2-dihydrobenz[j]aceanthrylene-1,2-dione (Dansi, 1937; Miller *et al.*, 1984). Friedel–Crafts acylation of BA with acetic anhydride and AlCl$_3$ is less regiospecific, furnishing 7-, 9-, and 10-acetoxy-BA and two additional monoacetoxy-BA products (Fieser & Hershberg, 1938; Cook & Hewett, 1933). Reaction of BA with methylformanilide and POCl$_3$ yields 7-formyl-BA (Fieser & Hartwell, 1939).

Oxidation of BA with either chromic acid (Graebe, 1905) or periodic acid (Fatiadi, 1967) takes place in the meso region to furnish BA 7,12-dione. Reaction of BA with OsO$_4$ occurs in the K-region to provide the *cis*-5,6-dihydrodiol of BA (Harvey *et al.*, 1975; Cook & Schoental, 1948).

Reduction of BA may be controlled to yield a variety of hydroaromatic products. The initial reduction of BA with Li or Na in liquid ammonia takes place in the meso region in accord with MO theoretical prediction to furnish 7,12-dihydro-BA (Harvey & Urberg, 1968; Harvey *et al.*, 1969; Harvey, 1970) . The same dihydro isomer (**22**) is obtained from methanolysis of the disodio adduct of BA (Bachmann, 1936). Further stepwise reduction of **22** with Li/NH$_3$ yields **23** and **24**. Reduction of BA with Na and amyl alcohol yields hexahydro-BA (**25**) which is reduced by Li/NH$_3$ to octahydro-BA (**26**) and by lithium in methylamine to dodecahydro-BA (**27**) (Harvey & Urberg, 1968). Hydrogenation of BA over a Pd catalyst occurs regiospecifically in the K-region under mild conditions to yield 5,6-dihydro-BA (**28**), while hydrogen addition in the presence of a Pt catalyst takes place in the terminal ring to provide tetrahydro-BA (**29**) (Fu *et al.*, 1980).

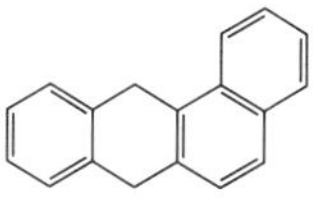

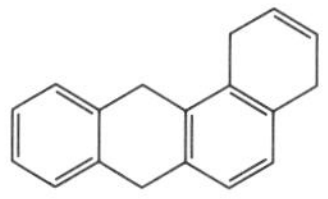

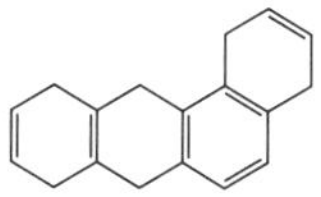

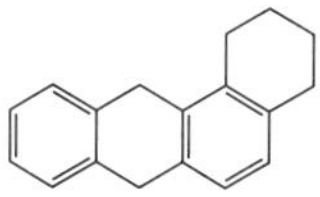

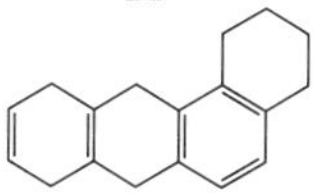

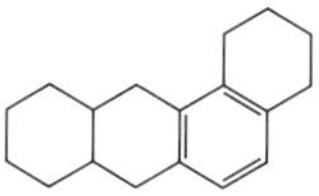

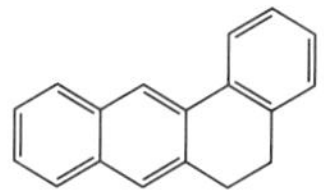

Diels–Alder cycloadditions with dienophiles, such as maleic anhydride, take place in the meso region of BA. Sublimation of the BA–maleic anhydride adduct regenerates BA (Clar, 1932). In sunlight, BA forms a photodimer covalently linked at the 7,12-positions which dissociates on heating to regenerate BA (Schoenberg *et al.*, 1948).

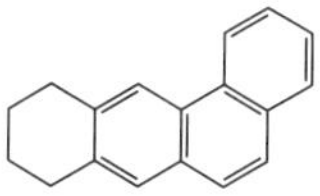

All of the isomeric monomethyl-BAs and numerous di- and trimethyl-BAs are known, and many of these are carcinogenic (Chap. 3, Tables 3.5 and 3.6).

8.5   7,12-Dimethylbenz[a]anthracene

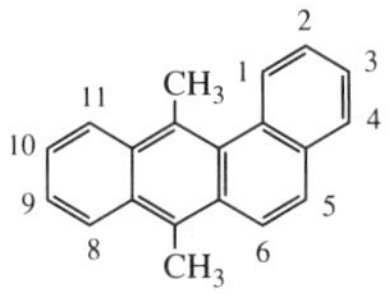

***Other names: 9,10-dimethyl-1,2-benzanthracene* (DMBA)**

Physical and spectral properties $C_{20}H_{16}$, mol. wt. 256.36, thin plates, mp 122-23 °C, sublimes. Dissolves in most common solvents more readily than BA. X-ray crystal structure data on DMBA is available (Klein *et al.*, 1987). Spectral data: UV (Karcher, 1988; TRC, 1983a; Friedel & Orchin, 1951; Sadtler), IR (Karcher, 1988; Pouchert, 1981; Sadtler), ^{1}H-NMR (Karcher, 1988; Memory & Wilson, 1982; TRC, 1983), ^{13}C-NMR (Karcher, 1988; Ozubuku *et al.*, 1974), mass spectrum (Karcher, 1988; Stenhagen *et al.*, 1974), PE spectrum (Akiyama *et al.*, 1981).

Occurrence and carcinogenicity Despite claims to the contrary, DMBA probably does not occur as an environmental pollutant. In any case, it is unlikely that it would survive very long due to the facility of its conversion to its photooxide and ease of decomposition by other pathways. For the same reason, DMBA should always be purified prior to use in chemical and biological studies by chromatography on alumina or silica gel and protected from air and light. Since appropriate precautions were not always observed in the early biological studies, the data must be treated with caution. DMBA is one of the most potent carcinogenic PAHs known (Table 3.6). This has led to its wide use in experimental investigations of mouse skin and rat mammary gland tumorigenesis. The DMBA-induced rat mammary developed by Huggins is the standard laboratory animal model in the study of breast cancer (Welsch, 1985).

Synthesis The most convenient syntheses of DMBA are based upon BA-7,12-dione which is commercially available. Addition of methyllithium or methylmagnesium bromide to the quinone affords the dimethyldiol adduct (Fig. 8.9) which may be converted to DMBA by various procedures. Fieser's method entails treatment of the adduct with HI in methanol to form 7-iodomethyl-12-methyl-BA and reduction of this with $SnCl_2$ and HCl (Sandin

& Fieser, 1940). Subsequent modifications employ anhydrous HCl in place of HI and yield the analogous 7-chloromethyl adduct which is reduced to DMBA with SnCl$_2$ (Newman *et al.*, 1978) or NaBH$_4$ (Sukumaran & Harvey, 1980). More recently it was found that the adduct may be reduced directly to DMBA in a single step by treatment with HI in acetic acid (Konieczny & Harvey, 1980) or TiCl$_3$·LiAlH$_4$ (Harvey & Cortez, 1986).

Reactions DMBA is highly susceptible to various modes of oxidation. On exposure to air and light, DMBA undergoes photooxidation to yield the 7,12-epidioxide along with other oxidized products (Cook & Martin, 1940; Logani *et al.*, 1977). Reaction with OsO$_4$ takes place in the K-region to yield the *cis*-5,6-dihydrodiol (Harvey *et al.*, 1975). Oxidation of DMBA with periodate and catalytic amount of OsO$_4$ provides the dialdehyde **30** arising from cleavage of the 5,6-bond (Fig. 8.10) (Harvey *et al.*, 1975). The latter on treatment with hexamethylphosphorus triamide undergoes cyclization to yield DMBA-5,6-oxide (**31**). The reactions of DMBA with other oxidants takes place primarily on the methyl groups. For example, reaction with lead tetraacetate in acetic acid affords the 7- and 12-acetoxymethyl and 7,12-bis(acetoxymethyl) derivatives which on treatment with KOH in methanol are converted to the corresponding hydroxymethyl derivatives (Boyland & Sims, 1965). Reaction of DMBA with one-electron oxidants, such as MnO$_2$ and ceric ammonium nitrate, yields a mixture of 12-methyl-12-hydroxybenz[a]anthrone, 7-methyl-7-hydroxybenz[a]anthrone, 7-methyl-12-formyl-BA, BA-7,12-dione, and other oxidized products (Fried & Schumm, 1967). One-electron oxidation with I$_2$ in pyridine affords a mixture

Fig. 8.9. Synthesis of 7,12-dimethylbenz[a]anthracene.

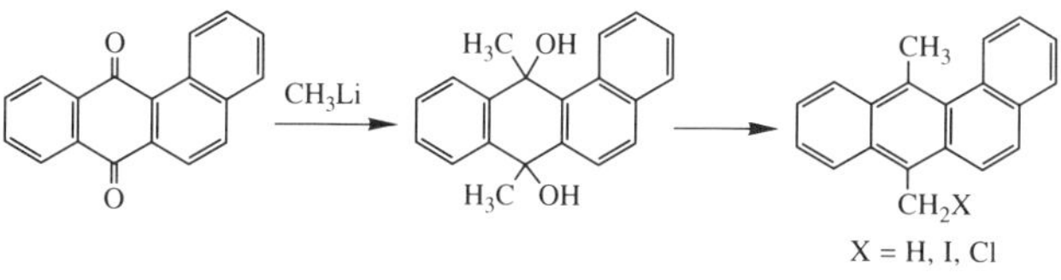

Fig. 8.10. Synthesis of DMBA 5,6-oxide via direct oxidation of DMBA.

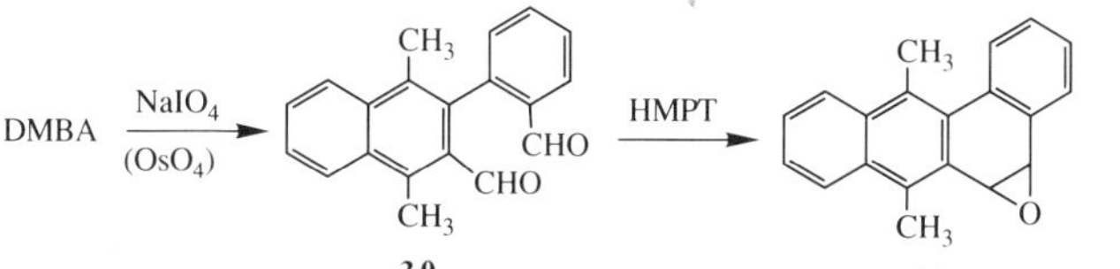

of three pyridinium salts in which the nitrogen atom is attached to the 7-methyl-, 12-methyl-, or 5-positions of DMBA (Cavalieri & Roth, 1976).

DMBA also reacts with bromine in CS_2 to yield 7,12-bis(bromomethyl)-BA (Badger & Cook, 1939) and enters into Diels–Alder cycloaddition reactions with maleic anhydride and other dienophiles more readily than BA (Bachmann & Chemerda, 1938).

Catalytic hydrogenation of DMBA over a palladium catalyst gives 5,6-dihydro-DMBA (80%) and 7,12-dihydro-DMBA (20%), while hydrogenation over platinum provides 8,9,10,11-tetrahydro-BA (Fu *et al.*, 1980). Reduction with Li/NH_3 is similar to that of BA, affording 7,12-dihydro-BA as the product in the initial stage (Harvey, 1970).

8.6   3-Methylcholanthrene

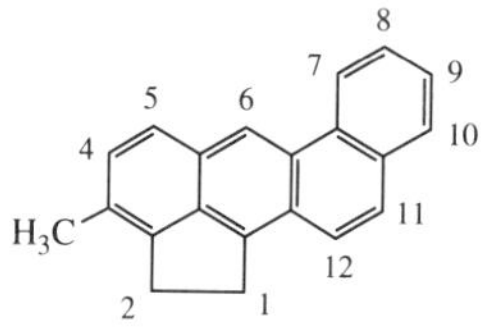

***Other names: 1,2-dihydro-3-methylbenz[j]aceanthrylene* (3-MC)**
Physical and spectral properties $C_{21}H_{16}$, mol. wt. 268.37, pale yellow prisms, mp 179-80 °C. Soluble in most common organic solvents. Spectral data: UV (Karcher, 1988; TRC, 1983a), UV fluorescence (Karcher, 1988; Sawicki *et al.*, 1960), IR (Karcher, 1988; Sadtler), ^{1}H-NMR (Karcher, 1988; TRC, 1983), ^{13}C-NMR (Karcher, 1988; Ozubu *et al.*, 1974), mass spectrum (Karcher, 1988; Stenhagen *et al.*, 1974).

Occurrence and carcinogenicity Like DMBA, 3-MC is not formed in the combustion of fossil fuels and it is unlikely that it would survive long in the environment because of its high chemical reactivity. 3-MC is one of the most potent carcinogenic PAHs known, exhibiting activity similar to that of DMBA.

Synthesis The classical synthetic approach to 3-MC involves Elbs pyrolysis of the ketone obtained from reaction of naphthoyl chloride with the Grignard reagent of 7-bromo-4-methylindane (Fig. 7.23). A more modern synthesis, which is adaptable to the preparation of the carcinogenic 9,10-dihydrodiol metabolite of 3-MC, involves condensation of 4-methylindanone with the lithium salt of *N,N*-diethylnaphthamide (Fig. 7.7). Reduction of the lactone product with zinc and alkali and cyclization of the resulting carboxylic acid with Ac$_2$O-AcOH yields 6-acetoxy-3-MC which is converted to 3-MC on treatment with HI in propionic acid (Harvey *et al.*, 1982). This approach is readily modified for the preparation of cholanthrene itself and the highly carcinogenic 6-methylcholanthrene (Harvey & Cortez, 1987). 9-Methoxy-3-MC, the synthetic precursor of the carcinogenic 9,10-dihydrodiol metabolite of 3-MC has also been synthesized via this route (Jacobs *et al.*, 1983).

Syntheses of cholanthrene and 1-, 2-, 4-, 5-, 6-, 7-, and 11-methylcholanthrene have also been described (Harvey & Cortez, 1987; Newman *et al.*, 1966; Bachmann *et al.*, 1941; Fieser *et al.*, 1940).

Reactions 3-MC tends to react predominantly in the meso region. Oxidation with chromic acid under mild conditions affords 3-MC-1-one (Fieser & Hershberg, 1938a) and under more vigorous conditions provides 9-methyl-BA-7,12-dione-8-carboxylic acid (Cook & Haselwood, 1934). Reaction of 3-MC with Pb(OAc)$_4$ yields 1-acetoxy-3-MC along with other oxidized products (Sims, 1966; Fieser & Hershberg, 1938a). Reaction of 3-MC with Br$_2$ followed by dehydrobromination with pyridine furnishes 3-methylbenz[j]aceanthrylene (Sims, 1966; Cavalieri *et al.*, 1978). However, reaction with OsO$_4$ takes place in the K-region to yield the *cis*-11,12-dihydrodiol (Cook & Schoental, 1948).

Hydrogenation of 3-MC over a Pd/C catalyst also occurs in the K-region to provide 11,12-dihydro-3-MC (Fu *et al.*, 1980), while hydrogenation over a mixed Pd/Pt catalyst furnishes 6,7,8,9,10,12b-hexahydro-3-MC (Fieser & Hershberg, 1938b). Reduction of 3-MC with Li/NH$_3$ affords mainly the product of addition in the meso region, 6,12b-dihydro-3-MC (Harvey *et al.*, 1969; Harvey, 1970). Reductive methylation with Na/CH$_3$I followed by dehydrogenation with sulfur yields 3,6-dimethylcholanthrene (Newman & Sujeeth, 1983).

8.7   Naphthacene

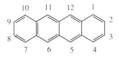

Other names: tetracene, 2,3-benzanthracene

Physical and spectral properties C$_{18}$H$_{12}$, mol. wt. 228.28, orange–yellow leaflets (xylene), mp 357 °C, sublimes. Poorly soluble in most common solvents. Spectral data: UV (Karcher, 1988; TRC, 1985; Jaffe & Orchin, 1962; Friedel & Orchin, 1951), UV fluorescence (Karcher, 1988; Berlman, 1971; Schoental & Scott, 1949), IR (Karcher, 1988; Sadtler;

Karcher *et al.*, 1985), ^{1}H-NMR (Karcher, 1988; TRC, 1986; Karcher *et al.*, 1985), ^{13}C-NMR (Karcher, 1988; Vysotskii & Mestechkin, 1975), mass spectrum (Karcher, 1988; Stenhagen *et al.*, 1974).

Occurrence and carcinogenicity Naphthacene is found in coal tar and low levels are detected as an environmetal pollutant. It is generally considered to be inactive as a carcinogen.

Synthesis The classical synthetic approaches to naphthacene entail cyclodehydration of carboxylic acid intermediates (Fig. 8.11). Condensation of phthalic anhydride with tetralin and AlCl3 takes place in the 2-position to form the keto acid **32** which is cyclized in sulfuric acid to yield a mixture of the quinones **33** and **34** (Clar, 1942). Compare the analogous synthesis of BA in which condensation of phthalic anhydride with naphthalene takes place in the 1-position (Fig. 7.3). Distillation of **33** with zinc dust and copper powder furnishes naphthacene (Clar, 1932). Naphthacene may also be obtained by reduction of **32** with zinc and alkali to a mixture of the phthalide **35** and the free acid **36**, followed by fusion of the mixture with ZnCl2 and NaCl to yield 5,12-dihydronaphthacene which may be dehydrogenated to naphthacene (Clar, 1942). Other variations of this approach include cyclization of 3-benzoyl-2-naphthoic acid or o-naphthoylbenzoic acid with AlCl3–NaCl to naphthacene-5,12-dione (Waldmann & Mathiowetz, 1931; Weizmann *et al.*, 1935).

Several newer synthetic approaches to naphthacene make use of Diels–Alder cycloaddition (Fig. 8.12). Reaction of 2-methylisoindole with 2,3-naphthyne (generated from 2,3-dibromonaphthalene and phenyllithium) provides an adduct which on treatment with *m*-chloroperbenzoic acid yields naphthacene (LeHoullier & Gribble, 1983). Similar reaction of 1,3-bis(trimethylsilyl)isobenzofuran with 2,3-naphthyne affords an adduct which is

Fig. 8.11.   Synthetic routes to naphthacene derivatives involving cyclohydration.

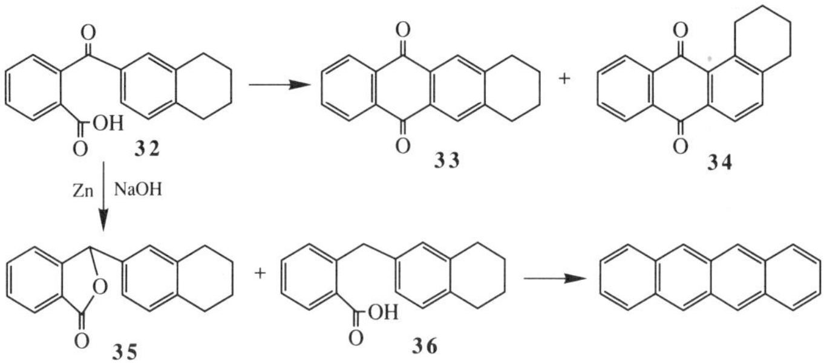

also readily transformed to naphthacene (Netka *et al.*, 1986). Reaction of furan with 2,6-naphthodiyne yields a bis adduct which on catalytic hydrogenation and acidic dehydration furnishes naphthacene (Gribble *et al.*, 1985a). Also, reaction of isobenzofuran with 1,4-naphthoquinone affords naphthacene-5,12-dione (Smith & Dibble, 1983), and reaction of naphtho[2,3-c]furan with *p*-benzoquinone gives naphthacene-1,4-dione in poor yield (Smith *et al.*, 1986).

Additional syntheses of naphthacene and its derivatives are surveyed by Clar, 1964.

Reactions The chemistry of naphthacene parallels that of anthracene. Electrophilic reactions take place mainly in the central rings, with preferential monosubstitution in the 5-position and disubstitution in the 5,11-positions. Bromination with $CuBr_2$ yields 5-bromonaphthacene, while reaction with bromine affords 5,11-dibromonaphthacene (Marschalk & Stumm, 1948). Reaction with sulfuryl chloride yields 5-chloro- and 5,11-dichloronaphthacene (Marschalk & Stumm, 1948; Martynoff, 1954). Vilsmeier reaction of naphthacene provides 5-formylnaphthacene (Meek & Dewey, 1970).

Diels–Alder cycloadditions take place in the 5,12-positions of naphthacene more readily than they do with anthracene (Meek *et al.*, 1967). Diels–Alder reactions of 5-bromo-, 5-cyano-, 5-formyl-, and 5,12-diacetoxynaphthacene occur preferentially at the 6,11-positions (Meek & Dewey, 1970).

Naphthacene undergoes photooxidation in air to yield a transannular epidioxide (Dufraisse & Horclois, 1936). Irradiation of naphthacene in the absence of air yields a mixture of the 5,12 + 5,12 and 5,12 + 6,11

Fig. 8.12. Diels–Alder synthetic routes to naphthacene.

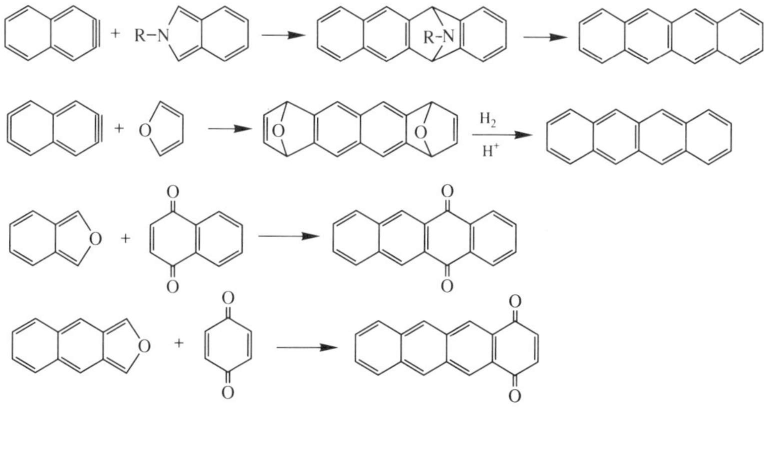

photodimers (LaPouyade *et al.*, 1980). Oxidation with chromic acid or periodic acid gives naphthacene-5,12-dione (Fatiadi, 1967). The latter is also a product of ozonolysis of naphthacene along with anthraquinone-2,3-dicarboxylic acid (Copeland *et al.*, 1961).

Reduction of naphthacene by Li/NH_3 (Harvey *et al.*, 1969) or by hydrazine and sodium hydrazide (Kauffmann *et al.*, 1963) both afford 5,12-dihydronaphthacene.

8.8   Pyrene

Physical and spectral properties $C_{16}H_{10}$, mol. wt. 202.24, colorless plates (alcohol), mp 156° C, sublimes. Soluble in most solvents with pale blue fluorescence. Spectral data: UV (Karcher *et al.*, 1985; TRC, 1982a; Jaffe & Orchin, 1962; Friedel & Orchin, 1951), UV fluorescence (Berlman, 1971; Schoental & Scott, 1949), PE (Clar & Schmidt, 1979a), IR (Pouchert, 1981; Karcher *et al.*, 1985), ^{1}H- and ^{13}C-NMR (Karcher *et al.*, 1985; Memory & Wilson, 1982; TRC, 1982), mass spectrum (Stenhagen *et al.*, 1974; Karcher *et al.*, 1985).

Occurrence and carcinogenicity Pyrene is found in relatively high levels in coal tar and is commonly obtained from this source. Pyrene and methylpyrenes are common atmospheric pollutants which are also present in carbon black, engine exhaust, and cigarette and marijuana smoke (Grimmer, 1979; IARC, 1983). It is generally considered to be noncarcinogenic.

Synthesis Pyrene itself is readily available, so that syntheses are of interest mainly for the preparation of substituted pyrenes or as models for the construction of larger polycyclic ring systems. A classical synthesis entails Reformatski reaction of 4-oxo-1,2,3,4-tetrahydrophenanthrene, followed by hydrogenation and cyclodehydration to yield a cyclized ketone convertible to pyrene by standard methods (Bachmann & Edgerton, 1940) (Fig. 8.13).

Other syntheses include: Jutz synthesis involving condensation of phenalene with a 'vinamidinium salt' followed by thermal electrocyclic ring closure (Jutz, 1978); cyclization of 2,2'-biphenyldiacetic acid and reduction with zinc dust (Chatterjee *et al.*, 1947); photocyclization of 2,2'-divinylbiphenyl (Padwa & Mazzu, 1974) and 4-vinylphenanthrene (Horgan *et al.*, 1973); reductive cyclization of 2,2',6,6'-tetraformylbiphenyl with hydrazine (Bacon & Lindsay, 1958), dehydrogenation of 2,2-metacyclophane over palladium (Baker *et al.*, 1951), and treatment of 4,5-bis(bromomethyl)-phenanthrene with phenyllithium (Marvel & Wilson, 1958) (Fig. 7.28).

Reactions Electrophilic substitutions take place predominantly in the 1-position of pyrene. Chlorination, nitration, and formylation afford 1-chloro-, 1-nitro-, and 1-formylpyrene, respectively (Vollmann *et al.*, 1937). Further reaction gives the 1,6- and 1,8-disubstituted, 1,6,8-trisubstituted, and 1,3,6,8-tetrasubstituted products. Chlorination with sulfuryl chloride in CCl_4 affords tetrachloropyrene as the main product. 1-Bromopyrene is conveniently synthesized from pyrene by reaction with NBS in CCl_4 (Buu-Hoi & LeCocq, 1948) or dimethylformamide (Mitchell *et al.*, 1979) or $CuBr_2$ in chlorobenzene (Nonhebel, 1963). 1-Bromopyrene on treatment with bromine furnishes a mixture of 1,6- and 1,8-dibromopyrene which on further reaction with bromine is converted to 1,3,6-tribromopyrene (Grimshaw & Trocha-Grimshaw, 1972). While direct reaction of pyrene with iodine affords 1-iodopyrene in only low yield, this compound may be efficiently synthesized by treatment of pyrene with ICN and $AlCl_3$ (Radner, 1989). Iodination of pyrene with I_2–HIO_3–H_2SO_4 gives a mixture of 1,6- and 1,8-diiodopyrene, with the former predominating at lower temperature and the latter at higher temperature (Chaikovskii & Novikov, 1984). Nitration of pyrene with dinitrogen tetroxide in CH_2Cl_2 furnishes 1-nitropyrene virtually quantitatively (Radner, 1983). 1-Nitropyrene is also obtained in high yield from an oxidative nucleophilic substitution reaction of pyrene with sodium peroxydisulfate as the oxidizing agent and nitrite as the nucleophile (van den Braken-van Leersum *et al.*, 1987)

Friedel–Crafts reactions also occur preferentially in the 1-position. Reaction of pyrene with carbamyl chloride and $AlCl_3$ affords 1-pyrenecarboxylic amide which on saponification gives 1-pyrenecarboxylic acid (Vollmann *et al.*, 1937). This acid is obtained directly from reaction of pyrene with oxalyl chloride and $AlCl_3$; however, the major product is $(C_{16}H_9C=O)_2$ formed from reaction of oxalyl chloride on two pyrenes

Fig. 8.13. Synthesis of pyrene via Reformatski reaction and acidic cyclization.

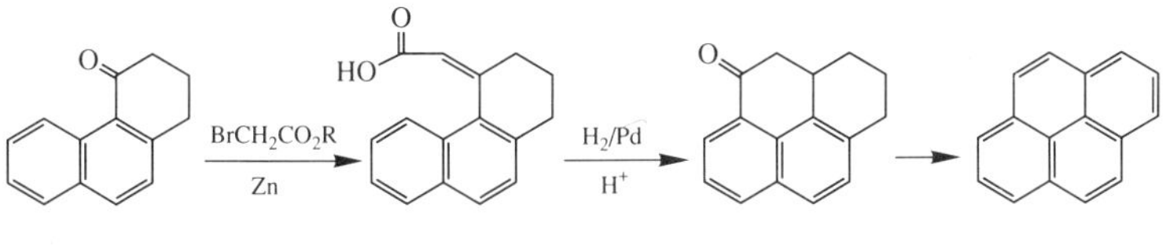

(Miller *et al.*, 1984). The reactions of pyrene with acetyl chloride and propionyl chloride in nitrobenzene yield 1-acetyl- and 1-propionylpyrene, respectively (Vollmann *et al.*, 1937), while acetylation of pyrene with acetyl chloride and AlCl$_3$ in CS$_2$ affords 1,3-, 1,6-, and 1,8-diacetylpyrene in the ratio of 1:1:3 (Harvey *et al.*, 1984). Analogous benzoylation and chloroacetylation of pyrene provides a mixture of the corresponding 1,6- and 1,8-disubstituted products (Harvey *et al.*, 1984). Vilsmeier reaction of pyrene with formylmethylaniline and POCl$_3$ gives 1-pyrenecarboxaldehyde (Rieche *et al.*, 1960), and reaction of pyrene with chloroacetic acid in dichlorobenzene yields pyrenyl-1-acetic acid (Vollmann *et al.*, 1937). The Friedel–Crafts reactions of pyrene with succinic and phthalic anhydrides afford the corresponding 1-substituted products (Barker *et al.*, 1955) which are useful synthetic precursors of polyarenes with one or two additional rings.

While 2- and 4-substituted pyrenes are not formed by direct substitution, they are readily accessible from reactions of 4,5,9,10-tetrahydro- and 1,2,3,6,7,8-hexahydropyrene, respectively (Fig. 6.5). Thus, nitration of tetrahydropyrene followed by dehydrogenation affords 2-nitropyrene, and acetylation of tetrahydropyrene with acetyl chloride in CS$_2$ followed by DDQ dehydrogenation furnishes 2-acetylpyrene (Bolton, 1964; Harvey *et al.*, 1983; van den Bracken-van Leersum, 1987). Similar acetylation in CH$_2$Cl$_2$ yields 2,7-diacetyl-4,5,9,10-tetrahydropyrene (Harvey *et al.*, 1983). Treatment of tetrahydropyrene with bromine in aqueous dimethylformamide and dehydrogenation affords 2-bromopyrene (Harvey *et al.*, 1988), whereas similar reaction in an aqueous medium furnishes principally 2,7-dibromopyrene (Lee & Harvey, 1986a). Bromination (Konieczny & Harvey, 1979), acetylation (Vollmann *et al.*, 1937), and nitration (Bavin, 1959) of

Fig. 8.14. Ozonolysis of pyrene.

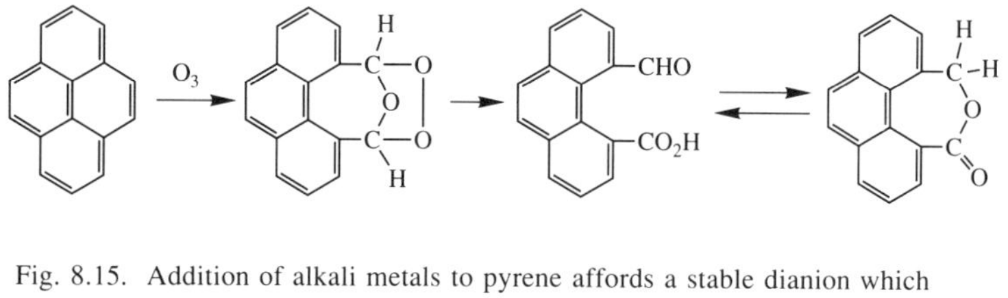

Fig. 8.15. Addition of alkali metals to pyrene affords a stable dianion which undergoes proton addition in the 1,9-positions.

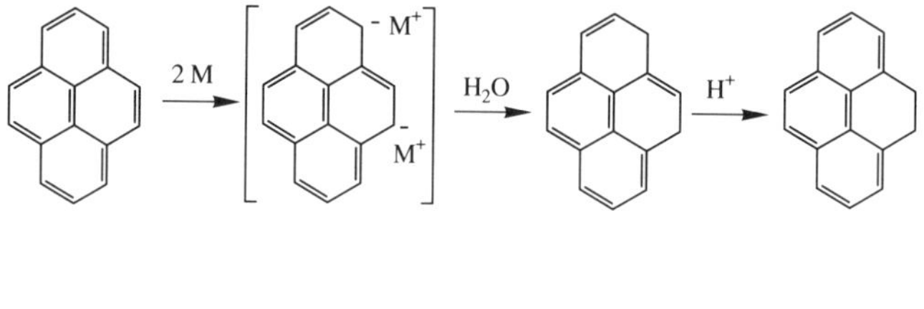

hexahydropyrene followed by dehyrogenation give 4-bromo-, 4-acetyl-, and 4-nitropyrene, respectively.

Oxidation of pyrene with sodium dichromate in acetic anhydride–acetic acid gives a mixture of the pyrene 1,6- and 1,8-diones which are separable only by careful chromatographic procedures (Cho & Harvey, 1976). Ozonolysis of pyrene furnishes a monoozonide which rearranges to 5-formylphenanthrene-4-carboxylic acid (Sturrock & Duncan, 1968) (Fig. 8.14). The latter acid is obtained in low yield along with pyrene-4,5-dione from oxidation of pyrene with OsO_4 and periodate (Oberender & Dixon, 1959). Oxidation of pyrene with OsO_4 alone furnishes the *cis*-4,5-dihydrodiol (Cook & Schoental, 1948). The reaction of pyrene with iodoxybenzene also occurs in the K-region to provide mainly pyrene-4,5-dione (Ranganathan *et al.*, 1984). Oxidation of 4,5-dihydropyrene with sodium dichromate in acetic anhydride–acetic acid under mild conditions yields pyrene-4,5-dione (Cho & Harvey, 1974). Oxidative coupling of pyrene to form 1,1'-bipyrene occurs on treatment of pyrene with periodic acid (Fatiadi, 1967) or $AlCl_3$–$CuCl_2$ (Guenther & Kovacic, 1984); the latter reagent also affords the products of further cyclodehydrogenation, 1.10',10.1'-bipyrene and 1.1',10.10'-bipyrene.

The reaction of pyrene with alkali metals affords a stable dianion. Protonation yields 1,9-dihydropyrene which rearranges with acid to 4,5-dihydropyrene (Harvey & Rabideau, 1970) (Fig. 8.15). Alkylation of the dianion occurs preferentially in the 9-position, providing a convenient synthesis of 4-methyl-4,5-dihydropyrene which on treatment with DDQ is converted to 4-methylpyrene (Tintel *et al.*, 1983). Low pressure hydrogenation of pyrene provides 4,5,9,10-tetrahydropyrene essentially quantitatively (Harvey *et al.*, 1983); with shorter reaction time, 4,5-dihydropyrene may be isolated (Fu *et al.*, 1980). Hydrogenation of pyrene over a copper chromite catalyst under more vigorous conditions affords a mixture of the symmetrical 1,2,3,6,7,8- and the asymmetrical 1,2,3,3a,4,5-hexahydropyrene isomers (Triebs & Mann, 1958; Cameron *et al.*, 1945). The reaction of pyrene with sodium in amyl alcohol provides a mixture of the same hexahydropyrene isomers (Cook & Hewett, 1933a; Coulson, 1937).

Pyrene also undergoes nucleophilic addition of alkyllithium reagents. Addition of methyllithium to pyrene and dehydrogenation of the product with iodine gives 4-methylpyrene (Peake *et al.*, 1983).

8.9   References

Akiyama, I., LeBreton, P. R. & Harvey, R. G. (1981). Ultraviolet photoelectron studies of methyl substituted benz[a]anthracene. *J. Amer. Chem. Soc.* **103**, 6330–2.

Amer, I., Amer, H., Ascher, R., Blum, J., Sasson, Y., and Vollhardt, K. P. (1987).

Hydrogenation of arenes by the RhCl$_3$-ALIQUAT™336 catalyst. Part 3. Selective reduction of polycyclic compounds. *J. Mol. Catalysis*, **39**, 185–94.

Bachmann, W. E. (1936). The reactions of alkali metals with polycyclic hydrocarbons: 1,2-benzanthracene, 1,2,5,6-dibenzanthracene and methylcholanthrene. *J. Org. Chem.* **1**, 347–53.

Bachmann, W. E. & Chemerda, J. (1938). The synthesis of 9,10-dimethyl-1,2-benzanthracene, 9,10-diethyl-1,2-benzanthracene and 5,9,10-trimethyl-1,2-benzanthracene. *J. Amer. Chem. Soc.* **60**, 1023–6.

Bachmann, W. E. & Chemerda, J. (1941). The synthesis of 4-methylcholanthrene and 5-methylcholanthrene. *J. Org. Chem.* **6**, 50–3.

Bachmann, W. E. & Edgerton, O. (1940). The synthesis of 3,4-benzphenanthrene and 1-methylpyrene. *J. Amer. Chem. Soc.* **62**, 2970–3.

Bacon, R. G. & Lindsay, W. S. (1958). Cyclisations with hydrazine. Part I. The preparation of phenanthrene compounds and of pyrene from aldehydes. A variation in reductions of the Wolff–Kishner type. *J. Chem. Soc.* 1375–81.

Badger, G. M. (1948). A modified synthesis of chrysene. *J. Chem. Soc.* 999–1001.

Badger, G. M. & Cook, J. W. (1939). The synthesis of growth-inhibitory polycyclic compounds. Part I.. *J. Chem. Soc.* 802–6.

Badger, G. M. & Cook, J. W. (1940). The synthesis of growth-inhibitory polycyclic compounds. Part II. *J. Chem. Soc.* 409–12.

Baker, W., McOmie, J. F. & Norman, J. M. (1951). Eight- and higher-membered ring compounds. Part IV. Di-*m*-xylylene, tri-*p*-xylylene, and new syntheses of pyrene and coronene. *J. Chem. Soc.* 1114–18.

Barker, C. C., Emmerson, R. G. & Periam, J. D. (1955). The monosubstitution of triphenylene. *J. Chem. Soc.* 4482–5.

Barton, J. M. & McOmie, J. F. W. (1956). Triphenylene and 2-methyltriphenylene. *J. Chem. Soc.* 796–7.

Bavin, P. M. (1959). 4-Nitropyrene. *Canad. J. Chem.* **37**, 1614–15.

Bax, A., Ferretti, J. A., Nashed, N. & Jerina, D. M. (1985). Complete ^{1}H and ^{13}C NMR assignment of complex polycyclic aromatic hydrocarbons. *J. Org. Chem.* **50**, 3029–34.

Bergmann, E. & Blum-Bergmann, O. (1937). Synthesis of triphenylene. *J. Am. Chem. Soc.* **59**, 1441–2.

Berlman, I. B. (1971). *Handbook of Fluorescence Spectra of Aromatic Molecules*, New York: Academic Press.

Beyer, H. (1938). The condensation of chrysene with succinic anhydride. *Chem. Ber.* **71**, 915–22.

Bolton, R. (1964). Tetrahydropyrene as a source of 2-pyrenyl derivatives. *J. Chem. Soc.* 4637–8.

Bolton, R., de la Mare, P. B. D. & Main, L. (1969). The kinetics and mechanisms of aromatic halogen substitution. Part XXVII. Substitution products in the chlorination of triphenylene. *J. Chem. Soc.* 170–2.

Boyland, E. & Sims, P. (1965). Metabolism of polycyclic compounds. The metabolism of 7,12-dimethylbenz[a]anthracene by rat liver homogenates. *Biochem. J.* **95**, 780–7.

Browne, C. E., Dobbs, T. K., Hecht, S., S. & Eisenbraun, E. J. (1978). Stereochemical assignment of (E)- and (Z)-2-(1-naphthyl)-1-phenylpropene and their photocyclization to 5-methylchrysene. *J. Org. Chem.* **43**, 1656–60.

Buchta, E. & Zollner, R. (1968). Benzo[a]pyrene and benz[a]anthracene. *Liebigs Ann.Chem.* **716**, 102–5.

Buu-Hoi, N. P .& Jacquignon, P. (1953). Friedel–Crafts reactions of triphenylene. *J. Chem. Soc.* 941–2.

Buu-Hoi, N. P. & Le Cocq, J. (1948). Action of *N*-bromosuccinimide on some polycyclic hydrocarbons. *C.R. Acad. Sci., Ser. B*, **226**, 87–9.

Cameron, J. M. L., Cook, J. W. & Graham, W. (1945). Catalytic hydrogenation of pyrene. *J. Chem. Soc.* 286–8.

Carruthers, W. (1953). Friedel–Crafts acetylation of chrysene. *J. Chem. Soc.* 3486–89.

Carruthers, W. (1967). Photocyclisation of some stilbene analogues. Synthesis of dibenzo[a,l]pyrene. *J. Chem. Soc.* 1525–7.

Cavalieri, E. & Roth, R. (1976). Reactions of methylbenzanthracenes and pyridine by one-electron oxidation. A model for metabolic activation and binding of carcinogenic aromatic hydrocarbons. *J. Org. Chem.* **41**, 2679–84.

Cavalieri, E., Roth, R., Althoff, J., Grandjean, C., Patil, K., Marsh, S. & McLaughlin, D. (1978). Carcinogenicity and metabolic profiles of 3-methylcholanthrene oxygenated derivatives at the 1 and 2 positions. *Chem.–Biol. Interact.* **22**, 69–81.

Cerfontain, H., Khosrow, L., Lembrechts, H. J. A. (1982). Aromatic sulfonation. 84. Sulfonation of bi- and triphenylene. *Recl.: J.R.Neth. Chem. Soc.* **101**, 313–16.

Chaikovskii, V. & Novikov, A. N. (1984). Synthesis of pyrene derivatives. *Zh. Org. Khim.* **20**, 1482–5.

Chao, C. S., Cheng, C. H. & Chang, C. T. (1983). New methods for the preparation of activated nickel and cobalt powders and their application in biaryl synthesis. *J. Org. Chem.* **48**, 4904–7.

Chatterjee, N. N., Bose, A. & Roy, H. (1947). Synthesis of pyrene. *J. Indian Chem. Soc.* **24**, 169–72.

Cho, H. & Harvey, R. G. (1974). Synthesis of 'K-region' quinones and arene oxides of polycyclic aromatic hydrocarbons. *Tetrahedron Lett.* 1491–4.

Cho, H. & Harvey, R. G. (1976). Synthesis of hydroquinone diacetates from polycyclic aromatic quinones. *J. Chem. Soc. Perkin I,* 836–9.

Clar, E. (1964). *Polycyclic Hydrocarbons*, New York: Academic.

Clar, E. (1942). A new synthesis of tetracene. *Chem. Ber.* **75**, 1271–3.

Clar, E. (1948). Aromatic hydrocarbons. Part XLIV. Synthesis of 1.2,3.4-dibenztetracene. *Chem. Ber.* **81**, 68–71.

Clar, E. (1932). Localization of double bonds in condensed aromatic hydrocarbons. *Chem. Ber.* **65**, 503–19.

Clar, E. & Schmidt, W. (1979). Correlations between photoelectron and UV absorption spectra of polycyclic hydrocarbons. The pyrene series. *Tetrahedron,* **35**, 1027–32.

Clar, E. & Schmidt, W. (1979a). Localized *vs* delocalized molecular orbitals in aromatic hydrocarbons. *Tetrahedron,* **35**, 2673–80.

Cook, J. W. (1931). Polycyclic aromatic hydrocarbons. Part VI. 3;4-benzphenanthrene and its quinone. *J. Chem. Soc.* 2524–8.

Cook, J. W. & Haslewood, G. A. (1934). The synthesis of 5:6-dimethyl-1:2-benzanthraquinone, a degradation product of deoxycholic acid. *J. Chem. Soc.* 428–33.

Cook, J. W. & Hewett, C. L. (1933). Polycyclic aromatic hydrocarbons. Part XI. The acetylation of 1:2-benzanthracene. *J. Chem. Soc.* 1408–10.

Cook, J. W. & Hewett, C. L .(1933). The isolation of a cancer-producing hydrocarbon from coal tar. Part III. Synthesis of 1:2- and 4:5-benzpyrene. *J. Chem. Soc.* 398–405.

Cook, J. W. & Martin, R. H. (1940). Polycyclic aromatic hydrocarbons. Part XXIV. *J. Chem. Soc.* 1125–7.

Cook, J. W. & Robinson, A. M. (1938). Polycyclic aromatic hydrocarbons. Part XVII. Completion of the synthesis of the twelve monomethyl-1:2-benzanthracenes. *J. Chem. Soc.* 505–13.

Cook, J. W. & Schoental, R. (1948). Oxidation of carcinogenic hydrocarbons by osmium tetroxide. *J. Chem. Soc.* 170–3.

Copeland, P. G., Dean, R. E. & McNeil, D. (1960). The cyclodehydrogenation of p-terphenyl and 1-2'-biphenyl-3,4-dihydronaphthalene. *J. Chem. Soc.* 1687–9.

Copeland, P. G., Dean, R. E. & McNeil, D. (1961). The ozonolysis of polycyclic hydrocarbons. Part II. *J. Chem. Soc.* 1232–8.

Copeland, P. G., Dean, R. E. & McNeil, D. (1961a). Ozonolysis of polycyclic hydrocarbons. III. *J. Chem. Soc.* 3858–60.

Coulson, E. A. (1937). Studies in tar hydrocarbons. Part 1. Reduction products of pyrene. *J. Chem. Soc.* 1298–305.

Crump, S. L., Netka, J. & Rickborn, B. (1985). Preparation of isobenzofuran–aryne cycloadducts. *J. Org. Chem.* **50**, 2746–50.

Dallinga, G., Stuart, A. A., Smit, P. J., Mackor, E. L. (1957). Hydrogen–deuterium exchange in polynuclear aromatics. *Z. Electrochem.* **61**, 1019–27.

Dansi, A. (1937). Friedel–Crafts reactions of oxalyl chloride with 1:2-benzanthracene. *Gazz. Chem. Ital.* **67**, 85–8.

Davies, W. & Porter, Q. (1957). The synthesis of polycyclic aromatic compounds. Part III. The reaction of quinones with vinylnaphthalenes and related dienes. *J. Chem. Soc.* 4967–70.

Dewar, M. J. S., Mole, T., Urch, D. S. & Warford, E. W. (1956). Electrophilic substitution. Part IV. The nitration of diphenyl, chrysene, benzo[a]pyrene, and anthanthrene. *J. Chem. Soc.* 3572–5.

Diels, O. & Karstens, A. (1927). Dehydrogenation with selenium. *Chem. Ber.* **60**, 2323–4.

Di Raddo, P. & Harvey, R. G. (1988). A new synthesis of polycyclic aromatic hydrocarbons via titanium (IV)-catalyzed aldol-type condensation of silyl enol ethers with 2-arylacetaldehydes. *Tetrahedron Lett.* **29**, 3885–6.

Dufraisse, C. & Horclois, R. (1936). Naphthacene is the prototype of the rubrenes. *Bull. Soc. Chim. Fr.* **3**, 1880–93.

Fatiadi, A. J. (1967). Periodic acid, a novel oxidant of polycyclic aromatic hydrocarbons. *J. Chem. Soc. Chem. Commun.* 1087–8.

Fatiadi, A. J. (1967a). A novel, facile preparation of 1,1'-bipyrene. *J. Org. Chem.* **32**, 2903–4.

Fieser, L. F. (1942). The Elbs reaction. *Org. Reactions*, **1**, 129–54.

Fieser, L. F. & Bowen, D. M. (1941). New methyl and dimethyl derivatives of cholanthrene. *J. Am. Chem. Soc.* **62**, 2103–8.

Fieser, L. F. & Hartwell, J. L. (1938). Meso aldehydes of anthracene and 1,2-benzanthracene. *J. Amer. Chem. Soc.* **60**, 2555–9.

Fieser, L. F. & Hershberg, E. B. (1938). Substitutions of meso derivatives of 1,2-benzanthracene. *J. Org. Chem.* **60**, 1893–6.

Fieser, L. F. & Hershberg, E. B. (1938a). The oxidation of methylcholanthrene and 3,4-benzpyrene with lead tetraacetate; further derivatives of 3,4-benzpyrene. *J. Amer. Chem. Soc.* **60**, 2542–8.

Fieser, L. F. & Hershberg, E. B. (1938b). Reduction and hydrogenation of methylcholanthrene. *J. Org. Chem.* **60**, 940–7.

Fonken, G. J. (1962). Photochemical formation of polynuclear aromatic compounds from diaryl polyarenes. *Chem. & Ind.* 1327.

Fried, J. & Schmunn, D. E. (1967). One electron transfer oxidation of 7,12-dimethyl-benz[a]anthracene, a model for the metabolic activation of carcinogenic hydrocarbons. *J. Org. Chem.* **89**, 5508–9.

Friedel, R. A. & Orchin, M. (1951). *Ultraviolet Spectra of Aromatic Compounds*. New York: Wiley.

Fu, P. P., Cortez, C., Sukumaran, K. B. & Harvey, R. G. (1979). Synthesis of the isomeric phenols of benz[a]anthracene from benz[a]anthracene. *J. Org. Chem.* **44**, 4265–71.

Fu, P. P. & Harvey, R. G. (1974). A convenient dehydrogenation reagent: trityl trifluoroacetate generated *in situ*. *Tetrahedron Lett.* 3217–20.

Fu, P. P. & Harvey, R. G. (1979). Synthesis of the dihydrodiols and diolepoxides of chrysene from chrysene. *J. Org. Chem.* **44**, 3778–4.

Fu, P. P., Lee, H. M. & Harvey, R. G. (1980). Regioselective catalytic hydrogenation of polycyclic aromatic hydrocarbons under mild conditions. *J. Org. Chem.* **45**, 2797–803.

Graebe, C. (1905). Naphthoylbenzoic acid. *Liebigs Ann.* **340**, 249–59.

Graebe, C. & Honigsberger, F. (1900). *Liebigs Ann.* **311**, 257–5.

Gribble, G. W., LeHoullier, C. S., Sibi, M. P. & Allen, R. W. (1985). Synthesis and deamination of 7,12-dihydrobenz[a]anthracen-7,12-imines. A new benz[a]anthracene synthesis. *J. Org. Chem.* **50**, 1611–16.

Gribble, G. W., Perni, R. B. & Onan, K. D. (1985a). Twin benzoannulation of naphthalene via

1,3-, 1,6-, and 2,6-naphthdiyne synthetic equivalents. New syntheses of triphenylene, benz[a]anthracene, and naphthacene. *J. Org. Chem.* **50**, 2934–9.

Grimmer, G. (1979). *Environmental Carcinogens - Selected Methods of Analysis,* III, 31–61. Lyon, France: International Agency for Research on Cancer.

Grimshaw, J. & Trocha-Grimshaw, J. (1972). Characterisation of 1,6- and 1,8-dibromopyrenes. *J. Chem. Soc. Perkin I,* 1622–3.

Guenther, H. & Kovacic, P. (1984). Oxidative coupling of 9,10-dihydrophenanthrene and polynuclear hydrocarbons by aluminum chloride–cupric chloride. *Syn. Commun.* **14**, 413–27.

Haigh, C. W. & Mallion, R. B. (1971). Proton magnetic resonance of nonplanar condensed benzenoid hydrocarbons. I. Spectra of 3,4-benzophenanthrene, pentahelicene, and hexahelicene. *Molec. Phys.* **22**, 945–53.

Harvey, R. G. (1971). Metal–ammonia reduction. XI. Regiospecific and stereoselective reduction in the chrysene series. *J. Org. Chem.* **36**, 3306–11.

Harvey, R. G. (1970). Metal–ammonia reduction of aromatic molecules. *Synthesis,* 161–72.

Harvey, R. G., Arzadon, L., Grant, J. & Urberg, K. (1969). Metal–ammonia reduction. IV. Single-stage reduction of polycyclic aromatic hydrocarbons. *J. Amer. Chem. Soc.* **91**, 4535–41.

Harvey, R. G. & Cortez, C. (1987). Synthesis of cholanthrene and 6-methylcholanthrene, biologically active analogs of the potent carcinogen 3-methylcholanthrene. *J. Org. Chem.* **52**, 283–4.

Harvey, R. G. & Cortez, C. (1986). Synthesis of 7,12-dimethylbenz[a]anthracene and its 1,2,3,4-tetrahydro derivative. *J. Org. Chem.* **51**, 5023–4.

Harvey, R. G., Cortez, C. & Jacobs, S. (1982). Synthesis of polycyclic hydrocarbons via a novel annelation method. *J. Org. Chem.* **47**, 2120–5.

Harvey, R. G., Fu, P. P. & Rabideau, P. W. (1976). Stereochemistry of 1,3-cyclohexadienes: Conformational preferences in 9-substituted 9,10-dihydrophenanthrenes. *J. Org. Chem.* **41**, 3722–5.

Harvey, R. G., Goh, S. H. & Cortez, C. (1975). 'K-region' oxides and related oxidized metabolites of carcinogenic aromatic hydrocarbons. *J. Amer. Chem. Soc.* **97**, 3468–79.

Harvey, R. G., Konieczny, M. & Pataki, J. (1983). Synthesis of the isomeric mono- and bisoxiranylpyrenes. *J. Org. Chem.* **48**, 2930–2.

Harvey, R. G., Lee, H. & Shyamasundar, N. (1979). Synthesis of the dihydrodiols and diol epoxides of benzo[e]pyrene and triphenylene. *J. Org. Chem.* **44**, 78–83.

Harvey, R. G., Pataki, J. & Lee, H. (1984). The Friedel–Crafts acylation and benzoylation of pyrene. *Org. Prep. Proc. Internat.* **16**, 144–8.

Harvey, R. G. & Rabideau, P. W. (1970). Regiospecific reduction of pyrene to 1,9-dihydropyrene. *Tetrahedron Lett.* 3695–8.

Harvey, R. G., Schmolka, S., Cortez, C. & Lee, H. (1988). Convenient syntheses of 2-bromopyrene and 2-hydroxypyrene. *Syn. Commun.* **18**, 2207–9.

Harvey, R. G. & Urberg, K. (1968). Metal–ammonia reduction. III. Stepwise transformation of polycyclic aromatic hydrocarbons. *J. Org. Chem.* **33**, 2206–11.

Hauptmann, S. & Hartig, S. (1963). The mechanism of the reaction of oxalyl bromide with aromatic hydrocarbons in the absence of catalysts. *J. Prakt. Chem.* **20**, 197–201.

Heaney, H. & Millar, I. T. (1973). Triphenylene. *Org. Syn.* **Coll. Vol. V**, 1120–3.

Herbstein, F. H. & Schmidt, G. M. J. (1954). The structure of overcrowded aromatic compounds. Part III. The crystal structure of 3:4-benzophenanthrene. *J. Chem. Soc.* 302–13.

Horgan, S. W., Morgan, D. D. & Orchin, M. (1973). The photochemistry of 2-vinylbiphenyl and 4-vinylphenanthrene. *J. Org. Chem.* **38**, 3801–3.

Hunt, S. E. & Lindsey, A. S. (1958). Metallation and carboxylation of chrysene. *J. Chem. Soc.* 2227–30.

IARC (1973). *Monograph on the Evaluation of Carcinogenic Risk of the Chemical to Man: Certain Polycyclic Aromatic Hydrocarbons and Heterocyclic Compounds*, 3, Lyon, France: International Agency for Research on Cancer.

IARC (1983). *Monograph on the Evaluation of Carcinogenic Risk of the Chemical to Man: Certain Polycyclic Aromatic Hydrocarbons and Heterocyclic Compounds*, 32, Lyon, France: International Agency for Research on Cancer.

Ittah, Y. & Jerina, D. M. (1980). Synthesis of monofluorobenzo[c]phenanthrenes. *J. Fluorine Chem.* **16**, 137–44.

Iversen, B., Sydnes, L. K. & Greibrokk, T. (1985). Characterization of nitrobenzanthracenes and nitrodibenzanthracenes. *Acta Chem. Scand.* **B39**, 837–47.

Jacobs, S., Cortez, C. & Harvey, R. G. (1983). Synthesis of proximate and ultimate carcinogenic metabolites of 3-methylcholanthrene. *Carcinogenesis*, **4**, 519–22.

Jaffe, H. H. & Orchin, M. (1962). *Theory and Applications of Ultraviolet Spectroscopy*, New York: Wiley.

Jutz, J. C. (1978). Aromatic and heteroaromatic compounds by electrocyclic ring closure. *Topics in Current Chem.* **73**, 127–230.

Karcher, W. (1988). *Spectral Atlas of Polycyclic Aromatic Compounds,* Vol. 2, Dordrecht, Netherlands: Kluwer.

Karcher, W., Fordham, R., DuBois, J. & Gloude, P. (1985). *Spectral Atlas of Polycyclic Aromatic Compounds.* Dordrecht, Netherlands: D. Reidel.

Kauffmann, T., Kosel, C. & Schoeneck, W. (1963). Metalhydrazides. IV. The reduction of unsaturated and polynuclear aromatic hydrocarbons with the system sodium hydrazide–hydrazine. *Chem. Ber.* **96**, 999–1010.

Kharasch, N., Alston, T. G., Lewis, H. B. & Wolf, W. (1965). The photochemical conversion of o-terphenyl into triphenylene. *J. Chem. Soc. Chem. Commun.* 242–3.

Klein, C. L., Stevens, E. D., Zacharias, D. E. & Glusker, J. P. (1987). 7,12-Dimethyl-benz[a]anthracene: Refined structure, electron density distribution, and endoperoxide structure. *Carcinogenesis*, **8**, 5–18.

Konieczny, M. & Harvey, R. G. (1979). Synthesis of cyclopenta[c,d]pyrene. *J. Org. Chem.* **44**, 2158–60.

Konieczny, M. & Harvey, R. G. (1979a). Efficient reduction of polycyclic quinones, hydroquinones, and phenols to polycyclic aromatic hydrocarbons with hydriodic acid. *J. Org. Chem.* **44**, 4813–16.

Konieczny, M. & Harvey, R. G. (1980). Reductive methylation of polycyclic aromatic quinones. *J. Org. Chem.* **45**, 1308–10.

Konieczny, M. & Harvey, R. G. (1984). Reduction of polycyclic quinones with hydriodic acid: Synthesis of benz[a]anthracene. *Org. Syn.* **62**, 165–9.

Konieczny, M. & Harvey, R. G. (1990). Reduction of quinones with hydriodic acid: Benz[a]anthracene. *Org. Syn.* Coll. Vol. VII, 18–22.

Lang, K. F., Buffleb, H., Froitzheim, M. & Kalowy, J. (1965). Hydrogenation of chrysenes. *Chem. Ber.* **98**, 593–6.

LaPouyade, R., Nourmamode, A. & Bouas-Laurent, H. (1980). Photocycloaddition of polynuclear aromatic hydrocarbons in solution. The photodimerizations of tetrahydro-1,2,3,4 naphthacene and the two photodimers of naphthacene. *Tetrahedron*, **36**, 2311–16.

Lee, H. & Harvey, R. G. (1986). Synthesis of 2,7-dibromopyrene. *J. Org. Chem.* **51**, 2847–8.

Lee, H. M. & Harvey, R. G. (1979). Synthesis of biologically active metabolites of 7-methylbenz[a]anthracene. *J. Org. Chem.* **44**, 4948–53.

Lee-Ruff, E., Hopkinson, A. C. & Dao, L. H. (1981). Acid-catalyzed rearrangement of cyclobutanones. VI. Syntheses of chrysenes and steroid-like substances. *Can. J. Chem.* **59**, 1675–9.

LeHoullier, C. S. & Gribble, G. W. (1983). A convenient generation of 2,3-naphthalyne. Linear annulation of naphthalene and a new naphthacene series. *J. Org. Chem.* **48**, 2364–6.

Levin, W., Wood, A. W., Chang, R. L., Ittah, Y., Croisy-Delcey, M., Yagi, H., Jerina, D. M. & Conney, A. H. (1980). Exceptionally high tumor-initiating activity of benzo(c)phenanthrene bay-region diol-epoxides on mouse skin. *Cancer Res.* **40**, 391–4.

Levy, L. A. & Pruitt, L. (1980). An expeditious synthesis of benz[a]anthracene and some of its oxygenated derivatives. *J. Chem. Soc. Chem. Commun.* 227–8.

Levy, L. A. & Sashikumar, V. P. (1985). Synthesis of chrysene, 5-methylchrysene, and chrysene derivatives via intramolecular cycloaddition reactions. *J. Org. Chem.* **50**, 1760–3.

Logani, M. K., Austin, W. A. & Davies, R. E. (1977). Photooxygenation of 7,12-dimethylbenz[a]anthracene. *Tetrahedron Lett.* 2467–70.

Lyle, T. A. & Daub, G. H. (1979). Synthesis of some tetrahydrochrysenes as potential ultraviolet laser dyes. *J. Org. Chem.* **44**, 4933–8.

Mabille, P. & Buu-Hoi, N. P. (1960). Orientation in Friedel–Crafts acylations of 6-substituted chrysenes. *J. Org. Chem.* **25**, 1092–6.

Mannich, C. (1907). Triphenylene. *Chem. Ber.* **40**, 159–65.

Marschalk, C. & Stumm, C. (1948). The structural problem of the tetracene series. *Bull. Soc. Chim. Fr.* 418–28.

Martin, R. H., Moriau, J. & Defay, N. (1974). 13C-NMR spectroscopy: Isotope shifts and couplings in mono- and dideuterated polycyclic aromatic hydrocarbons. XIX. *Tetrahedron*, **30**, 179–85.

Martynoff, M. (1954). Research in the naphthacene group. I. Monosubstituted functional derivatives. 9-Formyl- and 9-cyanonaphthacenes. *C. R. Acad. Sci. Paris*, **238**, 249–51.

Marvel, C. S. & Wilson, B. D. (1958). Synthetic studies in the dihydropyrene series. *J. Org. Chem.* **23**, 1483–8.

Meek, J. S. & Dewey, F. M. (1970). Diels–Alder reactions of 5-substituted naphthacenes. *J. Org. Chem.* **32**, 1315–18.

Meek, J. S., Dewey, F. M. & Hanna, M. W. (1967). Some Diels–Alder reactions of naphthacene. *J. Org. Chem.* **32**, 69–72.

Memory, J. D. & Wilson, N. K. (1982). *NMR of Aromatic Compounds*. New York: Wiley–Interscience.

Mikhailov, B. M. & Kozminskaya, T. K. (1951). Action of phosphorus pentahalides on benz[a]anthracene and its derivatives. *J. Gen. Chem. USSR*. **21**, 2184–8.

Miller, D. W., Freeman, J. P., Evans, F. E., Fu, P. P. & Yang, D. T. C. (1984). Reaction of pyrene, benz[a]anthracene, and phenanthrene with oxalyl chloride. *J. Chem. Res. (S)*, 418–19.

Mitchell, R. H., Lai, Y. & Williams, R. V. (1979). N-Bromosuccinimide-dimethylformamide: A mild, selective nuclear monobromination reagent for reactive aromatic compounds. *J. Org. Chem.* **44**, 4733–5.

Mukherji, S. M., Handa, R. N. & Sharma, K. S. (1967). Polynuclear aromatic hydrocarbons. X. Synthesis of tetraphene by the Robinson–Mannich reaction. *Tetrahedron*, **23**, 3859–62.

Muller, A. & Hanke, F. G. (1949). Structure analogs of carcinogenic compounds. III. 10-chloro-1,2-benzanthracene. *Monatsh*, **80**, 435–7.

Muschik, G. M., Tomaszewski, J. E., Sato, R. I. & Manning, W. B. (1979). Synthesis of the 1-, 2-, 3-, and 4-hydroxy isomers of benz[a]anthracene-7,12-dione, benz[a]anthracene, and 7,12-dimethylbenz[a]anthracene. *J. Org. Chem.* **44**, 2150–3.

Nagel, D., Kupper, R., Antonson, K. & Wallcave, L. (1977). Excited states. I. Direction of photocyclization of naphthalene-substituted ethylenes. *J. Org. Chem.* **42**, 3626–8.

Netka, J., Crump, S. L. & Rickborn, B. (1986). Isobenzofuran-aryne cycloadducts: Formation and regioselective conversion to anthrones and substituted polycyclic aromatics. *J. Org. Chem.* **51**, 1189–99.

Newman, M. S., Anderson, H. V. & Takemura, K. H. (1953). The synthesis of polynuclear aromatic hydrocarbons. II. Methylbenzo[c]phenanthrenes. *J. Amer. Chem. Soc.* **75**, 347–9.

Newman, M. S. & Joshel, L. M. (1938). A new synthesis of 3,4-benzphenanthrene. *J. Amer. Chem. Soc.* **60**, 485–8.

Newman, M. S., Khanna, J. M., Kanakarajan, K. & Kumar, S. (1978). Syntheses of 1-,2-,3-,4-, 6-, 9-, and 10-hydroxy-7,12-dimethylbenz[a]anthracene. *J. Org. Chem.* **43**, 2553–7.

Newman, M. S. & Kosak, A. I. (1949). The orientation of benzo[c]phenanthrene. *J. Org. Chem.* **14**, 375–81.

Newman, M. S. & Lilje, K. C. (1979). Synthesis of 7-fluorobenz[a]anthracene. *J. Org. Chem.* **44**, 1347–8.

Newman, M. S. & Sujeeth, P. K. (1983). Synthesis of 3,6-dimethylcholanthrene. *J. Org. Chem.* **48**, 2426–7.

Newman, M. S., Tierney, B. & Veeraraghavan, S. (1988). *The Chemistry and Biology of Benz[a]anthracenes,* eds M. M. Coombs, J. Ashby & H. Baxter. Cambridge: Cambridge University Press.

Newman, M. S. & Wheatley, W. B. (1948). Optical activity of the 4,5-phenanthrene type: 4-(1-methylbenzo[c]phenanthryl)acetic acid and 1-methylbenzo[c]phenanthrene. *J. Amer. Chem. Soc.* **70**, 1913–16.

Newman, M. S., Wotring, R. W., Jr., Pandit, A. & Chakrabarti, P. M. (1966). The synthesis and resolution of 1- and 2-methylcholanthrene. *J. Org. Chem.* **31**, 4293–6.

Nonhebel, D. C. (1963). Copper (II) halides as halogenating agents. *J. Chem. Soc.* 1216–20.

Oberender, F. G. & Dixon, J. A. (1959). Osmium and ruthenium tetroxide-catalyzed oxidations of pyrene. *J. Org. Chem.* **24**, 1226–9.

Ozubuko, R. S., Buchanan, G. W. & Smith, I. C. (1974). Carbon-13 nuclear magnetic resonance spectra of carcinogenic polynuclear hydrocarbons. I. 3-Methylcholanthrene and related benzanthracenes. *Canad. J. Chem.* **52**, 2493–501.

Padwa, A. & Mazzu, A. (1974). Photocyclization of substituted 2,2'-divinylbiphenyl derivatives to tetrahydropyrenes. *Tetrahedron Lett.* 4471–4.

Pataki, J., Di Raddo, P. & Harvey, R. G. (1989). An efficient synthesis of the highly tumorigenic *anti*-diol epoxide derivative of benzo[c]phenanthrene. *J. Org. Chem.* **54**, 840–4.

Pataki, J. & Harvey, R. G. (1982). Benzo[c]phenanthrene and its oxidized metabolites. *J. Org. Chem.* **47**, 20–2.

Peake, D. A., Oyler, A. R., Heikkila, K. E., Liukkonen, R. J., Engroff, E. C. & Carlson, R. M. (1983). Alkyl aromatic synthesis: Nucleophilic alkyl lithium addition. *Syn. Commun.* **13**, 21–6.

Platt, K. L. & Oesch, F. (1981). Reductive cyclization of keto acids to polycyclic aromatic hydrocarbons by hydroiodic acid–red phosphorus. *J. Org. Chem.* **46**, 2601–3.

Pouchert, C. E. (1981). *Aldrich Library of Infrared Spectra, Edit. III,* Milwaukee, Wisc.: Aldrich Chemical Co.

Pouchert, C. E. & Campbell, J. R. (1983). *Aldrich Library of NMR Spectra, Edit. II,* Milwaukee, Wisc.: Aldrich Chemical Co.

Radner, F. (1983). Nitration of polycyclic aromatic hydrocarbons with dinitrogen tetroxide. A simple and selective synthesis of mononitro derivatives. *Acta Chem. Scand. B,* **37**, 65–7.

Radner, F. (1989). Iodine cyanide promoted iodination of aromatic compounds. A simple synthesis of 1-iodopyrene. *Acta Chem. Scand.* **43**, 481–484.

Ranganathan, S., Ranganathan, D. & Ramachandran, P. V. (1984). Iodoxybenzene. *Tetrahedron,* **40**, 3145–51.

Reppe, W. (1955). Triphenylene. *Liebigs Ann.* **596**, 135.

Rieche, A., Gross, H. & Hoeft, E. (1960). Synthesis of aromatic halides with dichloromethyl alkyl ethers. *Chem. Ber.* **93**, 88–94.

Sadtler. *The Sadtler Standard Spectra,* Philadelphia: Sadtler Research Laboratories, serial publication.

Sammes, P. G. & Dodsworth, D. J. (1979). Simple one-step route to substituted anthraquinones. *J. Chem. Soc. Chem. Comm.* 33–34.

Sandin, R. B. & Fieser, L. F. (1940). Synthesis of 9,10-dimethyl-1,2-benzanthracene and of a thiophene isolog. *J. Amer. Chem. Soc.* **62**, 3098–105.

Sawicki, E., Hauser, R. T. & Stanley, T. W. (1960). Ultraviolet, visible, and fluorescence spectral analysis of polynuclear hydrocarbons. *Int. J. Air Pollution,* **2**, 253–72.

Schoenberg, A., Mustafa, A., Barakat, M. Z., Latif, N., Moubashec, R. & Mustafa, A. (1948). Photochemical reactions. Part XIII. (a) Photochemical reactions of ethylenes with phenanthroquinone and with 1:2:3-triketones. (b) Dimerisation reactions in sunlight. *J. Chem. Soc.* 2126–9.

Schoental, R. & Scott, E. J. (1949). Fluorescence spectra of polycyclic aromatic hydrocarbons in solution. *J. Chem. Soc.* 1683–96.

Scholz, M., Muhlstadt, M. & Dietz, F. (1967). Excited states. I. Direction of photocyclization of naphthalene-substituted ethylenes. *Tetrahedron Lett.* 665–8.

Sims, P. (1966). The metabolism of 3-methylcholanthrene and some related compounds by rat liver homogenates. *Biochem. J.* **98**, 215–28.

Smith, J. G. & Dibble, P. W. (1983). 2-(Dimethoxymethyl)benzyl alcohol: A convenient isobenzofuran precursor. *J. Org. Chem.* **48**, 5361–2.

Smith, J. G., Dibble, P. W. & Sandborn, R. E. (1986). The preparation and reactions of naphtho[2,3-c]furan. *J. Org. Chem.* **51**, 3762–8.

Smuszkovicz, J. & Modest, E. J. (1948). Condensation of phenylcycloalkenes with maleic anhydride. I. Synthesis of 7-methoxy-3,4-benzphenanthrene. *J. Amer. Chem. Soc.* **70**, 2542–5.

Snook, M. E., Severson, R. F., Arrendale, R. F., Higman, H. C. & Chortyk, O. (1977). The identification of high molecular weight polynuclear aromatic hydrocarbons in a biologically active fraction of cigarette smoke condensate. *Beitr. Tabakforsch.* **9**, 79–101.

Stenhagen, E., Abrahamsson, S. & McLafferty, F. W. (1974). *Registry of Mass Spectral Data.* New York: Wiley.

Studt, P. & Win, T. (1983). Synthesis of benzo[ghi]fluoranthene. *Liebigs Ann.* **519**.

Sturrock, M. G. & Duncan, R. A. (1968). The ozonation of pyrene. A monomeric monoozonide formed in polar solvents. *J. Org. Chem.* **33**, 2149–52.

Sugiyama, T. (1982). The reaction involving one electron transfer in key step. NO_2-catalyzed halogenation of polycyclic aromatic compounds with metal halides. *Bull. Chem. Soc. Jpn.* **55**, 1504–8.

Sukumaran, K. B. & Harvey, R. G. (1980). Synthesis of the o-quinones and dihydrodiols of polycyclic aromatic hydrocarbons from the corresponding phenols. *J. Org. Chem.* **45**, 4407–13.

Sukumaran, K. B. & Harvey, R. G. (1981). A novel annelation reaction: Synthesis of polycyclic hydrocarbons from o-quinones. *J. Org. Chem.* **46**, 2740–5.

Tintel, C., Cornelisse, J. & Lugtenburg, J. (1983). Convenient synthesis of cyclopenta[c,d]pyrene and 3,4-dihydrocyclopenta[c,d]pyrene. The reactivity of the pyrene dianion. *Rec. Trav. Chim. Pays-Bas,* **102**, 14–20.

TRC (1982). *Selected Nuclear Magnetic Resonance Spectral Data.* Suppl. Vol. F–26, College Station, Texas: Thermodynamics Research Center, Texas A & M University.

TRC (1982a). *Selected Ultraviolet Spectral Data.* Suppl. Vol. C–48, College Station, Texas: Thermodynamics Research Center, Texas A & M University.

TRC Hydrocarbon Project (1983). *Selected Nuclear Magnetic Resonance Spectral Data.* Suppl. Vol. F–27, College Station, Texas: Thermodynamics Research Center, Texas A & M University.

TRC (1983a). *Selected Ultraviolet Spectral Data.* Suppl. Vol. C–49, College Station, Texas: Thermodynamics Research Center, Texas A & M University.

TRC (1985). *TRC Spectral Data. Ultraviolet,* Suppl. No. 1, College Station, Texas: Thermodynamics Research Center, Texas A & M University.

TRC (1986). *TRC Spectral Data. ^1H Nuclear Magnetic Resonance,* Suppl. No. 2, College Station, Texas: Thermodynamics Research Center, Texas A & M University.

Treibs, W. & Mann, G. (1958). Autooxidation of polynuclear, partially hydrogenated aromatic hydrocarbons. III. *Chem. Ber.* **91**, 1910–16.

van Bladeren, P. J. & Jerina, D. M. (1983). Facile synthesis of K-region arene oxides. *Tetrahedron Lett.* **24**, 4903–6.

van den Bracken-van Leersum, A. M., Tintel, C., van't Zelfde, M., Cornelisse, J., Lugtenburg, J. (1987). Spectroscopic and photochemical properties of mononitropyrenes. *Rec. Trav. Chim. Pays-Bas,* **106**, 120–8.

Vickery, E. H. & Eisenbraun, E. J. (1979). Benzo[c]phenanthrene. *Org. Prep. Proc. Internat.* **11**, 261–3.

Vollmann, H., Becker, H., Corell, M. & Streeck, H. (1937). Pyrene and its derivatives. *Liebigs Ann.* **531**, 1–159.

Vysotskii, Y. B. & Mestechkin, M. M. (1975). Effect of π-electron currents on chemical shifts in carbon-13. *Zh. Struht. Khim.* **16**, 303–6.

Waldmann, H. & Mathiowetz, H. (1931). A new synthesis in the *lin*-benzanthraquinone series. *Chem. Ber.* **64**, 1713–24.

Ward, J. J., Kirner, W. R. & Howard, H. C. (1945). Alkaline permanganate oxidation of certain condensed cyclic compounds including coal. *J. Amer. Chem. Soc.* **67**, 246–53.

Weizmann, C., Blum-Bergmann, E. & Bergmann, F. (1935). Grignard reactions with phthalic anhydrides. *J. Chem. Soc.* 1367–70.

Welsch, C. W. (1985). Host factors affecting the growth of carcinogen-induced rat mammary carcinomas: A review and tribute to Charles Brenton Huggins. *Cancer Res.* **45**, 3415–43.

Wittig, G. & Pohmer, L. (1956). The formation of dehydrobenzene as an intermediate. *Chem. Ber.* **89**, 1334–51.

Wittig, G., Uhlenbrock, W. & Weinhold, P. (1962). Formation and properties of 9,10-dehydrophenanthrene. *Chem. Ber.* **95**, 1692–702.

Wood, A. W., Chang, R. L., Huang, M., Levin, W., Lehr, R. E., Kumar, S., Thakker, D. R., Yagi, H., Jerina, D. M. & Conney, A. H. (1980). Mutagenicity of benzo(e)pyrene and triphenylene tetrahydroepoxides and diol-epoxides in bacterial and mammalian cells. *Cancer Res.* **40**, 1985–9.

Wood, C. S. & Mallory, E. B. (1964). Photochemistry of stilbenes. IV. The preparation of substituted phenanthrenes. *J. Org. Chem.* **29**, 3373–7.

9

Alternant pentacyclic polyarenes

The chemistry of the alternant PAHs with five rings is summarized in this chapter. As in the previous chapter, information is provided on the physical, chemical, and spectral properties, environmental occurrence, and carcinogenicity of each hydrocarbon along with a review of methods of synthesis and chemical reactivity. While the chemical and biological properties of pentacyclic polyarenes which are important in carcinogenesis research, such as benzo[a]pyrene and dibenz[a,h]anthracene, have received considerable attention, surprisingly little is known concerning the properties of most other PAHs of this class.

9.1   Picene

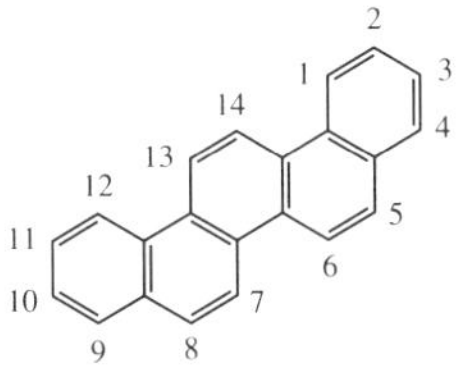

Other names: benzo[a]chrysene, 1,2,7,8-dibenzophenanthrene
Physical and spectral properties $C_{22}H_{14}$, mol. wt. 278.33, colorless plates (ethyl acetate), mp 366 °C. Sparingly soluble in hot benzene, chloroform, and acetic acid. Spectral data: UV (Karcher, 1988; Friedel & Orchin, 1951), UV fluorescence (Karcher, 1988; Schoental & Scott, 1949), PE (Clar & Schmidt, 1979), IR (Karcher, 1988; Pouchert, 1981), NMR (Karcher, 1988; Cobb & Memory, 1967), mass spectrum (Karcher, 1988; Shushan & Boyd, 1980).

Occurrence and carcinogenicity Picene is obtained from petroleum fractionation residues and high-boiling coal tar distillates. Only trace amounts are commonly detected in airborne atmospheric pollutants (Lao *et al.*, 1973). Limited tests to date indicate that picene is noncarcinogenic (Hartwell, 1951).

Synthesis Synthetic approaches to picene are summarized in Fig. 9.1. The most convenient syntheses are cyclodehydrogenation of 1,2-di-(1-naphthyl)ethane (**1**) with AlCl₃ (Buu-Hoi & Hoan, 1949) and photocyclization of 1,2-di-(1-naphthyl)ethylene (**2**) (Dietz & Scholtz, 1968). Photocyclization of 1,2-distyrylbenzene (**3**), or 1-styrylphenanthrene (**4**) affords picene in lower yield (Levi & Orchin, 1966). Another practical route involves double Haworth synthesis of 9,10-dihydrophenanthrene with succinic anhydride and AlCl₃, followed by reduction and dehydrogenation of the diketone product (**5**) (Phillips, 1953). Other syntheses include addition of maleic anhydride to tetrahydrobinaphthyl, followed by dehydrogenation and decarboxylation of the adduct (**6**) (Weidlich, 1938) and Diels–Alder reaction between 1-vinylnaphthalene and 1,2-naphthyne (Corbett & Porter, 1965).

Reactions The chemical properties of picene are relatively unexplored. Electrophilic substitution is predicted by MO theory to take place preferentially in the central K-region 13,14-bond. Oxidation of picene

Fig. 9.1. Synthetic routes to picene.

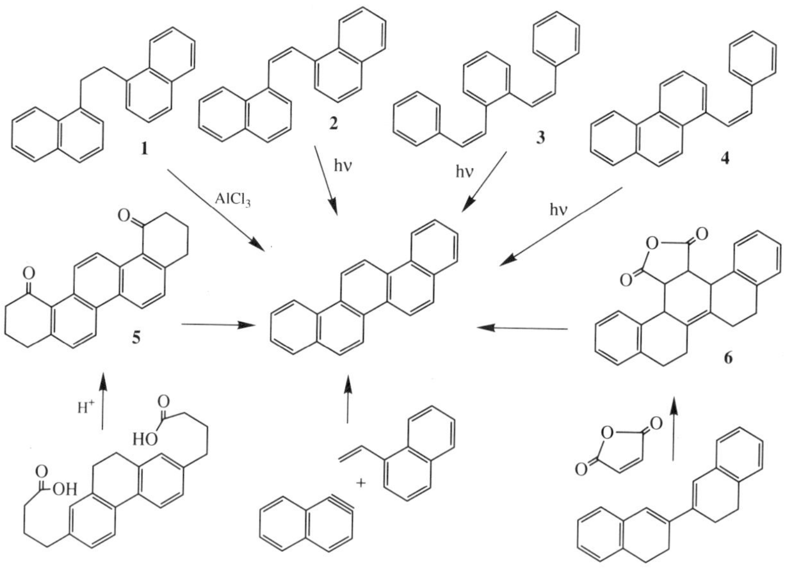

with chromic acid in acetic acid provides picene-5,6-dione and a lesser amount of picene-13,14-dione (Davies & Ennis, 1959).

9.2   Dibenz[a,c]anthracene

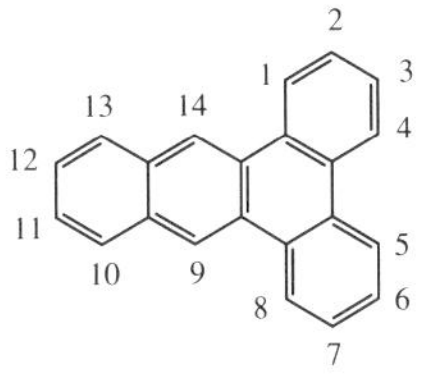

Other names: 1,2,3,4-dibenzanthracene (DBacA)

Physical and spectral properties $C_{22}H_{14}$, mol. wt. 278.33, colorless needles (acetic acid), mp 205 °C. Moderately soluble in benzene and toluene. Spectral data: UV (Karcher *et al.*, 1985; TRC, 1982a; Friedel & Orchin, 1951), UV fluorescence (Perin-Roussel *et al.*, 1972), PE (Clar & Schmidt, 1979), IR (Karcher *et al.*, 1985; Pouchert, 1981; Perin-Roussel *et al.*, 1972), ^{1}H-NMR (Karcher *et al.*, 1985; TRC, 1982; Cobb & Memory, 1967), ^{13}C-NMR (Karcher *et al.*, 1985; Ozubuku *et al.*, 1974), mass spectrum (Shushan & Boyd, 1980).

Occurrence and carcinogenicity Dibenz[a,c]anthracene occurs ubiquitously in products of incomplete combustion, and is a common atmospheric pollutant (Lao *et al.*, 1973). It occurs in fossil fuels, in crude oil, and used motor oil; it is also detected in cigarette smoke, and marijuana smoke (IARC, 1983). Dibenz[a,c]anthracene is inactive or only weakly active as a complete carcinogen on mouse skin (Hartwell, 1951; IARC, 1983), but shows significant tumor-initiating activity with TPA promotion (Slaga *et al.*, 1980).

Synthesis Synthetic approaches to dibenz[a,c]anthracene are summarized in Fig. 9.2. The most efficient synthesis involves reaction between phthalic anhydride and 9-phenanthrylmagnesium bromide to yield the keto acid **7** followed by reductive cyclization of the latter with HI in acetic acid (Harvey *et al.*, 1978). With excess HI and longer reaction, 9,14-dihydro-DBacA is the major product. Another relatively convenient method involves Haworth reaction of triphenylene with succinic anhydride and AlCl$_3$ to give a keto acid which on reduction and acid-catalyzed cyclodehydration yields the ketone **8**. Reduction and dehydrogenation of **8** with selenium provides DBacA (Buu-Hoi *et al.*, 1959). DBacA is also available from BA-5,6-dione by reaction with lithium acetylide to form a diacetylenic diol which is reduced with LiAlH$_4$ to the divinyl diol **9** (Sukumaran & Harvey, 1981). Treatment of **9** with III in acetic acid yields DBacA. Other syntheses include: Elbs pyrolysis of 9-(*o*-toluoyl)phenanthrene (**10**) (Bachmann, 1934); bis-Wittig reaction of **11** with phenanthrene-9,10-dione (Minsky & Rabinovitz, 1983); and condensation of *o*-bis(cyanomethyl)benzene with phenanthrene-9,10-dione to furnish 9,14-dicyano-DBacA (**12**), followed by hydrolysis and decarboxylation (Moureu *et al.*, 1948).

9,14-Dimethyl-DBacA was synthesized by reductive methylation of DBacA-9,14-dione (DiGiovanni *et al.*, 1983; Konieczny & Harvey, 1980).

Reactions Electrophilic substitution is predicted by MO theory to take place preferentially in the meso region, i.e. the 9,14-positions of DBacA. However, there is a dearth of published information on this point, and steric crowding may be expected to interfere with substitution in this site. Nitration of DBacA gives mainly 9-nitro-DBacA based on analysis of the high resolution ^{1}H-NMR spectrum (Iversen *et al.*, 1985). It has recently been shown in the author's laboratory that bromination of DBacA with N-bromosuccinimide affords 9-bromo-DBacA as the major product, while reaction of DBacA with Br$_2$ in CH$_2$Cl$_2$ gives mainly 10-bromo-DBacA (unpublished studies). Diels–Alder reaction of DBacA with maleic anhydride takes place in the meso region, in agreement with expectation (Biermann & Schmidt, 1980).

Fig. 9.2. Synthetic routes to dibenz[a,c]anthracene.

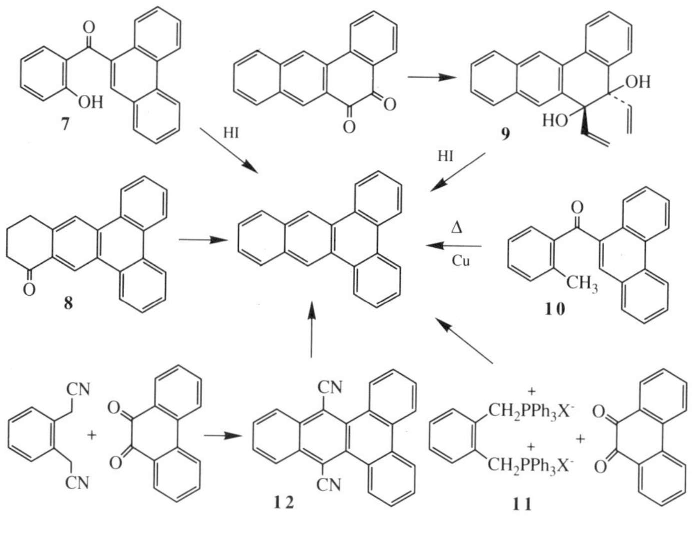

Oxidation of DBacA with chromic acid furnishes DBacA-9,14-dione (Clar, 1929). Reduction of DBacA with Na or Li and methanol affords 9,14-DBacA (Bachmann & Pence, 1937). Reduction of DBacA with Li/NH₃ also provides 9,14-DBacA (Harvey, 1970). Reductive methylation of DBacA-9,14-dione with methyllithium followed by treatment with HI furnishes 7,14-dimethyl-DBacA in high yield (Konieczny & Harvey, 1980). Hydrogenation of DBacA over a platinum catalyst at low pressure provides the terminal ring saturated product 10,11,12,13-tetrahydro-DBacA quantitatively (Fu *et al.*, 1980).

9.3   Dibenz[a,h]anthracene

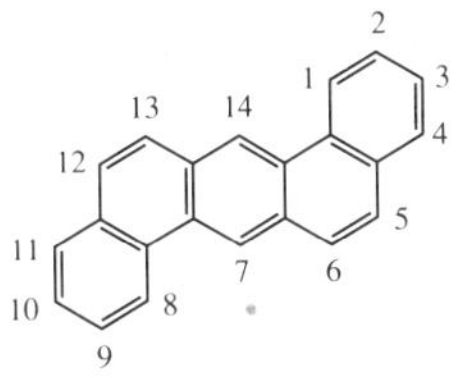

Other names: 1,2,5,6-dibenzanthracene (DBA)

Physical and spectral properties $C_{22}H_{14}$, mol. wt. 278.33, monoclinic and orthorhombic crystals, the crystal structure has been shown to be centrosymmetric and planar (Iball & Morgan, 1975), mp 266 °C, sublimes. DBA is soluble in most common organic solvents, but is only slightly soluble in ethanol and diethyl ether. Spectral data: UV (Karcher *et al.*, 1985; TRC, 1982a; Perkamper *et al.*, 1967; Friedel & Orchin, 1951), UV fluorescence (Karcher *et al.*, 1985; Schoental & Scott, 1949; Perin-Roussel *et al.*, 1972), PE (Clar & Schmidt, 1979a), IR (Karcher *et al.*, 1985; Pouchert, 1981; Perin-Roussel *et al.*, 1972), ^{1}H-NMR (Karcher *et al.*, 1985; Memory & Wilson, 1982; TRC, 1982), ^{13}C-NMR (Karcher *et al.*, 1985; Memory & Wilson, 1982), mass spectrum (Karcher *et al.*, 1985; Shushan & Boyd, 1980; Stenhagen *et al.*, 1974).

Occurrence and carcinogenicity Dibenz[a,h]anthracene is found in the atmosphere, soil, auto exhaust, and cigarette smoke at levels lower than BA or BaP (IARC, 1983). It was the first synthetic PAH shown to be carcinogenic, and its biological properties have been studied extensively. It is moderately active as a carcinogen between BA and BaP in activity (Hartwell, 1951; IARC, 1983).

Synthesis Synthetic approaches to DBA are summarized in Fig. 9.3. One of the newest methods entails reaction of 2-lithio-*N*,*N*-diethyl-1-

naphthamide with 1-naphthaldehyde to furnish the lactone **13** (Harvey *et al.*, 1982). Reduction of **13** with zinc and alkali gives the free acid which undergoes cyclization with $ZnCl_2$ and acetic anhydride; reduction of 7-acetoxy-DBA with HI in acetic acid yields DBA. Another interesting new synthesis involves reaction of 1-bromonaphthalene with a lithium–amine salt in tetrahydrofuran which provides a mixture of DBA and dibenz[a,j]anthracene. The mechanism involves reaction of naphthyne with the lithium enolate of acetaldehyde generated *in situ* by retro-cycloaddition of the lithium salt of tetrahydrofuran; the resulting naphthocyclobutane is in equilibrium with a quinodimethane intermediate which undergoes cycloaddition of a second naphthyne to yield the product; thus, the meso carbon atoms derive from the solvent (Fleming & Mah, 1975). Other syntheses include reductive cyclization of the ketoacid **14** with HI (Platt & Oesch, 1981), and Elbs pyrolysis of the ketones **15** or **16** (Cook, 1931, 1932). In the reaction of **16** a rearrangement is evidently involved.

The phenolic derivatives of DBA are synthetically accessible by Diels–Alder reaction of styrene with the appropriate methoxy-substituted derivative of phenanthrene-1,4-dione in the presence of chloranil, followed by reduction of the resulting DBA-7,14-dione (**17**) with Zn/HOAc (Muschik *et al.*, 1982). The analogous DBajA-7,14-dione is a coproduct of the Diels–Alder cycloaddition. The seven isomeric phenols of DBA are also available by reductive cyclization of *o*-naphthoylnaphthoic acids with HI/P (Platt & Oesch, 1982). The 7,14-dimethyl derivative of DBA, which is a more potent carcinogen than DBA, is obtainable by reductive methylation of DBA-7,14-dione (DiGiovanni *et al.*, 1983; Konieczny & Harvey, 1980).

Fig. 9.3. Synthetic routes to dibenz[a,h]anthracene.

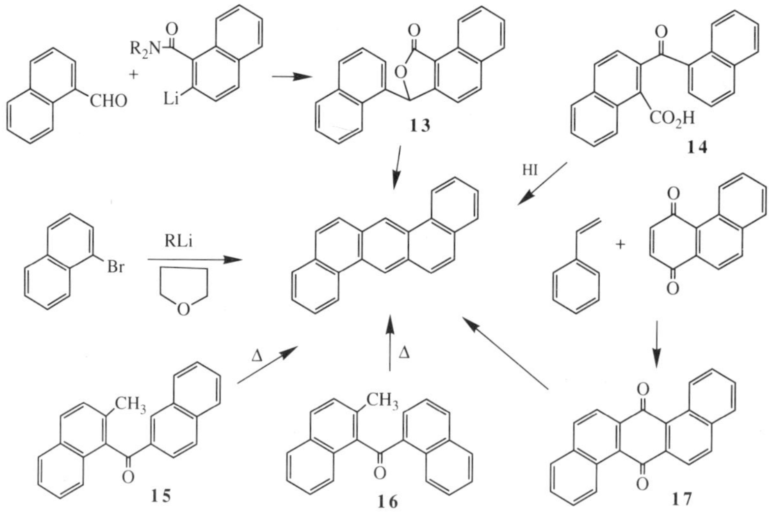

Reactions The chemistry of DBA resembles that of anthracene more closely than that of phenanthrene. Electrophilic substitutions are predicted theoretically to occur in the 7,14-positions. However, steric hindrance interferes with reactions in this region. As a consequence, bromination yields no identifiable products (Cook, 1931), and DBA is not attacked by $Pb(OAc)_4$ in acetic acid (Fieser & Hershberg, 1938a). Nitration takes place with nitric acid in acetic acid to yield 7-nitro-DBA (Cook, 1931). DBA reacts with maleic anhydride more slowly than does anthracene to give the meso region Diels–Alder adduct (Cook, 1931).

Oxidation of DBA with chromic acid yields DBA-7,14-dione (Clar, 1929), while ozonolysis affords the K-region mono- and diozonides (Moriconi *et al.*, 1960; Agarwal & Van Duuren, 1975). Oxidation of the latter gives the corresponding di- and tetracarboxylic acids, while their reduction furnishes the corresponding di- and tetraaldehydes. Oxidation of DBA with peracetic acid gave a high yield of the K-region oxidation product 2-phenylphenanthrene-3, 2'-dicarboxylic acid along with a small amount of the 7,14-5,6-diones (Van Duuren *et al.*, 1964). Reaction of DBA with OsO_4 also takes place in the K-region to yield the *cis*-5,6-dihydrodiol of DBA (Harvey, 1986).

Reduction with Li/NH_3 takes place regiospecifically in accord with theoretical prediction to yield 7,14-dihydro-DBA (Harvey, 1970). Hydrogenation over a Pd/C catalyst affords 5,6-dihydro-DBA (Fu *et al.*, 1980), while hydrogenation over a Pt catalyst yields a mixture of polyhydrogenated products (Lijinsky, 1961).

9.4   Dibenz[a,j]anthracene

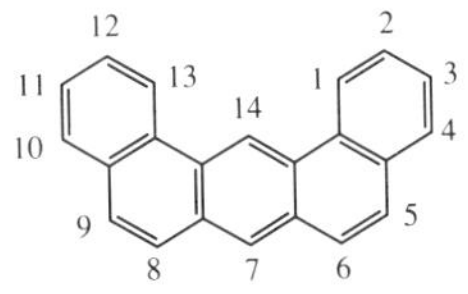

Other names: 1,2,7,8-dibenzanthracene (DBajA)
Physical and spectral properties $C_{22}H_{14}$, mol. wt. 278.33, colorless needles (acetic acid), mp 196 °C. Spectral data: UV (Karcher *et al.*, 1985; TRC, 1982a; Friedel & Orchin, 1951), UV fluorescence (Perin-Roussel *et al.*, 1972; Schoental & Scott, 1949), PE (Clar & Schmidt, 1979a), IR (Karcher *et al.*, 1985; Perin-Roussel *et al.*, 1972), ^{1}H-NMR (Karcher *et al.*, 1985; TRC, 1982; Memory & Wilson, 1982), ^{13}C-NMR (Karcher *et al.*, 1985), mass spectrum (Karcher *et al.*, 1985).

Occurrence and carcinogenicity Occurs in the high boiling fraction of coal tar. Trace levels of DBajA are detected in cigarette smoke (IARC, 1983). DBajA is a weak skin-tumor-initiator in mice, less active than DBahA (DiGiovanni *et al.*, 1983).

Synthesis Methods for the synthesis of DBajA are summarized in Fig. 9.4. A convenient synthesis involves coupling of 2-naphthaldehyde with 2-lithio-*N,N*-diethyl-1-naphthamide to furnish the lactone **18**. Reduction of **18** with zinc and alkali gives the free acid which undergoes acidic cyclization and reduction with HI to yield DBajA (Harvey *et al.*, 1982). Another interesting new synthesis entails photocyclization of 2-styryl-9,10-dihydro-phenanthrene (**19**); dehydrogenation of the product affords a mixture of DBajA and benzo[c]chrysene (Diederich *et al.*, 1984). It is necessary to employ the dihydro compound **19** for this purpose, since photocyclization of 2-styrlphenanthrene affords exclusively benzo[c]chrysene (Dietz & Scholz, 1968). DBajA is also synthetically accessible via cyclodehydration of the acid **21** followed by reduction (Cook, 1932). The acid **21** is obtained from reduction of the keto acid **20** which itself is prepared by SeO_2 oxidation of 2-methyl-1,1'-dinaphthyl ketone. Other syntheses include: reductive cyclization of the keto acid **22** with HI (Platt & Oesch, 1981); reaction of 1-bromonaphthalene with a lithium–amine salt in tetrahydrofuran which provides a mixture of DBa,jA and dibenz[a,j]anthracene (Fleming & Mah, 1975); and cyclodehydrogenation of **23** (Studt, 1978).

7,14-Dimethyl-DBajA, which is a highly potent carcinogen, is obtainable

Fig. 9.4. Methods for the synthesis of dibenz[a,j]anthracene.

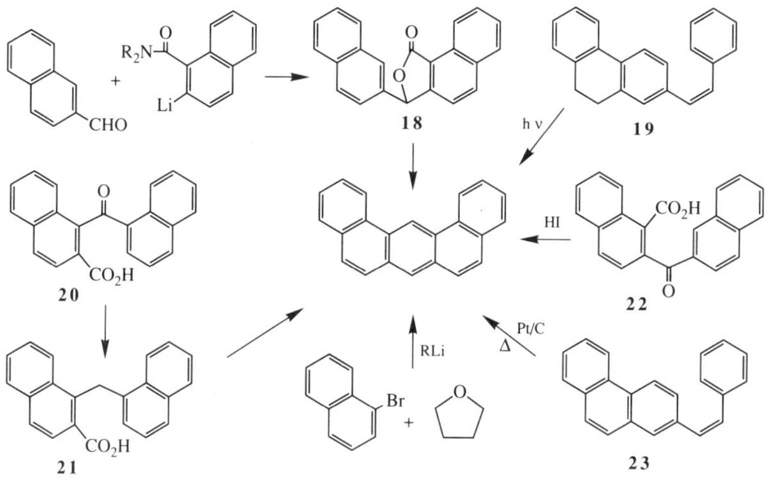

by reductive methylation of DBa,jA-7,14-dione (DiGiovanni *et al.*, 1983; Konieczny *et al.*, 1980). The 3-hydroxy derivative of 7,14-dimethyl-DBajA was obtained by a similar route and converted to the 3,4-dihydrodiol (Harvey *et al.*, 1988). Other phenolic derivatives of DBajA are synthetically accessible by reduction of methoxy-substituted DBajA-7,14-diones with Zn/HOAc (Muschik *et al.*, 1982). These quinones are obtained through Diels–Alder reaction of styrene with the appropriate methoxy-substituted derivatives of phenanthrene-1,4-dione in the presence of chloranil.

Reactions The chemistry of DBajA is relatively unexplored. Reaction with maleic anhydride yields a Diels–Alder meso region adduct. Oxidation with CrO_3 in acetic acid affords DBajA-7,14-dione (Clar, 1929). Ozonolysis of DBajA followed by oxidation with alkaline hydrogen peroxide provides mainly the dicarboxylic acid arising from oxidation in the K-region (Moriconi *et al.*, 1962).

9.5   Pentaphene

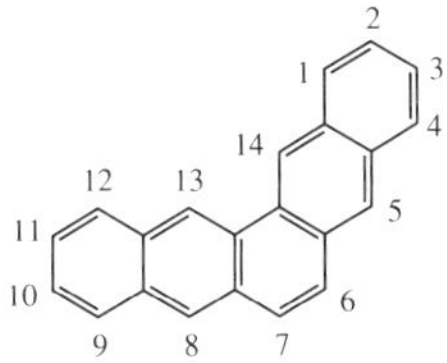

Other names: 2,3,6,7-dibenzophenanthrene, dibenzo[b,h]phen- anthrene, 2'3'-naphtho-1,2-anthracene
Physical and spectral properties $C_{22}H_{14}$, mol. wt. 278.33, pale yellow needles, mp 264 °C, sublimes. Spectral data: UV (Friedel & Orchin, 1951), PE (Clar & Schmidt, 1979), ^{1}H-NMR (Memory & Wilson, 1982).

Occurrence and carcinogenicity Occurs in the high boiling fraction of coal tar and automobile exhaust. The limited data available indicate it to be noncarcinogenic (Hartwell, 1951).

Synthesis Methods for the synthesis of pentaphene are summarized in Fig. 9.5. The first practical synthesis to be developed utilized Elbs pyrolysis of the ketones **24, 25**, and **26** (Clar & John, 1931). 6,13-Dihydropentacene, formed by partial rearrangement, is separated from the product mixture by its dehydrogenation with *o*-chloranil to form the sparingly soluble pentacene which precipitates from solution. The newest synthesis of pentaphene involves Diels–Alder addition of 1,3-bis(trimethylsilyl)isobenzofuran with 1,2-anthracyne and reduction of the adduct **27** with Zn/HOAc (Camenzind & Rickborn, 1986). Other syntheses include reaction of bis-bromomethyl compound **28** with phenyllithium followed by catalytic dehydrogenation over palladium (Bergmann & Ikan, 1958; Badger *et al.*, 1957), and treatment of the dialdehyde **29** with hydrazine (Bacon & Bankhead, 1963). Pentaphene is also synthetically accessible from Friedel–Crafts reaction of phthalic anhydride with 2-benzylbenzoic acid via the intermediate **30** (Franck & Zander, 1966).

Reactions Although little is known concerning the patterns of electrophilic substitution of pentaphene, it behaves in most respects as an anthracene derivative. Pentaphene combines with maleic anhydride to form a bis-adduct in the 5,8,13,14-positions (Clar, 1931). Oxidation with chromic acid takes place in the same molecular regions to provide pentaphene-5,8,13,14-tetraone (Clar & John, 1931). On the other hand, ozonolysis occurs preferentially in the K-region (Moriconi & Salce, 1967); reductive workup of the product furnishes the dialdehyde **29**. Reaction with OsO4 also takes place on this bond to yield the *cis*-6,7-dihydrodiol.

Fig. 9.5. Synthetic routes to pentaphene.

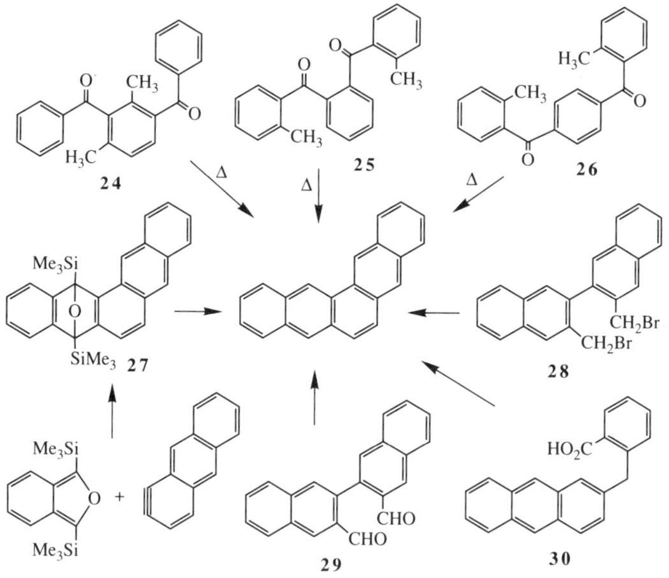

9.6   Benzo[b]chrysene

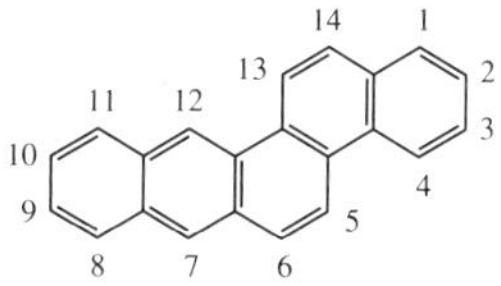

Other names: 3,4-benzotetraphene, 1,2-6,7-dibenzophenanthrene, 2'3'-naphtho-1,2-phenanthrene

Physical and spectral properties $C_{22}H_{14}$, mol. wt. 278.33, pale greenish-yellow plates or needles (xylene), mp 294° C, solutions exhibit blue fluorescence. Spectral data: UV (Karcher *et al.*, 1985; Clar & Stewart, 1952), UV fluorescence (Karcher *et al.*, 1985; Schoental & Scott, 1949), IR (Karcher *et al.*, 1985), ^{1}H-NMR (Karcher *et al.*, 1985; Cobb & Memory, 1967), ^{13}C-NMR (Karcher *et al.*, 1985), mass spectrum (Karcher *et al.*, 1985; Shushan & Boyd, 1980; Stenhagen *et al.*, 1974).

Occurrence and carcinogenicity Present as a minor component of coal tar (Wise *et al.*, 1988) and airborne pollution (Lao *et al.*, 1973). The limited data available indicate it to be noncarcinogenic (Hartwell, 1951).

Synthesis Synthetic routes to benzo[b]chrysene are summarized in Fig. 9.6. The Diels–Alder reaction of 1-vinylnaphthalene with 1,4-naphtho-quinone provides benzo[b]chrysene-7,12-dione (**31**) reduction of which yields benzo[b]chrysene (Davies & Porter, 1957). The Haworth synthesis with chrysene affords the keto acid **32** which is transformed to benzo[b]-chrysene by conventional methods (Cook & Graham, 1944). The reaction of *o*-toluoyl chloride with phenanthrene and AlCl₃ affords a mixture of **33**, **34**, and other *o*-toluoylphenanthrene isomers (Clar, 1929a; Bachmann & Pence,

Fig. 9.6.   Synthetic routes to benzo[b]chrysene.

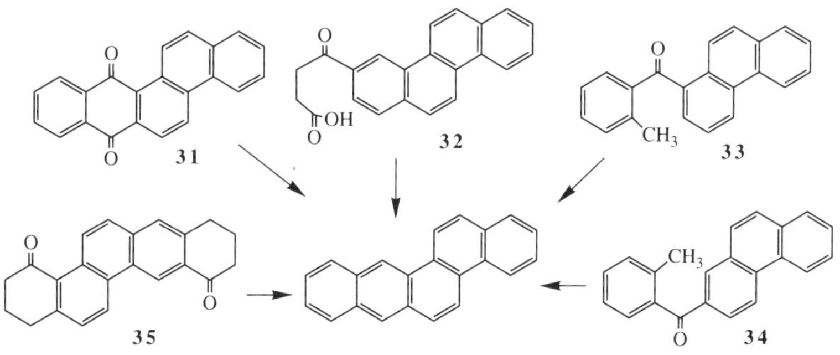

1935). Elbs pyrolysis of this mixture furnishes a mixture of benzo[b]-chrysene, benzo[a]naphthacene, and dibenz[a]anthracene, separable by their differences in reactivity with maleic anhydride or by chromatographic methods. Benzo[b]chrysene is also obtained from the reduction and dehydrogenation of the diketone **35** obtained as a secondary product from cyclization of its dicarboxylic acid precursor (Phillips, 1953). Although no modern synthetic approaches to benzo[b]chrysene have been reported, compounds of this class should be accessible by some of the newer methods of PAH synthesis, such as the enamine alkylation route (Chap. 7).

Reactions The chemistry of benzo[b]chrysene is relatively un-explored. Oxidation with chromic acid in acetic acid initially affords **31**, and further reaction yields benzo[b]chrysene-7,12,13,14-tetraone (Clar, 1929a).

9.7   Benzo[c]chrysene

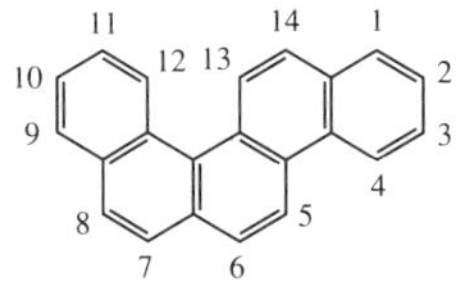

Other names: 5,6-benzochrysene, 1,2:5,6-dibenzophenanthrene
Physical and spectral properties $C_{22}H_{14}$, mol. wt. 278.33, colorless needles (acetic acid), mp 127 °C; the low mp contrasts with those of the more symmetrical 5-ring PAHs, such as picene and benzo[b]chrysene. Spectral data: UV (Karcher *et al.*, 1985; Snatzke & Kunde, 1973), UV fluorescence (Karcher *et al.*, 1985), IR (Karcher *et al.*, 1985), ^{1}H-NMR (Bax *et al.*, 1985; Karcher *et al.*, 1985; Snatzke & Kunde, 1973), ^{13}C-NMR (Bax *et al.*, 1985; Karcher *et al.*, 1985), mass spectrum (Shushan & Boyd, 1980).

Occurrence and carcinogenicity Occurs in coal tar and crude oil. Limited data indicate benzo[c]chrysene to be a weak carcinogen on mouse skin (Hartwell, 1951).

Synthesis Synthetic routes to benzo[c]chrysene are summarized in Fig. 9.7. Photocyclization of 1,3-distyrylbenzene (**36**) or 1-(1-naphthyl)-2-(2-naphthyl)ethylene (**37**) affords benzo[c]chrysene directly in good yield (Dietz & Scholz, 1968; Levi & Orchin, 1966). Diels–Alder reaction of maleic anhydride with the diene **38** yields the adduct **39** which is transformed to benzo[c]chrysene by dehydrogenation and decarboxylation (Wiedlich, 1938).

Other syntheses include cyclodehydrohalogenation of **40** with KOH followed by decarboxylation (Hewett, 1938a) and reaction of **41** with AlCl$_3$ and dehydrogenation of the cyclized adduct with selenium (Bergmann, 1938).

Reactions The chemical properties of benzo[c]chrysene are unexplored.

9.8   Benzo[g]chrysene

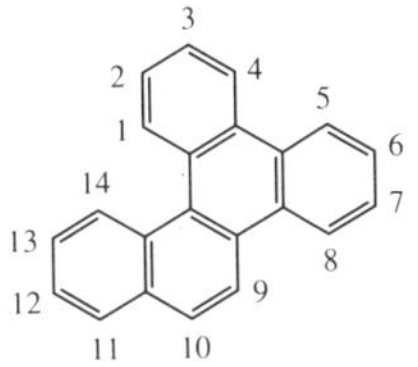

Other names: 5,6-benzochrysene, 1,2:5,6-dibenzophenanthrene

Physical and spectral properties C$_{22}$H$_{14}$, mol. wt. 278.33, colorless needles (acetic acid), mp 114.5 °C. Spectral data: UV (Clar & Stewart, 1952), UV fluorescence (McKay & Latham, 1973), ^{1}H-NMR (Bax *et al.*, 1985; Cobb & Memory, 1967), ^{13}C-NMR (Bax *et al.*, 1985).

Occurrence and carcinogenicity Occurs in coal tar and petroleum distillates (McKay & Latham, 1973). Limited data indicate benzo[g]chrysene to be a moderately potent carcinogen on mouse skin or injected subcutaneously (Harris & Bradsher, 1946; Hartwell, 1951).

Fig. 9.7. Synthetic routes to benzo[c]chrysene.

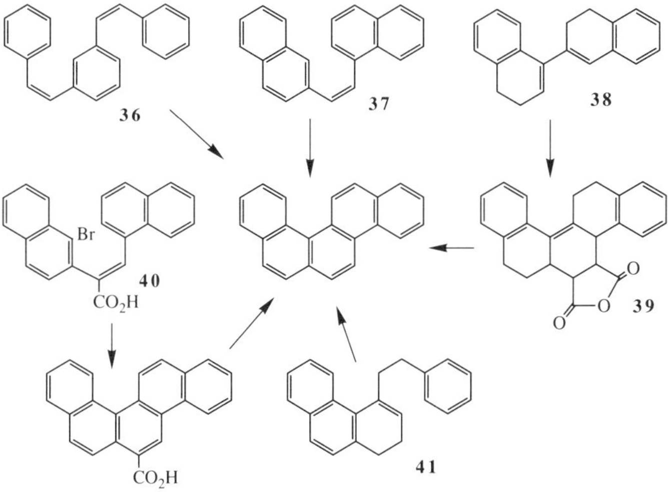

Synthesis Synthetic routes to benzo[g]chrysene are summarized in Fig. 9.8. Haworth synthesis based on reaction of chrysene with succinic anhydride and AlCl₃ gives the adduct **42** which is readily transformed to benzo[g]chrysene by the usual methods (Agarwal *et al.*, 1985). A more unusual synthetic approach entails acid-catalyzed cyclodehydration of the epoxide intermediate **43** followed by dehydrogenation (Bradsher & Rapoport, 1943); it is likely that isomerization of **43** to the corresponding ketone precedes cyclization. Benzo[g]chrysene is also conveniently prepared from chrysene-5,6-dione by reaction with lithium acetylide followed by reduction with LiAlH₄ to furnish the divinyl diol **44** which undergoes cyclization and dehydration on treatment with HI (Sukumaran & Harvey, 1981). Other syntheses include photochemical cyclization of 9-styrylphenan-threne (**45**) (Carruthers, 1967); the Pschorr reaction of **46** (Hewett, 1938); Diels–Alder reaction between 1,1'-bicyclohexenyl and 1,2-naphthyne to furnish the adduct **47** which on catalytic dehydrogenation provides benzo[g]chrysene in low yield (Corbett & Porter, 1965); and Diels–Alder cycloaddition of maleic anhydride to cyclohexenylphenanthrene to form the adduct **48** followed by dehydrogenation and decarboxylation (Bergmann & Smuszkovicz, 1947).

Reactions The chemical properties of benzo[g]chrysene are virtually unexplored. Oxidation with chromic anhydride yields the 9,10-dione (Clar,

Fig. 9.8. Synthetic routes to benzo[g]chrysene.

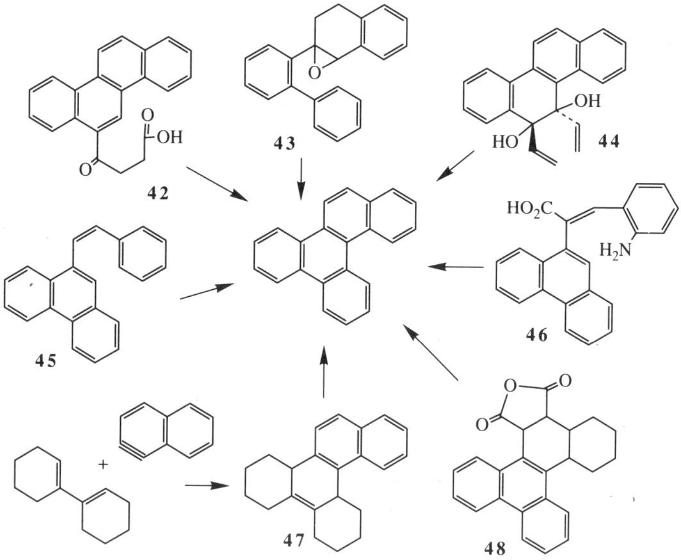

1964), while ozonolysis yields the 9,10-dione and the dicarboxylic acid arising from further oxidation in the K-region (Copeland *et al.*, 1961).

9.9   Benzo[a]pyrene

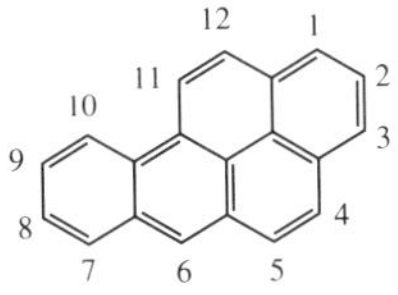

Other names: 1,2-benzopyrene, 3,4-benzpyrene, benzo[def]chry-sene (BaP)

Physical and spectral properties $C_{20}H_{12}$, mol. wt. 252.32, pale yellow needles or plates, mp 179-80 °C; soluble in benzene, toluene, chloroform, tetrahydrofuran; moderately soluble in acetone; sparingly soluble in ethanol; aqueous solubility is enhanced by purines and DNA (Boyland & Green, 1962). Spectral data: UV (Karcher *et al.*, 1985; TRC, 1982a; Friedel & Orchin, 1951), UV fluorescence (Schoental & Scott, 1949; Sawicki *et al.*, 1960), IR (Karcher *et al.*, 1985; Pouchert, 1981), PE (Clar & Schmidt, 1979), ^{1}H-NMR (Karcher *et al.*, 1985; Unkefer *et al.*, 1983; TRC, 1982; Memory & Wilson, 1982), ^{13}C-NMR (Karcher *et al.*, 1985; Unkefer *et al.*, 1983; Memory & Wilson, 1982; Ozubuku *et al.*, 1974), mass spectrum (Shushan & Boyd, 1980; Stenhagen *et al.*, 1974).

Occurrence and carcinogenicity BaP was first isolated from coal tar and was subsequently identified as a widespread environmental pollutant (IARC, 1983). It is also a component of cigarette and marijuana smoke (Lee *et al.*, 1976) and automobile exhaust (Grimmer, 1979), and significant levels are present in many common foods (Baum, 1978). It is a relatively potent carcinogen whose biological properties have been extensively documented (IARC, 1983).

Synthesis Synthetic approaches to BaP and its derivatives are summarized in Fig. 9.9. The most frequently employed method is Haworth synthesis involving reaction of pyrene with succinic anhydride and $AlCl_3$ (Schlude, 1971; Cook & Hewett, 1933). Wolff–Kishner reduction of the keto acid adduct and acid-catalyzed cyclization provides 7-oxo-7,8,9,10-tetrahydro-BaP (**49**) which is readily transformed to BaP by reduction with $NaBH_4$, dehydration, and dehydrogenation. Compound **49** is an important intermediate for the synthesis of the carcinogenic diol epoxide and other oxidized metabolites of BaP (Harvey, 1986; Harvey & Fu, 1978). Another practical synthesis of BaP entails reaction of dihydrophenalenone with benzoyl chloride and AlCl₃ to give 6-benzoyldihydrophenalene (**50**); this product undergoes cyclodehydrogenation to yield **51** which is converted to BaP on heating with zinc dust (Fieser & Hershberg, 1938b). A new synthetic approach involves reaction of 2-lithio-*N*,*N*-diethylbenzamide with perinaphthanone followed by reduction of the lactone product **52** with zinc and alkali, reductive cyclization with HI, and dehydrogenation with DDQ; this method has been employed to prepare 11-*tert*-butyl-BaP (Pataki *et al.*, 1982). BaP has also been prepared from 1-oxo-1,2,3,4-tetrahydro-BA by Reformatski reaction with bromoacetic ester and zinc to provide **53**; dehydration and dehydrogenation of **53** yields 11-hydroxy-BaP from which BaP is obtained by reduction with zinc (Fieser & Heymann, 1941). Contrary to an earlier claim (Jutz, 1978), BaP is not a coproduct along with BeP from the reaction of benzanthrene with the vinamidinium salt Me₂N=CH-CH=CH-NMe₂ X⁻ followed by thermal electrocyclic ring closure (Lee & Harvey, 1981; Lee *et al.*, 1981). Other methods of synthesis are reviewed by Osborne & Crosby, 1987 and Clar, 1964.

All 12 of the isomeric monomethyl-BaPs and numerous dimethyl-BaPs have been synthesized and tested for tumorigenic activity (Osborne & Crosby, 1987). All of the isomeric BaP phenols are also known (Yagi *et al.*, 1976; Fu & Harvey, 1981, 1983; Harvey & Fu, 1982; Harvey & Cho, 1975).

Reactions Electrophilic substitutions take place mainly in the 6-position of BaP, in accord with theoretical prediction. BaP reacts with N-

Fig. 9.9. Synthetic routes to benzo[a]pyrene.

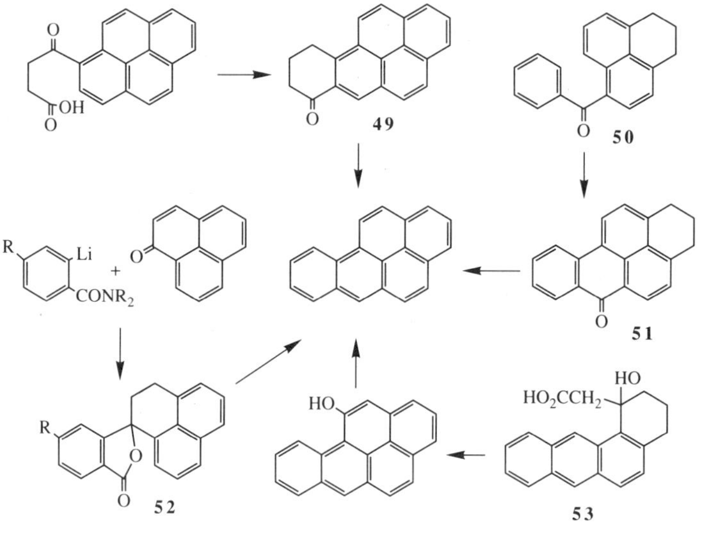

bromosuccinimide and sulfuryl chloride to afford 6-bromo- and 6-chloro-BaP, respectively (Dewhurst & Kitchen, 1972). The reaction of BaP with Br_2 in pyridine also furnishes 6-bromo-BaP, while its reaction with Br_2 in chlorobenzene yields 1,3,6-tribromo-BaP, and further reaction under more vigorous conditions provides a heptabromo-BaP derivative (Lang & Zander, 1964). Nitration gives 6-nitro-BaP along with lesser amounts of the 1-nitro and 3-nitro isomers (Dewar *et al.*, 1956; Fieser & Hershberg, 1939). Vilsmeier reaction of BaP with methylformanilide yields 6-formyl-BaP (Fieser & Hershberg, 1938, see Chap. 8), and reaction of BaP with $Pb(OAc)_4$ affords 6-acetoxy-BaP (Fieser & Hershberg, 1939). On the other hand, acetylation with acetic anhydride and $AlCl_3$ provides 1-acetyl-BaP from which BaP 1-carboxylic acid is obtained by oxidation with hypochlorite (Windaus & Raichle, 1938). Apparently, acetylation takes place initially in the 6-position, but is reversible leading to ultimate formation of the thermodynamically more stable 1-acetyl-BaP (Gore, 1955). Direct *tert*-butylation of BaP with *tert*-butanol in refluxing trifluoroacetic acid proceeds contrary to the normal pattern of substitution, affording instead 11-*tert*-butyl-BaP as the major product (Pataki *et al.*, 1982).

Oxidation of BaP with chromic acid was reported by Vollmann *et al.*, 1937 to give the 1,6- and 3,6-diones as the primary products. However, the wide range of melting points found by subsequent investigators prompted a reinvestigation by Cho & Harvey, 1976 who isolated by careful chromatography the pure 1,6-, 3,6-, and 6,12-diones in yields of 40, 20, and 7%, respectively. Oxidation of BaP with ceric ammonium sulfate gave a mixture of the 1,6- and 3,6-diones (Balanikas *et al.*, 1988). Ozonolysis of BaP affords the 1,6- and 3,6-diones in 1:3 ratio along with a trace of the 4,5-dione and other oxidized products (Moriconi *et al.*, 1961). Oxidation of BaP with OsO_4 yields the K-region *cis*-4,5-dihydrodiol; the crude dihydrodiol

Fig. 9.10. Hydrogenation of benzo[a]pyrene.

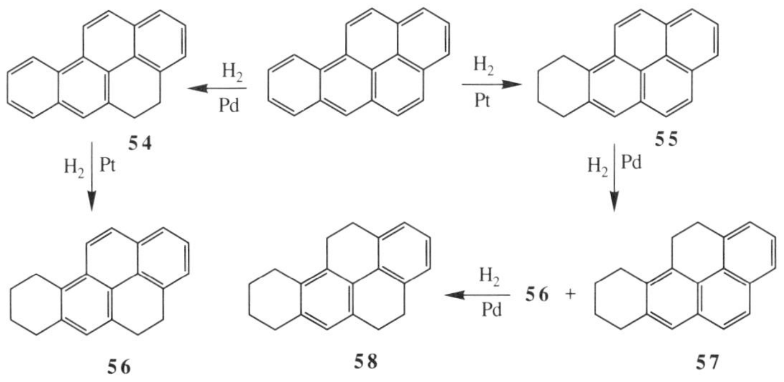

decomposes in air and is most conveniently isolated and purified as its diacetate (Harvey *et al.*, 1975).

Hydrogenation of BaP over a Pd catalyst occurs regiospecifically in the K-region to yield 4,5-dihydro-BaP (**54**), whereas similar reaction in the presence of a Pt catalyst takes place in the benzo ring to provide 7,8,9,10-tetrahydro-BaP (**55**), in accord with the usual regioselectivities of these catalysts (Fu *et al.*, 1980) (Fig. 9.10). Further hydrogenation of **54** over Pt affords the hexahydro derivative **56**, while further hydrogenation of **55** over Pd initially provides **56** and the hexahydro isomer **57**, and with longer reaction time the sole product is the octahydro derivative **58** (Fu *et al.*, 1980).

9.10   Benzo[e]pyrene

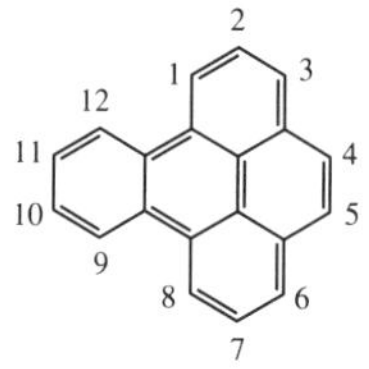

Other names: 1,2-benzopyrene, 4,5-benzpyrene (BeP)

Physical and spectral properties $C_{20}H_{12}$, mol. wt. 252.32, colorless prisms (benzene), mp 178-79 °C. Spectral data: UV (Karcher *et al.*, 1985; TRC, 1982a; Friedel & Orchin, 1951), UV fluorescence (Karcher *et al.*, 1985; Berlman, 1971), PE (Clar & Schmidt, 1979), IR (Karcher *et al.*, 1985; Pouchert, 1981), ^{1}H-NMR (Karcher *et al.*, 1985; Memory & Wilson, 1982; TRC, 1982; Perin-Roussel, 1972), ^{13}C-NMR (Karcher *et al.*, 1985), mass spectrum (Shushan & Boyd, 1980; Stenhagen *et al.*, 1974).

Occurrence and carcinogenicity Occurs in coal tar from which it was isolated (Cook & Hewett, 1933). Common environmental contaminant occurring at levels generally lower than the more carcinogenic BaP (IARC, 1983) and is also a component of cigarette and marijuana smoke (IARC, 1983; Lee *et al.*, 1976). BeP is not active as a complete carcinogen and is a weak tumor initiator with TPA promotion (IARC, 1983).

Synthesis Synthetic approaches to BeP are summarized in Fig. 9.11. The first successful synthesis of BeP was based on the Haworth synthesis with 1,2,3,6,7,8-hexahydropyrene, succinic anhydride and AlCl$_3$ (Cook & Hewett, 1933). The cyclized ketone (**59**) obtained by this route is readily converted to BeP via reduction with NaBH$_4$, acidic dehydration, and dehydrogenation (Harvey *et al.*, 1979). Compound **59** is also a useful starting compound for the preparation of the 9,10-dihydrodiol and the corresponding diol epoxide derivatives of BeP (Harvey *et al.*, 1979; Harvey, 1985). Photocyclization of either 1-ß-naphthyl-4-phenyl-1,3-butadiene (**60**) or 4-phenylphenanthrene (**61**) provides BeP in fewer steps, but is more suitable for small scale preparations (Hayward *et al.*, 1972). An interesting new synthesis is the dialkylation of the pyrene 'dianion' in liquid ammonia with 1,4-diiodobutane to yield hexahydro-BeP (**62**) which is dehydrogenated with DDQ to BeP (Tintel *et al.*, 1983). Since the pyrene dianion is likely to undergo protonation to form the monoanion in ammonia, it is likely that the mechanism involves alkylation of this monoanion, followed by generation of a second monoanion by reaction with amide anion and cyclization (Harvey, 1970). BeP is also synthetically accessible from pyrene-4,5-dione by reaction with lithium acetylide, followed by reduction with LiAlH4 to the divinyl diol **63** and reaction of the latter with HI (Sukumaran & Harvey, 1981). BeP may also be prepared from 7*H*-benzanthrene by the Jutz synthesis with a vinamidinium salt, followed by thermal electrocyclic ring closure of the adduct **64** (Jutz, 1978; Lee & Harvey, 1981). This method has been utilized to prepare otherwise unobtainable derivatives of BeP, such as 1- and 2-methyl-BeP and 2-hydroxy-BeP (Lee & Harvey, 1981; Lee *et al.*, 1981, 1981a). Other methods of synthesis of BeP and its derivatives are reviewed by Osborne & Crosby, 1987 and by Clar, 1964.

Syntheses of the complete sets of six isomeric monomethyl derivatives and

Fig. 9.11. Synthetic routes to benzo[e]pyrene.

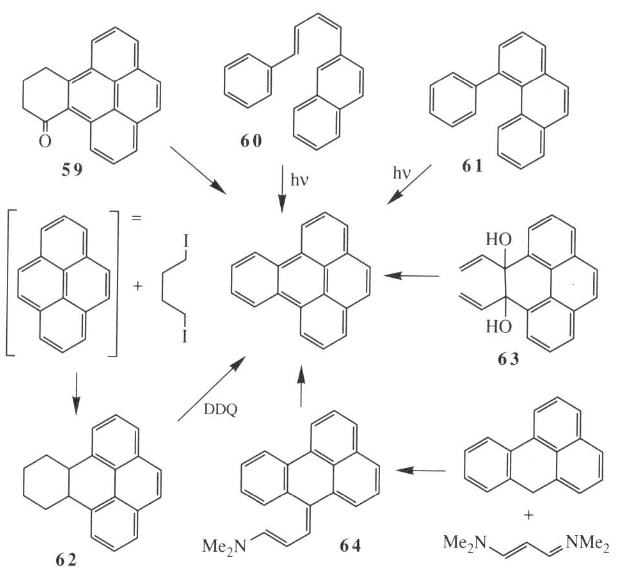

phenols of BeP have also been reported (Lee & Harvey, 1981; Lee *et al.*, 1981, 1981a).

Reactions The electrophilic reactions of BeP resemble those of pyrene. Bromination affords initially 3-bromo-BeP (Lee *et al.*, 1981), and further reaction with excess Br_2 yields 3,6-dibromo-BeP (Lee *et al.*, 1981; Lang & Zander, 1964). Chlorination proceeds all the way to 1,3,6,8-tetrachloro-BeP (Lang & Zander, 1964). This difference is evidently a consequence of the smaller steric demand of the chlorine atom. Chlorination of 3,6-dibromo-BeP provides 3,6-dibromo-1,8-dichloro-BeP which was utilized to prepare 1,8-dichloro-BeP by reaction with magnesium and hydrolysis (Lee *et al.*, 1981a).

Oxidation of BeP with OsO_4 takes place in the K-region to provide the *cis*-4,5-dihydrodiol (Lee *et al.*, 1981a; Lehr *et al.*, 1978). Acid treatment of the diacetate of this diol converts it to 4-hydroxy-BeP (Lee *et al.*, 1981a) which is transformed to BeP-4,5-dione by oxidation with DDQ (Lehr *et al.*, 1978). Reduction of BeP with Na and amyl alcohol gives a somewhat impure 1,2,3,6,7,8-hexahydro-BeP which on further reduction yields 1,2,3,6, 7,8,9,10,11,12-decahydro-BeP (Lang & Zander, 1964).

9.11   Dibenzo[c,g]phenanthrene

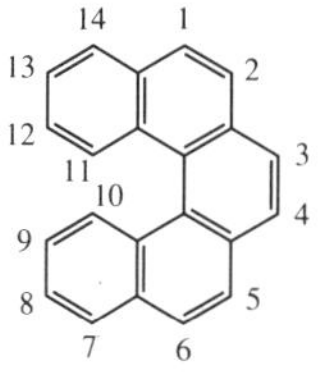

Other names: [5]helicene, pentahelicene

Physical and spectral properties $C_{22}H_{14}$, mol. wt. 278.33, colorless needles (alcohol), mp 181-82 °C. The loss of delocalization energy due to the distortion of the molecule from planarity is calculated to be 18 kcal/mol. Its relative instability may partially account for the fact that it does not appear to occur as an environmental pollutant. The crystal structures of the two racemic modifications of [5]helicene have been determined (Kuroda, 1982) as have those of the racemate and S-(+)-enantiomer of its 3,4-dihydro derivative (Kuroda & Mason, 1981). The optically active isomers of dibenzo[c,g]phenanthrene have been resolved (Bestmann & Both, 1974; Goedke & Stegemeyer, 1970). Spectral data: UV (Clar, 1964), UV fluorescence (Schoental & Scott, 1949), ^{1}H-NMR (Perin-Roussel, 1972;

Haigh & Mallion, 1971), ^{13}C-NMR (Defay *et al.*, 1971), mass spectrum (Ueda *et al.*, 1985), CD (Goedke & Stegemeyer, 1970).

Occurrence and carcinogenicity No information could be found on the occurrence of this hydrocarbon. On the basis of limited data, it appears to be inactive as a tumorigen on mouse skin (Hartwell, 1951).

Synthesis Synthetic routes to dibenzo[c,g]phenanthrene are summarized in Fig. 9.12. Dibenzo[c,g]phenanthrene is synthetically accessible from 2,2'-bis(bromomethyl)-1,1'-binaphthyl (**65**) by treatment with phenyllithium followed by dehydrogenation over a Pd/C catalyst (Bergmann & Smuszkovicz, 1951) or by reaction of its diphosphonium salt **66** with sodium ethoxide (Bestmann *et al.*, 1969). Diels–Alder reaction of the diene **67** with maleic anhydride gives the adduct **69** which on dehydrogenation and decarboxylation yields dibenzo[c,g]phenanthrene (Altman & Ginsburg, 1959). This hydrocarbon is also obtained by irradiation of dinaphthylethene **68** in the presence of an amine followed by dehydrogenation (LaPouyade *et al.*, 1982).

Reactions The chemistry of dibenzo[c,g]phenanthrene is relatively unknown. Ozonolysis yields the tetracarboxylic acid arising from oxidation of the 1,2- and 5,6-bonds (Copeland *et al.*, 1961).

Fig. 9.12. Synthetic routes to dibenzo[c,g,] phenanthrene.

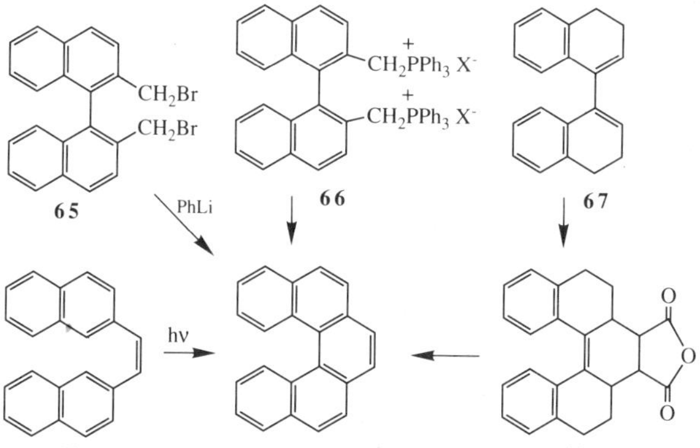

9.12   Perylene

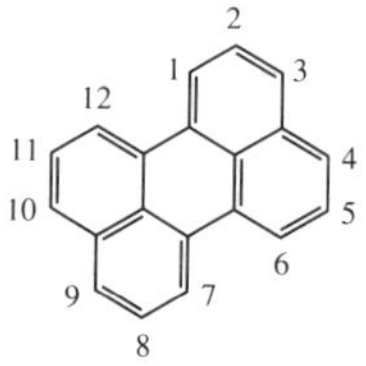

Other names: peri-dinaphthalene
Physical and spectral properties $C_{20}H_{12}$, mol. wt. 252.30, dimorphous crystals α-form yellow plates, mp 140 °C, ß-form greenish-yellow plates, mp 279 °C; freely soluble in CS_2, chloroform, moderately soluble in benzene, slightly soluble in ether, acetone, alcohol. Solutions show strong blue fluorescence. Spectral data: UV (Karcher, 1988; TRC, 1982; Sawicki *et al.*, 1960; Friedel & Orchin, 1951), UV fluorescence (Karcher, 1988; Sawicki *et al.*, 1960; Schoental & Scott, 1949), IR (Karcher, 1988; Pouchert, 1981), PE (Clar & Schmidt, 1979), ^{1}H-NMR (Karcher, 1988; Memory & Wilson, 1982; TRC, 1982), [13]H-NMR (Karcher, 1988; Minsky *et al.*, 1982), mass spectrum (Karcher, 1988; Shushan & Boyd, 1980; Stenhagen *et al.*, 1974).

Occurrence and carcinogenicity Perylene is obtained from coal tar and has been detected in petroleum, carbon black, and airborne pollutants (IARC, 1983; Lao *et al.*, 1973). Perylene exhibits essentially no activity as a complete carcinogen or a tumor initiator (Hartwell, 1951; IARC, 1983).

Synthesis Synthetic routes to perylene are summarized in Fig. 9.13. The first reported synthesis, albeit in low yield, was from heating naphthalene with $AlCl_3$ (Scholl *et al.*, 1910). A more efficient method involves heating 1,8-naphthalimide with KOH in ethanol to obtain the diimide **70** (Bradley & Pexton, 1954). Hydrolysis of **70** gives the corresponding tetracarboxylic acid, decarboxylation of which yields perylene. Perylene can also be prepared from anthracene via bis-chloromethylation in the 9,10-positions and reaction of the product with sodiomalonic ester to provide **71** (R = CO_2H); saponification and decarboxylation of this furnishes the dicarboxylic acid **71** (R = H). Acid-catalyzed cyclization of the latter gives the ketone **72** which is converted to perylene by reduction and dehydrogenation (Postovskii & Bednyagina, 1937). Additional syntheses of perylene are described by Clar, 1964.

Reactions Electrophilic substitution of perylene takes place predominantly in the 3-position, and to a lesser extent in the 1-position, in accord with MO theoretical prediction. Nitration with dilute nitric acid in dioxane affords 3-nitro- and 1-nitroperylene in 7:3 ratio (Looker, 1972), while nitration with nitric acid in acetic anhydride is more selective, providing the 1- and 3-nitro isomers in the ratio of 97:3 (Nordbotten *et al.*, 1984). Further nitration with this reagent gives a mixture of dinitro isomers consisting mainly of 3,6-, 3,9-, and a lesser amount of 3,7-dinitroperylene (Nordbotten *et al.*, 1984). The reaction of perylene with conc. nitric acid yields 3,4,9,10-tetranitroperylene (Zinke *et al.*, 1925). In keeping with the trend to develop milder, more selective reagents, it has been found recently that nitration of perylene with dinitrogen tetroxide at room temperature affords 3-nitroperylene (95%) with high regioselectivity (99%) (Radner, 1983). Bromination and chlorination yield the corresponding 3,9- and 3,10-dihaloperylenes (Uchida *et al.*, 1979; Ware & Bochert, 1961; Zinke *et al.*, 1925). Sulfonylation of perylene with SO_3 under mild conditions yields perylene 3-sulfonic acid (Cerfontain *et al.*, 1983), while reaction with sulfuric acid in acetic acid furnishes a mixture of the 3,9- and 3,10-disulfonic acid derivatives (Marschalk, 1927).

Formylation of perylene with *N*-methylformanilide and phosphoryl chloride yields 3-formylperylene (Buu-Hoi & Long, 1956), and reaction of perylene with acetyl chloride and $AlCl_3$ furnishes 3-acetylperylene (Zieger, 1966). However, the site of substitution can be effectively controlled by prior hydrogenation. Thus, hydrogenation of perylene over a copper chromite catalyst affords 1,2,3,10,11,12-hexahydroperylene which undergoes acetylation preferentially in the 5-position; dehydrogenation of this product yields 2-acetylperylene (Zieger, 1966). In contrast, addition of alkyllithium reagents

Fig. 9.13. Synthetic routes to perylene.

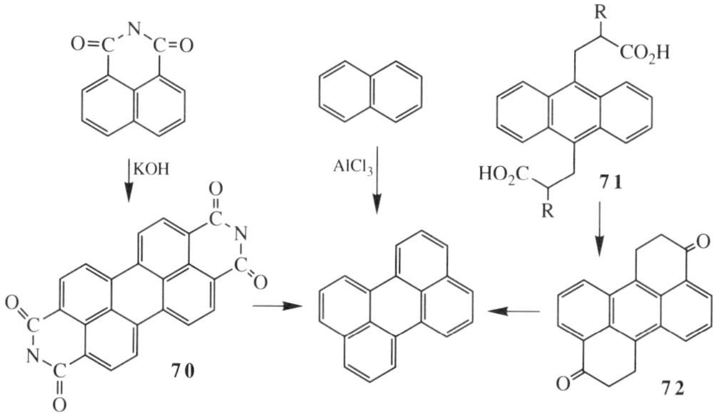

to perylene takes place in the 1-position (to form the relatively more stable 3-anion); treatment of the adducts with iodine provides the corresponding 1-alkylperylenes (Peake *et al.*, 1983; Zieger & Rosenkranz, 1964). Although not subsequently exploited, this reaction potentially allows synthetic access to other 1-substituted derivatives of perylene (e.g. through oxidation of the alkyl group to carboxyl with subsequent conversion to various other functions).

Perylene undergoes Diels–Alder cycloaddition of maleic anhydride in the presence of chloranil to yield benzo[g,h,i]perylene dicarboxylic anhydride, providing a convenient synthesis of this polycyclic ring system (Clar & Zander, 1957) (Fig. 7.10). Similarly, Diels–Alder reaction of perylene with dialkyl diazenedicarboxylates takes place in the same molecular region to furnish adducts which are decarboxylated to the corresponding pyridazines (Tokita *et al.*, 1982).

Oxidation of perylene with aqueous chromic acid furnishes perylene-3,10-dione (Zinke & Unterkreuter, 1919). Ozonolysis of perylene affords anthraquinone-1,5-dicarboxylic acid in low yield (Copeland *et al.*, 1959).

Reduction of perylene provides a range of hydroaromatic products. As already stated, hydrogenation over a copper chromite catalyst affords the hexahydro derivative **73** (R = H) which has a UV spectrum similar to that of phenanthrene (Zieger, 1966). Reduction with HI and phosphorus yields a hexahydroperylene isomer identified as **73** or **74** (Zinke & Unterkreuter, 1919). Reduction of perylene with sodium and ethanol is reported in one study to provide **74** and the octahydro product **75** (Zinke & Bendorf, 1934), while in another study the main product is decahydroperylene **76** (Read *et al.*, 1959). Reduction of perylene with sodium in amyl alcohol furnishes **75** and **77** (Zinke & Bendorf, 1932).

$$73 \qquad 74 \qquad 75 \qquad 76 \qquad 77$$

9.13   Benzo[a]naphthacene

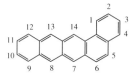

Other names: 1,2-benzotetracene, dibenz[a,i]anthracene
Physical and spectral properties $C_{22}H_{14}$, mol. wt. 278.33, golden

leaflets, mp 270-71 °C (263-64 °C) (xylene or AcOH). Solutions exhibit deep green fluorescence. Spectral data: UV (Friedel & Orchin, 1951; Clar & Lombardi, 1932), UV fluorescence (Schoental & Scott, 1949), ^{1}H-NMR (Pollart & Rickborn, 1986), mass spectrum (Pollart & Rickborn, 1986).

Occurrence and carcinogenicity No reliable data could be found.

Synthesis Synthetic routes to benzo[a]naphthacene are summarized in Fig. 9.14. The oldest preparative method is Elbs pyrolysis of the ketones **78** and **79** in the presence of copper powder (Clar, 1929a; Bachmann & Pence, 1935). A superior modification of this method is the pyrolysis of the partially saturated ketones **80** and **81**; dehydrogenation takes place concurrently to give benzo[a]naphthacene directly (Clar, 1929a). The reaction of naphthalene-2,3-dicarboxylic anhydride and naphthalene in the presence of AlCl$_3$ affords a mixture of two naphthoyl-*o*-naphthoic acids

Fig. 9.14. Synthetic routes to benzo[a]naphthacene.

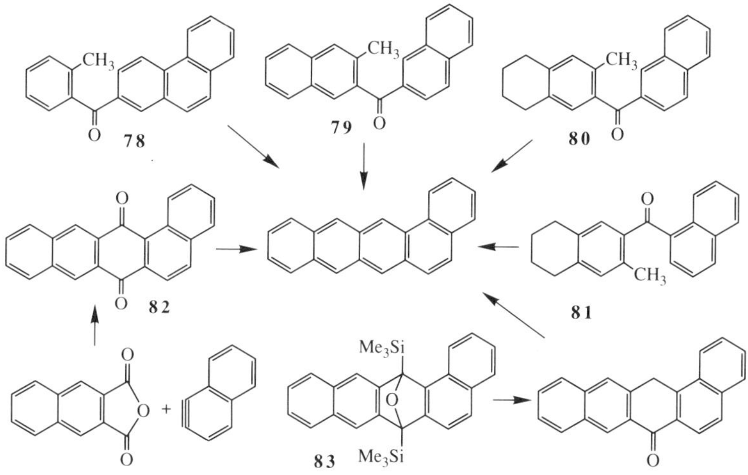

Fig. 9.15. Synthesis of benzo[a]naphthacene 8,13-dione via a quinodimethane intermediate.

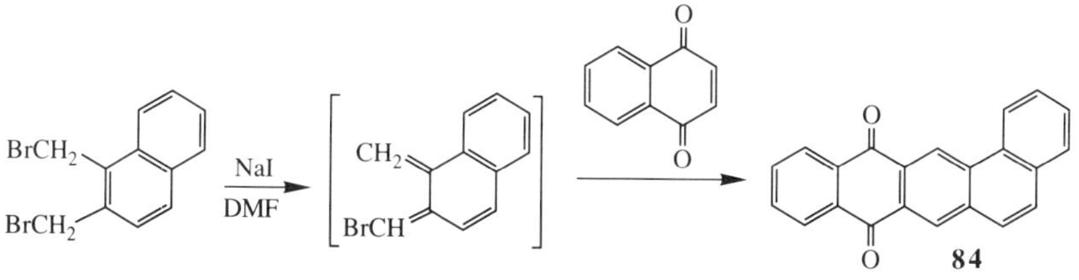

which yield on ring closure a mixture of benzo[a]naphthacene-7,14-dione (**82**) and pentacene-6,13-dione (Weizmann *et al.*, 1935). A newer synthetic approach involves the reaction of 2,3-naphthalyne generated *in situ* with 1,3-bis(trimethylsilyl)naphtho[1,2-c]furan to form the adduct **83**; treatment of **83** with trifluoroacetic acid gave the anthrone, which was reduced by LiAlH$_4$ and dehydrated to the hydrocarbon (Pollart & Rickborn, 1986). Another potentially useful synthesis involves reaction of 2'-bromo-1,2-naphtho-quinodimethane (generated *in situ*) with 1,4-naphthoquinone (Fig. 9.15) to yield benzo[a]naphthacene-8,13-dione (**84**) (Gribble *et al.*, 1977); presumably the primary product is dehydrogenated by the quinone reagent.

Reactions Electrophilic substitutions take place preferentially in the 8,13-positions of benzo[a]naphthacene. Diels–Alder cycloaddition with maleic anhydride also occurs in this region; the adduct is useful for the purification of the hydrocarbon (Clar & Lombardi, 1932). Oxidation with chromic acid yields benzo[a]naphthacene-8,13-dione, and further reaction affords benzo[a]naphthacene-5,6,8,13-dione (Clar, 1929a). Methanolysis of the disodio or dilithio adducts of benzo[a]naphthacene furnishes a mixture of 7,14- and 8,13-dihydrobenzo[a]naphthacene (Bachmann & Pence, 1937).

9.14   References

Agarwal, S. C. & Van Duuren, B. L. (1975). Synthesis of diepoxides and diphenol ethers of pyrene and dibenz[a,h]anthracene. *J. Org. Chem.* **40**, 2307–10.

Agarwal, S. K., Boyd, D. R. & Jennings, W. B. (1985). Synthesis of benzo[g]chrysene, benzo[g]chrysene 9,10-oxide and benzo[g]chrysene 1,2:9,10-dioxide. *J. Chem. Soc. Perkin I*, 857-60.

Altman, Y. & Ginsburg, D. (1959). Alicyclic studies. Part XVI. An improved synthesis of 3:4-5:6-dibenzophenanthrene and 1:2-benzoperylene. *J. Chem. Soc.* 466-8.

Bachmann, W. E. (1934). Syntheses of phenanthrene derivatives. I. Reactions of 9-phenanthryl-magnesium bromide. *J. Amer. Chem. Soc.* **56**, 1363-7.

Bachmann, W. E. & Pence, L. H. (1935). Synthesis of phenanthrene derivatives. III. *o*-Toluoyl- and ß-methylnaphthoylphenanthrenes. *J. Amer. Chem. Soc.* **57**, 1130-1.

Bachmann, W. E. & Pence, L. H. (1937). The reaction of alkali metals with polycyclic hydrocarbons. II. *J. Amer. Chem. Soc.* **59**, 2339-42.

Bacon, R. G. & Bankhead, R. (1963). Cyclisations with hydrazine. Part III. Syntheses of pentaphene and dinaphtho[2,1-d:1',2'-f][1,l2]diazocine. *J. Chem. Soc.* 839-45.

Badger, G. M., Jefferies, P. R. & Kimber, R. W. (1957). The synthesis of polycyclic aromatic hydrocarbons. Part I. A synthesis of optically active 9:10-dihydrodinaphtho(2':3'-3:4)-(2":3"-5:6)phenanthrene, and a new synthesis of pentaphene. *J. Chem. Soc.* 1837-41.

Balanikas, G., Hussain, N., Amin, S. & Hecht, S. (1988). Oxidation of polynuclear aromatic hydrocarbons with ceric ammonium sulfate: Preparation of quinones and lactones. *J. Org. Chem.* **53**, 1007-10.

Baum, E. J. (1978). Occurrence and surveillance of polycyclic aromatic hydrocarbons. *Polycyclic Hydrocarbons and Cancer*, **1**, eds H. V. Gelboin & P. O. P. Ts'o, pp. 45-70. New York: Academic Press.

Bax, A., Ferretti, J. A., Nashed, N. & Jerina, D. M. (1985). Complete ^{1}H and ^{13}C NMR assignment of complex polycyclic aromatic hydrocarbons. *J. Org. Chem.* **50**, 3029-34.

Bergmann, D. (1938). 1:2:5:6-Dibenzphenanthrene. *J. Chem. Soc.* 1291-2.

Bergmann, D. & Ikan, R. (1958). A new synthesis of 2,3,6,7-dibenzophenanthrene. *J. Amer. Chem. Soc.* **80**, 208-9.

Bergmann, E. D. & Smusckovicz, J. (1951). A new synthesis of 3,4,5,6-dibenzphenanthrene. *J. Amer. Chem. Soc.* **73**, 5153–5.

Bergmann, F. & Szmuszkovicz, J. (1947). 1,2,3,4-Dibenzphenanthrene and its derivatives. III. Synthesis of 1,2-dimethyl-3,4-benzphenanthrene. *J. Amer. Chem. Soc.* **69**, 1367–70.

Berlman, I. B. (1971). *Handbook of Fluorescence Spectra of Aromatic Molecules,* New York: Academic.

Bestmann, H. J., Armsen, R. & Wagner, H. (1969). Oxidation of phosphinalkenes with periodate. Synthetic application to α,ß-dicarbonyl compounds, olefins and polycyclic compounds. *Chem. Ber.* **102**, 2259–69.

Bestmann, H. J. & Both, W. (1974). Synthesis and absolute configuration of (+)-pentahelicene. *Chem. Ber.* **107**, 2923–5.

Biermann, D. & Schmidt, W. (1980). Diels–Alder reactivity of polycyclic aromatic hydrocarbons. 1. Acenes and benzologs. *J. Amer. Chem. Soc.* **102**, 3163–73.

Boyland, E. & Green, B. (1962). The interaction of polycyclic hydrocarbons and purines. *Brit. J. Cancer,* **16**, 347–60.

Bradley, W. & Pexton, F.W. (1954). Nuclear substitution by anions and self union in 1:8-naphthalimide and its N-methyl derivative. *J. Chem. Soc.* 4432–5.

Bradsher, C. K. & Rapoport, L. (1943). Aromatic cyclodehydration. XIII. 1,2,3,4-dibenzophenanthrene. *J. Amer. Chem. Soc.* **65**, 1646–7.

Buu-Hoi, N. P. & Hoan, N. (1949). The reaction of α-halogenated arylalkanes with metal powders in hydroxylated media. *J. Org. Chem.* **14**, 1023–35.

Buu-Hoi, N. P., Lavit, D. & Lamy, J. (1959). A new synthesis of dibenz[a,c]anthracene, benzo[k]fluoranthene, and benzo[b]fluoranthene. *J. Chem. Soc.* 1845–9.

Buu-Hoi, N. P. & Long, C. T. (1956). Polycyclic aromatic hydrocarbons. II. The formylation of perylene and 3-methylperylene. *Rec. Trav. Chim.* **75**, 1221–6.

Camenzind, R. & Rickborn, B. (1986). Pentaphene via 1,2-anthracyne: An application of repeated aryne-isobenzofuran methodology. *J. Org. Chem.* **51**, 1914–16.

Carruthers, W. (1967). Photocyclisation of some stilbene analogues. Synthesis of dibenzo[a,l]pyrene. *J. Chem. Soc.(C),* 1525–7.

Cerfontain, H., Laali, K. & Lambrechts, H. J. (1983). Aromatic sulfonation 86. Sulfonation of pyrene, 1-methylpyrene and perylene. *Recl. J. R. Neth. Chem. Soc.* **102**, 210–14.

Cho, H. & Harvey, R. G. (1976). Synthesis of hydroquinone diacetates from polycyclic aromatic quinones. *J. Chem. Soc. Perkin I,* 836–9.

Clar, E. (1929). Polynuclear aromatic hydrocarbons and their derivatives. I. Dibenzanthracenes and their quinones. *Chem. Ber.* **62**, 350–9.

Clar, E. (1929a). Polynuclear aromatic hydrocarbons and their derivatives. Part IV. Naphthophenanthrene and its quinones. *Chem. Ber.* **62**, 1574–90.

Clar, E. (1931). Polynuclear aromatic hydrocarbons and their derivatives. XI. Constitution of anthracene. 2. Remarks on a paper of Otto Diels and Kurt Alder. *Chem. Ber.* **64**, 2194–200.

Clar, E. (1964). *Polycyclic Hydrocarbons.* New York: Academic.

Clar, E. & John, F. (1931). Polynuclear aromatic hydrocarbons and their derivatives. VIII. Naphtho-2',3':1,2-anthracenes, 2,3,6,7-dibenzanthracene-9,10-diyls and their oxidation products. *Chem. Ber.* **64**, 981–8.

Clar, E. & Lombardi, L. (1932). Polynuclear aromatic hydrocarbons. XV. Constitution of phenanthrene, of the polynuclear ring systems derived from it, and a new method for the separation of hydrocarbons. *Chem. Ber.* **65**, 1411–20.

Clar, E. & Schmidt, W. (1979). Correlations between photoelectron and UV absorption spectra of polycyclic hydrocarbons. The pyrene series. *Tetrahedron,* **35**, 1027–32.

Clar, E. & Schmidt, W. (1979a). Localized vs delocalized molecular orbitals in aromatic hydrocarbons. *Tetrahedron,* **35**, 2673–80.

Clar, E. & Stewart, D. G. (1952). Aromatic hydrocarbons. LVIII. Resonance restriction and absorption spectra of aromatic hydrocarbons. *J. Amer. Chem. Soc.* **74**, 6235–8.

Clar, E. & Zander, M. (1957). Syntheses of coronene and 1:2–7:8-dibenzocoronene. *J. Chem. Soc.* 4616–19.

Cobb, T. B. & Memory, J. B. (1967). High resolution NMR spectra of polycyclic hydrocarbons. II. Pentacyclic compounds. *J. Chem. Phys.* **47**, 2020–5.

Cook, J. W. (1931). Polycyclic aromatic hydrocarbons. Part VIII. The chemistry of 1:2:5:6-dibenzanthrene. *J. Chem. Soc.* 3273–9.

Cook, J. W. (1932). Polycyclic aromatic hydrocarbons. Part X. 1:2:7:8-dibenzanthracene. *J. Chem. Soc.* 1472–84.

Cook, J. W. & Graham, W. (1944). The condensation of chrysene with succinic anhydride. *J. Chem. Soc.* 329–30.

Cook, J. W. & Hewett, C. L. (1933). The isolation of a cancer-producing hydrocarbon from coal tar. Part III. Synthesis of 1:2- and 4:5-benzpyrenes. *J. Chem. Soc.* 398–405.

Copeland, P. E., Dean, R. E. & McNeil, D. (1961). The ozonolysis of polycyclic hydrocarbons. Part II. *J. Chem. Soc.* 1232–8.

Copeland, P. G., Dean, R. E. & McNeil, D. (1959). The ozonolysis of polycyclic hydrocarbons. *Chem. & Ind.* 329–30.

Corbett, T. G. & Porter, Q. N. (1965). Reaction of benzyne and 1,2-naphthyne with some dienes. *Aust. J. Chem.* **18**, 1781–5.

Davies, W. & Ennis, H. C. (1959). The synthesis of polycyclic aromatic compounds. Part II. Picene-5:6- and -13:14-quinone and picene-5:6:7:8-diquinone. *J. Chem. Soc.* 915–18.

Davies, W. & Porter, Q. (1957). The synthesis of polycyclic aromatic compounds. Part III. The reaction of quinones with vinylnaphthalenes and related dienes. *J. Chem. Soc.* 4967–70.

Defay, N., Zimmermann, D. & Martin, R. H. (1971). ^{13}C NMR spectroscopy in the helicene series: heptahelicene, hexahelicene and the lower benzologues. *Tetrahedron Lett.* 1871–4.

Dewar, M. J. S., Mole, T., Urch, D. S. & Warford, E. W. (1956). Electrophilic substitution. Part IV. The nitration of diphenyl, chrysene, benzo[a]pyrene, and anthanthrene. *J. Chem. Soc.* 3572–5.

Dewhurst, F. & Kitchen, D. A. (1972). Synthesis and properties of 6-substituted benzo[a]pyrene derivatives. *J. Chem. Soc. Perkin I*, 710–12.

Diederich, F., Schneider, K. & Staab, H. A. (1984). Dibenz[a,j]anthracene via photocyclodehydrogenation of 9,10-dihydro-2-styrylphenanthrene. *Chem. Ber.* **117**, 1255–8.

Dietz, F. & Scholz, M. (1968). Chemistry of excited states. IV. The photocyclization of three isomeric distyrylbenzenes. *Tetrahedron*, **24**, 6845–9.

DiGiovanni, J., Diamond, L., Harvey, R. G. & Slaga, T. J. (1983). Enhancement of the skin tumor-initiating activity of polycyclic aromatic hydrocarbons by methyl substitution of nonbenzo'bay-region' positions. *Carcinogenesis*, **4**, 403–7.

Fieser, L. F. & Hershberg, E. B. (1938). The oxidation of methylcholanthrene and 3,4-benzpyrene with lead tetraacetate; further derivatives of 3,4-benzpyrene. *J. Amer. Chem. Soc.* **60**, 2542–8.

Fieser, L. F. & Hershberg, E. B. (1938a). Substitution reactions of meso derivatives of 1,2-benzanthracene. *J. Amer. Chem. Soc.* **60**, 2555–9.

Fieser, L. F. & Hershberg, E. B. (1938b). A new synthesis of 3,4-benzpyrene derivatives. *J. Amer. Chem. Soc.* **60**, 1658–65.

Fieser, L. F. & Hershberg, E. B. (1939). The orientation of 3,4-benzpyrene in substitution reactions. *J. Amer. Chem. Soc.* **61**, 1565–74.

Fieser, L. F. & Heymann, H. (1941). Synthesis of 2-hydroxy-3,4-benzpyrene and 2-methyl-3,4-benzpyrene. *J. Amer. Chem. Soc.* **63**, 2333–40.

Fleming, I. & Mah, T. (1975). A simple synthesis of anthracenes. *J. Chem. Soc. Perkin I*, 964–5.

Franck, H. G. & Zander, M. (1966). A new synthesis of pentaphenes. *Chem. Ber.* **99**, 396–8.

Friedel, R. A. & Orchin, M. (1951). *Ultraviolet Spectra of Aromatic Compounds.* New York: Wiley.

Fu, P. P. & Harvey, R. G. (1981). Synthesis of benzo[a]pyren-12-ol. *Org. Prep. Proc. Int.* **13**, 152–5.

Fu, P. P. & Harvey, R. G. (1983). Synthesis of 4-hydroxybenzo[a]pyrene. *J. Org. Chem.* **48**, 1534–6.

Fu, P. P., Lee, H. M. & Harvey, R. G. (1980). Regioselective catalytic hydrogenation of polycyclic aromatic hydrocarbons under mild conditions. *J. Org. Chem.* **45**, 2797–803.

Goedke, C. & Stegemeyer, H. (1970). Resolution and racemization of pentahelicene. *Tetrahedron Lett.* 937–40.

Gore, P. H. (1955). The Friedel–Crafts acylation reaction and its application to polycyclic aromatic hydrocarbons. *Chem. Rev.* **55**, 229–81.

Gribble, G. W., Holubowitch, E. J. & Venuti, M. C. (1977). Generation and Diels–Alder reaction of α'-bromo-1,2-naphthoquinodimethane. A new phenanthrene synthesis. *Tetrahedron Lett.* 2857–60.

Grimmer, G. (1979). *Environmental Carcinogens–Selected Methods of Analysis*, II, 31–61. Lyon, France: International Agency for Research on Cancer.

Haigh, C. W. & Mallion, R. B. (1971). Proton magnetic resonance spectra of nonplanar condensed benzenoid hydrocarbons. I. Spectra of 3,4-benzophenanthrene, pentahelicene, and hexahelicene. *Mol. Phys.* **22**, 945–53.

Harris, P. N. & Bradsher, C. K. (1946). Observations on the carcinogenicity of 1,2,3,4-dibenzophenanthrene and its 9-methyl and 10-methyl derivatives. *Cancer Res.* **6**, 671–3.

Hartwell, J. L. (1951). *Survey of Compounds which have been Tested for Carcinogenic Activity*, U.S. Public Health Service Publ. No. 149. Washington, DC: Superintendent of Documents, U.S. Government Printing Office.

Harvey, R. G. (1970). Metal–ammonia reduction of aromatic molecules. *Synthesis*, 161–72.

Harvey, R. G. (1985). Synthesis of the dihydrodiol and diol epoxide metabolites of carcinogenic polycyclic hydrocarbons. In *Polycyclic Hydrocarbons and Carcinogenesis*, Mono. No.283, ed. R. G. Harvey, pp. 35–62. Washington, DC: American Chemical Society.

Harvey, R. G. (1986). Synthesis of oxidized metabolites of carcinogenic hydrocarbons. *Synthesis*, 605–19.

Harvey, R. G. & Cho, H. (1975). Improved synthesis of benzo[a]pyrene-1-ol and isolation of a covalent benz[a]pyrene lead compound. *J. Chem. Soc. Chem. Comm.* 373-4.

Harvey, R. G., Cortez, C. & Jacobs, S. A. (1982). Synthesis of polycyclic hydrocarbons via a novel annelation method. *J. Org. Chem.* **47**, 2120–5.

Harvey, R. G., Cortez, C., Sawyer, T. W. & DiGiovanni, J. (1988). Synthesis of the tumorigenic 3,4-dihydrodiol metabolites of dibenz[a,j]anthracene and 7,14-dimethyldibenz[a,j]anthracene. *J. Med. Chem.* **31**, 1308–12.

Harvey, R. G. & Fu, P. P. (1978). Synthesis and reactions of diolepoxides and related metabolites of carcinogenic hydrocarbons. *Polycyclic Hydrocarbons and Cancer*, **1**, ed. H. V. Gelboin & P. O. P. Ts'o, pp. 133–65. New York: Academic Press.

Harvey, R. G. & Fu, P. P. (1982). Synthesis of 7-hydroxybenzo[a]pyrene. *Org. Proc. Prep. Int.* **14**, 414–17.

Harvey, R. G., Goh, S. H. & Cortez, C. (1975). 'K-region' oxides and related oxidized metabolites of carcinogenic aromatic hydrocarbons. *J. Amer. Chem. Soc.* **97**, 3468–79.

Harvey, R. G., Lee, H. M. & Shyamasundar, N. (1979). Synthesis of the dihydrodiols and diolepoxides of benzo[e]pyrene and triphenylene. *J. Org. Chem.* **44**, 78–83, 5006.

Harvey, R. G., Leyba, C., Konieczny, M., Fu, P. P. & Sukumaran, K. B. (1978). A novel and convenient synthesis of dibenz[a,c]anthracene. *J. Org. Chem.* **43**, 3423–5.

Hayward, R. J., Hopkinson, A. C. & Leznoff, C. C. (1972). Photocyclization reactions of arylpolyenes. VI. The photo cyclization of 1,4-diaryl-1,3-butadienes. *Tetrahedron*, **28**, 439–47.

Hewett, C. L. (1938). Polycyclic aromatic hydrocarbons. Part XVI. 1:2:3:4-dibenzphenanthrene. *J. Chem. Soc.* 193–96.

Hewett, C. L. (1938a). Polycyclic aromatic hydrocarbons. Part XVIII. A general method for the synthesis of 3:4-benzphenanthrene derivatives. *J. Chem. Soc.* 1286–91.

IARC (1983). *Monograph on the Evaluation of the Carcinogenic Risk of the Chemical to man: Certain Polycyclic Aromatic Hydrocarbons and Heterocyclic Compounds*, **32**, Lyon, France: International Agency for Research on Cancer.

Iball, J., Morgan, C. H. & Zacharias, D. E. (1975). Refinement of the crystal structure of orthorhombic dibenz[a,h]anthracene. *J. Chem. Soc. Perkin II*, 1271–2.

Iversen, B., Sydnes, L. K. & Greibrokk, T. (1985). Characterization of nitrobenzanthracenes and nitrodibenzanthracenes. *Acta Chem. Scand.* **B 39**, 837–47.

Jutz, J. C. (1978). Aromatic and heteroaromatic compounds by electrocyclic ring-closure with elimination. *Topics in Current Chem.* **73**, 127–230.

Karcher, W. (1988). *Spectral Atlas of Polycyclic Aromatic Compounds*, Vol. 2, Dordrecht, Netherlands: Kluwer.

Karcher, W., Fordham, R., DuBois, J. & Gloude, P. (1985). *Spectral Atlas of Polycyclic Aromatic Compounds*, Dordrecht, Netherlands: D. Reidel.

Konieczny, M. & Harvey, R. G. (1980). Reductive methylation of polycyclic aromatic quinones. *J. Org. Chem.* **45**, 1308–10.

Kuroda, R. (1982). Crystal and molecular structure of [5]helicene: Crystal packing modes. *J. Chem. Soc. Perkin II*, 789–94.

Kuroda, R. & Mason, S. F. (1981). The crystal and molecular structure of (S)-(+)- and racemic 9,10-dihydrodibenzo[c,g]phenanthrene. *J. Chem. Soc. Perkin II*, 870–6.

Lang, K. F. & Zander, M. (1964). 1,2- and 3,4-benzopyrene. *Chem. Ber.* **97**, 218–24.

Lao, R. C., Thomas, R. S., Oja, H. & Dubois, L. (1973). Application of gas chromatograph–mass spectrometer–data processor combination to the analysis of the PAH content of airborne pollutants. *Anal. Chem.* **45**, 908–15.

Lapouyade, R., Veyres, A., Hanafi, N., Coutoure, A. & Lablache-Combier, A. (1982). Photocyclization of 1,2–diarylethylenes in primary amines. A convenient method for the synthesis of dihydro aromatic compounds and a means of reducing the loss of methyl groups during the cyclization of *o*-methylstilbenes. *J. Org. Chem.* **47**, 1361–4.

Lee, H. & Harvey, R. G. (1981). Reinvestigation of the Jutz synthesis of benzo[e]pyrene and benzo[a]pyrene derivatives from benzanthrene. *Tetrahedron Lett.* **22**, 995–6.

Lee, H. M., Shymasundar, N. & Harvey, R. G. (1981). The monomethyl and dimethyl derivatives of benzo[e]pyrene. *Tetrahedron,* **37**, 2563–8.

Lee, H. M., Shymasundar, N. & Harvey, R. G. (1981a). Synthesis of the isomeric phenols of benzo[e]pyrene. *J. Org. Chem.* **46**, 288–95.

Lee, M. L., Novotny, M. & Bartle, K. D. (1976). Gas chromatography/mass spectrometric and nuclear magnetic resonance spectrometric studies of carcinogenic polynuclear aromatic hydrocarbons in tobacco and marijuana smoke condensates. *Anal. Chem.* **48**, 405–16.

Lehr, R. E., Taylor, C. W., Kumar, S., Mah, H. D. & Jerina, D. M. (1978). Synthesis of the non-K-region and K-region *trans*-dihydrodiols of benzo[e]pyrene. *J. Org. Chem.* **43**, 3462–6.

Levi, E. J. & Orchin, M. (1966). Photocyclization–aromatization of stilbenes using selenium radicals. A synthesis of 2,4,5,7-tetramethylphenanthrene. *J. Org. Chem.* **31**, 4302–3.

Levin, W., Wood, A. W., Chang, R. L., Ittah, Y., Croisy-Delcey, M., Yagi, H., Jerina, D. M. & Conney, A. H. (1980). Exceptionally high tumor-initiating activity of benzo[c]phenanthrene bay-region diol-epoxides on mouse skin. *Cancer Res.* **40**, 3910–3914.

Lijinsky, W. J. (1961). The catalytic hydrogenation of dibenz[a,h]anthracene. *J. Org. Chem.* **26**, 3230–7.

Looker, J. J. (1972). Mononitration of perylene. Preparation and structure proof of 1 and 3 isomers. *J. Org. Chem.* **37**, 3379–81.

Marschalk, C. (1927). Action of sulfuric acid on perylene. *Bull. Soc. Chim. Fr.* **41**, 74–8.

McKay, J. F. & Latham, D. R. (1973). Polyaromatic hydrocarbons in high-boiling petroleum distillates. *Anal. Chem.* **45**, 1050–5.

Memory, J. D. & Wilson, N. K., (1982). *NMR of Aromatic Compounds,* New York: Wiley-Interscience.

Minsky, A., Meyer, A. Y. & Rabinovitz, M. (1982). Super-charged polycyclic π systems: Pyrene and perylene tetraanions. *J. Amer. Chem. Soc.* **104**, 2475–82.

Minsky, A. & Rabinowitz, M. (1983). A facile synthesis of some polycyclic hydrocarbons: Application of phase transfer catalysis in the bis-Wittig reaction. *Synthesis*, 497–8.

Moriconi, E. J., O'Connor, W. F., Schmitt, W. J., Cogswell, G. W. & Furer, B. P. (1960). Ozonolysis of polycyclic aromatics. VII. Dibenz[a,h]anthracene. *J. Amer. Chem. Soc.* **82**, 3441–6.

Moriconi, E. J., Rakoczny, B. & O'Connor, W. F. (1961). Ozonolysis of polycyclic aromatics. VIII. Benzo[a]pyrene. *J. Amer. Chem. Soc.* **83**, 4618–23.

Moriconi, E. J., Rakoczny, B. & O'Connor, W. F. (1962). Ozonolysis of polycyclic aromatics. IX. Dibenz[a,j]anthracene. *J. Org. Chem.* **27**, 3618–19.

Moriconi, E. J. & Salce, L. (1967). Ozonolysis of polycyclic aromatics. XIV. Ozonation of pentaphene and benzo[rst]pentaphene. *J. Org. Chem.* **32**, 2829–37.

Moureu, H., Chovin, P. & Rivoal, G. (1948). The condensation of o-bis(cyanomethyl)benzene with 1,2-dicarbonyl compounds; the preparation of 2,3,1′,8′-binaphthylene. *Bull. Soc. Chem. Fr.* **15**, 99–103.

Muschik, G. M., Kelly, T. P. & Manning, W. B. (1982). Simple synthesis of 1-,2-,3-, and 4-hydroxydibenz[a,j]anthracenes and 2-,3-, and 4-hydroxydibenz[a,h]anthracenes. *J. Org. Chem.* **47**, 4709–12.

Nordbotten, A., Sydnes, L. K. & Greibokk, T. (1984). Preparation and characterization of dinitroperylenes. *Acta Chem. Scand.* **B 38**, 701–6.

Osborne, M. & Crosby, N. T. (1987). *Benzopyrenes*, Cambridge, England: Cambridge University Press.

Ozubuko, R. S., Buchanan, G. W. & Smith, I. C. (1974). Carbon-13 nuclear magnetic resonance spectra of carcinogenic polynuclear hydrocarbons. I. 3-Methylcholanthrene and related benzanthracenes. *Can. J. Chem.* **52**, 2493–501.

Pataki, J., Konieczny, M. & Harvey, R. G. (1982). Synthesis of *tert*-butylarenes from acetylarenes. *J. Org. Chem.* **47**, 1133–6.

Peake, D. A., Oyler, A. R., Heikkila, K. E., Liukkonen, R. J., Engroff, E. C. & Carlson, R. M. (1983). Alkyl aromatic synthesis: Nucleophilic alkyl lithium addition. *Syn. Comm.* **13**, 21–26.

Perin-Roussel, O., Jacquignon, P., Saperas, B. & Viallet, P. (1972). Vibrational and electronic spectra of three dibenzanthracenes. *C.R. Acad. Sci. Paris*, **274**, 1593–6.

Perkamper, H. H., Sanderman, I. & Timmores, C. J. (1967). *DMS UV Atlas of Organic Compounds*, Vol. III, London: Butterworths.

Phillips, D. D. (1953). Polynuclear aromatic hydrocarbons. I. A new synthesis of picene. *J. Amer. Chem. Soc.* **75**, 3223–6.

Platt, K. L. & Oesch, F. (1981). Reductive cyclization of keto acids to polycyclic aromatic hydrocarbons by hydroiodic acid–red phosphorus. *J. Org. Chem.* **45**, 2601–3.

Platt, K. L. & Oesch, F. (1982). Synthesis and properties of the seven isomeric phenols of dibenz[a,h]anthracene. *J. Org. Chem.* **47**, 5321–6.

Pollart, D. J. & Rickborn, B. (1986). Cycloadducts of arynes with 1,3-bis(trimethylsilyl)-naphtho[1,2-c]furan: Formation of novel polycyclic aromatic derivatives and related reactions. *J. Org. Chem.* **51**, 3155–61.

Postovskii, I. & Bednyagina, N. P. (1937). Synthesis of perylene from anthracene. *Zhur. Obschei Chem. USSR*, **7**, 2919–25.

Pouchert, C. E. (1981). *Aldrich Library of Infrared Spectra, Edit. III,* Milwaukee, Wisc.: Aldrich Chemical Co.

Radner, F. (1983). Nitration of polycyclic aromatic hydrocarbons with dinitrogen tetroxide. A simple and selective synthesis of mononitro derivatives. *Acta Chem. Scand.* **B 37**, 65–7.

Read, G., Shu, P., Vining, L. C. & Haskins, R. H. (1959). Mycochrysone I. Isolation, properties, and preliminary characterization. *Can. J. Chem.* **37**, 731–6.

Sawicki, E., Hauser, T. R. & Stanley, T. W. (1960). Ultraviolet, visible and fluorescence spectral analysis of polynuclear hydrocarbons. *Int. J. Air Poll.* **2**, 253–72.

Schlude, H. (1971). Two improvements in the synthesis of 3,4-benzpyrene according to Cook and Hewett. *Chem. Ber.* **104**, 3995–6.

Schoental, R. & Scott, E. J. (1949). Fluorescence spectra of polycyclic aromatic hydrocarbons in solution. *J. Chem. Soc.* 1683–96.

Scholl, R., Seer, C. & Weitzenbock, R. (1910). Perylene, a highly condensed aromatic hydrocarbon, $C_{20}H_{12}$. *Chem. Ber.* **43**, 2202–9.

Shushan, B. & Boyd, R. K. (1980). Unimolecular and collision induced fragmentations of molecular ions of polycyclic aromatic hydrocarbons. *Org. Mass Spectr.* **15**, 445–53.

Slaga, T. J., Gleason, G. L., Mills, G., Ewald, L., Fu, P. P., Lee, H. M. & Harvey, R. G. (1980). Comparison of the skin tumor-initiating activities of dihydrodiols and diol-epoxides of various polycyclic aromatic hydrocarbons. *Cancer Res.* **40**, 1981–4.

Snatzke, G. & Kunde, K. (1973). Synthesis of 2-substituted dibenz[a,j]anthracene derivatives. *Chem. Ber.* **106**, 1341–62.

Stenhagen, E., Abrahamsson, S. & McLafferty, F. W. (1974). *Registry of Mass Spectral Data*, New York: Wiley.

Studt, P. (1978). Synthesis of dibenz[a,j]anthracene. *Ann. Chem.* 2105–6.

Sukumaran, K. B. & Harvey, R. G. (1981). A novel annelation reaction: Synthesis of polycyclic hydrocarbons from *o*-quinones. *J. Org. Chem.* **46**, 2740–5.

Tintel, C., Lugtenburg, J., van Amsterdam, G. A. J., Erkelens, C. & Cornelisse, J. (1983). A two-step synthesis of benzo[e]pyrene via the pyrene dianion. *Recl. Trav. Chim. Pays-Bas*, **102**, 228–31.

Tokita, S., Hiruta, K., Kitahara, K. & Nishi, H. (1982). Diels–Alder reaction of diazenedicarboxylates with perylenes; a new synthesis of polycyclic aromatic pyridazines. *Synthesis*, 229–31.

TRC (1982). *Selected Nuclear Magnetic Resonance Spectral Data*, Suppl. Vol. F–26, College Station, Texas: Thermodynamics Research Center, Texas A & M University.

TRC (1982a). *Selected Ultraviolet Spectral Data,* Suppl. Vol. C–48, College Station, Texas: Thermodynamics Research Center, Texas A & M University.

Uchida, T., Kozawa, K., Nagao, Y. & Misonoo, T. (1979). The crystal and molecular structure of an isomer of dibromoperylenes. *Bull. Chem. Soc. Jpn.* **52**, 1547–8.

Ueda, T., Yano, R., Ohno, M., Iwashima, S., Takekawa, M., Aoki, J. & Kan, T. (1985). Effect of overcrowding on mass spectra of aromatic molecules. *J. Chem. Soc. Perkin Trans. II*, 1195–8.

Unkefer, C. J., London, R. E., Whaley, T. W. & Daub, G. H. (1983). ^{13}C and ^{1}H NMR analysis of isotopically labeled benzo[a]pyrenes. *J. Amer. Chem. Soc.* **105**, 733–5.

Van Duuren, B. L., Berkersky, I. & Le Far, M. (1964). The peracid oxidation of dibenz[a,h]anthracene. *J. Org. Chem.*, **29**, 686–689.

Vollmann, H., Becker, H., Corell, M. & Streeck, H. (1937). Pyrene and its derivatives. *Liebigs Ann.* **531**, 1–159.

Ware, J. C. & Borchert, E. E. (1961). Chlorination of aromatic hydrocarbons by cupric chloride. II. Reactivity of some polynuclear compounds. *J. Org. Chem.* **26**, 2267–70.

Weidlich, H. A. (1938). Synthesis of condensed-ring systems. I. *Chem. Ber.* **71**, 1203–9.

Weizmann, C., Blum-Bergmann, O. & Bergmann, F. (1935). Grignard reactions with phthalic anhydrides. *J. Chem. Soc.* 1367–70.

Windaus, A. & Raichle, R. (1938). Derivatives of 3,4-benzopyrene. *Leibigs Ann.* **537**, 157–70.

Wise, S. A., Benner, B., Byrd, G. D., Chesler, S. N., Bebbert, R. E. & Schantz, M. M. (1988). Determination of polycyclic aromatic hydrocarbons in a coal tar standard reference material. *Anal. Chem.* **60**, 887–94.

Yagi, H., Holder, G. M., Dansette, P. M., Hernandez, O., Yeh, H. J. C., LeMahieu, R. A. & Jerina, D. M. (1976). Synthesis and spectral properties of the isomeric hydroxybenzo[a]pyrenes. *J. Org. Chem.* **41**, 977–85.

Zeiger, H. E. (1966). Alkylperylenes. The isomeric ethylperylenes. *J. Org. Chem.* **31**, 2977–81.

Zeiger, H. E. & Rosenkranz, J. E. (1964). Alkylation and metalation of perylene with n-butyllithium. 1-*n*-Butylperylene. *J. Org. Chem.* **29**, 2469–71.

Zinke, A. & Benndorf, O. (1932). Perylene and its derivatives. Part 34. Hydrogenation of perylene. *Monatsh.* **59**, 241–55.

Zinke, A. & Benndorf, O. (1934). Perylene and its derivatives. Part 40. *Monatsh.* **64**, 87–96.

Zinke, A., Pongratz, A. & Funke, K. (1925). Perylene and its derivatives. *Chem. Ber.* **58**, 330–2.

Zinke, A. & Unterkreuter, E. (1919). New derivatives of perylene. *Monatsh.* **40**, 405–10.

10

Alternant hexacyclic polyarenes

The number of alternant polyarenes with six rings is considerably greater than the combined number of alternant PAHs with fewer rings. According to graph theory, there are 37 possible cata-condensed PAHs and 15 possible peri-condensed polyarenes with six fused aromatic rings (Dias, 1987) (Tables 10.1 and 10.2). Although the synthesis of approximately 40 of these polyarenes have been reported, surprisingly little is known concerning the chemistry of the majority of them. This chapter reviews the chemistry of eight representative alternant six-ring polyarenes selected primarily for their importance in carcinogenesis research. As in the preceding chapters, information is provided on the physical, chemical, and spectral properties, environmental occurrence, and carcinogenic properties, in so far as information is available, of each hydrocarbon along with a review of methods for their synthesis and chemical reactivity.

10.1 Dibenzo[def,mno]chrysene

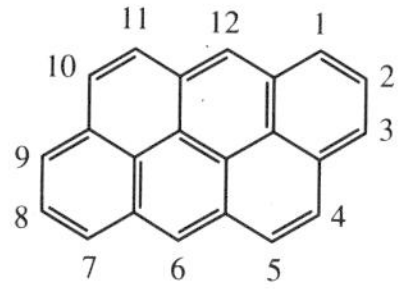

Other names: anthanthrene

Physical and spectral properties $C_{22}H_{12}$, mol. wt. 276.31, golden yellow plates (xylene), mp 264 °C. Sparingly soluble in benzene, toluene, dioxane, and other organic solvents. Spectral data: UV (Karcher *et al.*, 1985; Friedel & Orchin, 1951), UV fluorescence (Pierce & Katz, 1975; Berlman, 1971; Schoental & Scott, 1949), PE (Boschi *et al.*, 1974), IR (Buu-Hoi & Lavit, 1958), NMR (Karcher *et al.*, 1985), mass spectrum (Ansell *et al.*, 1976).

Table 10.1. *Cata-condensed polycyclic hydrocarbons with six rings*

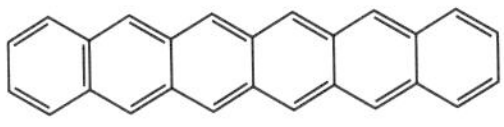

hexacene

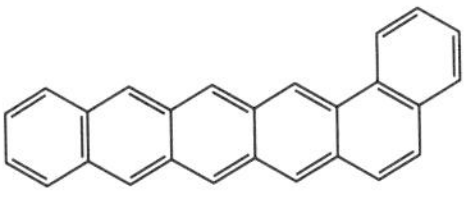

benzo[a]pentacene

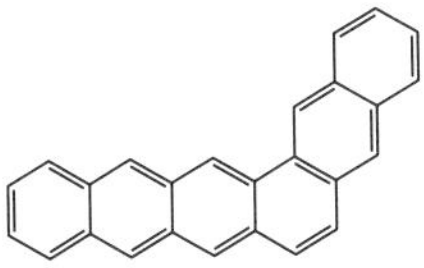

hexaphene

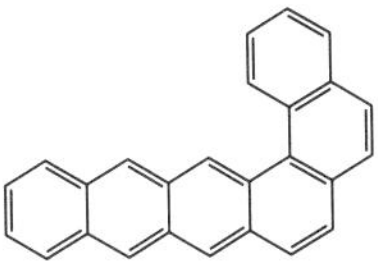

naphtho[1,2-a]naphthacene

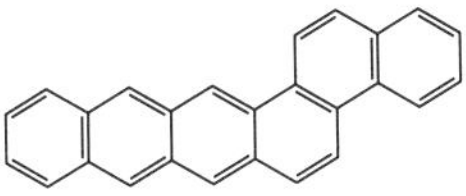

naphtho[2,1-a]naphthacene

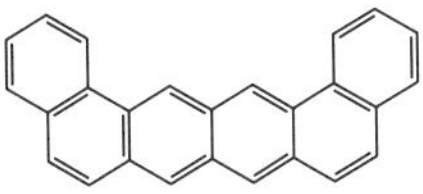

dibenzo[a,l]naphthacene

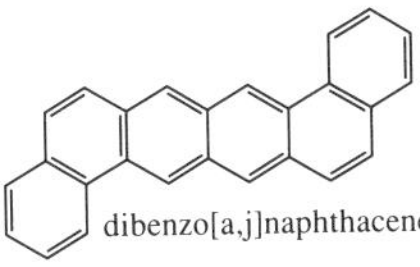

dibenzo[a,j]naphthacene

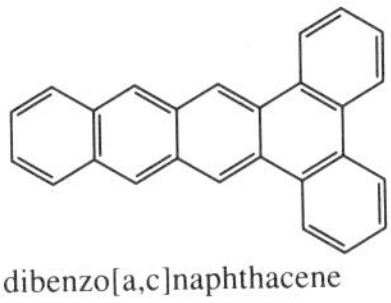

dibenzo[a,c]naphthacene

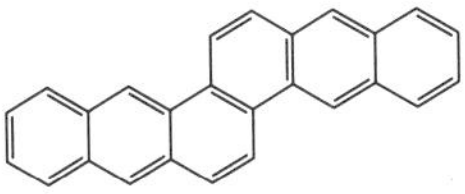

dibenzo[b,k]chrysene

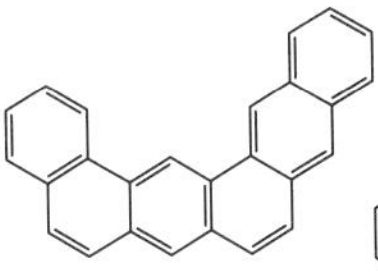

benzo[a]pentaphene

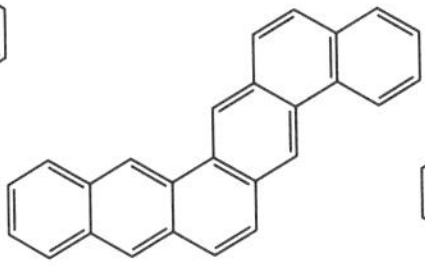

benzo[c]pentaphene

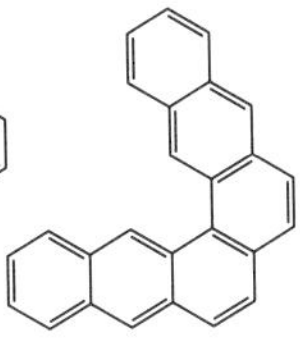

anthra[1,2-a]anthracene

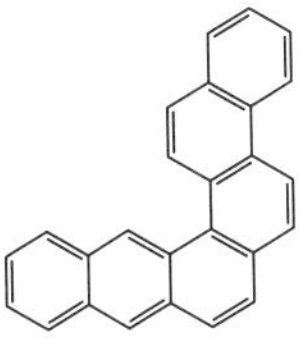

naphtho[2,3-c]chrysene

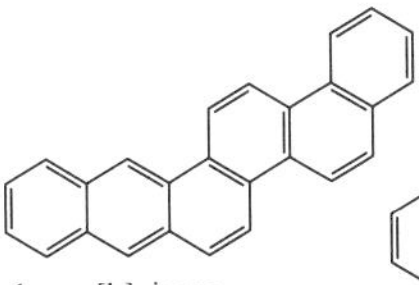

benzo[b]picene

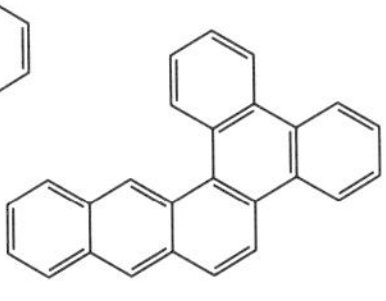

dibenzo[b,g]chrysene

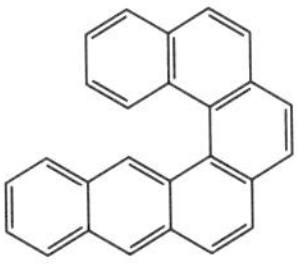

phenanthro[4,3-a]anthracene

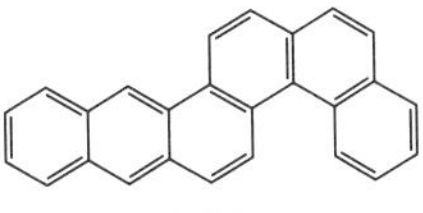

dibenzo[b,l]chrysene

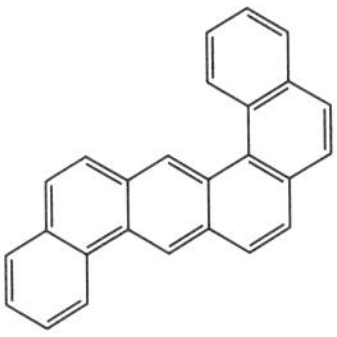

benzo[a]naphth[1,2-h]-
anthracene

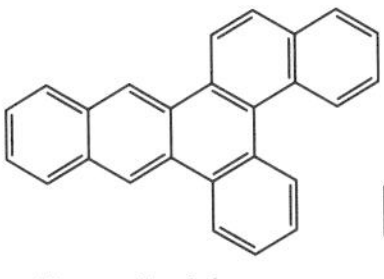

dibenzo[b,p]chrysene

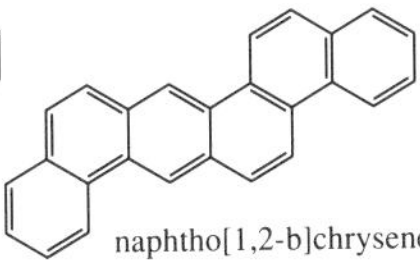

naphtho[1,2-b]chrysene

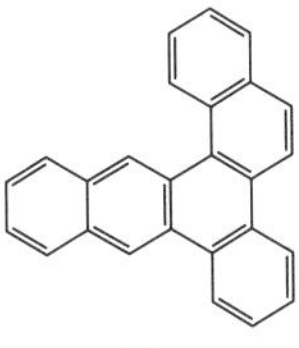

naphtho[2,3-g]chrysene

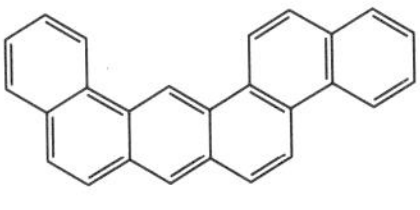

naphtho[2,1-b]chrysene

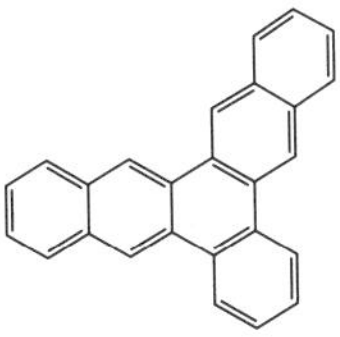

benzo[h]pentaphene

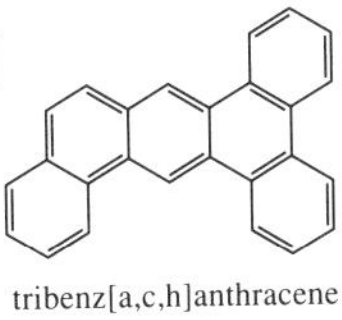

tribenz[a,c,h]anthracene

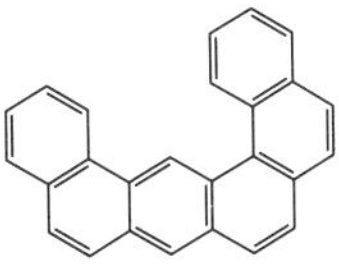

benzo[a]naphth[2,1-j]anthracene

Table 10.1. continued

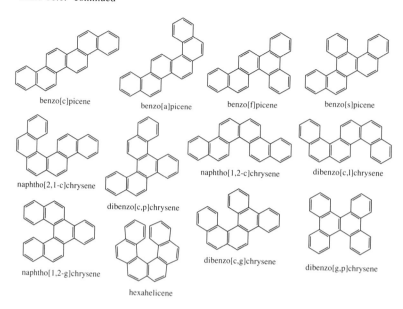

benzo[c]picene

benzo[a]picene

benzo[f]picene

benzo[s]picene

naphtho[2,1-c]chrysene

dibenzo[c,p]chrysene

naphtho[1,2-c]chrysene

dibenzo[c,l]chrysene

naphtho[1,2-g]chrysene

hexahelicene

dibenzo[c,g]chrysene

dibenzo[g,p]chrysene

Table 10.2. *Peri-condensed polycyclic hydrocarbons with six rings*

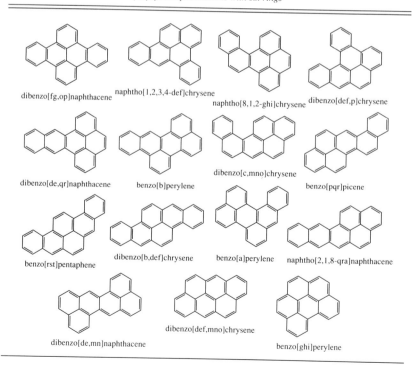

dibenzo[fg,op]naphthacene

naphtho[1,2,3,4-def]chrysene

naphtho[8,1,2-ghi]chrysene

dibenzo[def,p]chrysene

dibenzo[de,qr]naphthacene

benzo[b]perylene

dibenzo[c,mno]chrysene

benzo[pqr]picene

benzo[rst]pentaphene

dibenzo[b,def]chrysene

benzo[a]perylene

naphtho[2,1,8-qra]naphthacene

dibenzo[de,mn]naphthacene

dibenzo[def,mno]chrysene

benzo[ghi]perylene

Occurrence and carcinogenicity Occurs in relatively high concentrations in coal tar and carbon black and is a minor component of atmospheric pollution (IARC, 1983; Grimmer, 1979; Sawicki, 1977). It is also found in tobacco and marijuana smoke (Grimmer, 1979; Seversen *et al.*, 1976). In tests for skin carcinogenicity it exhibited no activity in three out of four tests, and only minimal activity in the mouse skin initiation-promotion assay (IARC, 1983).

Synthesis The available methods for the synthesis of anthanthrene involve the double cyclization of appropriately substituted dinaphthyl derivatives (Fig. 10.1). Acid-catalyzed double cyclization of 1,1'-dinaphthyl-2,2'-dicarboxylic acid or 1,1'-dinaphthyl-8,8'-dicarboxylic acid affords anthanthrone (**1**) (Ansell *et al.*, 1976; Kalb, 1914). Reduction of **1** with aluminum alkoxide yields anthanthrene directly (Coffey & Boyd, 1954). Alternatively, reduction of **1** with a large excess of HI and red phosphorus provides 1,2,3,7,8,9-hexahydroanthanthrene (**2**) which is converted to anthanthrene by catalytic dehydrogenation (Ansell *et al.*, 1976). However, it is likely that **2** could be obtained more directly by the use of a lower ratio of HI to **1** (Konieczny & Harvey, 1979). Acid-catalyzed cyclization of 8,8'-diformyl-1,1'-dinaphthyl (**3**) is claimed to afford anthanthrene directly (Vorozhtsov *et al.*, 1979), although the most likely anticipated product of this reaction is 6-hydroxyanthanthrene; identification is based solely on melting point and IR spectrum. These authors also report that electrochemical

Fig. 10.1. Synthetic routes to dibenzo[def,mno]chrysene.

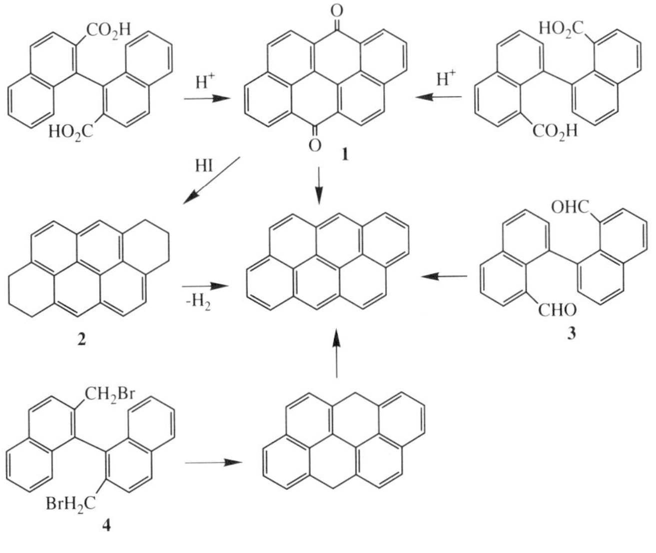

reduction of **3** furnishes anthanthrene quantitatively. Anthanthrene is also synthetically accessible by treatment of 8,8'-bis-bromomethyl-1,1'-dinaphthyl (**4**) with phenyllithium to give 6,12-dihydroanthanthrene (Badar *et al.*, 1972) which may be expected to furnish the fully aromatic parent hydrocarbon by dehydrogenation.

Reactions Electrophilic substitutions take place primarily in the meso region. Thus, chlorination with sulfuryl chloride gives 6,12-dichlorodibenzo[def,mno]chrysene (Buu-Hoi & Lavit, 1957). Vilsmeier reaction yields 6-formyldibenzo[def,mno]chrysene which may be converted to the 6-methyl derivative by Wolff–Kishner reduction (Buu-Hoi & Lavit, 1957). Nitration affords two mononitro derivatives tentatively assigned as the 6-nitro- and 1- or 3-nitro isomers (Dewar *et al.*, 1956). Oxidation of this hydrocarbon with chromic acid provides the meso region quinone **1**. Hydrogenation of dibenzo[def,mno]chrysene over a Pt catalyst furnishes a mixture of the 4,5-dihydro- derivative and the hexahydro derivative **2** (Lijinsky *et al.*, 1972).

10.2   Benzo[ghi]perylene

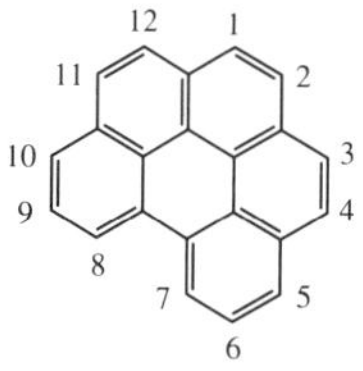

Other names: 1,12-benzoperylene
Physical and spectral properties $C_{22}H_{12}$, mol. wt. 276.31, yellow plates, mp 282-83 °C. Solutions show a blue fluorescence. Spectral data: UV (TRC, 1985; Karcher *et al.*, 1985; Friedel & Orchin, 1951), UV fluorescence (Pierce & Katz, 1975; Berlman, 1971), IR (Karcher *et al.*, 1985; Pouchert, 1981), NMR (TRC, 1986; Karcher *et al.*, 1985; Pouchert, 1983), mass spectrum (Karcher *et al.*, 1985; Shushan & Boyd, 1980).

Occurrence and carcinogenicity It is a major constituent of coal tar pitch and hydrogenated tars. Significant levels are also found in carbon black (Peaden *et al.*, 1980), automobile exhaust (Grimmer, 1979), atmospheric pollution (IARC, 1983; Pierce & Katz, 1975; Sawicki, 1977), and tobacco and marijuana smoke (Severson *et al.*, 1976). The finding from several assays indicate it to be noncarcinogenic (IARC, 1983).

Synthesis Benzo[ghi]perylene may be prepared from perylene by Diels–Alder cycloaddition of maleic anhydride in the presence of chloranil (Clar & Zander, 1957) (Fig. 10.2). The resulting dicarboxylic anhydride (**5**) is decarboxylated to benzo[ghi]perylene by heating with soda-lime. A modification of this approach involves similar Diels-Alder reaction of the diene **6** followed by decarboxylation of the adduct with lead dioxide and dehydrogenation (Altman & Ginsburg, 1959). Treatment of 7,7'-bis-bromomethyl-1,1'-binaphthyl (**7**) with sodium gives not the expected bridged binaphthyl derivative, but a mixture of benzo[ghi]perylene and its dihydro derivative which is dehydrogenated over Pd-C to benzo[ghi]perylene (Sato *et al.*, 1976). Photocyclization of 1,2-di-ß-naphthylethylene (**8**), 3-styryl-phenanthrene (**9**), 1,4-styrylbenzene (**10**), or the biphenylparacyclophane-diene **11** also affords benzo[ghi]perylene (Carruthers, 1967; Dietz & Scholz, 1968; Jessup & Reiss, 1976).

Reactions Quantum mechanical calculations yield different predictions of the relative reactivity of the molecular sites of benzo[ghi]-perylene. According to HMO calculations the positional order of reactivity is 4 > 5 > 7 > 3 > 1; by the SCF method it is 5 > 4 > 7 > 1 > 3; and by the Dewar method it is 5 > 7 > 4 > 1 > 3 > 6 (Ivanenko, 1983). Nitration of benzo[ghi]perylene has recently been reinvestigated and shown to afford a 3:2 mixture of the 5- and 7-nitro derivatives of benzo[ghi]perylene (Johansen

Fig. 10.2. Synthetic routes to benzo[ghi]perylene.

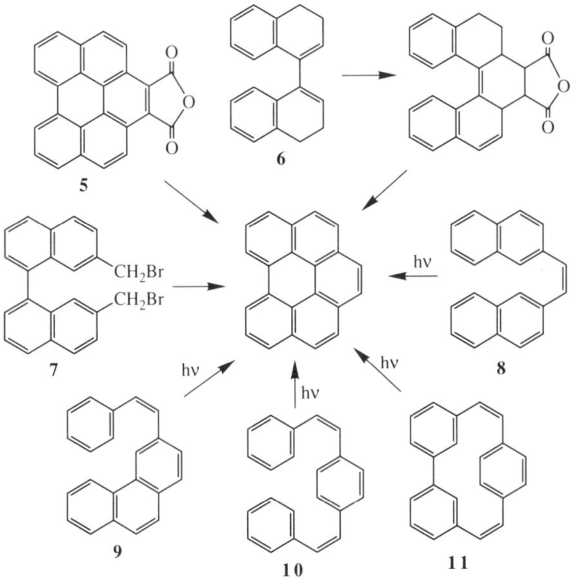

et al., 1984), in best agreement with the prediction by the Dewar method. Acetylation of benzo[ghi]perylene with various acylating reagents and various conditions gives 5-acetylbenzo[ghi]perylene, and further acetylation yields 5,10-diacetylbenzo[ghi]perylene (Ivanenko *et al.*, 1983). Formylation with *n*-butyl dichloromethyl ether and TiCl$_4$ furnishes 5-formylbenzo[ghi]-perylene which is reduced with hydrazine and pyridine to 5-methylbenzo[ghi]perylene (Clar et al., 1968). Reaction of benzo[ghi]-perylene with maleic anhydride affords a Diels–Alder adduct useful for the preparation of coronene (Clar & Zander, 1957).

10.3   Benzo[rst]pentaphene

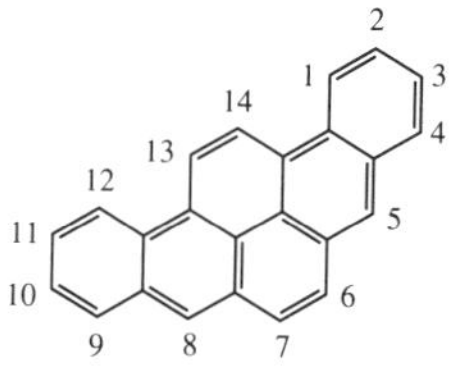

Other names: *dibenzo[a,i]pyrene, benzo[ghi]picene, 3,4:9,10-dibenzopyrene*

Physical and spectral properties C$_{24}$H$_{14}$, mol. wt. 302.35, greenish-yellow crystals, mp 281.5-82 °C. Solutions in organic solvents show a blue fluorescence. Spectral data: UV (Karcher, 1988; Friedel & Orchin, 1951), UV fluorescence (Karcher, 1988; Pierce & Katz, 1975), PE (Clar & Schmidt, 1979), IR (Karcher, 1988; Pouchert, 1981), NMR (Karcher, 1988; Mitchell *et al.*, 1982), mass spectrum (Karcher, 1988; Thomas & Lao, 1978).

Occurrence and carcinogenicity Occurs in coal tar (Lang & Eigen, 1967), atmospheric pollution (Sawicki, 1977; Pierce & Katz, 1975), auto exhaust (Hoffmann & Wynder, 1962), and tobacco and marijuana smoke (Lee *et al.*, 1976). Exhibits exceptional potency in the induction of sarcomas in mice (Buu-Hoi, 1964); it is less active than BaP in the induction of skin tumors in mice (IARC, 1973).

Synthesis The high tumorigenic activity of this hydrocarbon has stimulated the development of a number of syntheses (Fig. 10.3). Acid-catalyzed cyclization of 1,4-dibenzoylnaphthalene or 4-benzoylbenzanthrone affords benzo[rst]pentaphene-5,8-dione (**12**) reduction of which yields benzo[rst]pentaphene (Scholl & Neumann, 1922). Benzo[rst]pentaphene is synthetically accessible from benzo[a]pyrene by the Haworth synthesis via the intermediate **13** (Buu-Hoi & Lavit, 1960). Similar double Haworth synthesis from pyrene affords the diketone **14** which is readily converted to benzo[rst]pentaphene (Rahman et al., 1976). Another practical synthesis involves reaction of 3-keto-1,2,3,11b-tetrahydro-7*H*-benzanthrene with *o*-tolylmagnesium bromide and dehydration to provide **15** which is cyclodehydrogenated with Pd-C to benzo[rst]pentaphene (Daub & Smith, 1960). Reaction of picene with maleic anhydride and I$_2$ furnishes the adduct **16** which is decarboxylated to benzo[rst]pentaphene (Clar, 1973).

Reactions Electrophilic substitutions occur predominantly in the 5- and 8-positions of benzo[rst]pentaphene in accord with theoretical prediction. Chlorination with sulfuryl chloride gives 5,8-dichlorobenzo[rst]pentaphene, and nitration gives 5,8-dinitrobenzo[rst]pentaphene (Buu-Hoi & Lavit, 1956; Unseren & Fieser, 1962). Reaction of benzo[rst]pentaphene with *N*-methyl-formanilide and POCl$_3$ yields the 5-formyl derivative which is reduced by the Wolff–Kishner method to 5-methylbenzo[rst]pentaphene (Buu-Hoi & Lavit, 1956). Repetition of this sequence furnishes 5,8-dimethylbenzo-[rst]pentaphene.

Oxidation of benzo[rst]pentaphene with chromic acid provides the quinone **12** (Unseren & Fieser, 1962). Reaction with Pb(OAc)$_4$ yields 5,8-diacetoxybenzo[rst]pentaphene (Unseren & Fieser, 1962). Ozonolysis of benzo[rst]pentaphene gives **12** along with other oxidation products (Moriconi & Salce, 1967).

Fig. 10.3. Synthetic routes to benzo[rst]pentaphene.

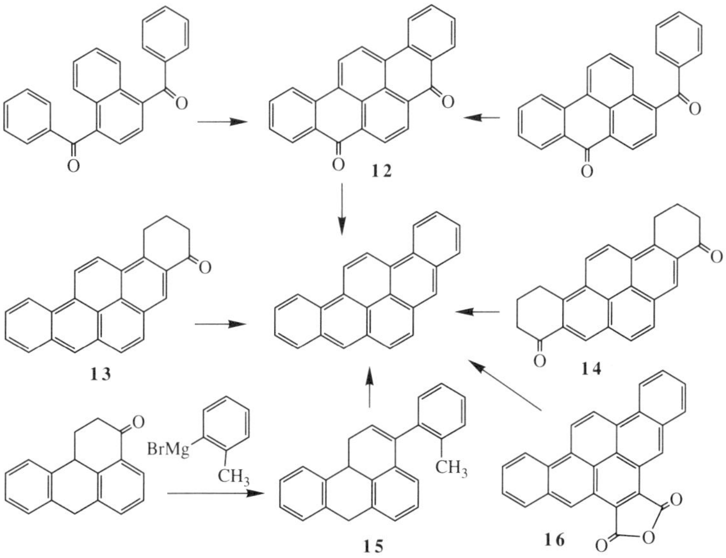

Reduction with sodium and amyl alcohol gives 6,7,13,14-tetrahydrobenzo[rst]pentaphene identified by its UV spectrum which resembles that of 2,2'-binaphthyl (Unseren & Fieser, 1962). Hydrogenation over an Adam's catalyst affords 6,7-dihydrobenzo[rst]pentaphene, and further hydrogenation furnishes the octahydro derivative with two saturated terminal rings (Unseren & Fieser, 1962).

10.4   Dibenzo[def,p]chrysene

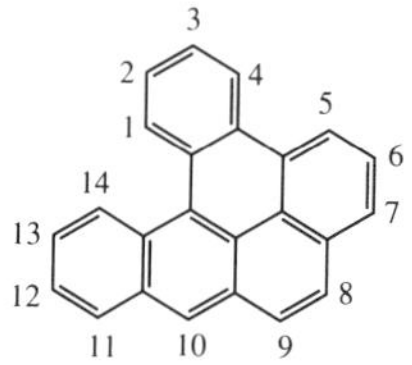

Other names: dibenzo[a,l]pyrene, 1.2,3.4-dibenzopyrene
Physical and spectral properties $C_{24}H_{14}$, mol. wt. 302.35, pale yellow plates, mp 162–3 °C. Spectral data: UV (Karcher *et al.*, 1985), UV fluorescence (Karcher *et al.*, 1985; Pierce & Katz, 1975; Van Duuren, 1960), PE (Clar & Schmidt, 1979), IR (Karcher *et al.*, 1985), NMR (Karcher *et al.*, 1985), mass spectrum (Karcher *et al.*, 1985).

Occurrence and carcinogenicity Occurs in coal tar (Wise *et al.*, 1988). It has also been identified in cigarette smoke (Snook *et al.*, 1977). Tumorigenicity studies reported to have been conducted with this hydrocarbon prior to 1966 were in fact done with dibenzo[a,e]fluoranthene (Lavit-Lamy ·& Buu-Hoi, 1966). More recent tests indicate that

Fig. 10.4. Synthetic routes to dibenzo[def,p]chrysene.

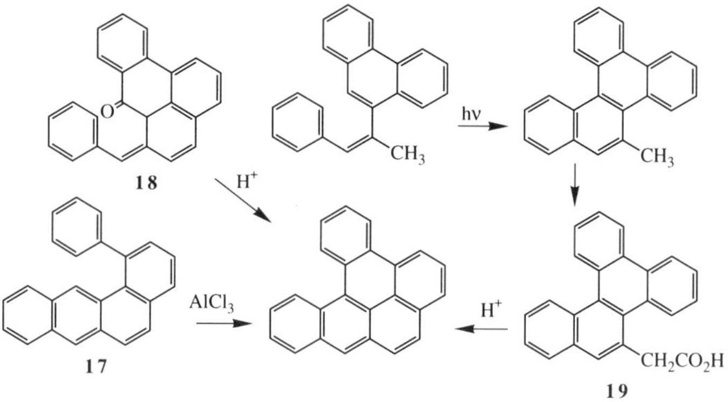

dibenzo[def,p]chrysene is a relatively potent carcinogen on mouse skin comparable in activity to BaP (IARC, 1983).

Synthesis Synthetic routes to dibenzo[def,p]chrysene are summarized in Fig. 10.4. The earlier claims of synthesis of dibenzo[def,p]-chrysene by $AlCl_3$-catalyzed cyclization of 12-phenylbenzanthrone (Clar & Stewart, 1951), cyclization and reduction of 3-phenyl-3-naphthylphthalide (Clar, 1930), and reaction of benzene with benz[a]anthracene in the presence of $AlCl_3$–$SnCl_4$ (Zander, 1959) have been shown to be incorrect and the product has been identified as dibenz[a,e]fluoranthene (Lavit-Lamy & Buu-Hoi, 1966). Successful synthesis of dibenzo[def,p]chrysene was achieved by cyclodehydrogenation of 1-phenylbenz[a]anthracene (**17**) with $AlCl_3$ (Vingiello *et al.*, 1971). A more convenient preparation entails cyclodehydration of 6-benzylbenzanthrone (**18**) with polyphosphoric acid (Masuda & Kagawa, 1972). Dibenzo[def,p]chrysene is also synthetically accessible from 9-methyl[g]chrysene (obtained by photocyclization) by conversion to benzo[g]chrysene-9-acetic acid (**19**), cyclodehydration, and reduction with zinc dust (Carruthers, 1967).

Reactions Electrophilic substitution may be expected to occur preferentially in the 10-position of dibenzo[def,p]chrysene. The only example is the Vilsmeier reaction which yields the 10-carboxaldehyde (Perin-Roussel *et al.*, 1975). Reduction of this aldehyde furnishes 10-methyldibenzo[def,p]chrysene.

10.5   Dibenzo[b,def]chrysene

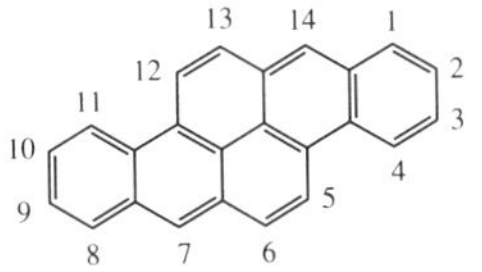

Other names: *dibenzo[a,h]pyrene, 3.4,8.9-dibenzopyrene*
Physical and spectral properties $C_{24}H_{14}$, mol. wt. 302.35, golden orange leaflets, mp 320-20.5 °C. Spectral data: UV (Karcher, 1988; Friedel & Orchin, 1951), UV fluorescence (Karcher, 1988; Pierce & Katz, 1975; Van Duuren, 1960; Schoental & Scott, 1949), PE (Clar & Schmidt, 1979), IR (Karcher, 1988), NMR (Karcher, 1988; Mitchell *et al.*, 1982), mass spectrum (Karcher, 1988; Thomas & Lao, 1978).

Occurrence and carcinogenicity Occurs in coal tar (Wise *et al.*, 1988), atmospheric pollution (Pierce & Katz, 1975), and tobacco and marijuana smoke (Grimmer, 1979; Lee *et al.*, 1976). Dibenzo[b,def]chrysene is tumorigenic on mouse skin at a lower level of activity than BaP (IARC, 1973; Hartwell, 1951).

Synthesis Dibenzo[b,def]chrysene is synthetically accessible by photocyclization of **20** in the presence of I$_2$ (Hayward *et al.*, 1972) or by AlCl$_3$-catalyzed cyclodehydration of 3-benzoylbenzanthrone or 1,5-dibenzoylnaphthalene to dibenzo[b,def]chrysene-7,14-dione (**21**) followed by reduction with zinc dust (Vollman *et al.*, 1937) (Fig. 10.5). Syntheses of several mono- and difluorinated derivatives of dibenzo[b,def]chrysene have been described (Sardella *et al.*, 1982).

Reactions Electrophilic substitution takes place in the 7,14-positions of dibenzo[b,def]chrysene. Reaction with sulfuryl chloride yields the 7,14-dichloro derivative (Buu-Hoi & Lavit, 1957), and nitration with nitric acid in nitrobenzene furnishes 7-nitro- and 7,14-dinitrodibenzo[b,def]chrysene (Ioffe & Efros, 1946). Vilsmeier reaction gives the 7-aldehyde which is reduced by the Wolff–Kishner method to 7-methyldibenzo[b,def]chrysene (Buu-Hoi & Lavit, 1957a). Repetition of this sequence yields 7,14-dimethyldibenzo-[b,def]chrysene.

10.6   Naphtho[1,2,3,4-def]chrysene

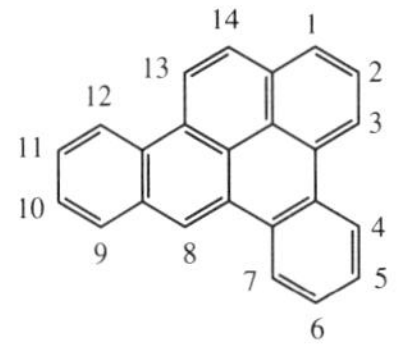

Other names: *dibenzo[a,e]pyrene, 1.2,4.5-dibenzopyrene*
Physical and spectral properties C$_{24}$H$_{14}$, mol. wt. 302.35, yellow

Fig. 10.5.   Synthetic routes to dibenzo[b,def]chrysene.

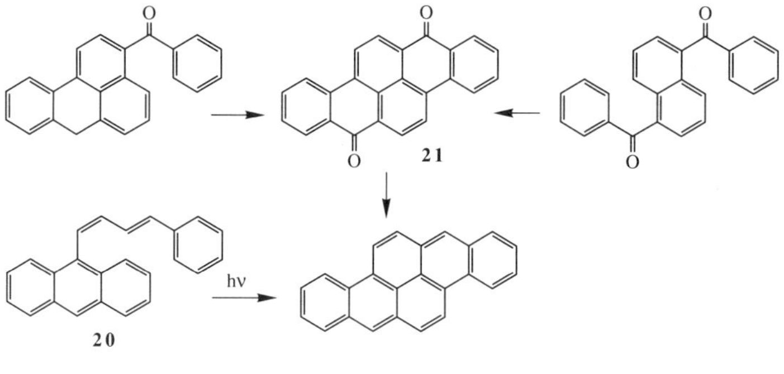

needles (xylene), mp 234 °C. Slightly soluble in organic solvents; solutions exhibit a blue fluorescence. Spectral data: UV (Karcher *et al.*, 1985), UV fluorescence (Karcher *et al.*, 1985; Pierce & Katz, 1975), PE (Clar & Schmidt, 1979), NMR (Karcher *et al.*, 1985), mass spectrum (Thomas & Lao, 1978).

Occurrence and carcinogenicity Present in carbon black (Peaden *et al.*, 1980), atmospheric pollution (Pierce & Katz, 1975), coal tar (Wise *et al.*, 1988), and tobacco smoke (Seversen *et al.*, 1976). Exhibits strong sarcomagenic activity in mice (Buu-Hoi, 1964), but is less active than BaP in the induction of skin tumors in this species (IARC, 1973).

Synthesis Naphtho[1,2,3,4-def]chrysene is obtained from reaction of chrysene with benzene in the presence of $AlCl_3$ (Zinke *et al.*, 1951). Similar reaction with toluene in place of benzene affords 5- and 6-dimethylnaphtho[1,2,3,4-def]chrysene (Buu-Hoi & Lavit-Lamy, 1963). Other syntheses are reviewed by Clar,1964.

Reactions The chemistry of naphtho[1,2,3,4-def]chrysene is relatively unknown. Oxidation with $Na_2Cr_2O_7$ in acetic acid yields the 8,9-dione initially, and further oxidation gives a carboxylic acid arising from ring cleavage (Fig. 10.6) (Ott, 1955). Decarboxylation of this acid furnishes dibenz[a,c]anthracene-7,14-dione.

10.7   Dibenzo[fg,op]naphthacene

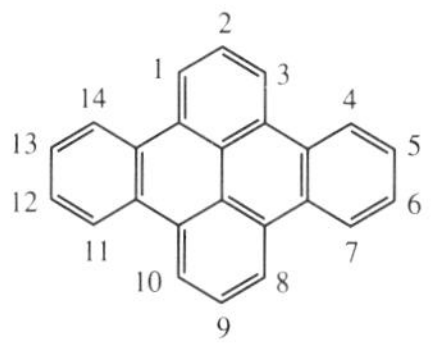

Other names: dibenzo[e,l]pyrene, 1.2,6.7-dibenzopyrene
Physical and spectral properties $C_{24}H_{14}$, mol. wt. 302.35, pale yellow crystals, mp 351–2 °C. Solutions in organic solvents show a blue

Fig. 10.6.   Chromic acid oxidation of naphtho[1,2,3,4-def]chrysene.

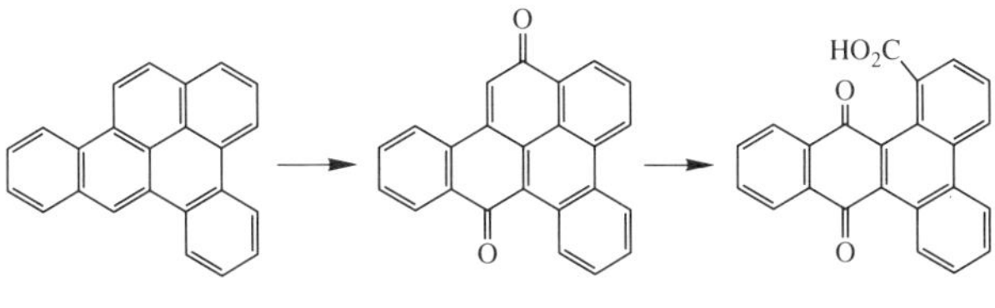

fluorescence. Spectral data: UV (Clar, 1964), UV fluorescence (Schoental & Scott, 1949), PE (Boschi *et al.*, 1974), mass spectrum (Thomas & Lao, 1978).

Occurrence and carcinogenicity Occurs in coal tar (Wise *et al.*, 1988). Limited available data indicate that this hydrocarbon is not carcinogenic (Buu-Hoi, 1964).

Synthesis While a number of synthetic routes to dibenzo[fg,op]-naphthacene are available (Fig. 10.7), most give low yields. The most efficient methods involve photocyclization of *o*-quaterphenyl (**22**: R = H) or its dichloro derivative (**22**: R = Cl) (Sato *et al.*, 1971); the latter does not require an oxidant. Photo-reaction of 1,2,3-triphenylbenzene (**23**) affords dibenzo[fg,op]naphthacene in lower yield (Sato *et al.*, 1971). Other synthetic methods include: reaction of biphenylene with lithium metal in tetrahydrofuran (Goldberg et al., 1969), heating triphenylene with $AlCl_3$ in benzene (Buu-Hoi & Lavit-Lamy, 1966), treatment of quaterphenyl with lithium in ether (Wittig *et al.*, 1962), heating quaterphenyl with platinum at elevated temperature (Copeland *et al.*, 1960), treatment of 2,2'-dilithio-biphenyl with $TiCl_4$ (Wittig & Lehmann, 1957), and decomposition of the tetrazonium sulfate of **22**: R = N_2 (Sako, 1934).

Fig. 10.7. Synthetic routes to dibenzo[fg,op]naphthacene.

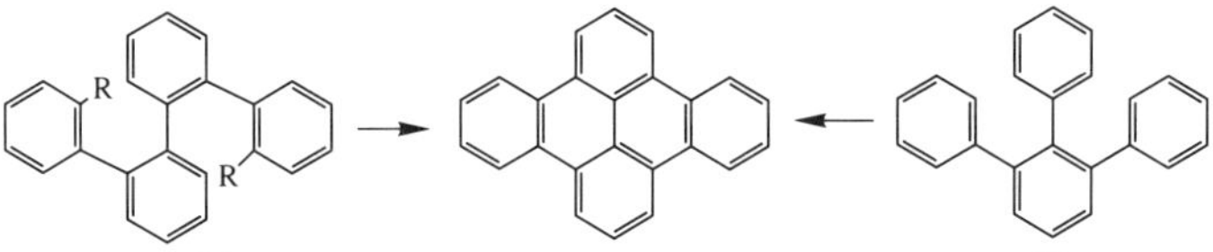

Fig. 10.8. Synthetic routes to dibenzo[b,k]chrysene.

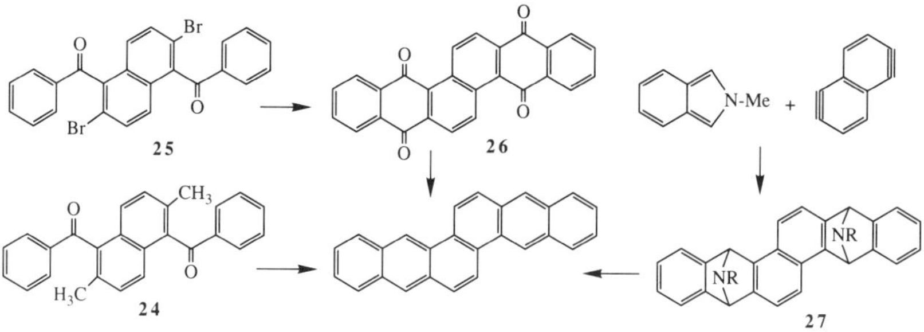

10.8 Dibenzo[b,k]chrysene

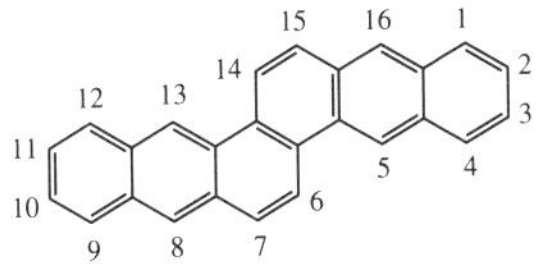

Other names: *anthraceno(2'.1':1.2)anthracene*
Physical and spectral properties $C_{26}H_{16}$, mol. wt. 328.39 yellow leaflets (xylene or nitrobenzene), mp 402-3 °C. Solutions in organic solvents exhibit deep blue fluorescence. Spectral data: UV (Clar *et al.*, 1929), PE (Boschi *et al.*, 1974), IR (LeHoullier & Gribble, 1983).

Occurrence and carcinogenicity No data could be found.

Synthesis This hydrocarbon was first synthesized by Elbs pyrolysis of the diketone **24** (Clar *et al.*, 1929) (Fig. 10.8). It has also been prepared from naphthalene by reaction with *o*-bromobenzoyl chloride and $AlCl_3$, followed by replacement of the bromine atoms of the diketone product **25** by nitrile groups by means of cuprous cyanide, hydrolysis, and cyclization to the diquinone **26** (Cook *et al.*, 1932). An elegant new method involves reaction of 1,5-naphthodiyne (generated *in situ* from 2,6-dibromo-1,5-bis[(*p*-tolyl-sulfonyl)oxy]naphthalene) with 2-methylisoindole to form the adduct **27** which is oxidized by *m*-CPBA to dibenzo[b,k]chrysene (LeHoullier & Gribble, 1983).

Reactions While the chemistry of dibenzo[b,k]chrysene is relatively unexplored, the molecule may be anticipated to behave like a double benz[a]anthracene. Oxidation with chromic acid yields the diquinone **26** arising from oxidation in the meso regions (Clar *et al.*, 1929).

10.9   References

Altman, Y. & Ginsburg, D. (1959). Alicyclic studies. Part XIV. An improved synthesis of 3:4-5:6-dibenzophenanthrene and 1:12-benzoperylene. *J. Chem. Soc.* 466–8.

Ansell, L. L., Rangarajan, T., Burgess, W. M., Eisenbraun, E. J., Keen, G. W. & Hamming, M. C. (1976). The synthesis of 1,2,3,7,8,9-hexahydrodibenzo[def,mno]chrysene and the use of hydriodic acid-red phosphorus in the deoxygenation of ketones. *Org. Prep. Proc. Int.* **8**, 133–40.

Badar, Y., Fatima, K., Siddiqui, M. S. & Hamdard, M. E. (1972). Synthesis of a new hydrocarbon 6,12-dihydroanthanthrene. *Pak. J. Sci. Ind. Res.* **15**, 18–20.

Berlman, I. B. (1971). *Handbook of Fluorescence Spectra of Aromatic Molecules,* New York: Academic.

Boschi, R., Clar, E. & Schmidt, W. (1974). Photoelectron spectra of polynuclear aromatics. III.

The effect of nonplanarity in sterically overcrowded aromatic hydrocarbons. *J. Chem. Phys.* **60**, 4406–18.

Buu-Hoi, N. P. (1964). New developments in chemical carcinogenesis by polycyclic hydrocarbons and related heterocycles: A review. *Cancer Res.* **24**, 1511–23.

Buu-Hoi, N. P. & Lavit, D. (1956). Polycyclic aromatic hydrocarbons. I. Substituted derivatives of 3,4-9,10-dibenzopyrene. *Rec. Trav. Chim.* **75**, 1194–8.

Buu-Hoi, N. P. & Lavit, D. (1957). Polycyclic aromatic hydrocarbons. III. Substitution products of anthanthrene. *Rec. Trav. Chim.* **76**, 200–4.

Buu-Hoi, N. P. & Lavit, D. (1957a). Polycyclic aromatic hydrocarbons. IV. The chemistry of dibenzo[a,h]pyrene. *Rec. Trav. Chim.* **76**, 321–4.

Buu-Hoi, N. P. & Lavit, D. (1958). Absorption in the ultraviolet, visible, and infrared of certain hexacyclic aromatic hydrocarbons and their methyl homologs. *Bull. Soc. Chim. Fr.* 1404–8.

Buu-Hoi, N. P. & Lavit, D. (1960). Synthesis of dibenzo[a,i]pyrene, tribenzo[a,e,i]pyrene, and new homologues of naphtho[2,3-a]pyrene. *Tetrahedron*, **8**, 1–6.

Buu-Hoi, N. P. & Lavit-Lamy, D. (1963). Action of aluminum chloride on aromatic hydrocarbons. The reaction of toluene on chrysene and picene. *Bull. Soc. Chim. Fr.* 341–3.

Buu-Hoi, N. P. & Lavit-Lamy, D. (1966). New method of synthesis of dibenzo[e,l]pyrene. *Bull. Soc. Chim. Fr.* 2500–1.

Carruthers, W. (1967). Photocyclisation of some stilbene analogues. Synthesis of dibenzo[a,l]pyrene. *J. Chem. Soc.* 1525–7.

Clar, E. (1930). Polynuclear aromatic hydrocarbons and their derivatives. VI. Synthesis of 1,2,3,4-dibenzopyrene and its derivatives. *Chem. Ber.* **63**, 112–20.

Clar, E. (1964). *Polycyclic Hydrocarbons*, New York: Academic Press.

Clar, E. (1973). The reaction of picene with maleic anhydride. *Tetrahedron Lett.* 3471–2.

Clar, E. & Stewart, D. (1951). Aromatic hydrocarbons. Part LIX. 1:2–3:4-Dibenzpyrene. *J. Chem. Soc.* 687–90.

Clar, E., Sanigok, U. & Zander, M. (1968). NMR studies of perylene and coronene derivatives. *Tetrahedron*, **24**, 2817–23.

Clar, E. & Schmidt, W. (1979). Correlations between photoelectron and UV absorption spectra of polycyclic hydrocarbons. The pyrene series. *Tetrahedron*, **35**, 1027–32.

Clar, E., Wallenstein, H. & Avenarius, R. (1929). Polynuclear aromatic hydrocarbons and their derivatives. III. Anthracenoanthracenes and their quinones. *Chem. Ber.* **62B**, 950–5.

Clar, E. & Zander, M. (1957). Synthesis of coronene and 1:2–7:8-dibenzocoronene. *J. Chem. Soc.* 4616–18.

Coffey, S. & Boyd, V. (1954). The reduction of anthraquinone and other polycyclic quinones with aluminum alkoxides (Meerwein–Pondorff reagent). *J. Chem. Soc.* 2468–70.

Cook, J. W., Hieger, I., Kennaway, E. L. & Mayneord, W. V. (1932). The production of cancer by pure hydrocarbons – Part II, *Proc. Roy. Soc.* **B111**, 455–84.

Copeland, P. G., Dean, R. E. & McNeil, D. (1960). Cyclodehydrogenation of *o,o'*-quaterphenyl and 4-(bicyclohex-1-en-2-yl)biphenyl. *J. Chem. Soc.* 4522–4.

Daub, G. H. & Smith, M. A. (1960). A new synthesis of dibenzo[a,i]pyrene. *J. Org. Chem.* **25**, 2043.

Dewar, M. J. S., Mole, T., Urch, D. S. & Warford, E. (1956). Electrophilic substitution. Part IV. The nitration of biphenyl, chrysene, and anthanthrene. *J. Chem. Soc.* 3572–5.

Dias, J. R. (1987). *Handbook of Polycyclic Hydrocarbons, Part A, Benzenoid Hydrocarbons*, Amsterdam: Elsevier.

Dietz, F. & Scholz, M. (1968). Chemistry of excited states. IV. The photocyclization of three distyrylbenzenes. *Tetrahedron*, **24**, 6845–9.

Friedel, R. A. & Orchin, M. (1951). *Ultraviolet Spectra of Aromatic Compounds*, New York: Wiley.

Goldberg, I. B., Borch, R. F. & Bolton, J. R. (1969). The synthesis of dibenzo[fg,op]naphthacene from biphenylene and lithium. *J. Chem. Soc. Chem. Commun.* 223–4.

Grimmer, G. (1979). *Environmental Carcinogens–Selected Methods of Analysis*, II, 31–61. Lyon, France: International Agency for Research on Cancer.

Hartwell, J. L. (1951). *Survey of Compounds which have been Tested for Carcinogenic Activity*, U.S. Public Health Service Publ. No 149. Washington, DC: Superintendent of Documents, U.S. Government Printing Office.

Hayward, R. J., Hopkinson, A. C. & Leznoff, C. C. (1972). Photocyclization reactions of aryl polyenes VI. The photocyclization of 1,4-diaryl-1,3-butadienes. *Tetrahedron*, **28**, 439–47.

Hoffmann, D. & Wynder, E. L. (1962). Analytical and biological studies on gasoline exhaust. *Natl. Cancer Inst. Monograph, No. 9*, 91–116.

IARC (1973). Monograph on the Evaluation of the Carcinogenic Risk of the Chemical to Man: Certain Polycyclic Aromatic Hydrocarbons and Heterocyclic Compounds, **3**, Lyon, France: International Agency for Research on Cancer.

IARC (1983). Monograph on the Evaluation of the Carcinogenic Risk of the Chemical to Man: Certain Polycyclic Aromatic Hydrocarbons and Heterocyclic Compounds, **32**, Lyon, France: International Agency for Research on Cancer.

Ioffe, I. S. & Efros, L. S. (1946). Nitro and amino derivatives of dibenzopyrene. *J. Gen. Chem. (USSR)*, **16**, 111–16.

Ivanenkov, A. A., Kuznetsov, V. S. & El'tsov, A. V. (1983). Acetylation of benzo[ghi]perylene. *Zhur. Obsch. Khim.* **53**, 2104–8.

Jessup, P. J. & Reiss, J. A. (1976). Cyclophanes. VI. The synthesis of [2,2](3,3')-biphenylparacyclophanes. *Aust. J. Chem.* **29**, 1267–75.

Johansen, E., Sydnes, L. K. & Greibrokk, T. (1984). Separation and characterization of mononitro derivatives of benzo[a]pyrene, benzo[e]pyrene and benzo[ghi]perylene. *Acta Chem. Scand.* **38B**, 309–18.

Kalb, L. (1914). Anthanthrone. I. Preparation. *Chem. Ber.* **47**, 1724–30.

Karcher, W. (1988). *Spectral Atlas of Polycyclic Aromatic Compounds*, Vol. 2, Dordrecht, Netherlands: Kluwer.

Karcher, W., Fordham, R., DuBois, J. & Gloude, P. (1985). *Spectral Atlas of Polycyclic Aromatic Compounds*, Dordrecht, Netherlands: D. Reidel.

Konieczny, M. & Harvey, R. G. (1979). Efficient reduction of polycyclic quinones, hydroquinones, and phenols to polycyclic aromatic hydrocarbons with hydriodic acid. *J. Org. Chem.* **44**, 4813–16.

Lang, K. F. & Eigen, I. (1967). Organic compounds detected in coal tar. *Fortschritte Chem. Forsch.* **8**, 91–170.

Lavit-Lamy, D. & Buu-Hoi, N. P. (1966). The true nature of 'dibenzo[a,l]pyrene' and its known derivatives. *J. Chem. Soc. Commun.* 92–4.

Lee, R. E., Novotny, M. & Bartle, K. D. (1976). Gas chromatography/mass spectrometric and nuclear magnetic resonance spectrometric studies of carcinogenic polynuclear aromatic hydrocarbons in tobacco and marijuana smoke condensates. *Anal. Chem.* **48**, 405–16.

LeHoullier, C. S. & Gribble, G. W. (1983). Twin annulation of naphthalene via a 1,5-naphthodiyne synthon. New syntheses of chrysene and dibenzo[b,k]chrysene. *J. Org. Chem.* **48**, 1682–5.

Lijinsky, W., Advani, G., Keefer, L., Ramahi, H. Y. & Stach, L. (1972). Catalytic hydrogenation of polynuclear hydrocarbons. *J. Chem. Eng. Data*, **17**, 100–4.

Masuda, Y. & Kagawa, R. (1972). Novel synthesis and carcinogenicity of dibenzo[a,l]pyrene. *Chem. Pharm. Bull.* **20**, 2736–7.

Mitchell, R. H., Williams, R. V. & Dingle, T. W. (1982). Toward the understanding of benzannelated annulenes: Synthesis and properties of [a,h]- and [a,i]-ring dibenzannelated dihydropyrenes. *J. Am. Chem. Soc.* **104**, 2560–71.

Moriconi, E. J. & Salce, L. (1967). Ozonolysis of polycyclic aromatics. XIV. Ozonation of pentaphene and benzo[rst]pentaphene. *J. Org. Chem.* **32**, 2829–37.

Ott, R. (1955). Synthesis of more highly condensed ring systems by intermolecular dehydrogenation. IX. 1,2,4,5-Dibenzopyrene-quinone. *Monatsh.* **86**, 622–36.

Peaden, P. A., Lee, M. L., Hirata, Y. & Novotny, M. (1980). High performance liquid chromatographic separation of high molecular weight polycyclic aromatic hydrocarbons in carbon black. *Anal. Chem.* **52**, 2268–71.

Perin-Roussel, O., Jacquignon, P. & Perin, F. (1975). Formylation of dibenzo[a,l]pyrene and dibenzo[a,e]fluoranthene and reduction of the resulting aldehydes. *C. R. Hebd. Seances Acad. Sci., Ser. C,* **280**, 1315–18.

Pierce, R. C. & Katz, M. (1975). Determination of atmospheric isomeric polycyclic arenes by thin-layer chromatography and fluorescence spectrophotometry. *Anal. Chem.* **47**, 1743–8.

Pouchert, C. E. (1981). *Aldrich Library of Infrared Spectra Edit. III.* Milwaukee, Wisc.: Aldrich Chemical Co.

Pouchert, C. E. (1983). *Aldrich Library of NMR Spectra, Edit. II.* Milwaukee, Wisc.: Aldrich Chemical Co.

Rahman, A., Tombesi, O. & Ollo, J. L. (1976). A total synthesis of 3,4,9,10-dibenzpyrene. *Chem. & Ind. (London),* 29–30.

Sako, S. (1934). The formation of cyclic compounds from derivatives of biphenyl. II. The formation of 4,5,9,10-dibenzopyrene and 4,5-diphenylbiphenylene oxide from 6,6'-diphenylbiphenyl-2,2'-tetrazonium sulfates. *Bull. Chem. Soc. Jpn.* **9**, 55–74.

Sardella, D. J., Ghoshal, P. K. & Boger, E. (1982). Synthesis of fluorinated derivatives of dibenzo[a,h]pyrene. *J. Fluorine Chem.* **20**, 459–73.

Sato, T., Matsui, H. & Komaki, R. (1976). Medium-sized cyclophanes. Part XIX. Bridged naphthalenes: Structural aspects, carbon-13 nuclear magnetic resonance, and benzoperylene formation. *J. Chem. Soc. Perkin I,* 2051–4.

Sato, T., Shimada, S. & Hata, K. (1971). A new route to polycondensed aromatics: Photolytic formation of triphenylene and dibenzo[fg, op]naphthacene ring systems. *Bull. Chem. Soc. Jpn.* **44**, 2484–90.

Sawicki, E. (1977). *Air Pollution and Cancer in Man.* IARC No. 16, 127–57. Lyon, France: International Agency for Research on Cancer.

Sawicki, E., Hauser, T. R. & Stanley, T. W. (1960). Ultraviolet, visible and fluorescence spectral analysis of polynuclear hydrocarbons. *Int. J. Air Poll.* **2**, 253–72.

Schoental, R. & Scott, E. J. (1949). Fluorescence spectra of polycyclic aromatic hydrocarbons in solution. *J. Chem. Soc.* 1683–96.

Scholl, R. & Neumann, H. (1922). Ring closure in doubly benzoylated naphthalenes. *Chem. Ber.* **55**, 118–26.

Seversen, R. F., Snook, M. E., Higman, H. C., Chortyk, O. T. & Akin, F. J. (1976). *Carcinogenesis,* vol. I, eds R. I. Freudenthal and P. W. Jones, 253–70. New York: Raven Press.

Shushan, B. & Boyd, R.K. (1980). Unimolecular and collision induced fragmentations of molecular ions of polycyclic aromatic hydrocarbons. *Org. Mass Spectr.* **15**, 445–53.

Thomas, R. S. & Lao, R. C. (1978). Mass spectra of isomeric dibenzopyrenes. *Adv. Mass Spectrom.* **7B**, 1709–12.

TRC (1985). *TRC Spectral Data: Ultraviolet. Suppl. 1,* College Station, Texas: Thermodynamics Research Center, Texas A & M University.

TRC (1986). *TRC Spectral Data: ^1H Nuclear Magnetic Resonance. Suppl. 2,* College Station, Texas: Thermodynamics Research Center, Texas A & M University.

Unseren, E. & Fieser, L. F. (1962). Investigation of the metabolism of 3,4,9,10-dibenzpyrene. *J. Org. Chem.* **27**, 1386–9.

Van Duuren, B. (1960). The fluorescence spectra of aromatic hydrocarbons and heterocyclic aromatic compounds. *Anal. Chem.* **32**, 1436–42.

Vingiello, F. A., Yanez, J. & Campbell, J.A. (1971). A new approach to the synthesis of dibenzo[a,l]pyrenes. *J. Org. Chem.* **36**, 2053–6.

Vollmann, H., Becker, H., Corell, M. & Streeck, H. (1937). Pyrene and its derivatives. *Liebigs Ann.* **531**, 1–159.

Vorozhtsov, G. N., Dokunikhin, N. S., Khmel'nitskaya, E. Y. & Romanova, K. A. (1979). Derivatives of 1,1'-binaphthyl. VIII. Synthesis and cyclization of 8,8'-diformyl-1,1'-binaphthyl. *Zhur. Org. Khim.* **15**, 1930–3.

Wise, S. A., Benner, B. A., Liu, H. & Byrd, G. D. (1988). Separation and identification of polycyclic aromatic hydrocarbon isomers of molecular weight 302 in complex mixtures. *Anal. Chem.* **60**, 630–7.

Wittig, G., Hahn, E. & Tochtermann, W. (1962). From *o*-triphenylenemercury to the 1-phenyltribenzocycloheptatrienyl radical. *Chem. Ber.* **95**, 437–42.

Wittig, G. & Lehmann, G. (1957). Syntheses of cyclopolyenes. IV. Reactions of 2,2'-dilithiobiphenyl with metal chlorides. Synthesis of poly-o-phenylenes. *Chem. Ber.* **90**, 875–92.

Zander, M. (1959). Synthesis of 1,2;3,4-dibenzopyrene and 1,2;4,5;8,9-tribenzopyrene. *Chem. Ber.* **92**, 2749–51.

Zinke, A., Zimmer, W., Ott, R. & Wiesenberger, E. (1951). Synthesis of benzpyrene from chrysene. II. 1,2,3,4-Dibenzpyrene. *Monatsh.* **82**, 348–58.

11

Nonalternant polyarenes

The polycyclic aromatic hydrocarbons discussed in previous chapters are exclusively alternant polyarenes that contain only fused six-membered aromatic rings. While carcinogenesis research has focused for historical reasons primarily on these alternant polyarenes, there is increasing recognition that other classes of PAHs may also play an important role in carcinogenesis. Polyarenes such as fluoranthene, cyclopenta[c,d]pyrene, benzofluorene, and indeno[1,2,3-cd]pyrene are relatively widespread environmental contaminants, and some of these exhibit significant tumorigenic activity.

This chapter surveys the chemistry of several classes of polyarenes that contain a five-membered ring in addition to fused polycyclic aromatic ring systems. The PAHs surveyed were selected on the basis of their established environmental prevalence and their importance or potential importance as carcinogenic hazards. All of the PAHs reviewed are derivatives of fluoranthene, acenaphthylene, or fluorene.

11.1   Fluoranthene

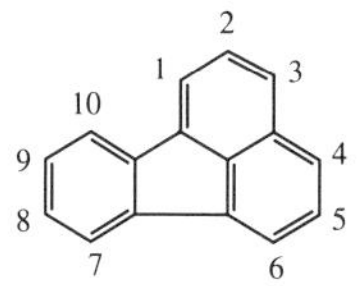

Physical and spectral properties $C_{16}H_{10}$, mol. wt. 202.24, colorless needles or plates, mp 110 °C. Solutions exhibit a bright green fluorescence. X-ray and neutron diffraction analyses of the crystal structure show a slight deviation from planarity on an axis through the central bond in the naphthalene molecular component (Hazell *et al.*, 1977). Spectral data: UV (Karcher *et al.*, 1985; Jaffe & Orchin, 1962; Friedel & Orchin, 1951),

UV fluorescence (Karcher, 1985; Berlman, 1971), IR (Karcher *et al.*,1985; Pouchert, 1981), ^{1}H-NMR (Karcher, 1985; Memory & Wilson, 1982; TRC, 1982; Pouchert & Campbell, 1983; Bartle *et al.*, 1967), ^{13}C-NMR (Karcher *et al.*, 1985; Memory & Wilson, 1982; Jones *et al.*, 1970), mass spectrum (Karcher, 1985).

Occurrence and carcinogenicity Fluoranthene is abundantly present in coal tar, and significant levels are found in urban atmospheres (Lee et al., 1976; Grimmer, 1979; IARC, 1983), auto exhaust (Grimmer, 1979), carbon black (Lee & Hites, 1976), tobacco and marijuana smoke (Lee *et al.*, 1976; Snook *et al.*, 1977), and sewage sludge (Grimmer, 1979). Fluoranthene is a relatively potent mutagen (Kaden *et al.*, 1979; Thilly *et al.*, 1980). Although it showed no activity on mouse skin or on subcutaneous injection (Buu-Hoi, 1964; Hoffmann *et al.*, 1972), it is tumorigenic in a newborn mouse lung bioassay (Busby *et al.*, 1984).

Synthesis Numerous syntheses of the fluoranthene ring system are available. Several of these are based on fluorene (Fig. 11.1). One of the earliest reported methods entails condensation of the sodium salt of ethyl fluorene-9-carboxylate (**1**) with β-chloropropionic ester, followed by hydrolysis, decarboxylation, and cyclization to yield the ketone **2** (von Braun & Anton, 1929). Clemmensen reduction of **2** and dehydrogenation yields fluoranthene. Modifications of this method include Michael addition of **1** to acrylonitrile and acrylic esters (Campbell & Tucker, 1949) and Michael

Fig. 11.1. Synthetic approaches to fluoranthene based upon fluorene and its derivatives.

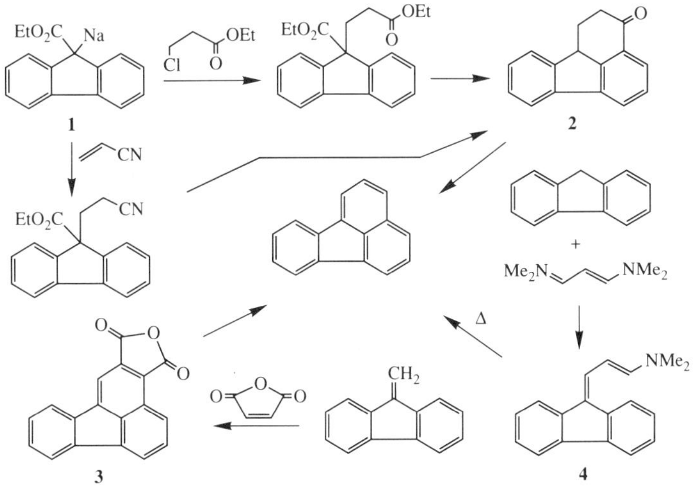

reaction of acrylonitrile with 9-fluorenol (Campbell & Fairfull, 1949). Diels–Alder reaction of 7-methylenefluorene, generated *in situ* from dehydration of 9-methylfluoren-9-ol, with maleic anhydride furnishes an adduct which undergoes spontaneous dehydrogenation to yield **3**. Decarboxylation of **3** provides fluoranthene (Campbell & Wang, 1949). Fluoranthene is also obtained by the Jutz synthesis involving reaction between fluorene and a vinamidinium salt to yield the adduct **4** which undergoes thermal electrocyclic ring closure (Jutz, 1978).

Fluoranthene derivatives are also synthetically accessible from acenaphthylene. Diels–Alder cycloaddition of butadiene affords tetrahydrofluoranthene (Kloetzel & Mertel, 1950) (Fig. 11.2). Reductive alkylation of acenaphthylene with lithium in ammonia and 1,4-dichlorobutane furnishes hexahydrofluoranthene as a minor product (**5**); the major product is 5-(ω-chlorobutyl)acenaphthylene (Neumann & Mullen, 1985). Maleic anhydride condenses with 1,2-dimethylacenaphthylene-1,2-diol in the presence of acetic anhydride (presumably via the diene intermediate **6**) to form an adduct (**7**) which is converted to fluoranthene by dehydrogenation and decarboxylation (Campbell & Gow, 1949). The spiro-indazole **8**, prepared by the cycloaddition of benzyne and 4-diazonaphthalen-1(4*H*)-one, undergoes thermal rearrangement with elimination of nitrogen to 3-hydroxyfluoranthene (Hirakawa *et al.*, 1980). Fluoranthene is also obtained, though in modest yield, from catalytic cyclodehydrogenation of 1-cyclohexenylnaphthalene or

Fig. 11.2. Additional syntheses of fluoranthene (R = OH in the product arising from **8**; R = H in all other cases).

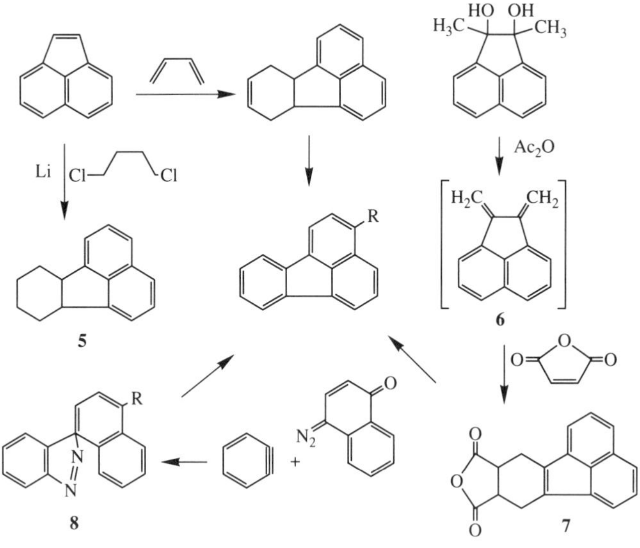

1-phenylnaphthalene (Orchin & Reggel, 1947) and from cyclodehydration of 2-(1-naphthyl)cyclohexanone (Orchin & Reggel, 1951). Other syntheses of fluoranthene are described by Clar, 1964.

Syntheses of all of the isomeric monomethyl derivatives (Tucker & Whalley, 1952) and phenol derivatives (Rice *et al.*, 1983) of fluoranthene have been reported.

Reactions The structure and properties of fluoranthene are of considerable theoretical interest. While fluoranthene is a nonalternant hydrocarbon with 16 π-electrons, it may also be regarded as a combination of benzene and naphthalene rings joined by formal single bonds. Support for this view is provided by semi-empirical MO calculations which indicate that the central ring supports negligible ring current (Bartle *et al.*, 1967). On the other hand, Huckel MO calculations are more consistent with a more delocalized structure (Michl & Zahradnik, 1966).

Electrophilic substitution occurs predominantly in the 3-position of fluoranthene. Nitration with nitric acid in acetic acid yields mainly 3-nitro- and 8-nitrofluoranthene (70% and 23%, respectively), whilst similar reaction in acetic anhydride is less selective providing the 3-, 8-, 7-, and 1-isomers in 43, 23, 18, and 11% yield, respectively (Streitweiser & Fahey, 1962), and nitration with dinitrogen tetroxide furnishes the 3-, 8- and other isomers in 63, 27, and 10 % yield, respectively (Radner, 1983). On the other hand, nitration with NO_2–N_2O_4 in CCl_4 gives 2-nitrofluoranthene as the main product at low conversion by what is assumed to be a homolytic rather than an ionic mechanism (Squaditro *et al.*, 1987). Protodetritiation in trifluoroacetic acid gives the positional order of reactivity $3 > 8 > 1 > 7 > 2$ (Bancroft & Howe, 1970). Bromination in CS_2 gives 3-bromofluoranthene initially (Allschuler & Berliner, 1966; von Braun & Manz, 1931), and further reaction yields the 3,8-dibromo derivative (Campbell *et al.*, 1950). The Friedel–Crafts reactions with acetyl or benzoyl chloride or with phthalic anhydride afford the products of substitution in both the 3- and 8-positions approximately equally (Campbell & Easton, 1949). The Friedel–Crafts reaction with oxalyl chloride provides fluoranthene-8-carboxylic acid and an unidentified dicarboxylic acid in 2:1 ratio (Campbell & Easton, 1949).

Oxidation of fluoranthene with chromic anhydride in acetic acid or ceric ammonium sulfate yields fluoranthene-2,3-dione, and further oxidation with the chromium reagent gives fluorenone-1-carboxylic acid (Periasamy & Bhatt, 1977; Campbell & Reid, 1958). Reaction of fluoranthene with Pb(OAc)4 provides 3-acetoxyfluoranthene (Shenbor & Cheban, 1969), and ozonolysis leads to formation of 1-formylfluorenone in good yield (Callighan *et al.*, 1960).

Reduction of fluoranthene with lithium in ammonia gives initially the theoretically predicted 3,10b-dihydro product (**9**) (Fig. 11.3) which under appropriately controlled conditions can be isolated in good yield (Harvey *et al.*, 1972). However, this olefin isomerizes readily into conjugation and undergoes further reduction to 1,2,3,10b-tetrahydrofluoranthene (**10**). The latter is the principal product of both the reaction of fluoranthene with sodium and alcohol and its hydrogenation over Raney nickel (Beaton & Tucker, 1952). Iodination of **10** with iodine and silver trifluoroacetate yields the 4-iodo derivative. Hydrogenation of fluoranthene under more strenuous conditions give decahydrofluoranthene and ultimately perhydrofluoranthene. Reductive methylation of fluoranthene with Li/NH_3 and methyl bromide affords 10b-methyl-3,10b-dihydrofluoranthene (**11**: R = H), whereas similar reaction with Na/NH_3 provides the 3,10b-dimethyl product (**11**: R = CH_3) (Harvey *et al.*, 1972). This difference was shown to be due to back reaction of $NaNH_2$ with **11**: R = H to form a second monoanionic intermediate which can be methylated; the low solubility of $LiNH_2$ effectively limits this pathway in the lithium reaction.

Nucleophilic addition of methyllithium to fluoranthene and treatment of the adduct with iodine furnishes 1-methylfluoranthene (5%) and *trans*-1,10b-dimethyl-1,10b-dihydro-fluoranthene (35%) (Peake *et al.*, 1983).

11.2   Benz[a]aceanthrylene

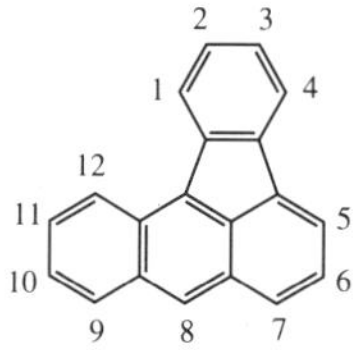

Other names: benzo[a]fluoranthene, 2,3-benzofluoranthene
Physical and spectral properties $C_{20}H_{12}$, mol. wt. 252.30, orange-

Fig. 11.3. Reduction and reductive methylation of fluoranthene.

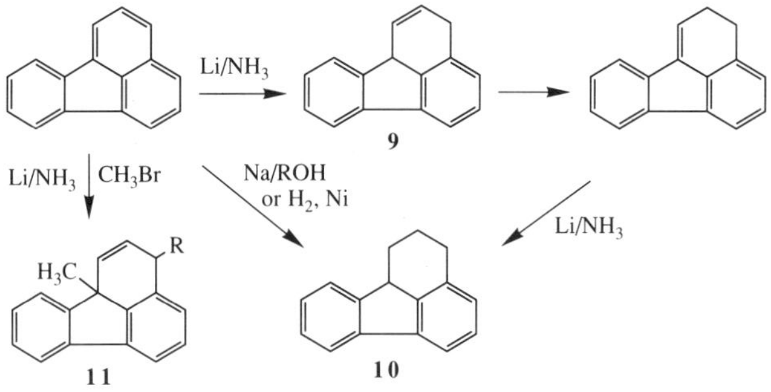

yellow needles, mp 144–5 °C. Solutions show a green fluorescence. Spectral data: UV (Karcher *et al.*, 1985; TRC, 1982a), UV fluorescence (Karcher *et al.*, 1985), IR (Karcher *et al.*, 1985), NMR (Cho & Harvey, 1987a; Karcher *et al.*, 1985; TRC, 1982), mass spectrum (Karcher *et al.*, 1985).

Occurrence and carcinogenicity Low levels have been recently shown to occur in coal tar (Wise *et al.*, 1988). Benz[a]aceanthrylene is a weak tumor-initiator less active than benzo[b]fluoranthene (Weyand *et al.*, 1990).

Synthesis An efficient new synthesis (Fig. 11.4) involves reaction of 9-lithioanthracene with cyclohexene oxide, oxidation of the alcohol product with 'periodane' to the ketone **12**, acid-catalyzed cyclodehydration, and dehydrogenation with DDQ (Cho & Harvey, 1987). Another interesting new synthesis involves reaction of fluorenone with 2-lithio-*N*,*N*-diethylbenzamide to provide the lactone **13** (Ray & Harvey, 1982). Reduction of **13** with zinc and alkali gives the carboxylic acid **14** which undergoes reductive cyclization with HF in the presence of the hydride donor triphenylmethane to yield benz[a]aceanthrylene. The lactone **13** may also be prepared by reaction of *o*-toluylmagnesium bromide with fluorenone to provide **15** and oxidation of the latter by MnO_2 and nitric acid (Stubbs & Tucker, 1951); zinc dust reduction of **13** gives benz[a]aceanthrylene. Another recent synthesis of

Fig. 11.4. Synthetic routes to benz[a]aceanthrylene.

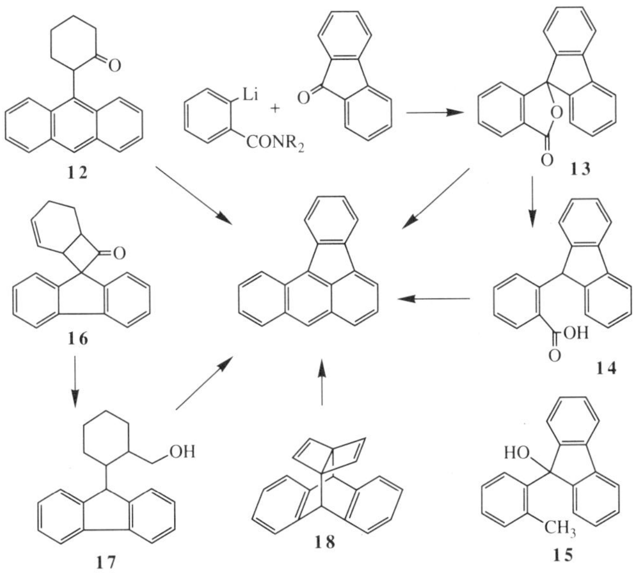

benz[a]aceanthrylene is based on the cyclobutanone **16** obtained from addition of 1,3-cyclohexadiene to the appropriate ketene (Chung *et al.*, 1987). Treatment of **16** with NaBH$_4$ gives the ring-opened alcohol **17** which is converted to benz[a]aceanthrylene by cyclization in HF and dehydrogenation. Benz[a]aceanthrylene may also be prepared by cyclodehydrogenation of 9-phenylanthracene over a platinum catalyst (Studt, 1979) and by the thermal rearrangement of **18** (Johnson & Bergman, 1979). Other syntheses are described by Clar, 1964.

Reactions The chemistry of benz[a]aceanthrylene is relatively unknown. Bromination takes place preferentially in the 8-position in accord with theoretical prediction by the DEWAR-PI method (Minabe *et al.*, 1989). Benz[a]aceanthrylene also forms a photo-oxide and reacts with maleic anhydride to form a colorless adduct (Clar, 1964).

11.3   Benz[e]acephenanthrylene

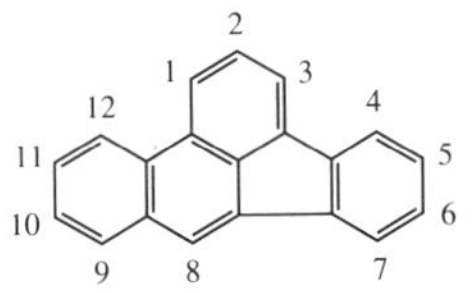

Other names: benzo[b]fluoranthene, 3,4-benzofluoranthene
Physical and spectral properties C$_{20}$H$_{12}$, mol. wt. 252.30, colorless needles, mp 168 °C. Spectral data: UV (Karcher *et al.*, 1985; Clar, 1964), UV fluorescence (Karcher *et al.*, 1985; Pierce & Katz, 1975), IR (Karcher *et al.*, 1985), ^{1}H-NMR (Cho & Harvey, 1987a; Karcher *et al.*, 1985), ^{13}C-NMR (Cho & Harvey, 1987a; Karcher *et al.*, 1985), mass spectrum (Karcher *et al.*, 1985).

Occurrence and carcinogenicity Occurs in coal tar (Wise *et al.*, 1988) and carbon black (Peaden *et al.*, 1980), and significant levels are detected in airborne pollutants (IARC, 1983; Grimmer, 1979), auto exhaust (IARC, 1983; Grimmer, 1979), tobacco and marijuana smoke (IARC, 1983; Seversen *et al.*, 1976; Lee *et al.*, 1976), and many foods (IARC, 1983; Grimmer, 1979). Benz[e]acephenanthrylene is more active than benzo[j]fluoranthene and much more active than benzo[b]fluoranthene as a tumor-initiator on mouse skin (Weyand *et al.*, 1990; LaVoie *et al.*, 1982).

Synthesis Benz[e]acephenanthrylene is conveniently prepared by reaction of 9-lithiophenanthrene with cyclohexene oxide, followed by oxidation to the ketone **19**, cyclodehydration, and dehydrogenation (Cho & Harvey, 1987) (Fig. 11.5). Benzyne generated from thermolysis of *o*-diazonitrobenzoate in the presence of excess benzofuran forms the bis-adduct **20** (Anthony & Wege, 1984). Treatment of **20** with acid results in rearrangement and dehydration to give benz[e]acephenanthrylene in good yield. Other syntheses of benz[e]acephenanthrylene include: the Jutz synthesis between benz[c]fluorene and a vinamidium salt and thermal cyclization of the adduct **21** (Jutz, 1978); photolysis of the fluorene-9-spiro-dihydrothiopyrane **22** and dehydrogenation (Praefcke & Weichsel, 1978); and acid-catalyzed rearrangement of the cyclobutanone adduct **16** to the pentacyclic ketone **23** followed by hydride reduction, dehydration, and dehydrogenation (Chung *et al.*, 1987).

Syntheses of all of the isomeric hydroxybenz[e]acephenanthrylenes (Amin *et al.*, 1986) and several mono- and dimethylbenz[e]acephenanthrylenes (Amin *et al.*, 1985a) have also been reported .

Reactions Surprisingly little is known concerning the chemical reactivity of benz[e]acephenanthrylene. Electrophilic substitution is predicted by the DEWAR-PI theoretical method to take place in the 8-position analogous to the 9-position of phenanthrene (Dewar & Dennington 1989). However, bromination affords a monobromo derivative identified on the basis of NMR analysis as 1-bromobenz[e]acephenanthrylene (Minabe *et al.*, 1989).

Fig. 11.5. Synthetic routes to benz[e]acephenanthrylene.

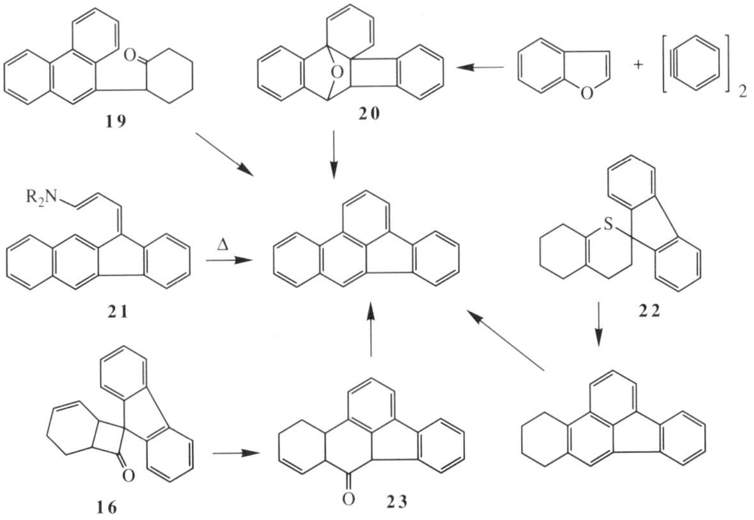

11.4   Benzo[j]fluoranthene

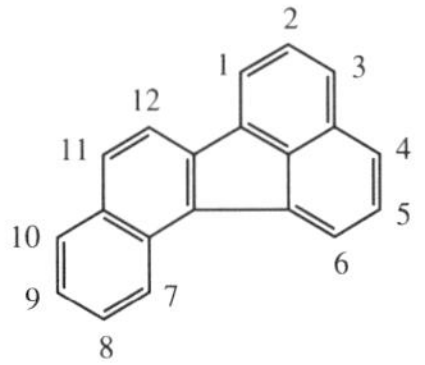

Other names: 10,11-benzofluoranthene
Physical and spectral properties $C_{20}H_{12}$, mol. wt. 252.30, yellow plates or needles, mp 165 °C. Spectral data: UV (Karcher *et al.*, 1985; Friedel & Orchin, 1951; Clar, 1964), UV fluorescence (Karcher *et al.*, 1985), IR (Karcher *et al.*, 1985), ^{1}H-NMR (Cho & Harvey, 1987a; Karcher *et al.*, 1985), ^{13}C-NMR (Cho & Harvey, 1987a; Karcher *et al.*, 1985), mass spectrum (Karcher *et al.*, 1985; Dobbs *et al.*, 1980).

Occurrence and carcinogenicity Occurs in coal tar (Wise *et al.*, 1988; IARC, 1983), soot (IARC, 1983), and carbon black (Lee & Hites, 1976), and significant levels are detected in urban atmospheres (IARC, 1983), auto exhaust (IARC, 1983), tobacco and marijuana smoke (IARC, 1983; Grimmer, 1979; Seversen *et al.*, 1976; Lee *et al.*, 1976), and foods (IARC, 1983; Grimmer, 1979). Benzo[j]fluoranthene is a weak tumor-initiator less active than benzo[b]fluoranthene (LaVoie *et al.*, 1982).

Synthesis A practical synthetic approach to benzo[j]fluoranthene is based on the tetrahydrobinaphthyl compound **24** obtained from pinacol condensation of α-tetralone (Dobbs *et al.*, 1984) (Fig. 11.6). Acid-catalyzed cyclization of **24** to hexahydrobenzo[j]fluoranthene **25** and dehydrogenation

Fig. 11.6.   Synthetic routes to benzo[j]fluoranthene.

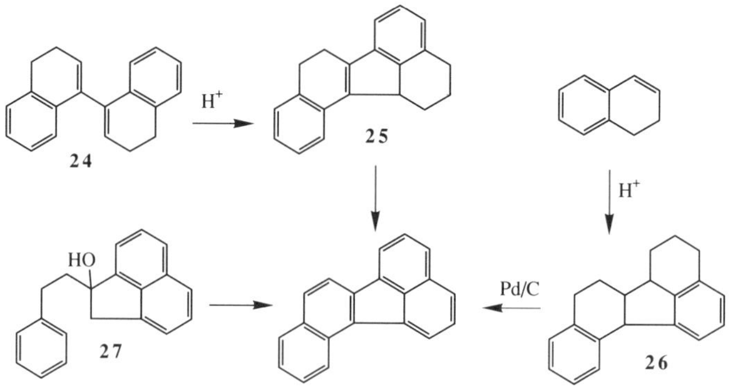

furnishes benzo[j]fluoranthene. A related route involves acid-catalyzed cyclodimerization of 1,2-dihydronaphthalene to yield a mixture of isomeric octahydrobenzo[j]fluoranthenes (**26**) which are readily dehydrogenated to benzo[j]fluoranthene (Dobbs *et al.*, 1980). This hydrocarbon is also synthetically accessible from reaction of phenylethylmagnesium bromide with acenaphthenone followed by cyclodehydration of the resulting alcohol **27** and dehydrogenation (Nenitzescu & Avram, 1950). Additional syntheses are described by Clar, 1964.

Reactions The chemistry of benzo[j]fluoranthene, like that of most polycyclic fluoranthene hydrocarbons, is virtually unknown. Its reaction with Na and alcohol gives 1,2, 3, 6b,11,12,12a,12b-octahydrobenzo[k]–fluoranthene (Nenitzescu & Avram, 1950).

11.5   Benzo[k]fluoranthene

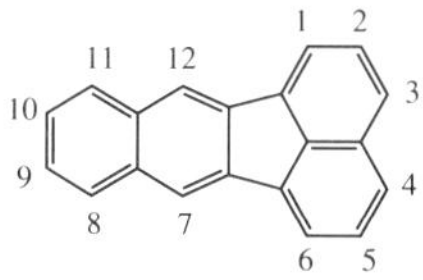

Other names: 11,12-benzofluoranthene
Physical and spectral properties $C_{20}H_{12}$, mol. wt. 252.30, colorless needles, mp 217 °C (benzene). Spectral data: UV (Karcher *et al.*, 1985; Friedel & Orchin, 1951), UV fluorescence (Karcher *et al.*, 1985; Pierce & Katz, 1975), IR (Karcher *et al.*, 1985), NMR (Karcher *et al.*, 1985; Bartle *et al.*, 1967), mass spectrum (Karcher *et al.*, 1985).

Occurrence and carcinogenicity Occurs in coal tar (Wise *et al.*, 1988) and carbon black (Peaden *et al.*, 1980; Lee & Hites, 1976), and significant levels are found in atmospheric pollution (IARC, 1983; Sawicki, 1977), tobacco and marijuana smoke (Seversen *et al.*, 1976; Lee *et al.*, 1976), sewage sludge (Grimmer, 1979), and common foods (Grimmer, 1979). Benzo[k]fluoranthene is listed as a priority pollutant by the Environmental Protection Agency and is one of several PAHs recommended for analysis in drinking water by the World Health Organization. Benzo[k]fluoranthene is mutagenic in S. typhimurium in the presence of microsomes (LaVoie *et al.*, 1980). However, it is inactive as a complete carcinogen on mouse skin, and it fails to induce lung or liver tumors in newborn mice (LaVoie *et al.*, 1987). On the other hand, it exhibits activity as a tumor initiator on mouse skin (LaVoie *et al.*, 1982), and it induces fibrosarcomas when administered by s.c. injection to mice (LaCassagne *et al.*, 1963).

Synthesis Condensation of *o*-phenylenediacetonitrile with accnaphthene-1,2-dione provides 7,12-dicyanobenzo[k]fluoranthene (**28**) (Fig. 11.7)(Orchin & Reggel, 1951a); hydrolysis and decarboxylation of **28** to benzo[k]fluoranthene may be accomplished in a single step by heating in polyphosphoric acid (Vickery & Eisenbraun, 1979). Benzo[k]fluoranthene may be obtained directly, albeit in modest yield, from the Wittig reactions of acenaphthene-1,2-dione with the diphosphonate **29** (Whitlock, Jr, 1964) or the bis-phosphonium salt **30** (Minsky & Rabinovitz, 1983). The Haworth synthesis involving Friedel–Crafts succinoylation of fluoranthene followed by reduction of the keto acid product, and AlCl₃-catalyzed cyclization affords the ketone **31** arising from cyclization to the 9-position; reduction and dehydrogenation of **31** provides benzo[k]fluoranthene (Buu-Hoi *et al.*, 1959). Benzo[k]fluoranthene-8,11-dione is synthetically accessible via Diels–Alder cycloaddition of 1,2-dimethyleneacenaphthylene (**6**), generated *in situ*, to *p*-benzoquinone (Campbell & Gow, 1949).

Reactions Oxidation of benzo[k]fluoranthene with ceric ammonium sulfate provides a mixture of the 2,3- and 7,12-diones (Balanikas *et al.*, 1988).

11.6   Benzo[ghi]fluoranthene

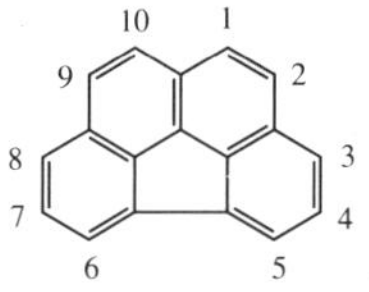

Other names: benzo[mno]fluoranthene, 2,13-benzofluoranthene
Physical and spectral properties C₁₈H₁₀, mol. wt. 226.26, yellow needles, mp 149 °C (alcohol). X-ray diffraction studies show the molecule to

Fig. 11.7. Synthetic routes to benzo[k]fluoranthene.

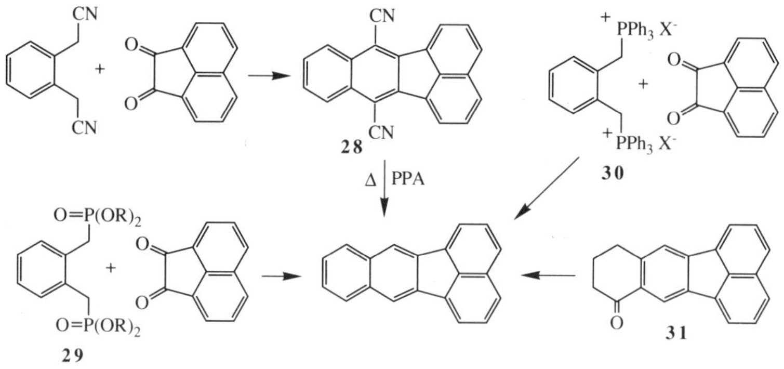

be flat, and all the bonds in the five-membered ring are long, whereas in the six-membered rings there is a Kekulé arrangement of alternating long and short bonds (Ehrlich & Beevers, 1956). Spectral data: UV (Clar, 1964), UV fluorescence (Berlman, 1971), ^{1}H-NMR (Bartle *et al.*, 1967), ^{13}C-NMR (Jones *et al.*, 1970).

Occurrence and carcinogenicity Occurs in coal tar (Wise *et al.*, 1988) and carbon black (Lee & Hites, 1976), and significant levels are commonly detected in urban atmospheres (IARC, 1983; Grimmer, 1979; Sawicki, 1977), auto exhaust (Grimmer, 1979), tobacco and marijuana smoke (Grimmer, 1979; Lee *et al.*, 1976; Seversen *et al.*, 1976), and many foods (Grimmer, 1979). Limited available data indicate that this PAH is inactive as a complete carcinogen on mouse skin (IARC, 1983).

Synthesis Several syntheses are based on cyclopenta[def]phenan-threne (Fig. 11.8). Michael addition of methyl cyclopenta[def]phenanthrene-4-carboxylate (**32**) to acrylonitrile followed by hydrolysis and cyclization furnishes the ketone **33** which undergoes reduction and dehydrogenation to yield benzo[ghi]fluoranthene (Campbell & Reid, 1952). 4-Methyl-enecyclopenta[def]phenanthrene, generated *in situ* from dehydration of 4-hydroxy-4-methylcyclopenta[def]phenanthrene (**34**), enters into a Diels–Alder reaction with maleic anhydride to give the adduct **35** which on hydrolysis and decarboxylation affords benzo[ghi]fluoranthene; however, the yield is low due to polymerization (Campbell & Reid, 1952). The Jutz synthesis between cyclopenta[def]phenanthrene and vinamidinium salts followed by thermal cyclization of the adduct **36** also provides synthetic access to benzo[ghi]fluoranthene derivatives (Jutz, 1978). Benzo[ghi]-fluoranthene may also be prepared directly from benzo[c]phenanthrene by dehydrogenation over a platinum catalyst at 400 °C (Studt, 1983) or from

Fig. 11.8. Synthetic routes to benzo[ghi]fluoranthene.

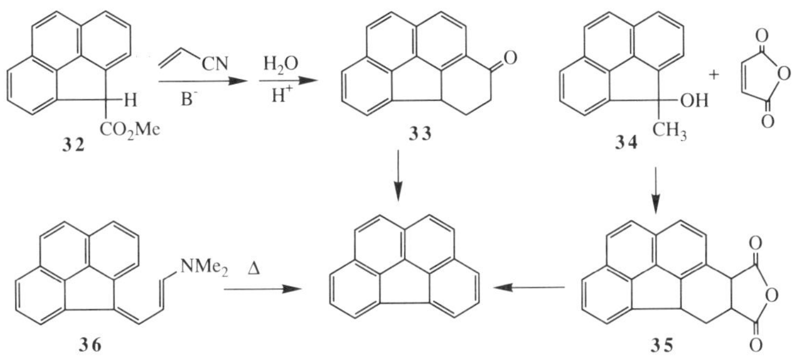

methyl fluorene-9-carboxylate by a multistep synthesis (Crombie & Shaw, 1969).

Reactions The chemical properties of benzo[ghi]fluoranthene are unexplored.

11.7   Indeno[1,2,3-cd]pyrene

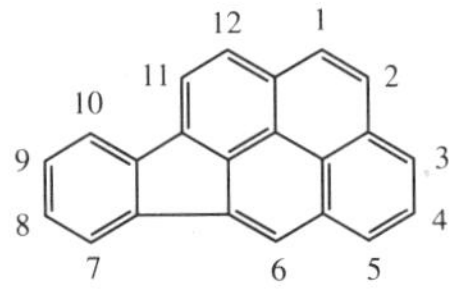

Other names: 2,3-o-phenylenepyrene
Physical and spectral properties $C_{22}H_{12}$, mol. wt. 276.32, yellow plates, mp 162.5–63.5 °C. Solutions show a greenish-yellow fluorescence. Spectral data: UV (Cho & Harvey, 1987; Karcher, 1988; Clar, 1964), UV fluorescence (Karcher, 1988; Berlman, 1971; Sawicki, 1960), IR (Karcher, 1988), NMR (Cho & Harvey, 1987a; Karcher, 1988), mass spectrum (Karcher, 1988).

Occurrence and carcinogenicity It is abundantly present in coal tar (Wise *et al.*, 1988; IARC, 1983), and carbon black (Lee & Hites, 1976), and significant levels are present in airborne pollutants (IARC, 1983; Grimmer, 1979; Sawicki, 1977), auto exhaust (IARC, 1983; Grimmer, 1979), tobacco smoke (IARC, 1983; Grimmer, 1979), sewage sludge (Grimmer, 1979), and foods (IARC, 1983). Indeno[1,2,3-cd]pyrene exhibits lower activity than BaP as a complete carcinogen on mouse skin (IARC, 1973).

Synthesis The newest synthesis entails reaction of 1-lithiopyrene with cyclohexene oxide (Fig. 11.9) and oxidation of the resulting alcohol with pyridinium dichromate to furnish the ketone **37** (Cho & Harvey, 1987). Acid-catalyzed cyclization of **37** and dehydrogenation provides indeno[1,2,3-cd]pyrene in good overall yield. Coupling of 1-iodopyrene with o-bromonitrobenzene and copper powder yields the nitro compound **38** which is converted to indeno[1,2,3-cd]pyrene by reduction of the nitro group to the amine followed by diazotization, and cyclization in the presence of copper (Aitken & Reid, 1956). This hydrocarbon is also synthetically accessible by the Diels–Alder reaction between indenoperinaphthene and maleic anhydride to yield the adduct **39** followed by dehydrogenation and decarboxylation (Aitken & Reid, 1956) and by cyclodehydrogenation of 1-phenylpyrene with NaAlCl$_4$ (Studt, 1978).

Reactions Bromination and acetylation of indeno[1,2,3-cd]pyrene furnish the 12-substituted derivatives (Minabe *et al.*, 1989) in agreement with MO theoretical prediction (Dewar & Dennington, 1989). The site of bromination was determined by conversion of the bromo compound to the monodeuterio analog and analysis of the high resolution ^{1}H- and ^{13}C-NMR spectra in comparison with those of the parent hydrocarbon. This method is potentially applicable to determination of the sites of substitution of other complex polyarenes. An earlier report that nitration of indeno[1,2,3-cd]pyrene yields its 8- or 9-nitro derivative (Bolger *et al.*, 1985) is inconsistent with these findings, and it is suggested that this product is probably the 12-nitro derivative.

11.8 Dibenz[a,e]aceanthrylene

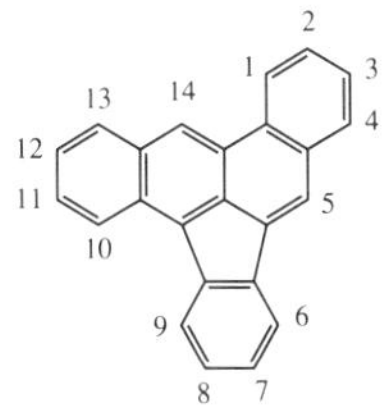

Other names: dibenzo[a,e]fluoranthene, 2,3,5,6-dibenzofluoranthene

Physical and spectral properties $C_{24}H_{14}$, mol. wt. 302.35, yellow needles, mp 232 °C, soluble in dioxane. Spectral data: UV (Karcher, 1988; Cho & Harvey, 1987; Jacquignon *et al.*, 1975; Lavit-Lamy & Buu-Hoi, 1966), UV fluorescence (Wise *et al.*, 1988a), IR (Karcher, 1988; Lavit-Lamy & Buu-Hoi, 1966), ^{1}H-NMR (Karcher, 1988; Cho & Harvey, 1987).

Fig. 11.9. Synthetic routes to indeno[1,2,3-cd]pyrene.

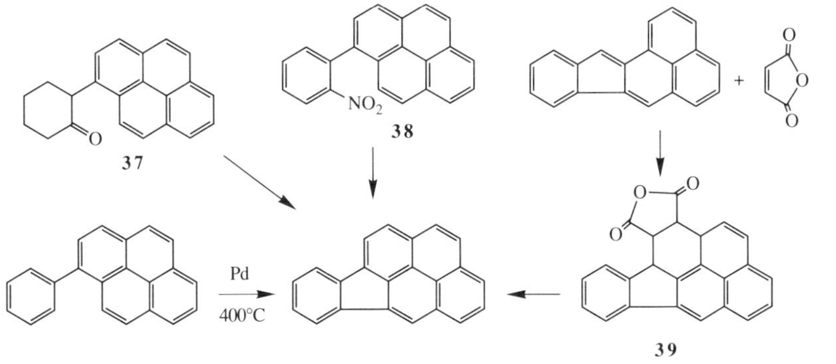

Occurrence and carcinogenicity Reported to occur in products of incomplete combustion; identified in tobacco smoke (Snook *et al.*, 1977). It occurs as a minor component of the total content of PAHs in the environment (IARC, 1983). There is limited evidence that dibenz[a,e]aceanthrylene is carcinogenic to experimental animals both as an initiator and a complete carcinogen (IARC, 1983).

Synthesis Lavit-Lamy & Buu-Hoi showed in 1966 that the polyarene formed by the action of AlCl₃ on 12-phenylbenz[a]anthracene and previously assumed to be dibenzo[a,l]pyrene was actually dibenz[a,e]aceanthrylene. The same hydrocarbon was shown to be formed by the cyclodehydrogenation of 7-phenylbenz[a]anthracene in the presence of AlCl₃ (Fig. 11.10). Dibenz[a,e]aceanthrylene is more conveniently obtained from the reaction of 7-lithiobenz[a]anthracene with cyclohexene oxide followed by oxidation with the Dess-Martin reagent, cyclodehydration of the resulting ketone **40**, and dehydrogenation with DDQ (Cho & Harvey, 1987); cyclization also occurs to the 8-position to afford dibenz[a,j]aceanthrylene as a major coproduct.

Reactions Formylation furnishes the 14-formyl derivative plus small amounts of two other aldehydes (Perin-Roussel *et al.*, 1975). Reaction with OsO₄ takes place on the substituted 5,5a-bond to yield the 5,5a-*trans*-dihydrodiol, but requires 40 days for completion (Jacquignon *et al.*, 1975).

Fig. 11.10.   Synthesis of dibenz[a,e]aceanthrylene.

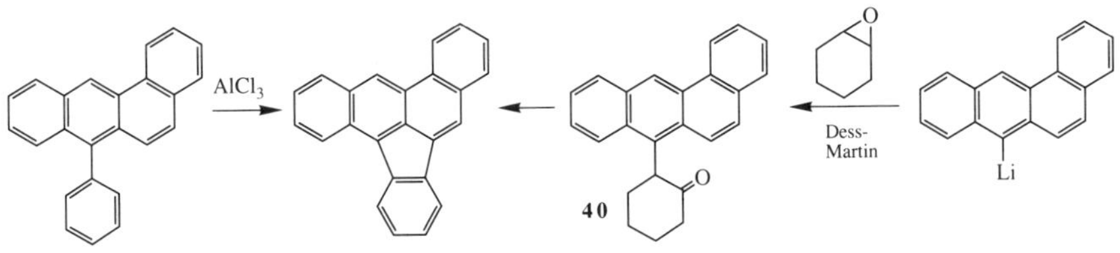

11.9   Dibenz[a,j]aceanthrylene

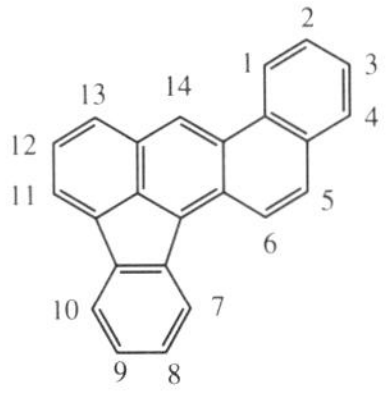

Other names: naphtho[2,1-a]fluoranthene, naphtho(2',1':2,3)-fluoranthene

Physical and spectral properties $C_{24}H_{14}$, mol. wt. 302.35, yellow needles, mp 181-81.3 °C (benzene), forms a brick red picrate, mp 174.5–175.5 °C. Spectral data: UV (Jacquignon *et al.*, 1975), NMR (Cho & Harvey, 1987).

Occurrence and carcinogenicity Recently identified as a component of coal tar (Wise *et al.*, 1988a). Dibenz[a,j]aceanthrylene was slightly more active than benz[a]aceanthrylene as a tumor initiator on mouse skin (Weyand *et al.*, 1990).

Synthesis The reaction between fluorene 1-carboxylic acid chloride and α-naphthylmagnesium bromide affords 1-(α-naphthoyl)fluorene (**41**) (Fieser & Seligman, 1935) which on pyrolysis gives dibenz[a,j]aceanthrylene (Fig. 11.11). Condensation of 9-fluorenone with the α-lithio salt of diethylbenzamide provides the lactone **42** which undergoes reduction with zinc and alkali to the free acid (Ray & Harvey, 1982). Treatment of the latter with liquid HF results in an unusual reductive cyclization to yield dibenz[a,j]aceanthrylene directly in a single step; the yield is doubled when this reaction is conducted in the presence of a hydride donor, such as triphenylmethane.

Fig. 11.11. Synthesis of dibenz[a,j]aceanthrylene.

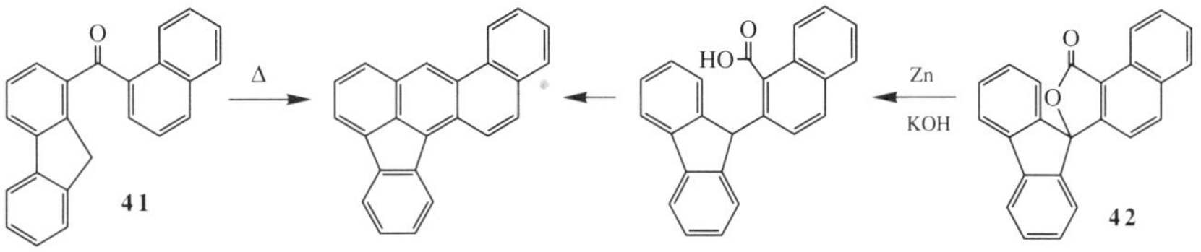

11.10   Aceanthrylene

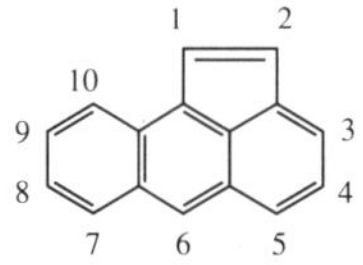

Physical and spectral properties $C_{16}H_{10}$, mol. wt. 202.24, scarlet plates, mps of 94–95 °C and 103-104 °C have been reported. Spectral data: UV (Plummer *et al.*, 1984; Sangaiah & Gold, 1985), IR (Plummer *et al.*, 1984), [1]NMR (Becker *et al.*, 1985; Sangaiah & Gold, 1985), [13]NMR (Plummer *et al.*, 1984), mass spectrum (Becker *et al.*, 1985; Plummer *et al.*, 1984).

Occurrence and carcinogenicity Despite numerous claims of the tentative identification of aceanthrylene as an environmental pollutant, even prior to its first reported synthesis in 1984, its environmental occurrence is not firmly established. Aceanthrylene is active as a frame-shift mutagen in *S. typhimurium* with micromal activation (Sangaiah *et al.*, 1986). No data on its carcinogenicity were found.

Synthesis Aceanthrylene is synthetically accessible from anthracene by reaction with oxalyl chloride and AlCl3 to give the diketone **43** (Fig. 11.12) followed by reduction with NaBH4 to the dihydrodiol, dehydration,

Fig. 11.12. Synthetic routes to aceanthrylene.

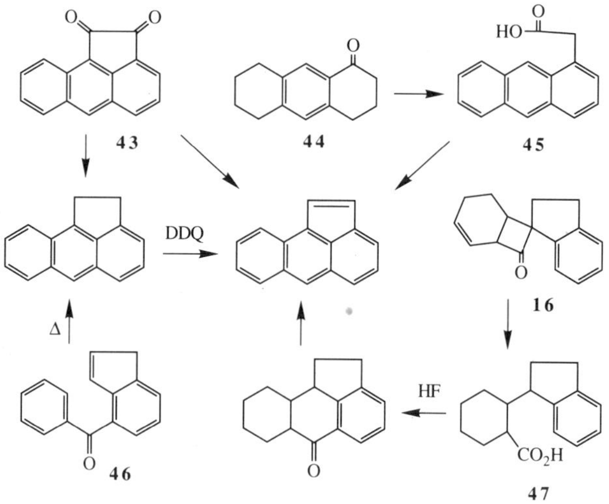

reduction, and a second dehydration (Plummer *et al.*, 1984; Becker *et al.*, 1985). More recently it has been shown that **43** may be reduced directly to aceanthrene by the Wolff–Kishner method which is converted to aceanthrylene by treatment with DDQ (Boerrigter *et al.*, 1989). Reformatski reaction of the ketone **44** followed by dehydration and dehydrogenation with DDQ yields 1-anthrylacetic acid (**45**) which is transformed into aceanthrylene by HF cyclization, Wolff–Kishner reduction, and dehydrogenation with DDQ (Sangaiah & Gold, 1985). Aceanthrene obtained from the pyrolysis of 4-indanyphenyl ketone (**46**) (Moriwake, 1966) is dehydrogenated with DDQ to aceanthrylene (Becker *et al.*, 1985). Hydrogenation of the cyclic ketone **16** followed by treatment with base gives the carboxylic acid **47** which is transformed to aceanthrylene by cyclization in HF, reduction of the resulting ketone with LiAlH$_4$, dehydration, and DDQ dehydrogenation (Chung *et al.*, 1987).

Reactions Aceanthrylene undergoes sensitized photo dimerization to produce both *syn* and *anti* head-to-head and head-to-tail stereoisomers (Plummer & Singleton, 1987). Lithium–ammonia reduction affords 2,6-dihydroaceanthrylene (Rabideau *et al.*, 1988), while catalytic hydrogenation takes place in the cyclopentano ring to yield aceanthrene (Becker *et al.*, 1985; Plummer *et al.*, 1984).

11.11   Acephenanthrylene

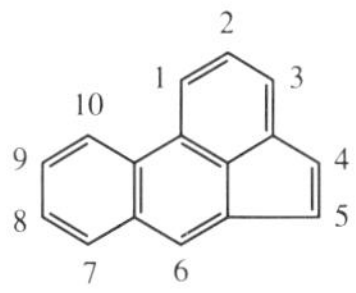

Other names: cyclopenta[j,k]phenanthrene
Physical and spectral properties C$_{16}$H$_{10}$, mol. wt. 202.24, yellow/red crystals (depending upon cooling rate), mp 141-42 °C. Spectral data: UV (Amin *et al.*, 1985; Scott *et al.*, 1985; Laarhoven & Cuppen, 1976), UV fluorescence (Amin *et al.*, 1985), IR (Scott *et al.*, 1985), [1]NMR (Scott *et al.*, 1985), [13]NMR (Scott *et al.*, 1985), mass spectrum (Scott *et al.*, 1985).

Occurrence and carcinogenicity Identified in carbon black, cigarette smoke condensate, and the combustion products from wood and coal (Wise *et al.*, 1988; Krishnan & Hites, 1981). Acephenanthrylene exhibits only marginal activity as a frame-shift mutagen in *S. typhimurium* with microsomal activation (Sangaiah *et al.*, 1986). No data on its carcinogenicity were found.

Synthesis Hexahydroacephenanthrylen-7-one (**48**) (Fig 11.13) obtained from acenaphthene by the Haworth synthesis is readily converted to acephenanthrylene by reduction with NaBH$_4$, acidic dehydration, and DDQ dehydrogenation (Scott *et al.*, 1985). Synthesis of acephenanthrylene by a similar route was reported earlier without experimental detail (Krishnan & Hites, 1981). Acephenanthrylene is also conveniently accessible from AlCl$_3$-catalyzed cyclization of 2-(9-phenanthryl)acetic acid (**49**) followed by reduction and dehydration (Amin *et al.*, 1985). Reductive alkylation of acenaphthylene with Li/NH$_3$ and 1,4-dichlorobutane gives **50** as the major product (Neumann & Mullen, 1985); intramolecular Friedel–Crafts alkylation of **50** with AlCl$_3$ followed by dehydrogenation with DDQ yields acephenanthrylene. Acephenanthrylene is also obtained from photocyclization of 1-(*o*-iodobenzylidene)indane (**51**) followed by dehydrogenation (Laarhoven *et al.*,1976) and from acidic rearrangement and dehydration of the ketone **16** to **52** followed by DDQ dehydrogenation (Chung *et al.*, 1987).

Reactions The cyclopentano ring of acephenanthrylene undergoes Diels–Alder cycloaddition with 2,3-dimethylbutadiene to yield 5,6-dimethylbenz[e]acephenanthrylene after dehydrogenation (Amin *et al.*, 1985). Diels–Alder reaction with 1-acetoxybutadiene has been used to prepare 4-hydroxy- and 7-hydroxybenz[e]acephenanthrylene (Amin *et al.*, 1986).

Fig. 11.13. Synthetic routes to acephenanthrylene.

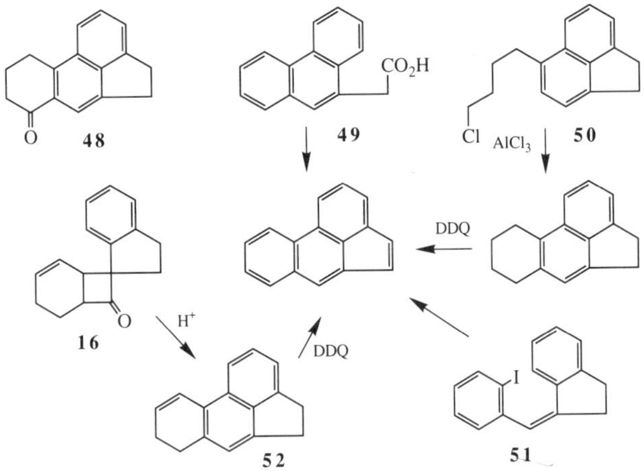

11.12   Cyclopenta[c,d]pyrene

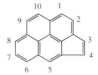

Physical and spectral properties $C_{18}H_{10}$, mol. wt. 226.26, orange crystals, mp 174-76 °C. Spectral data: UV (Karcher *et al.*, 1985; Tintel *et al.*, 1983), IR (Tintel *et al.*, 1983), [1]NMR (Jans *et al.*, 1986; Tintel *et al.*, 1983), [13]NMR (Jans *et al.*, 1986), mass spectrum (Tintel *et al.*, 1983).

Occurrence and carcinogenicity Widespread environmental contaminant found in carbon black (Wallcave *et al.*, 1975) and tobacco smoke (Snook *et al.*, 1977), and particularly high levels are detected in automobile exhaust (IARC, 1983). CPP was more mutagenic than BaP in bacterial mutation assays, but was considerably less active than BaP in *in vitro* rodent and human cell mutation assays (for leading references see Busby Jr *et al.*, 1988). CPP was also much less active than BaP as a tumor initiator and complete carcinogen on mouse skin (Wood *et al.*, 1980). CPP was also a potent tumorigen in the newborn mouse assay (Busby Jr. *et al.*, 1988).

Synthesis Several syntheses of cyclopenta[c,d]pyrene are based on cyclization of the key intermediate 4-pyrenylacetic acid (**53**) (Fig. 11.14). Attempted cyclization of the more readily accessible 1-pyrenylacetic acid failed to afford a cyclized product. It has been suggested that this is a consequence of the low reactivity of the 4-position (Gold *et al.*, 1978). However, this explanation does not appear tenable in view of the ease of acid-catalyzed cyclization of the closely related 1-pyrenylketone **37** into the 4-position (Cho & Harvey, 1987). Self-condensation and/or polymerization of 1-pyrenylacetic acid offer the most likely alternative explanations for its failure to cyclize. The ketone **54** obtained from cyclization of **53** is readily reduced with NaBH$_4$ and dehydrated to cyclopenta[c,d]pyrene (Konieczny & Harvey, 1979). Various modifications of this approach which differ mainly in the method of synthesis of **53** are available (Ittah & Jerina, 1978; Tintel *et al.*, 1983; Veeraraghavan *et al.*, 1987; Sagaiah & Gold, 1988). Recently, synthesis of **54** via photocyclization of 1-(bromoacetyl)pyrene has been described (Spijker *et al.*, 1990). Cyclopenta[c,d]pyrene is also obtained, albeit in low yield, from 1-acetylpyrene via reduction to the alcohol **55** and pyrolysis at 850 °C (Jacob & Grimmer, 1977).

Reactions Cyclopenta[c,d]pyrene is a relatively reactive hydro-carbon and nitration with NO$_2$ or nitric acid in acetic anhydride causes degradation. However, 4-nitrocyclopenta[c,d]pyrene can be prepared by reaction of the parent hydrocarbon with AgNO$_3$, NaNO$_2$, and I$_2$ in acetonitrile (van den Braken-van Leersum *et al.*, 1987). Nitration of partially hydrogenated derivatives of cyclopenta[c,d]pyrene affords mixtures of nitro derivatives that after separation and rearomatization furnish six additional isomeric mononitrocyclopenta[c,d]pyrenes. Hydrogenation takes place regiospecifically in the cyclopentano ring of cyclopenta[c,d]pyrene to yield the 4,5-dihydro derivative (Wallcave *et al.*, 1975).

11.13   Benz[e]aceanthrylene

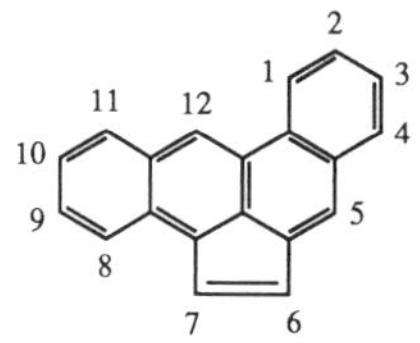

Physical and spectral properties C$_{18}$H$_{12}$, mol. wt. 252.30, mp 174-76 °C, orange needles (methanol). Spectral data: UV (Sangaiah *et al.*, 1983), NMR (Sangaiah *et al.*, 1983), mass spectrum (Sangaiah *et al.*, 1983).

Occurrence and carcinogenicity The environmental occurrence of this hydrocarbon is not documented. Benz[e]aceanthrylene exhibited greater

Fig. 11.14.   Synthetic routes to cyclopenta[c,d]pyrene.

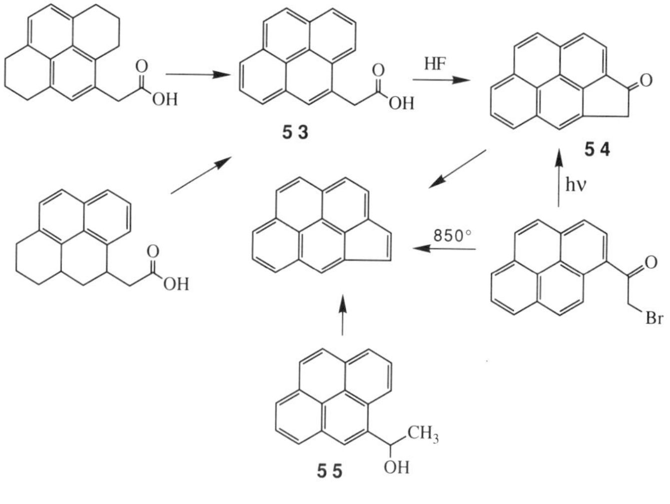

activity than BaP or benz[j]aceanthrylene as a frame-shift mutagen in *S. typhimurium* with micromal activation (Nesnow *et al.*, 1984a). It was as active as BaP as a mouse skin tumor initiator (Nesnow *et al.*, 1984).

Synthesis Reaction of benz[a]anthracene with paraformaldehyde and HCl affords 7-chloromethyl-BA which is transformed to 7-benz[a]anthrylacetic acid (**56**) by treatment with KCN and basic hydrolysis (Fig. 11.15). Cyclization of **56** by HF yields a mixture of the ketones **57** and **58** in 3:1 ratio (Sangaiah *et al.*, 1983). Reduction of **57** with NaBH4 and dehydration yields benz[e]aceanthrylene. Recently it has been shown in the author's laboratory that the low overall yield due to the unfavorable direction of cyclization of **56** may be counteracted by regiospecific hydrogenation in the terminal ring of **56** prior to cyclization (Lee & Harvey, 1990); reduction and dehydrogenation of the cyclized ketone **59** affords benz[e]aceanthrylene in good overall yield.

11.14   Benz[j]aceanthrylene

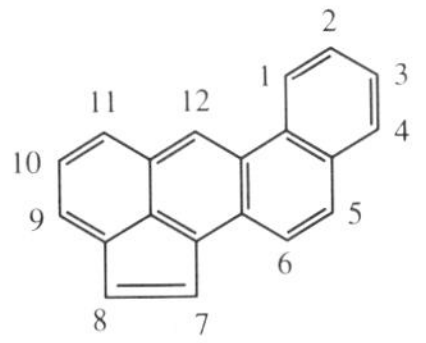

Other names: cholanthrylene
Physical and spectral properties $C_{18}H_{12}$, mol. wt. 252.30, mp 170-71 °C, orange plates (hexane). Spectral data: UV (Sangaiah *et al.*, 1983), NMR (Sangaiah *et al.*, 1983), mass spectrum (Sangaiah *et al.*, 1983).

Fig. 11.15. Synthesis of benz[e]aceanthrylene.

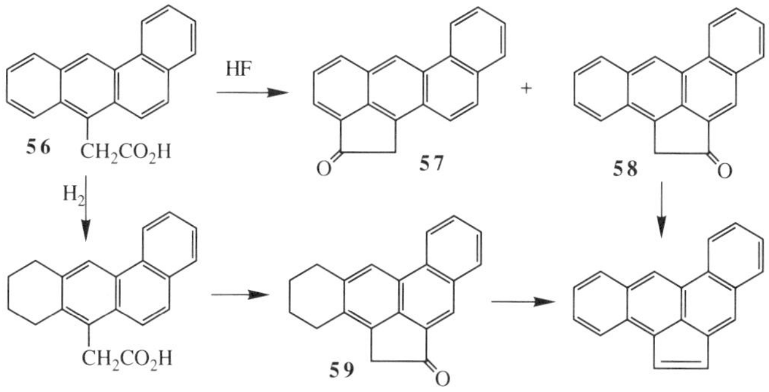

Occurrence and carcinogenicity The environmental occurrence of benz[j]aceanthrylene is not documented. It exhibited activity between that of BaP and benz[e]aceanthrylene as a frame-shift mutagen in *S. typhimurium* micromal activation (Nesnow *et al.*, 1984a).

Synthesis Benz[j]aceanthrylene may be obtained from reduction of the ketone **57** with NaBH$_4$ and dehydration (Sangaiah *et al.*, 1983) (Fig. 11.16). 6-Methylbenz[j]aceanthrylene has recently been synthesized by a modification of this approach (Lee & Harvey, 1990). The dihydro derivative of benz[j]aceanthrylene, known as cholanthrene (**60**), is conveniently synthesized by condensation of 2-lithio-*N,N*-diethyl-1-naphthamide with 2,2-dideuterioindan-1-one followed by reduction of the lactone product **61** with zinc and acetic acid, cyclization with ZnCl$_2$, and HI reduction (Harvey & Cortez, 1987). The use of the dideuterated ketone in this reaction affords higher yields than the parent ketone due to the isotope effect on the competing enolization reaction. Cholanthrene is readily converted to benz[j]aceanthrylene by DDQ dehydrogenation. Cholanthrene is also accessible by the Elbs pyrolysis of the ketone **62** (Fieser & Seligman, 1935).

11.15   4*H*-Cyclopenta[def]phenanthrene

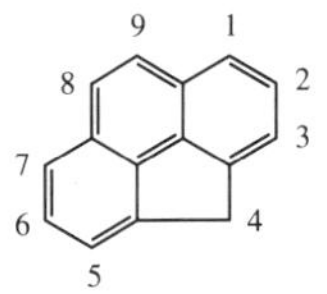

Other names: phenanthrindene
Physical and spectral properties C$_{15}$H$_{10}$, mol. wt. 190.22, mp 116 °C (EtOH). Spectral data: UV (Friedel & Orchin, 1951), NMR (Douris & Mathieu, 1971).

Fig. 11.16.   Synthetic routes to benz[j]aceanthrylene.

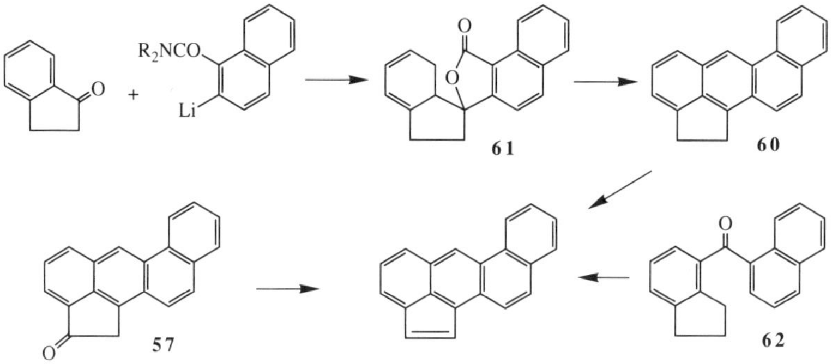

Occurrence and carcinogenicity Occurs in coal tar (Wise *et al.*, 1988), and significant levels are detected in carbon black (Lee & Hites, 1976), and tobacco and marijuana smoke (Lee *et al.*, 1976). No data on the carcinogenic properties of this hydrocarbon were found.

Synthesis 4*H*-Cyclopenta[def]phenanthrene is synthetically accessible from derivatives of its three structural components, phenanthrene, acenaphthylene, and fluorene (Fig. 11.17). Cyclization of phenanthrene-1-carboxylic acid with polyphosphoric acid yields 4*H*-cyclopenta[def]-phenanthren-4-one (**63**) (Rutherford & Newman, 1957). This ketone is also obtained from distillation of phenanthrene-4,5-dicarboxylic acid with barium hydroxide (Medenwald, 1953). Wolff–Kishner reduction of **63** gives the parent hydrocarbon. 3-(1-Acenaphthenyl)propionic acid (**64**) is obtained from 1-acenaphthenol in four steps and converted to the cyclic ketone **65** by reaction of its acid chloride with SnCl4 (Bachmann & Sheehan, 1941). Reduction and dehydration of **65** furnishes 4*H*-cyclopenta[def]phenanthrene. 4-Fluorenecarboxylic acid is transformed by a four-step standard sequence to 4-fluoreneacetic acid (**66**) which failed to undergo acid-catalyzed cyclization (Yoshida *et al.*, 1983). However, the acid chloride of **66** cyclized under Friedel–Crafts conditions to yield the expected 8-phenol accompanied by the 8,9-dione; reduction of the mixture with HI/P gave 4*H*-cyclopenta[def]phen-anthrene.

Reactions Nitration affords mainly the 1-nitro derivative accompanied by variable amounts of the 2-, 3-, and 8-nitro isomers depending upon

Fig. 11.17. Synthetic routes to 4*H*-cyclopenta[def]phenanthrene.

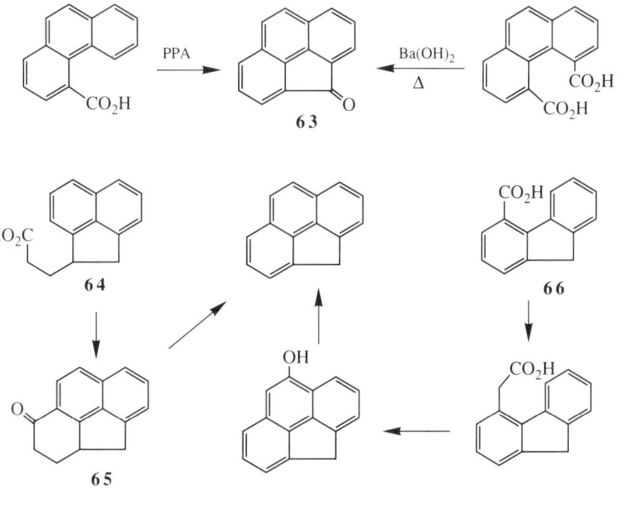

reaction conditions (Yoshida *et al.*, 1979b). Bromination of 4*H*-cyclopenta-[def]phenanthrene gives the 1-bromo derivative along with small amounts of the 3- and 8-bromo isomers (Yoshida *et al.*, 1979a). The site of substitution may be altered by conducting reactions on the 8,9-dihydro derivative of **63**. Bromination and nitration of the former yield exclusively the 2-substituted derivatives, while analogous reactions of **63** provide the 8-substituted derivatives (Yoshida *et al.*, 1979a, 1979b). Friedel–Crafts acetylation in CHCl$_3$ gives the 1-acetyl derivative, whereas similar reaction in nitrobenzene or nitromethane furnishes 1- and 3-acetyl-4*H*-cyclopenta[def]phenanthrene as the major products (Yoshida *et al.*, 1980).

The relative acidity of 4*H*-cyclopenta[def]phenanthrene may be used to advantage to prepare various derivatives in the 4-position such as the 4-carboxylic acid (Kimura *et al.*, 1978). The 4-hydroxymethyl derivative prepared via this route undergoes facile Wagner–Meerwein rearrangement to pyrene.

Hydrogenation of 4*H*-cyclopenta[def]phenanthrene over a Pd catalyst under mild conditions provides regioselectively the 8,9-dihydro derivative, whereas hydrogenation over Raney Ni affords the same dihydro derivative plus the 1,2,3,3a-tetrahydro product (Minabe *et al.*, 1984). Oxidation of 4*H*-cyclopenta[def]phenanthrene with dichromate takes place on the methylene bridge to yield the ketone **63**, while oxidation with iodic acid yields its 8,9-dione (Trost & Kinson, 1975). Ozonization (Fig. 11.18) gives a stable ozonide **67** which undergoes oxidative cleavage with alkaline peroxide to the corresponding diacid and reduction to the related dialdehyde, diol, and lactone by treatment with triphenylphosphine, LiAlH$_4$, and Na$_2$SO$_3$, respectively (Yoshida *et al.*, 1979).

Fig. 11.18. Products of ozonization of 4*H*-cyclopenta[def]phenanthrene.

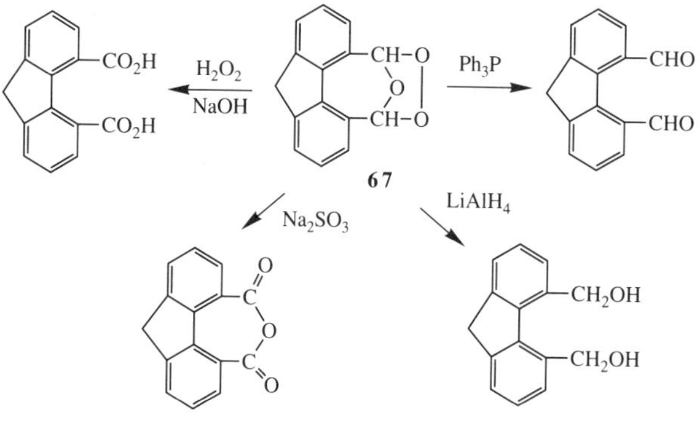

11.16   4*H*-Cyclopenta[def]chrysene

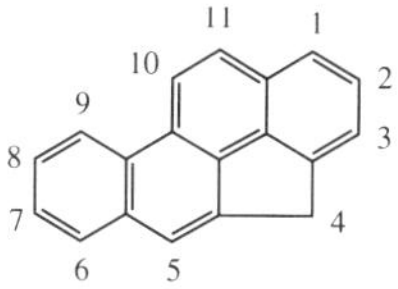

Other names: 4,5-methanochrysene, 4,5-methylenechrysene
Physical and spectral properties $C_{19}H_{12}$, mol. wt. 240.29, mp 174-76 °C. Spectral data: UV (Lee-Ruff *et al.*, 1984), IR (Lee-Ruff *et al.*, 1984), NMR (Lee-Ruff *et al.*, 1984).

Occurrence and carcinogenicity This hydrocarbon has been tentatively identified as a component of cigarette smoke (Snook *et al.*, 1977). 4*H*-Cyclopenta[def]chrysene exhibited activity as a complete carcinogen on subcutaneous injection in mice (Hartwell, 1951), and was somewhat less active than 5-methylchrysene as a tumor-initiator on mouse skin at similar dosage (Rice *et al.*, 1988).

Synthesis Friedel–Crafts succinoylation of cyclopent[def]phenan-threne occurs mainly in the 1-position to afford the ketoacid **68** (Fig. 11.19) which is transformed to 4*H*-cyclopenta[def]chrysene via reduction, HF cyclization, reduction, and dehydrogenation (Fieser & Cason, 1940). 4*H*-Cyclopenta[def]chrysene is also available by oxidative photocyclization of the stilbene carboxylic acid **69** followed by HF cyclization and HI/P reduction (Lee-Ruff *et al.*, 1984) and by photocyclization of the olefin **70** (Nagel *et al.*, 1977); however, the overall yield of **70** is low (8%).

Fig. 11.19. Synthetic routes to 4*H*-cyclopenta[def]chrysene.

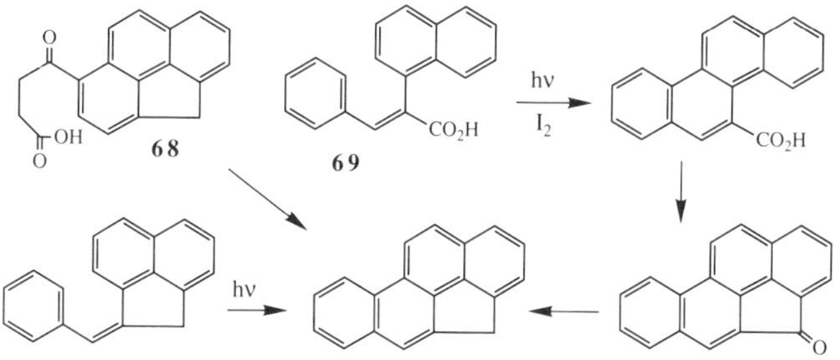

11.17   11*H*-Benz[bc]aceanthrylene

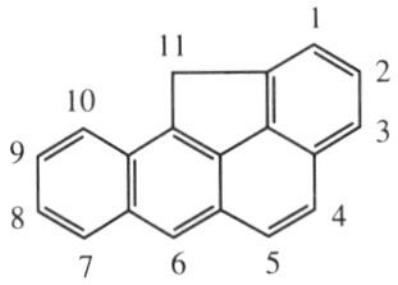

Other names: 1',9-methylene-1,2-benzanthracene, 1,12-methyl-enebenzanthracene
Physical and spectral properties $C_{19}H_{12}$, mol. wt. 240.29, mp 122-23 °C (EtOH), solutions show greenish-yellow fluorescence. Spectral data: UV (Sandorfy & Jones, 1956), NMR (Ray & Harvey, 1983).

Occurrence and carcinogenicity 11*H*-Benz[bc]aceanthrylene showed no activity as a complete carcinogen on subcutaneous injection in mice (Hartwell, 1951), but was found to be a moderately potent tumor-initiator, somewhat less active than 12-methyl-BA as a tumor-initiator on mouse skin at similar dosage (Rice *et al.*, 1988).

Synthesis Friedel–Crafts succinoylation of 8,9-dihydrocyclo-pent[def]phenanthrene occurs mainly in the 2-position to afford the ketoacid **71** (Fig. 11.20) which yields the ketone **72** via reduction, dehydrogenation over Pd/C, and HF cyclization (Fieser & Cason, 1940). Reduction and catalytic dehydrogenation of **72** affords 11*H*-benz[bc]aceanthrylene. Condensation of the monoketal of acenaphthylenedione with the 2-lithio salt of diethylbenzamide provides the lactone **73** (Ray & Harvey, 1983). Treatment of the latter with BF$_3$ etherate followed by reduction with zinc and alkali gave the keto acid **74** which underwent conversion by standard methods to 11*H*-benz[bc]aceanthrylene.

Fig. 11.20.   Synthetic routes to benzo[b,c]aceanthrylene.

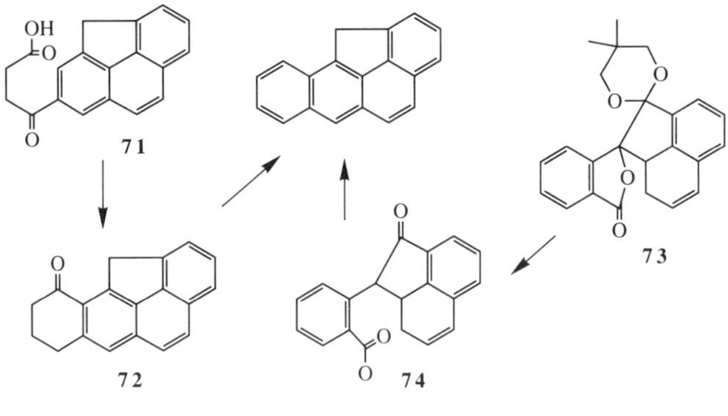

11.18   11*H*-Benzo[a]fluorene

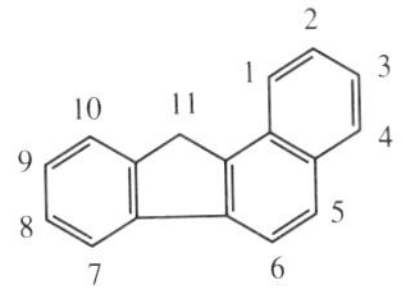

Other names: 1,2-benzofluorene, α-naphthofluorene

Physical and spectral properties $C_{17}H_{12}$, mol. wt. 216.17, mp 188-89 °C (EtOH), soluble in ethanol, $CHCl_3$, and hot benzene. Spectral data: UV (Jaffe & Orchin, 1962; Friedel & Orchin, 1951), UV fluorescence (Sawicki *et al.*, 1960), IR (Pouchert, 1981), NMR (Pouchert, 1983; Jones *et al.*, 1972).

Occurrence and carcinogenicity Occurs in coal tar (Wise *et al.*, 1988) and is an ubiquitous environmental pollutant. Significant concentrations are detected in urban atmospheres (IARC, 1983; Sawicki, 1977), sewage sludge (Grimmer, 1979), and tobacco and marijuana smoke (Lee *et al.*, 1976; Seversen *et al.*, 1976). The available data indicate that it is not active as a tumorigen (IARC, 1983).

Synthesis A convenient new synthesis of 11*H*-benzo[a]fluorene (Fig. 11.21) entails alkylation of the enamine of cyclohexanone with 1-

Fig. 11.21. Synthetic routes to 11*H*-benzo[a]fluorene.

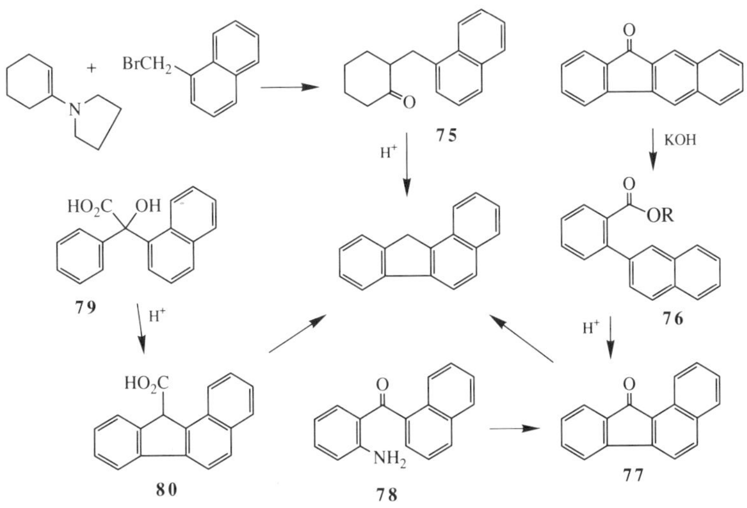

bromomethylnaphthalene followed by acidic cyclization of the ketone product **75** and DDQ dehydrogenation (Harvey *et al.*, 1991). Another interesting new synthesis entails condensation of indanone with phthalaldehyde to yield 11*H*-benzo[b]fluorenone which undergoes basic rearrangement to the carboxylic acid **76** (R = H) (Streitweiser & Brown, 1988). Subsequent reaction of **76** with polyphosphoric acid gives 11*H*-benzo[a]fluorenone (**77**) which is hydrogenolysed to 11*H*-benzo[a]fluorene. The phenyl ester **76** (R = Ph) obtained from the reaction of phenylmagnesium bromide on phenyl 2-methoxy-1-naphthoate cyclizes in H_2SO_4 to **77** (Fuson & Wassmund, 1956). This ketone is also obtained from treatment of 1-naphthyl 2'-aminophenyl ketone (**78**) with nitrous acid (Lothrup & Goodwin, 1943) and from the rhodium-catalyzed reaction of a mixture of 2-naphthoic anhydride and benzoic anhydride (Blum *et al.*, 1974). The ester **79** obtained from the reaction of methyl α-oxo-phenylacetate with 1-naphthylmagnesium bromide undergoes dehydration and cyclization on treatment with H_2SO_4 to furnish methyl benzo[a]fluorenecarboxylate (**80**) which on decarboxylation affords 11*H*-benzo[a]fluorene (Hopkinson *et al.*, 1986).

11.19   11*H*-Benzo[b]fluorene

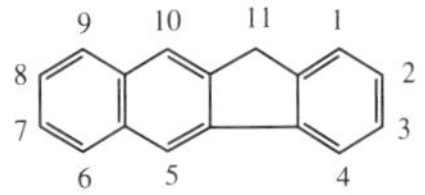

Other names: 2,3-benzofluorene
Physical and spectral properties $C_{17}H_{12}$, mol. wt. 216.17, mp 208 °C. Spectral data: UV (Jaffe & Orchin, 1962; Friedel & Orchin, 1951), UV fluorescence (Sawicki *et al.*, 1960), UV fluorescence (Sawicki *et al.*, 1960), IR (Pouchert, 1981), NMR (Pouchert, 1983; Jones *et al.*, 1972), mass spectrum (Guidugli *et al.*, 1987).

Occurrence and carcinogenicity Occurs in coal tar (Wise *et al.*, 1988) and is detected in airborne pollutants (IARC, 1983), and cigarette smoke (Lee *et al.*, 1976). The available data suggest that it may have marginal activity as a tumor-initiator on mouse skin (IARC, 1983).

Synthesis The most convenient synthesis (Fig. 11.22) entails condensation of indanone with phthalaldehyde to yield 11*H*-benzo[b]-fluorenone (**81**) followed by hydrogenolysis (Streitweiser & Brown, 1988). The ketone **81** is also obtained from rhodium-catalyzed reaction of a mixture of 2-naphthoic anhydride and benzoic anhydride (Blum *et al.*, 1974), from treatment of the diazonium salt **82** with sulfuric acid (Huisgen & Zahler, 1963), and from cyclization of 3-phenyl-2-naphthoic acid (**83**) (Huisgen & Rist, 1955).

Reactions Ozonolysis gives phthalic and homophthalic acids, indicative of attack mainly on the naphthalene ring adjacent to the 5-membered ring (Copeland *et al.*, 1960).

11.20   *7H*-Benzo[c]fluorene

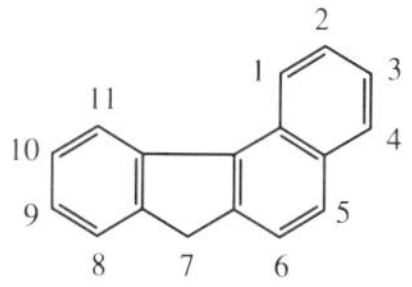

Other names: 3,4-benzofluorene
Physical and spectral properties $C_{17}H_{12}$, mol. wt. 216.17, mp 124-

Fig. 11.22. Synthetic routes to 11*H*-benzo[b]fluorene.

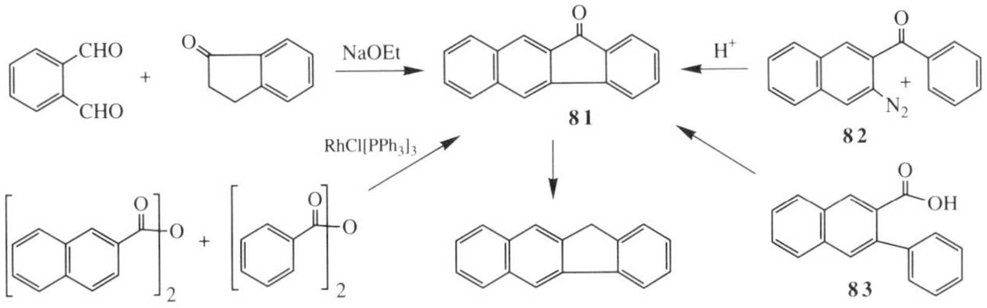

Fig. 11.23. Synthetic routes to 7*H*-benzo[c]fluorene.

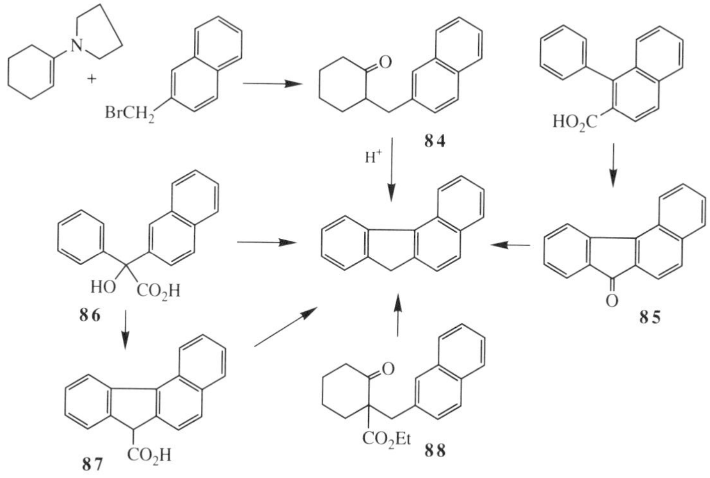

25 °C. Soluble in benzene and acetone. Spectral data: UV (Friedel & Orchin, 1951; Jaffe & Orchin, 1962), UV fluorescence (Sawicki *et al.*, 1960), NMR (Jones *et al.*, 1972).

Occurrence and carcinogenicity Occurs ubiquitously in products of incomplete combustion (IARC, 1983), and is detected in urban atmospheres (Sawicki, 1977), sewage sludge (Grimmer, 1979), and in mainstream cigarette smoke (IARC, 1983). The available data indicate only borderline activity as a tumor-initiator on mouse skin (IARC, 1983).

Synthesis Alkylation of the enamine of cyclohexanone with 2-bromomethylnaphthalene (Fig. 11.23) affords the ketone **84** which is transformed to 7*H*-benzo[c]fluorene by acidic cyclization and DDQ dehydrogenation (Harvey *et al.*, 1991). Cyclization of 1-phenyl-2-naphthoic acid furnishes 7*H*-benzo[c]fluorenone (**85**) (Huisgen & Rist, 1955) which may be reduced to 7*H*-benzo[c]fluorene. The ester **86** obtained from the reaction of methyl α-oxo-phenylacetate with 2-naphthylmagnesium bromide undergoes dehydration and cyclization on treatment with H_2SO_4 to furnish methyl benzo[c]fluorenecarboxylate (**87**) which on decarboxylation affords 7*H*-benzo[c]fluorene (Hopkinson *et al.*, 1986). Other methods of preparation include synthesis from indanone by a multistep sequence involving the Robinson–Mannich reaction (Keene & Schofield, 1958) and cyclization and aromatization of the keto ester **88** obtained from condensation of 2-bromomethylnaphthalene with ethyl cyclohexanone-2-carboxylate (Keene & Schofield, 1957).

11.21 References

Aitken, I. M. & Reid, D. H. (1956). The synthesis of indeno[2,1-a]perinaphthene. *J. Chem. Soc.* 3487–95.

Allschuler, L. & Berliner, E. (1966). Rates of bromination of polynuclear aromatic hydrocarbons. *J. Amer. Chem. Soc.* **88**, 5837–45.

Amin, S., Balanikas, G., Huie, K., Hussain, N., Geddie, J. E. & Hecht, S. S. (1985). Synthesis and fluorescence spectra of structural analogues of potential benzo[b]fluoranthene–DNA adducts. *J. Org. Chem.* **50**, 4642–6.

Amin, S., Huie, K., Hussain, N., Balanikas, G., Carmella, S. G. & Hecht, S. S. (1986). Synthesis of potential phenolic metabolites of benzo[b]fluoranthene. *J. Org. Chem.* **51**, 1206–11.

Amin, S., Huie, K., Hussain, N., Balanikas, G. & Hecht, S. S. (1985a). Synthesis of methylated benzo[b]fluoranthenes and benzo[k]fluoranthenes. *J. Org. Chem.* **50**, 1948–54.

Anthony, I. J. & Wege, D. (1984). The addition of benzyne to benzofuran. A ready route to benz[e]acephenanthrylene. *Aust. J. Chem.* **37**, 1283–92.

Bachmann, W. E. & Sheehan, J. C. (1941). The synthesis of 4,5-methylenephenanthrene. *J. Amer. Chem. Soc.* **63**, 204–6.

Balanikas, G., Hussain, N., Amin, S. & Hecht, S. S. (1988). Oxidation of polynuclear aromatic hydrocarbons with ceric ammonium sulfate: Preparation of quinones and lactones. *J. Org. Chem.* **53**, 1007–10.

Bancroft, K. C. & Howe, G. R. (1970). Reactivity parameters and aromatic systems. Part I. Detritiation rates in fluoranthene. *J. Chem. Soc.* 1541–3.

Bartle, K. D., Jones, D. W. & Pearson, J. E. (1967). High-resolution proton magnetic resonance spectra of fluoranthene, benzo[k]fluoranthene and benzo[ghi]fluoranthene. *J. Mol. Spectr.* **24**, 330–4.

Beaton, J. M. & Tucker, S. H. (1952). Synthesis of fluoranthenes. Part XI. Iodination of tetrahydrofluoranthenes leading to the synthesis of 3-methyl-l:2-5:6-dibenzopyracyclene. *J. Chem. Soc.* 3870–4.

Becker, H., Hansen, L. & Andersson, K. (1985). Aceanthrylene. *J. Org. Chem.* **50**, 277–9.

Berlman, I. B. (1971). *Handbook of Fluorescence Spectra of Aromatic Molecules,* New York: Academic Press.

Blum, J., Ashkenasy, M. & Pickholtz, Y. (1974). A simple, one-step synthesis of benzo- and dibenzofluorenes. *Synthesis,* 352–3.

Boerrigter, J. C. O., Mulder, P. J., vander Gen, A., Mohn, G. R., Cornelisse, J. & Lugtenburg, J. (1989). The use of a double Wolff–Kishner reduction in the preparation of aceanthrene and aceanthrylene. *Recl. Trav. Chim. Pays–Bas,* **108**, 79–80.

Bolgar, M., Hubball, J. A., Cunningham, J. T. & Smith, S. R. (1985). The separation and identification of nitro-PAHs and related compounds. *Polynuclear Aromatic Hydrocarbons: Mechanisms, Methods and Metabolisms,* ed, Cooke, M. & Dennis, A. J., pp. 199–214, Columbus, OH: Battelle Press.

Busby, W. F. Jr, Goldman, M. E., Newberne, P. M. & Woogan, G. N. (1984). Tumorigenicity of fluoranthene in newborn mouse lung adenoma bioassay. *Carcinogenesis,* **5**, 1311–16.

Buu-Hoi, N. P. (1964). New developments in chemical carcinogenesis by polycyclic hydrocarbons and related heterocycles: A review. *Cancer Res.* **24**, 1511–23.

Buu-Hoi, N. P., Lavit, D. & Lamy, J. (1959). New synthesis of dibenz[a,c]anthracene, benzo[k]fluoranthene, and benzo[b]fluoranthene. *J. Chem. Soc.* 1845–9.

Callighan, R. H., Tarker, M. F. & Wilt, M. H. (1960). Ozonolysis of fluoranthene. *J. Org. Chem.* **25**, 820–3.

Campbell, N., Easton, W. W., Rayment, J. L. & Wilshire, J. F. (1950). The orientation of disubstituted fluoranthene derivatives. *J. Chem. Soc.* 2784–7.

Campbell, N. & Fairfull, E. (1949). The condensation of fluorene derivatives with acrylonitrile. *J. Chem. Soc.* 1239–41.

Campbell, N. & Gow, R. S. (1949). Syntheses of fluoranthene and its derivatives from 7:8-dialkylacenaphthene-7,8-diols. *J. Chem. Soc.* 1555–9.

Campbell, N. & Reid, K. F. (1952). Syntheses of benzo[mno]fluoranthene and dibenzo[k,mno]fluoranthene. *J. Chem. Soc.* 3281–4.

Campbell, N. & Reid, K. F. (1958). The synthesis of properties of 2-azafluoranthene. *J. Chem. Soc.* 4743–6.

Campbell, A. & Tucker, S. H. (1949). Synthesis of fluoranthenes. II. Michael addition of vinyl cyanide to fluorene-9-carboxylic esters. *J. Chem. Soc.* 2623–6.

Campbell, A. & Wang, H. (1949). Syntheses in the fluoranthene series. *J. Chem. Soc.* 1513–15.

Cho, B. & Harvey, R. G. (1987a). Complete ^{1}H and ^{13}C NMR assignment of polycyclic aromatic fluoranthenes by long-range optimized homo- and heteronuclear correlation spectroscopy. *J. Org. Chem.* **52**, 5679–84.

Cho, H. & Harvey, R. G. (1987). Polycyclic fluoranthene hydrocarbons. 2. A new general synthesis. *J. Org. Chem.* **52**, 5668–78.

Chung, Y., Kruk, H., Barizo, M., Katz, M. & Lee-Ruff, E. (1987). Syntheses of cyclopentene-fused polynuclear aromatic hydrocarbons. *J. Org. Chem.* **52**, 1284–8.

Clar, E. (1964). *Polycyclic Hydrocarbons,* New York: Academic Press.

Copeland, P. G., Dean, R. E. & McNeil, D. (1960). The ozonolysis of polynuclear aromatic hydrocarbons. *J. Chem. Soc.* 3230–4.

Crombie, D. A. & Shaw, S. (1969). A new route to benzo[ghi]fluoranthene. *J. Chem. Soc.(C).* 2489–90.

Dewar, M. J. S. & Dougherty, R. C. (1989). DEWAR-PI study of electrophilic substitution in selected polycyclic fluoranthene hydrocarbons. *J. Amer. Chem. Soc.* **111**, 3804–8.

Dobbs, T. K., Hertzler, D. V., Keen, G. W., Eisenbraun, E. J., Fink, R., Hossain, M. B. & van der Helm, D. (1980). Regioselective acid-catalyzed cyclodimerization of 1,2-dihydronaphthalene. Mechanism of formation and single-crystal X-ray analysis of two octa-hydrobenzo[j]fluoranthenes. *J. Org. Chem.* **45**, 4769–74.

Dobbs, T. K., Taylor, A. R., Barnes, J. A., Iscimenler, B. D., Holt, E. M. & Eisenbraun, E. J. (1984). Acid-catalyzed cyclization of 3,3',4,4'-tetrahydro-1,1'-binaphthyl and single-crystal X-ray structure determination of a polycyclic stable ozonide. *J. Org. Chem.* **49**, 1030–3.

Douris, J. & Mathieu, A. (1971). Nuclear magnetic resonance study of condensed polycyclic hydrocarbons possessing a methylene group. *Bull. Chim. Fr.* 3365–73.

Ehrlich, H. W. & Beevers, C. A. (1956). The crystal structure of 2:13-benzofluoranthene. *Acta Cryst.* **9**, 602–6.

Fieser, L. F. & Cason, J. (1940). Synthesis of 4,5-methylenechrysene and 1',9-methylene-1,2-benzanthracene from 4,5-methylenephenanthrene. *J. Amer. Chem. Soc.* **62**, 1293–8.

Fieser, L. F. & Seligman, A. M. (1935). Cholanthrene and related hydrocarbons. *J. Amer. Chem. Soc.* **57**, 2174–6.

Friedel, R. A. & Orchin, M. (1951). *Ultraviolet Spectra of Aromatic Compounds,* New York: Wiley.

Fuson, R. C. & Wassmund, F. W. (1956). The reaction of phenyl 2-methoxy-1-naphthoate with Grignard reagents. A new route to fluorenones. *J. Amer. Chem. Soc.* **78**, 5409–13.

Gold, A., Schultz, J. & Eisenstadt, E. (1978). Relative reactivities of pyrene ring positions: cyclopenta[cd]pyrene via an intramolecular Friedel–Crafts acylation. *Tetrahedron Lett.* 4491–4.

Grimmer, G. (1979). *Environmental Carcinogens–Selected Methods of Analysis. II,* Lyon, France: International Agency for Research on Cancer.

Guidugli, F. H., Kavka, J., Garibay, M. E., Santillan, R. L. & Joseph-Nathan, P. (1987). Mass spectral studies of naphthoflavones. *Org. Mass Spectrom.* **22**, 479–85.

Hartwell, J. L. (1951). *Survey of Compounds which have been Tested for Carcinogenic Activity,* U.S. Public Health Service Publ. No. 149. Washington, DC: Superintendent of Documents, U.S. Government Printing Office.

Harvey, R. G. & Cortez, C. (1987). Synthesis of cholanthrene and 6-methylcholanthrene, biologically active analogues of the potent carcinogen 3-methylcholanthrene. *J. Org. Chem.* **52**, 283–4.

Harvey, R. G., Lindow, D. F. & Rabideau, P. W. (1972). Metal–ammonia reduction. XIV. Fluoranthene: correlation of primary product structure with HMO theoretical prediction. *Tetrahedron,* **28**, 2909–19.

Harvey, R. G., Pataki, J., Cortez, C., DiRaddo, P. & Yang, C. (1991). A new general synthesis of polycyclic aromatic compounds based on enamine chemistry. *J. Org. Chem.* **56**, 1210–17.

Hazell, A. C., Jones, D. W. & Sowden, J. M. (1977). The crystal structure of fluoranthene, $C_{16}H_{10}$: A study by X-ray and neutron diffraction. *Acta Cryst.* **B33**, 1516–22.

Hirakawa, K., Toki, T., Yamazaki, K. & Nakazawa, S. (1980). Reactions of spiro-indazoles containing keto-groups. Syntheses of benz[a]aceanthrylenes. Naphth[2,1-a]aceanthrylenes, and fluoranthenes. *J. Chem. Soc. Perkin I,* 1944–9.

Hoffmann, D., Rathkamp, G., Nesnow, S. & Wynder, E. (1972). Fluoranthenes: quantitative determination in cigarette smoke, formation by pyrolysis, and tumoor-initiating activity. *J. Natl. Cancer Inst.,* **49**, 1165–75.

Hopkinson, A. C., Lee-Ruff, E. & Maleki, M. (1986). An efficient synthesis of benzofluorenes via α-alkoxycarbonyldiarylmethyl cations. *Synthesis,* 366–71.

Huisgen, R. & Rist, H. (1955). Reaction of aromatic fluoro compounds with phenyl lithium. Rearrangements in nucleophilic aromatic substitutions. *Liebigs Ann. Chem.* **594**, 137–58.

Huisgen, R. & Zahler, W. D. (1963). Ionic and radical mechanisms of the intramolecular arylation via diazo compounds. *Chem. Ber.* **96**, 736–46.

IARC. (1983). *Monograph on the Evaluation of the Carcinogenic Risk of the Chemical to Man: Certain Polycyclic Aromatic Hydrocarbons and Heterocyclic Compounds*, Lyon, France: International Agency for Research on Cancer.

Ittah, Y. & Jerina, D. M. (1978). Cyclopenta[c,d]pyrene. *Tetrahedron Lett.* 4495–8.

Jacob, J. & Grimmer, G. (1977). Investigations on the carcinogenic burden by air pollution in man. *Chem. Abs.* **89**, 6143h.

Jacquignon, P., Perin-Roussel, O., Perin, F., Chalvet, O., Lhoste, J. M., Mathieu, A., Saperas, B., Viallet, P. & Zajdela, F. (1975). Oxidation of dibenzo[a,e]fluoranthene by osmium tetroxide. *Can. J. Chem.* **53**, 1670–6.

Jaffe, H. H. & Orchin, M. (1962). *Theory and Applications of Ultraviolet Spectroscopy*, New York: Wiley.

Jans, A. W. H., Tintel, C., Cornelisse, J. & Lugtenburg, J. (1986). [1]H and ^{13}C assignment of cyclopenta[cd]pyrene by two-dimensional NMR spectroscopy. *Mag. Res. Chem.* **24**, 101–4.

Johnson, G. C. & Bergman, R. G. (1979). Synthesis and thermal rearrangement of a potential butalene–anthracene adduct. *Tetrahedron Lett.* 2093–6.

Jones, A. J., Alger, T. D., Grant, D. & Litchman, W. M. (1970). Carbon-13 magnetic resonance. XV. Nonalternant hydrocarbons. *J. Amer. Chem. Soc.* **92**, 2386–94.

Jones, D. W., Matthews, R. S. & Bartle, K. D. (1972). High-resolution proton magnetic resonance spectra of fluorene and its derivatives. IV. The benzofluorenes. *Spectrochim. Acta*, **28A**, 2053–62.

Jutz, J. C. (1978). Aromatic and heteroaromatic compounds by electrocyclic ring closure. *Topics in Current Chem.* **73**, 127–30.

Kaden, D. A., Hites, R. A. & Thilly, W. G. (1979). Mutagenicity of soot and associated polycyclic aromatic hydrocarbons to *Salmonella typhimurium*. *Cancer Res.* **39**, 4152–9.

Karcher, W. (1988). *Spectral Atlas of Polycyclic Aromatic Compounds*, Dordrecht, Netherlands: Kluwer Academic.

Karcher, W., Fordham, R., DuBois, J. & Gloude, P. (1985). *Spectral Atlas of Polycyclic Aromatic Compounds*, Dordrecht, Netherlands: D. Reidel.

Keene, B. R. & Schofield, K. (1957). The synthesis of 3:4-benzofluorene and some of its monomethyl derivatives. *J. Chem. Soc.* 3181–6.

Keene, B. R. & Schofield, K. (1958). 5-Methyl-3:4-benzofluorene. *J. Chem. Soc.* 1080–84.

Kimura, T., Minabe, M. & Suzuki, K. (1978). Rearrangements and ring expansions of 4*H*-cyclopenta[def]phenanthrene derivatives. *J. Org. Chem.* **43**, 1247–8.

Kloetzel, M. C. & Mertel, H. E. (1950). Fluoranthene derivatives. II. The action of acenaphthylene with butadiene derivatives. *J. Amer. Chem. Soc.* **72**, 4786–91.

Konieczny, M. & Harvey, R. G. (1979). Synthesis of cyclopenta[c,d]pyrene. *J. Org. Chem.* **44**, 2158–60.

Krishnan, S. & Hites, R. A. (1981). Identification of acephenanthrylene in combustion effluents. *Anal. Chem.* **53**, 342–3.

Laarhoven, W. H. & Cuppen, T. J. (1976). Photodehydrocyclisations of stilbene-like compounds. XVI. Photoreactions of α-(9-phenanthryl)stilbene and 1-(9-phenanthryl)-1-phenylethylene. *Recl. Trav. Chim. Pays-Bas*, **95**, 165–8.

Lacassagne, A., Buu-Hoi, N. P., Zajdela, F., Lavit-Lamy, D. & Chalvet, O. (1963). Carcinogenic activity of polycyclic aromatic hydrocarbons with fluoranthene group. *Unio. Int. Contra Cancrum Acta*, **19**, 490–6.

Lavit-Lamy, D. & Buu-Hoi, N. P. (1966). Isomerization of polycyclic aromatic hydrocarbons by aluminum chloride. IV. Molecular rearrangement in the cyclodehydrogenation of 12-phenylbenzo[a]anthracene. *Bull. Chim. Soc. Fr.* 2613–9.

LaVoie, E., Amin, S., Hecht, S. S., Furuya, K. & Hoffmann, D. (1982). Tumor initiating activity of dihydrodiols of benzo[b]fluoranthene, benzo[j]fluoranthene, and benzo[k]fluoranthene. *Carcinogenesis*, **3**, 49–52.

LaVoie, E., Braley, J., Rice, J. E. & Rivenson, A. (1987). Tumorigenic activity of nonalternant polynuclear aromatic hydrocarbons in newborn mice. *Cancer Lett.*, **34**, 15–20.

LaVoie, E., Hecht, S. S., Amin, S., Bedenko, V. & Hoffmann, D. (1980). Identification of mutagenic dihydrodiols as metabolites of benzo[j]fluoranthene and benzo[k]fluoranthene. *Cancer Res.*, **40**, 4528–32.

Lee, H. & Harvey, R. G. (1990). Synthesis of cyclopentanobenz[a]aceanthracene compounds related to carcinogenic benz[a]anthracene and cholanthrene hydrocarbons. *J. Org. Chem.* **55**, 3787–91.

Lee, M. L. & Hites, R. A. (1976). Characterization of sulfur-containing polycyclic aromatic compounds in carbon black. *Anal. Chem.* **48**, 1890–3.

Lee, R. E., Novotny, M. & Bartle, K. D. (1976). Gas chromatography/mass spectrometric and nuclear magnetic resonance spectrometric studies of carcinogenic polynuclear aromatic hydrocarbons in tobacco and marijuana smoke condensates. *Anal. Chem.* **48**, 405–16.

Lee-Ruff, E., Kruk, H. & Katz, M. (1984). A short synthesis of 4,5-methanochrysene and 6-oxo-7-oxabenzo[a]pyrene, two benzo[a]pyrene analogues. *J. Org. Chem.* **49**, 553–5.

Lothrup, W. C. & Goodwin, P. R. (1943). New modification of the Ullmann synthesis of fluorene derivatives. *J. Amer. Chem. Soc.* **65**, 363–7.

Medenwald, H. (1953). Synthesis of 1-azapyrene and phenanthrylene-4,5-methane. *Chem. Ber.* **86**, 287–93.

Memory, J. D. & Wilson, N. K. (1982). *NMR of Aromatic Compounds,* New York: Wiley–Interscience.

Michl, J. & Zahradink, R. (1966). Electronic structure of nonalternant hydrocarbons, their analogues and derivatives. XI. HMO energy characteristics of fluoranthene-like hydrocarbons. *Coll. Czech. Chem. Commun.* **31**, 3442–52.

Minabe, M., Cho, B. & Harvey, R. G. (1989). Electrophilic substitution of polycyclic fluoranthene hydrocarbons. *J. Amer. Chem. Soc.* **111**, 3809–12.

Minabe, M., Yamamoto, Y., Nakada, K. & Suzuki, K. (1984). Catalytic reduction of 4H-cyclopenta[def]phenanthrene under mild conditions. *Bull. Chim. Soc. Jpn.* **57**, 725–8.

Minsky, A. & Rabinovitz, M. (1983). A facile synthesis of some polycyclic hydrocarbons: Application of phase transfer catalysis in the *bis*-Wittig reaction. *Synthesis* 497–8.

Moriwake, T. (1966). The syntheses of substituted 4-indanyl phenyl ketones and aceanthrenes. *Bull. Chem. Soc. Jpn.* **39**, 401–2.

Nagel, D. L., Kupper, R., Antonson, K. & Wallcave, L. (1977). Synthesis of alkyl-substituted benzo[c]phenanthrenes and chrysenes by photocyclization. *J. Org. Chem.* **42**, 3626–8.

Nenitzescu, D. & Avram, M. (1950). The polymerization of 1,2-dihydronaphthalene and the dehydrogenation condensation of 1,2,3,4-tetrahydronaphthalene. *J. Amer. Chem. Soc.* **72**, 3486–90.

Nesnow, S., Gold, A., Sangaiah, R., Triplett, L. L. & Slaga, T. J. (1984). Mouse skin tumor-initiating activity of benz(e)aceanthrylene and benz(l)aceanthrylene in SENCAR mice. *Cancer Lett.* **22**, 263–8.

Nesnow, S., Leavitt, S., Easterling, R., Watts, R., Toney, S. H., Claxton, L., Sangaiah, R., Toney, G. E., Wiley, J., Fraher, P. & Gold, A. (1984a). Mutagenicity of cyclopenta-fused isomers of benz(a)anthracene in bacterial and rodent cells and identification of the major rat liver microsomal metabolites. *Cancer Res.* **44**, 4993–5003.

Neumann, G. & Mullen, K. (1985). Reductive alkylation of acenaphthylene and synthesis of acephenanthrylene. *Chimia.* **39**, 269–70.

Orchin, M. & Reggel, L. (1947). Aromatic cyclodehydration. V. A synthesis of fluoranthene. *J. Amer. Chem. Soc.* **69**, 505–9.

Orchin, M. & Reggel, L. (1951). A synthesis of fluoranthene by cyclodehydration. *J. Amer. Chem. Soc.* **73**, 2955–6.

Orchin, M. & Reggel, L. (1951a). Synthesis of benzo[j]fluoranthene and benzo[k]fluoranthene. *J. Amer. Chem. Soc.* **73**, 436–42.

Peaden, P. A., Lee, M. L., Hirata, Y. & Novotny, M. (1980). High performance liquid chromotographic separation of high molecular weight polycyclic aromatic hydrocarbons in carbon black. *Anal. Chem.* **52**, 2268–71.

Peake, D. A., Oyler, A. R., Heikkila, K. E., Liukkonen, R. J., Engroff, E. C. & Carlson, R. M. (1983). Alkyl aromatic synthesis: Nucleophilic alkyl lithium addition. *Syn. Commun.* **13**, 21–6.

Periasamy, M. & Bhatt, V. (1977). A convenient method for the oxidation of polycyclic aromatic hydrocarbons to quinones. *Synthesis*, 330–2.

Perin-Roussel, O., Jacquignon, P. & Perin, F. (1975). Formylation of dibenzo[a,l]pyrene and dibenzo[a,e]fluoranthene and reduction of the resulting aldehydes. *C. R. Hebd. Seances Acad. Sci. Ser. C.* **280**, 1315–18.

Pierce, R. C. & Katz, M. (1975). Determination of atmospheric isomeric polycyclic arenes by thin-layer chromatography and fluorescence spectrophotometry. *Anal. Chem.* **47**, 1743–8.

Plummer, B. F., Al-Saigh, Z. Y. & Arfan, M. (1984). Synthesis of aceanthrylene. *J. Org. Chem.* **49**, 2069–71.

Plummer, B. F. & Singleton, S. F. (1987). The photodimerization of aceanthrylene. *Tetrahedron Lett.* **28**, 4801–4.

Pouchert, C. E. (1981). *Aldrich Library of Infrared Spectra Edit. III*, Milwaukee, WI: Aldrich Chemical Co.

Pouchert, C. E. & Campbell, J. R. (1983). *Aldrich Library of NMR Spectra. Edit. II*, Milwaukee, WI: Aldrich Chemical Co.

Praefcke, K. & Weichsel, C. (1978). Photochemical formation of fluoranthene from fluoren-9-spiro-dihydrothiopyran. *Liebigs Ann.* 1399–405.

Rabideau, P., Mooney, J. L., Smith, W. K., Sygula, A. & Paschal, J. W. (1988). Dissolving metal reduction of aceanthrylene and NMR analysis of a rigid boat-shaped 9,10-dihydroanthracene. *J. Org. Chem.* **53**, 589–91.

Radner, F. (1983). Nitration of polycyclic aromatic hydrocarbons with dinitrogen tetroxide. A simple and selective synthesis of mononitro derivatives. *Acta Chem. Scand. B.* **37**, 65–7.

Ray, J. K. & Harvey, R. G. (1982). Synthesis of benzo[a]fluoranthene and naphtho[2,1-a]-fluoranthene. *J. Org. Chem.* **47**, 3335–6.

Ray, J. K. & Harvey, R. G. (1983). Synthesis of methylene-bridged polycyclic hydrocarbons. *J. Org. Chem.* **48**, 1352–4.

Rice, J., Jordan, K., Little, P. & Hussain, N. (1988). Comparative tumor-initiating activity of methylene-bridged and bay-region methylated derivatives of benz[a]anthracene and chrysene. *Carcinogenesis*, **9**, 2275–8.

Rice, J., LaVoie, E. J. & Hoffmann, D. (1983). Synthesis of the isomeric phenols and the trans-2,3-dihydrodiol of fluoranthene. *J. Org. Chem.* **48**, 2360–3.

Rutherford, K. G. & Newman, M. S. (1957). A new synthesis and some reactions of 4-phenanthrenecarboxylic acid. *J. Amer. Chem. Soc.* **79**, 213–14.

Sandorfy, C. & Jones, R. N. (1956). The ultraviolet absorption spectra of methyl-1,2-benzanthracenes. *Can. J. Chem.* **34**, 888–905.

Sangaiah, R. & Gold, A. (1985). A synthesis of aceanthrylene. *Org. Prep. Proc. Internat.* **17**, 53–6.

Sangaiah, R. & Gold, A. (1988). Synthesis of cyclopenta[cd]pyrene and its benzannelated derivative naphtho[1,2,3-mno]acephenanthrylene. *J. Org. Chem.* **53**, 2620–2.

Sangaiah, R., Gold, A., Ball, L. M., Kohan, M., Bryant, B. J., Rudo, S. K., Claxton, L. & Nesnow, S. (1986). Biological activity and metabolism of aceanthrylene and acephenanthrylene. *Polynuclear Aromatic Hydrocarbons: Chemistry, Characterization and Carcinogenesis*, eds Cooke, M. & Dennis, A. J., pp 795–810, Columbus, OH: Battelle Press.

Sangaiah, R., Gold, A. & Toney, G. E. (1983). Synthesis of a series of novel polycyclic aromatic systems: Isomers of benz[a]anthracene containing a cyclopenta-fused ring. *J. Org. Chem.* **48**, 1632–8.

Sawicki, E. (1977). Chemical composition and potential 'genotoxic' aspects of polluted atmospheres. *Air Pollution and Cancer in Man*, **16**, eds U. Mohr, D. Schmähl & L. Tomatis, 127–57, Lyon, France: International Agency for Research on Cancer.

Sawicki, E., Hauser, T. R. & Stanley, T. W. (1960). Ultraviolet, visible and fluorescence spectral analysis of polynuclear hydrocarbons. *Int. J. Air Poll.* **2**, 253–72.

Schoental, R. & Scott, E. J. (1949). Fluorescence spectra of polycyclic aromatic hydrocarbons in solution. *J. Chem. Soc.* 1683–96.

Scott, L. T., Reinhardt, G. & Roelofs, N. H. (1985). Acephenanthrylene. *J. Org. Chem.* **50**, 5886–7.

Seversen, R. F., Snook, M. E., Higman, H. C., Chortyk, O. T. & Akin, F. J. (1976). Isolation, identification, and quantitation of the polynuclear hydrocarbons in tobacco smoke. *Carcinogenesis*, I, 253–70, New York: Raven Press.

Shenbor, M. I. & Cheban, G. A. (1969). Preparation of 3-fluoranthenol by the action of lead tetraacetate on fluoranthene. *Zhur. Org. Khim.* **5**, 143–4.

Snook, M. E., Seversen, R. F., Arrendale, R. F., Higman, H. C. & Chortyk, O. T. (1977). The identification of high molecular weight polynuclear aromatic hydrocarbons in a biologically active fraction of cigarette smoke condensate. *Beitr. Tabakforsch.* **9**, 79–101.

Spijker, N. M., van den Bracken-van Leersum, Lugtenburg, J. and Cornelisse, J. (1990). A very convenient synthesis of cyclopenta[cd]pyrene. *J. Org. Chem.*, **55**, 756–8.

Squadrito, G. L., Church, D. F. & Pryor, W. (1987). Anomalous nitration of fluoranthene with nitrogen dioxide in carbon tetrachloride. *J. Amer. Chem. Soc.* **109**, 6535–7.

Streitwieser, J. A. & Fahey, R. C. (1962). Partial rate factors for nitration of fluoranthene. *J. Org. Chem.* **27**, 2352–5.

Streitwieser, J. A. & Brown, S. (1988). Convenient preparation of 11*H*-benzo[a]fluorenone and 11*H*-benzo[b]fluorenone. *J. Org. Chem.* **53**, 904–6.

Stubbs, H. W. & Tucker, S. H. (1950). Synthesis of fluoranthene. Part VI. Utilization of the Mannich reaction. *J. Chem. Soc.* 3288–92.

Stubbs, H. W. & Tucker, S. H. (1951). Synthesis of fluoranthenes. Part VIII. 2:3-benzo-fluoranthene. *J. Chem. Soc.* 2939–41.

Studt, P. (1978). The synthesis of indeno[1,2,3-cd]pyrene. *Liebigs Ann.* 528–9.

Studt, P. (1979). Synthesis of benzo[a]fluoranthene. *Liebigs Ann.* 1443.

Studt, P. & Win, T. (1983). Synthesis of benzo[ghi]fluoranthene. *Liebigs Ann.* 519.

Thilly, W. G., DeLuca, J. G., Furth, E. E., Hoppe, H. I., Kaden, D. E., Krolewski, J. J., Liber, H. L., Skopek, T. R., Slapikoff, S. A., Tizard, R. J. & Penman, B. W. (1980). Gene locus mutation assays in diploid human lymphoblast lines. *Chemical Mutagens*. eds F. J. deSerres & A. Hollaender, 331–64, New York: Plenum Press.

Tintel, C., Cornelisse, J. & Lugtenburg, J. (1983). Convenient synthesis of cyclopenta[c,d]-pyrene and 3,4-dihydrocyclopenta[c,d]pyrene. The reactivity of the pyrene dianion. *Recl. J. Roy. Neth. Chem. Soc.* **102**, 14–20.

TRC (1982). *Selected Nuclear Magnetic Resonance Spectral Data,* College Station, Texas: Thermodynamics Research Center, Texas A & M University.

TRC (1982a). *Selected Ultraviolet Spectral Data*, College Station, Texas: Thermodynamics Research Center, Texas A & M University.

Trost, B. & Kinson, P. L. (1975). Perturbed [12]annulenes. Derivatives of dibenzo-[cd,gh]pentalene. *J. Amer. Chem. Soc.* **97**, 2438–48.

Tucker, S. H. (1949). Syntheses of fluoranthenes. Part I. Michael addition of fluorene and of methyl fluorene-9-carboxylate to crotonitrile. Synthesis of 2-methyl- and of 2:4-dimethylfluoranthene. *J. Chem. Soc.* 2182–6.

Tucker, S. H. & Whalley, M. (1952). The chemistry of fluoranthene. *Chem. Rev.* **52**, 483–538.

van den Braken-van Leersum, A. M., Spijker, N. M., Lugtenburg, J. & Cornelisse, J. (1987). Synthesis, purification and spectral analysis of mononitrocyclopenta[cd]pyrenes. *Recl. Trav. Chim. Pays-Bas*, **106**, 628–40.

Veeraraghavan, S., Jostmeyer, S., Myers, J. & Wiley, J. C. Jr. (1987). A convenient synthesis of cyclopentapyrene. *J. Org. Chem.* **52**, 1355–7.

Vickery, E. H. & Eisenbraun, E. J. (1979). An improved synthesis of benzo[k]fluoranthene. *Org. Proc. Prep. Internat.* **11**, 259–61.

von Braun, J. & Anton, E. (1929). Benzopolymethylene compounds. XV. Composition, constitution and synthesis of fluoranthene. *Chem. Ber.* **62**, 145–51.

von Braun, J. & Manz, G. (1931). Fluoranthene and its derivatives. *Liebigs Ann.* **488**, 111–26.

Wallcave, L., Nagel, D. L., Smith, J. W. & Waniska, R. D. (1975). Two pyrene derivatives of widespread environmental distribution. Cyclopenta(cd)pyrene and acepyrene. *Environ. Sci. Technol.* **9**, 143–5.

Weyand, E. H., Patel, S., LaVoie, E. J., Cho, B. & Harvey, R. G. (1990). Relative tumor-initiating activity of benzo[a]fluoranthene, benzo[b]fluoranthene, naphtho[1,2-b]fluoranthene, and naphtho[2,1-a]fluoranthene. *Cancer Lett.*, **52**, 229–33.

Whitlock, H. W. Jr (1964). A convenient preparation of benzo[k]fluoranthene. *J. Org. Chem.* **29**, 3129.

Wise, S. A., Benner, B. A., Byrd, G. D., Chesler, S. N., Rebbert, R. E. & Schantz, M. M. (1988). Determination of polycyclic aromatic hydrocarbons in a coal tar standard reference material. *Anal. Chem.* **60**, 887–94.

Wise, S. A., Benner, B. A., Liu, H. & Byrd, G. D. (1988a). Separation and identification of polycyclic aromatic hydrocarbon isomers of molecular weight 302 in complex mixtures. *Anal. Chem.* **60**, 630–7.

Wood, A. W., Levin, W., Chang, R. L., Huang, M.-T., Ryan, D. E., Thomas, P. E., Lehr, R. E., Kumar, S., Koreeda, M., Akagi, H., Ittah, Y., Dansette, P., Yagi, H., Jerina, D. M. & Conney, A. H. (1980). Mutagenicity and tumor-initiating activity of cyclopenta(c,d)pyrene and structurally related compounds. *Cancer Res.*, **40**, 642–9.

Yoshida, M., Hishida, K., Minabe, M. & Suzuki, K. (1980). Electrophilic substitution of 4*H*-cyclopenta[def]phenanthrene. Friedel–Crafts acetylation. *J. Org. Chem.* **45**, 1783–5.

Yoshida, M., Kadokura, A., Minabe, M. & Suzuki, K. (1979). Some reactions of stable ozonide derived from 4*H*-cyclopenta[def]phenanthrene. *Tetrahedron*, **35**, 2237–41.

Yoshida, M., Minabe, M., Nagayama, S. & Suzuki, K. (1979b). Electrophilic substitution of 4*H*-cyclopenta[def]phenanthrene. Nitration. *J. Org. Chem.* **44**, 1915–17.

Yoshida, M., Minabe, M. & Suzuki, K. (1979a). Electrophilic substitution of 4*H*-cyclopenta[def]phenanthrene. Bromination. *J. Org. Chem.* **44**, 3029–32.

Yoshida, M., Minabe, M. & Suzuki, K. (1983). Synthesis of 4*H*-cyclopenta[def]phenanthrene from the fluorene skeleton. *Bull. Chim. Soc. Jpn.* **56**, 2179–80.

12

Arene oxides and imines

Arene oxides have been identified as the primary metabolites of PAHs produced by mammalian cells (Chap. 4). Their biological importance has stimulated expanding interest in their chemistry. The related polycyclic imines (aziridines) have not been detected as metabolites. However, evidence has been presented that ß aminoalcohols may be transformed to arene imines via enzymatic formation of sulfate esters followed by mild base treatment (Bicker & Fischer, 1974). It has been suggested (Ittah *et al.*, 1978) that a similar process may lead to conversion of the amino-linked adducts of arene oxides with nucleic acids and proteins to arene imines in animal tissues. Polycyclic imines are found to exhibit exceptional mutagenic potencies (Glatt *et al.*, 1985, 1986). This chapter critically reviews the synthesis and chemical properties of the polycyclic arene oxides and imines.

12.1 Structure and stability

Arene oxides tend to be more reactive than aliphatic epoxides. The $4\pi + 2\sigma$ electron system of benzene oxide and its polycyclic analogs undergoes relatively facile rearrangement via at least two pathways (Fig. 12.1). Aromatization to yield the corresponding phenols may take place spontaneously or on gentle heating and is also catalyzed by acids and by various nucleophiles (Bruice & Bruice, 1976). This path is favored thermodynamically by the energy gain accompanying aromatization. A second

Fig. 12.1. Arene oxides undergo rearrangement by dual pathways to (A) phenols and (B) oxepins.

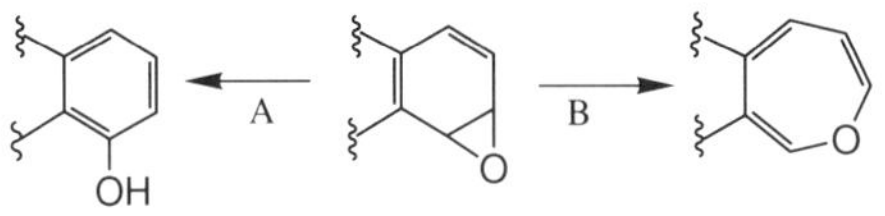

mode of isomerization entails rearrangement to the corresponding oxepins. While all arene oxides rearrange to phenols under appropriate conditions, the relative importance of the oxepin pathway is dependent upon the structure of the arene oxide. Some polycyclic arene oxides undergo facile rearrangement to yield stable oxepins, while others exhibit no tendency to rearrange by this pathway.

The arene oxide–phenol rearrangement often takes place with high regioselectivity to yield only one of the two possible isomeric phenols. The preferred direction of ring-opening is predictable by perturbational molecular orbital theory (Fu *et al.*, 1978). In all cases the predominant isomer is the one for which the calculated value of the reactivity number (N_t) of the intermediate carbocation (which is a zwitterion in neutral or basic solution and a protonated carbocation in acidic media) is minimum. For example, in the isomerization of benzo[a]pyrene 7,8-oxide (Fig. 12.2), opening of the epoxide ring in acidic media may afford two possible carbocations, **1a** and **1b**. The value of N_t for the structure **1a** is 1.55, while that for **1b** is 2.12. On this basis, intermediate **1a** is predicted to be more stable and 7-HO-BaP (**2a**) is predicted to be the predominant isomer. This agrees with the experimental observation that 7-HO-BaP is the sole phenolic product formed (Yagi & Jerina, 1975).

The mechanism of the arene oxide–phenol rearrangement is believed to involve hydride shift from the oxygenated carbon atom of the protonated ring-open epoxide intermediate to the carbocation site to form a keto intermediate (Fig. 12.3). Isomerization of [1-^{2}H]-naphthalene 1,2-oxide to [2-^{2}H]-1-naphthol was demonstrated to take place with 72% deuterium retention (Boyd *et al.*, 1972). Similar findings were obtained from a study of

Fig. 12.3. The mechanism of rearrangement of arene oxides to phenols involves a hydride shift to form a keto intermediate.

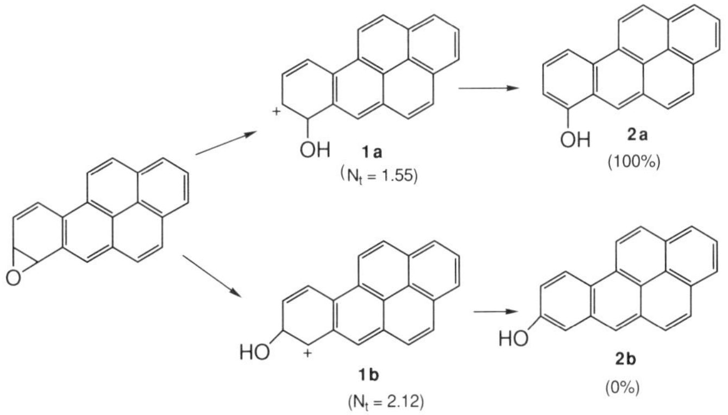

the microsomal conversion of [1-^{2}H]- and [2-^{2}H]-naphthalene to [2-^{2}H]-1-naphthol where both isomers were converted with 64% deuterium retention. These results suggest the formation of a common intermediate in the isomerization of either deuterated naphthalene 1,2-oxide. The keto intermediate which arises by hydride shift to the carbocation site (sometimes called the 'NIH shift') was proposed to be the common intermediate. The keto intermediates rearrange to the more thermodynamically favored phenol isomers. This mechanism is generally consistent with the available evidence.

The arene oxide–oxepin rearrangement has been studied extensively by Boyd and coworkers. They suggest on the basis of perturbational MO theory that polycyclic arene oxides may be classified by structural types which relate to their propensity to undergo isomerization to oxepins (Boyd & Stubbs, 1983). Certain arene oxides are predicted to be stable with respect to inversion to oxepin intermediates, while others are predicted to exhibit intermediate stability, or to be unstable with respect to the corresponding oxepins (Boyd *et al.*, 1987). Some examples of each of these types are shown in Figs.12.4. and 12.5. The types of arene oxides formed metabolically, both K-region and the non-K-region, do not conform in most cases to the structural types expected to lead to formation of stable oxepins, and oxepins are not generally detected as metabolites. However, these findings should be viewed with caution, since it is conceivable that in some cases oxepins are formed, but are not detected by the procedures usually employed for the isolation of more polar metabolites. Where the difference in resonance energy (ΔE_R) between the enantiomer of an optically active arene oxide and the related oxepin is sufficiently small (< 10 kcal/mol) racemization may be expected to take place via an unstable oxepin intermediate. Thus, attempts to isolate the optically active forms of BA 1,2- and 3,4-oxide, for which $\Delta E_R \cong$ 7 kcal/mol, have failed, although these compounds are definitely stable as the arene oxides rather than the tautomeric oxepins. On the other hand, BA 5,6-, 8,9-, and 10,11-oxide, for which $\Delta E_R > 17$ kcal/mol, have all been isolated in optically pure form. The stability of an arene oxide relative to that of the corresponding oxepin may be predicted qualitatively by the simple rule that *the isomer is favored whose structural formula contains the greatest number of benzenoid rings*, i.e. rings with three double bonds.

Evidence has also been obtained recently for an oxygen-walk mechanism

Fig. 12.3. The mechanism of rearrangement of arene oxides to phenols involves a hydride shift to form a keto intermediate.

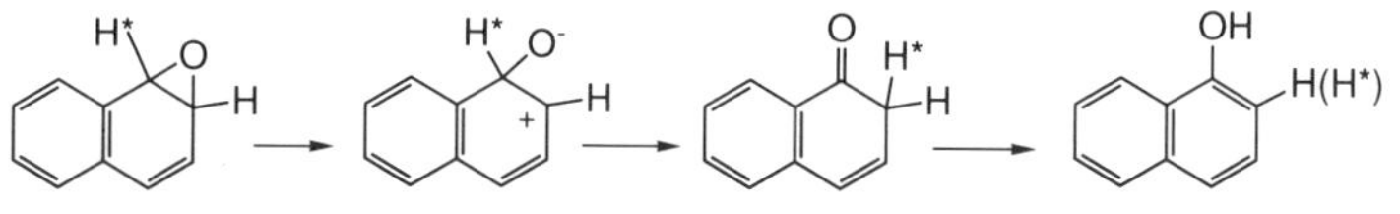

for the photoisomerization of the 1,2-oxide of dibenz[a,c]anthracene to a stable oxepin (Fig. 12.6: **B**) which is isomeric with the unstable oxepin intermediate (**A**) formed during racemization (Boyd & O'Kane, 1987; Griffin *et al.*, 1987a). This finding agrees with the prediction (Boyd & Stubbs, 1983) that those arene oxides with ΔE_R values < 7.9 kcal/mol should readily isomerize to an oxepin by an oxygen-walk process.

Fig. 12.4. Some examples of stable arene oxides and stable oxepins. The arene oxide–oxepin equilibrium tends to favor the former when the number of benzoid rings in the arene oxide structure exceeds that in the related oxepin structure, as in the case of the K-region arene oxides. Conversely, the oxepin structure is favored when the reverse is true.

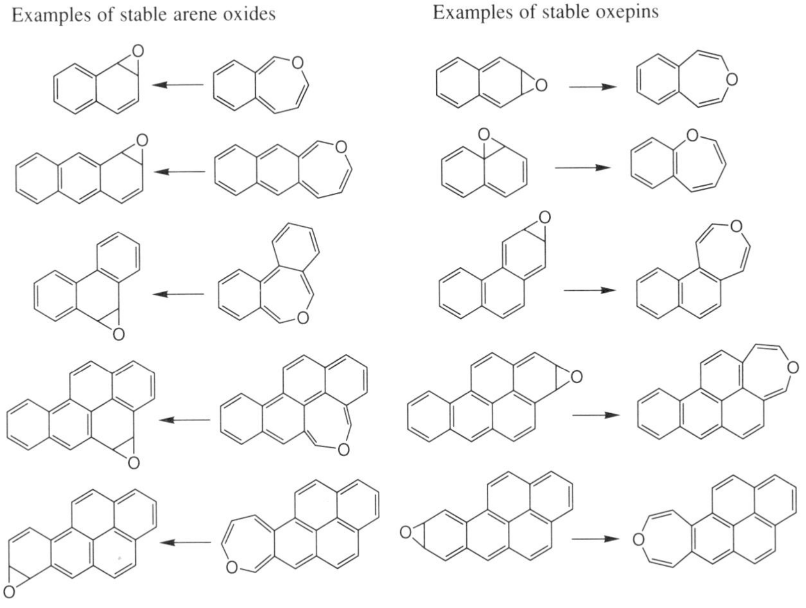

Examples of stable arene oxides   Examples of stable oxepins

Fig. 12.5. Examples of arene oxides which are predicted to exist as such but undergo inversion of configuration via an oxepin intermediate. This has been confirmed experimentally in the case of the BA 1,2-oxide.

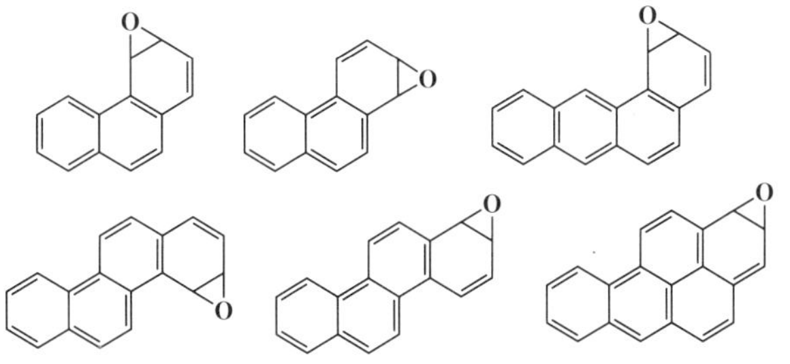

X-ray diffraction analysis of the structures of the K-region oxides of phenanthrene, BaP, and DMBA indicate the epoxide ring to lie almost perpendicular to the plane of the carbocyclic ring to which it is attached (Glusker, 1985). The lengths of the epoxide C-O bonds range from 1.43 to 1.45 Å, and the buckling of the ring system tends to be increased by presence of the oxide ring. On epoxidation of the K-region bonds of BaP and DMBA, the angle between the outer rings of BaP is increased 1° to 5°, while the related angle of DMBA is expanded from 24° to 35°.

12.2   Synthesis

It is convenient to consider the synthesis of the K-region and non-K-region arene oxides separately, since their methods of synthesis and relative stabilities differ. Because arene oxides may be mutagenic and/or tumorigenic, appropriate precautions (use of rubber gloves, well-ventilated hoods, face masks, etc.) should be employed when handling them. On the other hand, they tend to be only very weak carcinogens or inactive in animal assays, probably due to their facility of decomposition by multiple pathways and their tendency to react indiscriminately with proteins and other cellular components.

12.2.1   *K-region oxides*

The intramolecular coupling of dialdehydes with hexamethylphosphorous triamide was the first practical synthetic approach to be developed (Fig. 12.7) (Newman & Blum, 1964). The dialdehyde precursors are accessible from the parent polyarenes by ozonolysis (in the case of phenanthrene) or through reaction with OsO_4 to yield *cis*-dihydrodiols followed by oxidative cleavage with $NaIO_4$ (Harvey *et al.*, 1975). Early

Fig. 12.6. Racemization of dibenz[a,c]anthracene 1,2-oxide proceeds via the unstable oxepin intermediate A. The calculated loss of resonance energy is only 2.3 kcal/mol. Photo-isomerization of the 1,2-oxide affords the isomeric oxepin B via an oxygen-walk mechanism.

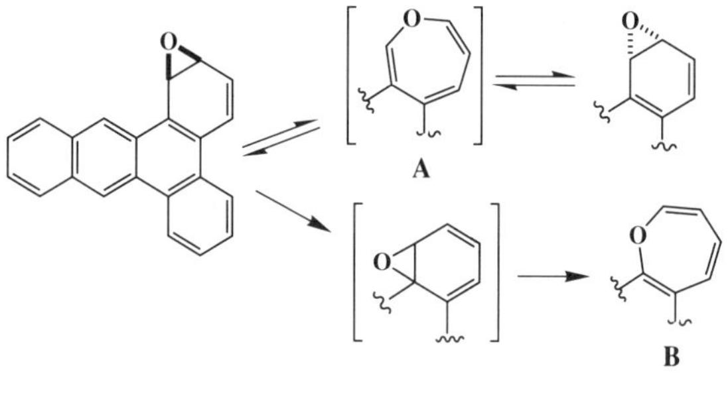

attempts to prepare the K-oxides of BaP and DMBA by this method were not successful, however, DMBA-5,6-oxide was subsequently obtained by the use of a modified procedure (Harvey *et al.*, 1975). The requisite dialdehyde precursor was obtained by oxidation of DMBA with $NaIO_4$ and a catalytic amount of OsO_4. The dialdehyde coupling method has been employed to synthesize the K-region oxides of chrysene (Boyland & Sims, 1967), DBA (Boyland & Sims, 1965), pyrene (Van Duuren *et al.*, 1974), the ^{3}H-labeled derivative of DMBA-5,6-oxide (Fu & Harvey, 1977), and several substituted derivatives of phenanthrene 9,10-oxide (Griffin *et al.*, 1976). It is worthy of note that the stabilities in storage of the polyarene oxides prepared by this route tend to be lower than those obtained by other methods. This is apparently a consequence of catalysis of decomposition by trace impurities.

Cyclodehydration of *trans*-dihydrodiols with the dimethyl acetal of dimethylformamide provides a more generally useful synthetic route to K-region oxides (Fig. 12.8) (Harvey *et al.*, 1975). It employs mild conditions and affords easily separable, water soluble byproducts. Another promising cyclodehydration reagent is diethoxytriphenylphosphorane [$Ph_3P(OEt)_2$]. With its use, phenanthrene 9,10-oxide was obtained virtually quantitatively from the corresponding dihydrodiol (Robinson *et al.*, 1985). Other less

Fig. 12.7. Synthesis of K-region oxides via the coupling of dialdehydes.

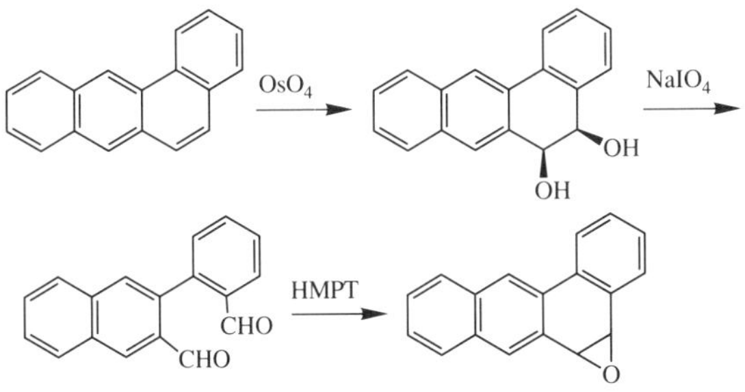

Fig 12.8. Synthesis of K-region oxides via the corresponding *trans*-dihydrodiols.

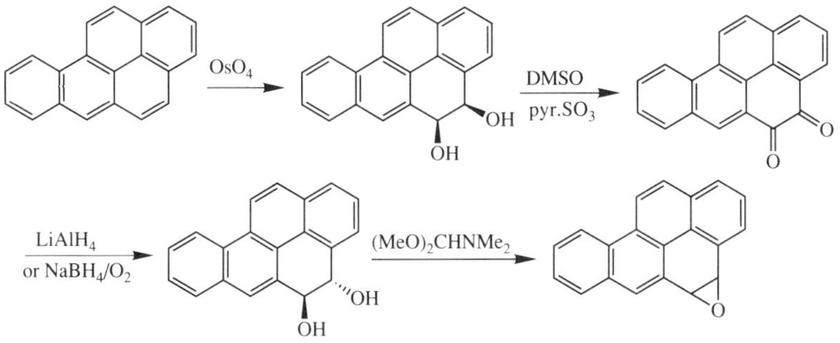

effective reagents for this purpose include diphenyl(1,1,1,3,3,3-hexafluoro-2-phenyl-2-propoxysulfurane), $Ph_2S[OC(CF_3)_2Ph]$ (Okamoto *et al.*, 1978), and *p*-toluenesulfonylchloride and NaH (Croisey-Delcey *et al.*, 1979). The *trans*-dihydrodiols are conveniently obtained from the corresponding quinones by reduction with $LiAlH_4$ in refluxing ether or with $NaBH_4$ in ethanol with O_2 bubbling through the solution (Platt & Oesch, 1982; Harvey, 1986) (Chap. 13).

Arene oxides synthesized by cyclization of *trans*-dihydrodiols include the K-region derivatives of phenanthrene, BaP, BA, DMBA, chrysene, DBA, pyrene, and 3-MC (Harvey *et al.*, 1975; Harvey, unpublished studies). Substituted K-region oxides have also been prepared by appropriate modification of this procedure. They include the 7-methyl, 9-acetoxy, 9-hydroxy, 9-methoxy, and 4,5-dimethyl analogs of BaP (Konieczny & Harvey, 1982; Harvey & Cortez, 1983; Harvey, unpublished studies), the 9,10-dimethyl- and 9,10-bis(*p*-chlorophenyl)phenanthrene 9,10-oxides (Avnir *et al.*, 1975), and 5,6-diphenylbenzo[c]phenanthrene 5,6-oxide (Avnir *et al.*, 1975). [3]H- and ^{13}C-labeled derivatives of BaP 4,5-oxide and its 8-methoxy and 9-methoxy analogs have also been synthesized by this method (Harvey & Fu, 1976; Engel *et al.*, 1978; Hylarides *et al.*, 1979; Silverman *et al.*, 1985).

K-region *cis*-dihydrodiols may be converted to polycyclic arene oxides via a three step reaction sequence involving initial treatment with trimethyl orthoacetate in refluxing benzene with a trace of benzoic acid (Dansette & Jerina, 1974) (Fig. 12.9). Reaction of the resulting mixture of 2-methyl-2-methoxy-1,3-dioxolane diastereomers with Me_3SiCl takes place with inversion to yield a mixture of *trans*-chlorohydrin acetate isomers. For PAHs

Fig. 12.9. Synthesis of K-region arene oxides from the corresponding *cis*-dihydrodiols via the mixtures of isomeric dioxolane and *trans*-chlorohydrin acetate intermediates.

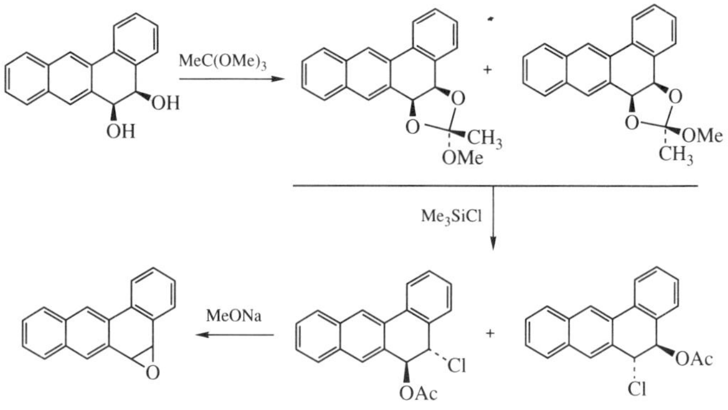

which undergo electrophilic substitution mainly in the K-region, e.g. chrysene, the *trans*-halohydrin acetates may be obtained directly from the PAHs by treatment with *N*-bromoacetamide in acetic acid (Van Bladeren & Jerina, 1983). Cyclization of the halohydrin esters with NaOMe affords the corresponding racemic arene oxides. The limitations of this synthetic method include the formation of mixtures of isomers in both the dioloxane and the halohydrin steps and the formation of phenol acetate byproducts by elimination of HCl from the halohydrin intermediate, all of which tend to complicate purification of intermediates and products.

Arene oxides synthesized by the halohydrin ester route include the K-oxides of pyrene, phenanthrene, BaP, BA, chrysene, benzo[c]phenanthrene, benzo[g]chrysene, 3-MC, and indeno[1,2,3-cd]pyrene (Dansette & Jerina, 1974; Van Bladeren & Jerina, 1983; Agarawal *et al.*, 1985; Rice *et al.*, 1985). This method has also been employed for the synthesis of 9-hydroxybenzo[a]-pyrene 4,5-oxide (Bochnitschek *et al.*, 1985) and the ^{3}H-labeled K-oxides of phenanthrene, BaP, and BA (Kolwyck *et al.*, 1976; Yagi *et al.*, 1976).

Direct oxidation of polyarenes to their K-region oxides is feasible for PAHs which do not undergo preferential oxidative attack elsewhere in the molecule. However, this excludes most of the biologically important PAHs, such as BaP and DMBA. The reagents most commonly employed for this purpose are peracids and sodium hypochlorite. Oxidations with *m*-chloroperbenzoic acid are usually conducted in a two-phase system with a large excess (10 fold) of the peracid in methylene chloride and aqueous NaHCO$_3$ (Isikawa *et al.*, 1977). The yields are moderate (10-60%). The K-region oxides of phenanthrene, 9,10-dimethylphenanthrene, 9-phenylphenan-threne, pyrene, and chrysene have been prepared by this method. The two-phase system serves to neutralize acidic products which otherwise might catalyze isomerization of the arene oxides to phenols.

Direct K-region oxidation of appropriate polyarenes may also be effected with sodium hypochlorite in aqueous chloroform in the presence of a phase transfer agent, e.g. benzyltrimethylammonium chloride (Krishnan *et al.*, 1977). The K-region oxides of chrysene, phenanthrene, pyrene, and several N-heterocyclic analogs of phenanthrene have been synthesized by this method. However, hypochlorite oxidation of 9-methylphenanthrene gave a mixture of the K-region oxide and 9-chloromethylphenanthrene 9,10-oxide (DiRaddo & Chan, 1982), and oxidation of naphthalene provided the *syn*-1,2,3,4-diepoxide (Krishnan *et al.*, 1977). The mechanism of these reactions is believed to involve a free radical pathway and the chloroxy radical (ClO·) (Fonouni *et al.*, 1983).

Other reagents employed for direct oxidation include dialkylcarbodiimides and hydrogen peroxide (Krishnan *et al.*, 1977a), superoxide and phosgene dimcr (Nagano *et al.*, 1983), and peroxymonosulfate (caroate)-acetone (Jeyaraman & Murray, 1984). The carbodiimide method requires an acidic medium, limiting its usefulness for sensitive arene oxides. These methods afford low yields and are of minimal practical utility.

12.2.2   Non-K-Region oxides

The relatively high reactivity and instability of the non-K-region arene oxides imposes practical limitations on methods for their synthesis. The first satisfactory method was developed by Vogel & Klarner (1968). It involves bromination of a tetrahydroarene epoxide with *N*-bromosuccinimide, followed by dehydrobromination with a suitable base, usually 1,5-diazobicyclo[4.3.0]nonane (Fig. 12.10). A useful modification of this method employs a bromohydrin ester in place of the tetrahydroepoxide (Yagi & Jerina, 1975). This modified procedure affords superior yields in most cases. Hydrolysis and cyclization of the bromohydrin ester and dehydrobromination are accomplished in a single step by base treatment.

The original Vogel method has been used to prepare phenanthrene 1,2-oxide (Yagi & Jerina, 1975), BA 8,9-oxide (Sims, 1971), dibenz[a,c]anthracene 10,11-oxide (Sims, 1972), and the BaP 7,8- and 9,10-oxides (Waterfall & Sims, 1972). The modified procedure has been employed for the synthesis of phenanthrene 3,4-oxide (Yagi & Jerina, 1975), BA 1,2-oxide (Boyd & Sharma, 1984), the BaP 7,8- and 9,10-oxides (Yagi & Jerina, 1975), chrysene 1,2-oxide (Boyd & Green, 1982), chrysene 3,4-oxide (Boyd *et al.*, 1983), benzo[c]phenanthrene 3,4-oxide (Balani *et al.*, 1984), benzo[e]pyrene 9,10-oxide (Agarawal *et al.*, 1988), and triphenylene 1,2-oxide (Boyd *et al.*, 1987a). Recently, the modified procedure has been employed to synthesize

Fig. 12.10.   Synthetic routes to non-K-region arene oxides.

Vogel Method

Jerina Method

R = CH$_3$CO, F$_3$CCO, Cl$_3$CCO

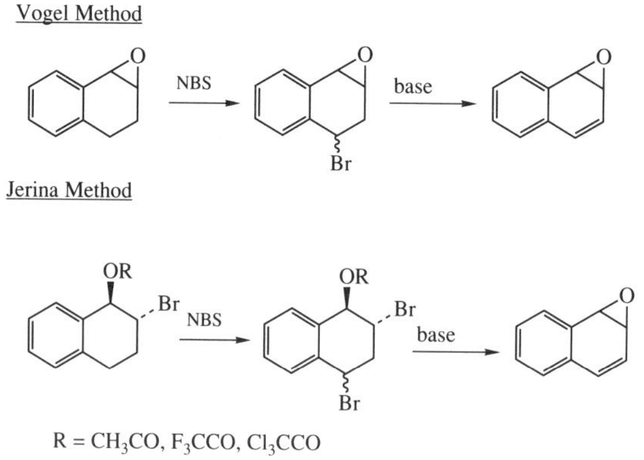

the BA 1,2- and 3,4-oxides, triphenylene 1,2-oxide, DBA 1,2- and 3,4-oxides, dibenz[a,j]anthracene 3,4-oxide, and benzo[e]pyrene 9,10-oxide (Boyd *et al.*, 1987; Platt *et al.*, 1989). It has also been demonstrated that small amounts of oxepins are produced by an oxygen-walk process during some of these syntheses (Boyd *et al.*, 1987).

12.2.3 Arene dioxides

A number of arene dioxides have been synthesized by adaptation of the methods employed for the synthesis of the related mono oxides. Thus, the K-region dioxides of pyrene, dibenz[a,h]anthracene, and benzo[a]pyrene were prepared by the intramolecular coupling of the appropriate tetraaldehyde precursors (Fig. 12.11) (Agarwal & Van Duuren, 1975, 1977; Moriarity *et al.*, 1975). The tetraaldehydes are synthetically accessible from the parent hydrocarbons via their respective diozonides or by reaction with OsO_4 followed by oxidative cleavage with periodic acid. The stereochemistry of these dioxides, which may be *anti* or *syn*, was not established. They underwent photochemical rearrangement, presumably to the corresponding oxepins, during measurement of their UV fluorescence spectra. Attempted synthesis of pyrene 4,5:9,10-dioxide (**3**) by the methoxydioxolane route was unsatisfactory. However, this dioxide was obtained in low yield by oxidation of pyrene 4,5-oxide with dimethyldioxirane (Agarawal *et al.*, 1989). The interesting 1,2: 9,10-dioxide of benzo-[g]chrysene (**4**), which has both K-region and non-K-region oxide rings, was synthesized by base treatment of the tribromodiacetate derivative (Fig. 12.11) (Agarwal *et al.*, 1985). A similar approach was utilized to synthesize the 5,6:8,9- and 5,6:10,11-dioxides of BA (**5** and **6**), the 5,6:9,10-dioxide of benzo[c]phenanthrene (**7**), and the 5,6:7,8-dioxide of chrysene (**8**) (Agarwal *et al.*, 1989). Oxidation of BA 8,9-oxide with dimethyldioxirane furnished

Fig. 12.11. Synthetic routes to polyarene dioxiranes.

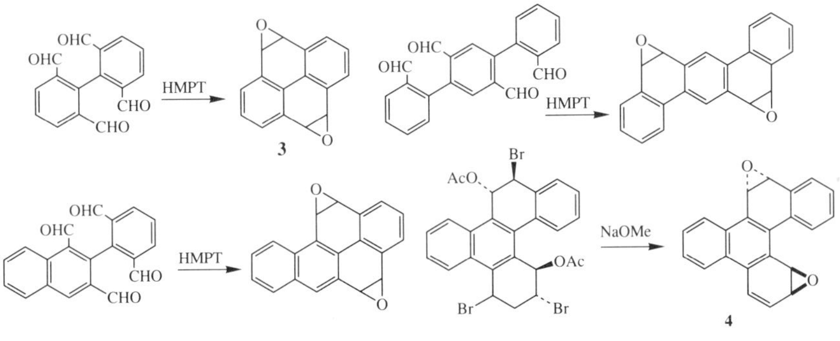

BA 8,9:10,11-dioxide (**9**) virtually quantitatively, while similar oxidation of BA 10,11-oxide gave only a low yield of **6** (Agarwal *et al.*, 1989).

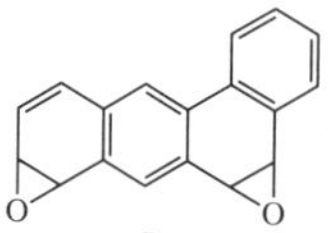

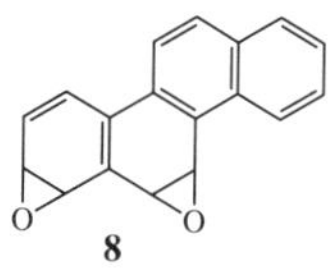

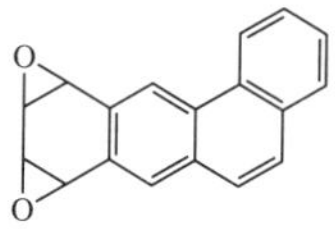

12.2.4 *Cyclopentano arene oxides*

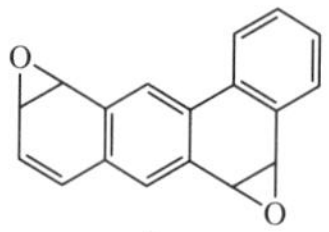

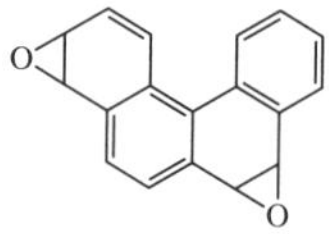

A third class of arene oxides is formed by PAHs which contain a cyclopentano ring, such as cyclopenta[c,d]pyrene. The cyclopentano arene oxides are distinguished by an unusually long carbon–carbon bond in the oxirane ring, resulting in a strained ring system. Molecular orbital calculations suggest that arene oxides of this type are more reactive than the diol epoxide derivatives of alternant PAHs (Fu *et al.*, 1980). The molecular structure of cyclopenta[c,d]pyrene 3,4-oxide has been determined by X-ray crystallography (Kuroda & Neidle, 1983). The plane of the epoxide ring is found to be tilted 71° to the aromatic ring system; this is smaller than the dihedral angle found for the K-region oxide of BaP (Glusker *et al.*, 1985).

Acenaphthylene 1,2-oxide is the only cyclopentano arene oxide that has been prepared by direct epoxidation. Treatment of acenaphthylene with *m*-chloroperbenzoic acid in a buffer system affords the 1,2-oxide in 90% yield (Kinstle & Ihrig, 1970). Attempts to extend this approach to the synthesis of higher polycyclic analogues have not met with success. This is probably a consequence of the facility of their rearrangement to the related ketones. The most commonly employed method for the synthesis of cyclopentano arene oxides, e.g. cyclopenta[cd]pyrene 3,4-oxide (**10**), is base-catalyzed cyclization of the corresponding halohydrins (Fig. 12.12) (Gold *et al.*, 1979; McCaustland *et al.*, 1980). The latter are most conveniently obtained by treatment of the parent PAHs with NBS in moist DMSO, although the dioxolane route has also been employed in one example (McCaustland *et al.*, 1980). Other cyclopentano arene oxides synthesized via the halohydrin route include the four isomeric cyclopenta-fused BA derivatives, benz-[e]aceanthrylene 5,6-oxide (**11**), benz[j]aceanthrylene-1,2-oxide (**12**), benz-[l]aceanthrylene-1,2-oxide (**13**), and benz[k]acephenanthrylene 4,5-oxide (**14**) (Bartczak *et al.*, 1987). Cyclopenta[cd]pyrene 3,4-oxide (**10**) has also been obtained from 3-oxo-3,4-dihydrocyclopenta[c,d]pyrene by oxidation with SeO$_2$ to the quinone, followed by reduction with NaBH$_4$ to the *trans*-dihydrodiol and cyclization with Ph$_3$P and (EtO)$_2$ (Fig. 12.12) (Sangaiah & Gold, 1985).

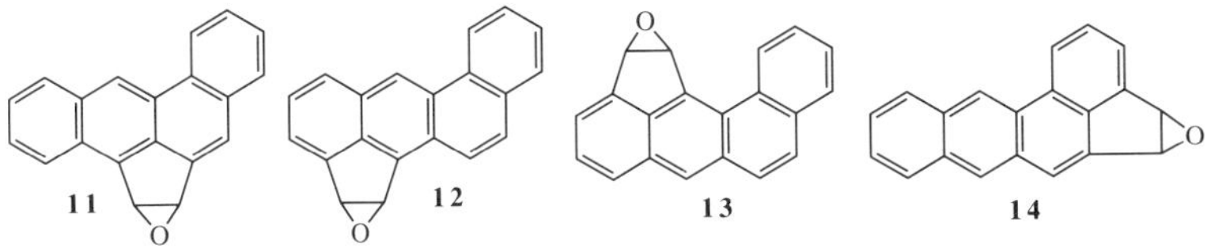

12.2.5 Optically active arene oxides

Since microsomal metabolism of polyarenes is generally highly stereoselective, the development of methods for the stereospecific synthesis and resolution of the optically pure enantiomers of arene oxides has attracted considerable interest. Optically active arene oxides of known absolute configuration can be used to define the stereoselectivity of the cytochromes P-450 which form such metabolites and to establish the mechanism and enantioselectivity of nonoxidative drug metabolizing enzymes, such as the microsomal epoxide hydrolases and glutathione S-transferases, which utilize arene oxides as substrates. In view of the relative reactivity and facility of rearrangement of many arene oxides, it is generally most practical to obtain the pure enantiomers by resolution of their synthetic precursors. Most suitable for this purpose are the dihydrodiol and halohydrin precursors. They can be readily converted to mixtures of diastereomers through reaction with the acid chlorides of suitable optically active acids, such as (−)-menthyloxyacetic acid (MAA) and (−)-methoxy(trifluoromethyl)phenylacetic acid (MTPAA). In the early studies, separations were effected by fractional crystallization or column chromatography; in more recent investigations, these techniques have been partially supplanted by more efficient HPLC methods. Methods for the direct resolution of racemic arene oxides by HPLC

Fig. 12.12. Synthetic routes to cyclopenta[c,d]pyrene 3,4-oxide.

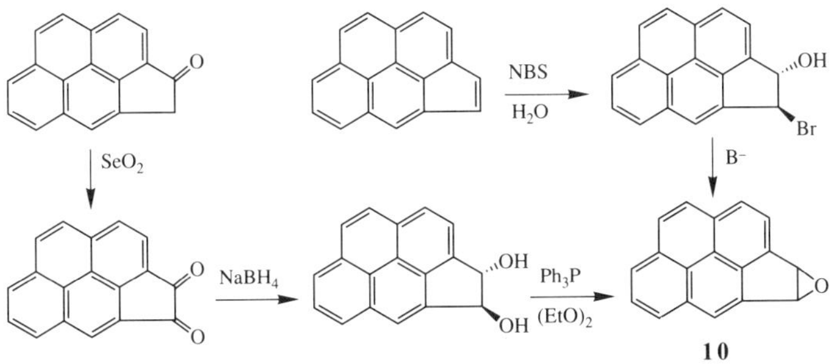

separation on chiral columns have also been developed. This technique has obvious important implications for metabolism studies.

The first reported example of stereospecific synthesis of an arene oxide is that of naphthalene 1,2-oxide (Fig. 12.13) (Aktar & Boyd, 1975; Aktar *et al.*, 1979). Reaction of (±)-*trans*-1-hydroxy-2-bromo-naphthalene with (–)-menthyloxyacetyl chloride in pyridine furnished the corresponding diastereomeric esters which were separated by column chromatography. Sequential treatment of the (1S,2S) diastereomer (**15**) with diborane and acetic anhydride gave the bromohydrin acetate which on treatment with NBS followed by NaOMe afforded (-)-naphthalene 1,2-oxide. The absolute configuration of the latter (1S,2S) was assigned by comparison with that of the known (2S)-2-hydroxytetrahydronaphthalene derived from the same (1S, 2S)-bromohydrin MAA ester. The (+)(1R,2R)-naphthalene 1,2-oxide was similarly prepared from the diastereomeric (1R,2R) MAA ester. While naphthalene 1,2-oxide showed poor thermal stability in the crystalline state, solutions of (+)-naphthalene 1,2-oxide in CHCl$_3$ showed little tendency to racemize at ambient temperature.

Similar methods were employed to prepare the enantiomers of anthracene 1,2-oxide (Aktar *et al.*, 1979), the phenanthrene 1,2- and 3,4-oxides (Boyd *et al.*, 1977), the chrysene 1,2- and 3,4-oxides (Boyd & Greene, 1982; Boyd *et al.*, 1983), the BA 8,9- and 10,11-oxides (Boyd *et al.*, 1981, 1981a), BaP 7,8-oxide (Boyd *et al.*, 1980), and benzo[c]phenanthrene 3,4-oxide (Balani *et al.*, 1984). Attempted resolution of BA 1,2-oxide by this method was not successful, apparently due to its conformational instability (Boyd & Sharma, 1984). Attempted preparation of the 9,10-oxide of BeP in optically active form by this method furnished a mixture of the oxepin **16** and the racemic

Fig. 12.13. Stereospecific synthesis of arene oxides from racemic halohydrin intermediates via the corresponding diastereomeric MAC esters (e.g. **15**) is illustrated for naphthalene (-)(1S,2S)-1,2-oxide.

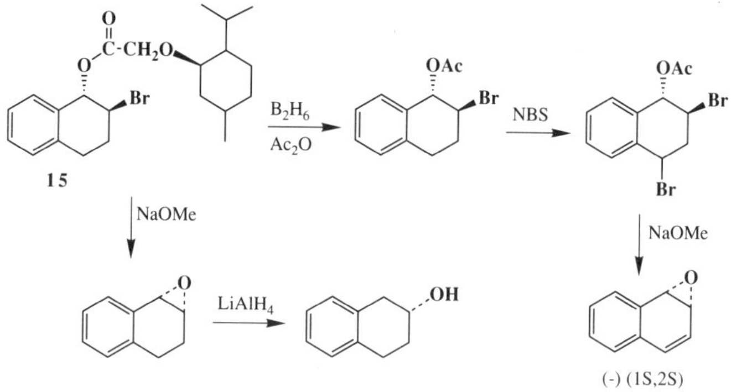

BeP 9,10-oxide (Fig. 12.14) (Agarwal *et al.*, 1988). These results are interpreted in terms of spontaneous thermal racemization of BeP 9,10-oxide (via the undetected oxepin intermediate **18**) and photoisomerization of the putative arene oxide intermediate **17** to yield **16**. This finding accords with the prediction of PMO calculations of the resonance energy changes associated with these reactions.

The chiral K-region oxides of BaP were synthesized from the racemic *cis*-4,5-dihydrodiols by treatment with (+)-MTPAA and separation of the mixed diastereomers by HPLC (Chang *et al.*, 1979). Alkaline hydrolysis gave the optically pure (+)- and (−)-*cis*-4,5-dihydrodiol enantiomers which were converted to the (+)- and (−)-4,5-oxides by sequential treatment with MeC(OMe)$_3$, Me$_3$SiCl, and MeONa (Dansette & Jerina, 1974). A similar synthetic approach was utilized to prepare the chiral K-region oxides of BA (Boyd *et al.*, 1981; Armstrong *et al.*, 1981), chrysene, DMBA, and benzo[c]phenanthrene (Balani *et al.*, 1987) from the related racemic K-region *cis*-dihydrodiols. Attempted synthesis of the enantiomers of triphenylene 1,2-oxide from the *cis*-1,2-diols of tetrahydrotriphenylene by modification of the same method gave only the racemic arene oxide in accord with PMO calculations which predict rapid racemization (Boyd *et al.*, 1987a).

The optically pure enantiomers of K-region oxides may also be obtained by resolution of the racemic K-region bromohydrins esterified with (−)-MAA. This method was employed for the synthesis of the (+)- and (−)-5,6-oxides of benzo[c]phenanthrene (Sayer *et al.*, 1986). The enantiomers of K-region arene oxides are also accessible, in principle, by resolution of the corresponding K-region *trans*-dihydrodiols, since the latter may be readily transformed to the former. The K-region *trans*-dihydrodiols of benzo[c]phenanthrene, chrysene, and pyrene have been resolved by chromatographic

Fig. 12.14. Attempted preparation of optically active BeP 9,10-oxide furnishes a mixture of the oxepin **16** (arising via photoisomerization of the arene oxide intermediate **17**) and racemic BeP 9,10-oxide (racemization occurs via the undetected isomeric oxepin **18**).

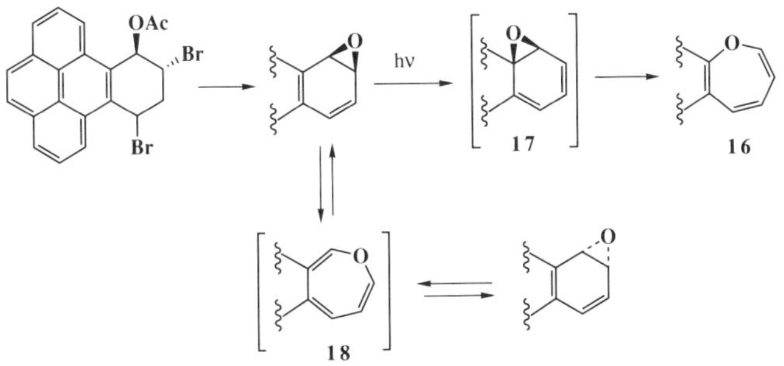

separation of their diastereomeric diesters with (−)-MAA (Balani *et al.*, 1986).

One of the most significant advances in this area is the development of methods for the direct resolution of the dihydrodiol and epoxide derivatives of PAHs by HPLC separation on chiral columns. This method was employed to resolve the enantiomers of the K-region *trans*-5,6-dihydrodiol of DMBA (Yang & Weems, 1984) and the DMBA 5,6-oxide (Mushtaq *et al.*, 1984); however, the absolute assignment of the latter was subsequently reversed (Balani *et al.*, 1987). The direct resolution of the K-region oxides of BA, BaP, 3-MC, 1-methyl-BA, 7-methyl-BA, 12-methyl-BA, chrysene, and

Fig. 12.15.   Absolute configurations of the enantiomers of optically active arene oxides. References: [a]Aktar *et al.*, 1979; [b]Balani *et al.*, 1983; [c]Boyd *et al.*, 1981a; [d]Armstrong *et al.*, 1981; [e]Weems *et al.*, 1987; [f]Weems *et al.*, 1985; [g]Boyd *et al.*, 1981; [h]Balani *et al.*, 1987; [i]Balani *et al.*, 1984; [j]Sayer *et al.*, 1986; [k]Boyd & Greene, 1982; [l]Boyd *et al.*, 1983; [m]Kedzierski *et al.*, 1981; [n]Boyd *et al.*, 1980.

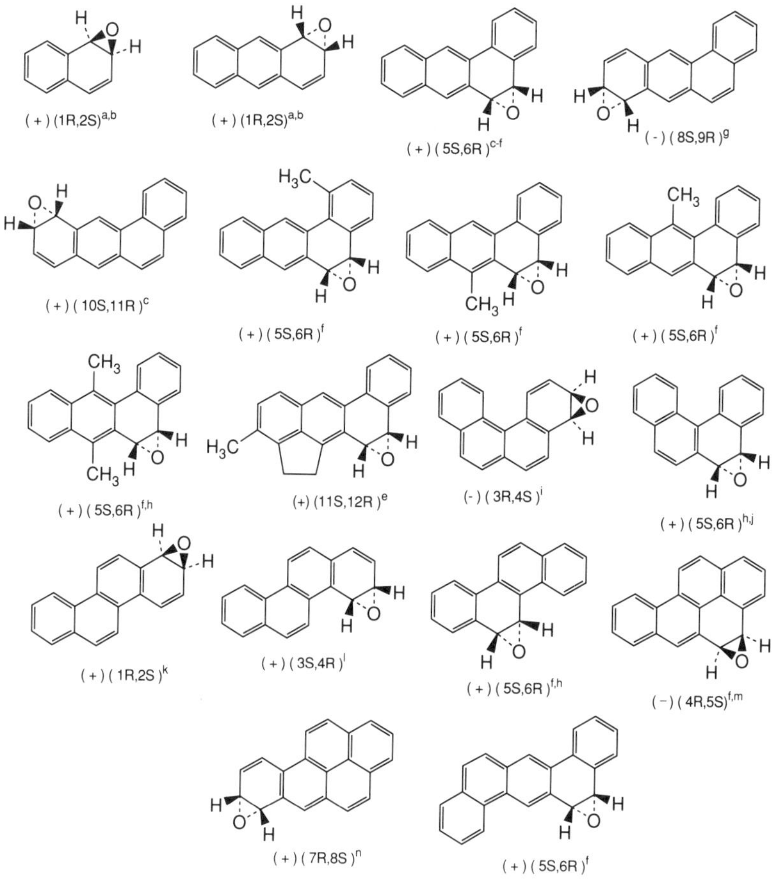

dibenz[a,h]anthracene, as well as the non-K-region 7,8-oxide of BaP and the 1,2- and 3,4-oxides of chrysene have also been achieved by direct separation on chiral columns (Yang & Chiu, 1985; Weems *et al.*, 1985; Yang & Bao, 1987).

The assignment of the absolute stereochemistry of arene oxides (Fig. 12.15) has been achieved by a variety of methods. In earlier studies, the method most commonly employed was to relate the configuration of a re-solved bromohydrin precursor of a non-K-region arene oxide to that of a related tetrahydro alcohol of established stereochemistry. In some cases the assignment of absolute stereochemistry has been made on the basis of crystal structure data. For example, analysis of the crystal structure of (+)-(7S,8S)-*trans*-8-bromo-7-menthyloxyacetoxy-7,8,9,10-tetrahydrobenzo[a]pyrene (**19**) indicated that the tetrahydro ring adopted a half-chair conformation with the bromine atom and the MA group in a *trans*-diequatorial relationship (Fig. 12.16) (Boyd *et al.*, 1980). The absolute configuration of the menthyl group is well established, and the configuration of **19** and the bromohydrin enantiomer from which it is derived were both assigned as 7S,8S. Base-catalyzed cyclization of the (–)-(7S,8S)-bromohydrin yielded the (–)-(7S,8S)-BaP 7,8-oxide. Similarly, the configuration of the (-)-enantiomer of BA 8,9-oxide was unequivocally assigned as (8S,9R) by configurational correlation with (+)-(9S,8S)-*trans*-9-bromo-8-menthyloxyacetoxy-8,9,10,11-tetrahy-drobenz[a]anthracene whose absolute stereochemistry was determined by X-ray crystal structure analysis.

The method of broadest scope and utility for the assignment of the absolute configurations of arene oxides, dihydrodiols and related oxidized metabolites of polyarenes involves application of the exciton chirality rule (Harada & Nakanishi, 1972) to the circular dichroism spectrum of an appropriate derivative. For example, absolute configuration was assigned to the (+)-*trans*-4,5-dihydrodiol of BaP by application of the exciton chirality rule to the CD spectrum of the bis-(*p-N,N*-dimethylamino)benzoate of its partially hydrogenated derivative **20**. The hydrogenated derivative was em-

Fig 12.16. The absolute configuration of the trans-7-bromo-8-methyloxy-acetoxy ester **19** was assigned by X-ray crystal structure analysis and utilized to assign the stereochemistry of the (-)-enantiomer of benzo[a]pyrene 7,8-oxide.

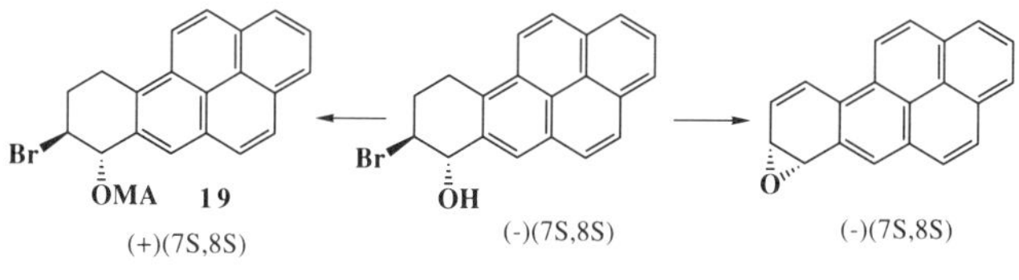

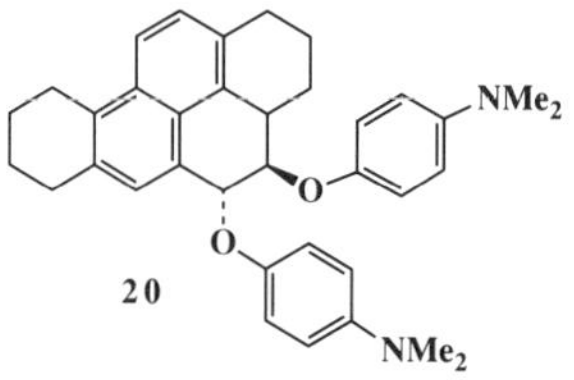

ployed in order to minimize undesirable interactions between the electric transition dipoles of the benzoate chromophores and the polycyclic aromatic ring system. The CD spectrum showed strong negative interaction bands at ~320-25 nm crossing through zero ~310-13 nm which requires (4R,5R) absolute configuration (Kedzierski *et al.*, 1981). Since the (+)-*trans*-4,5-dihydrodiol can be related to the (+)-4,5-oxide, the latter must have the (4S,5R) absolute configuration.

Although chirotopical methods are the most reliable, several additional more convenient criteria may be utilized to assign absolute configuration to K-region *trans*-dihydrodiols and, by inference, the corresponding K-region oxides. For a discussion of these topics with examples and leading references cf. Balani *et al*, 1986. They point out that significant correlations exist between absolute configuration and retention times on HPLC of the diastereomeric esters with MAA as well as with the sign of rotation of the CD band. Thus, the R,R-diastereomers of the MAA diesters of a series of K-region *trans*-dihydrodiols were less retained on silica gel HPLC columns on elution with cyclohexane–ether mixtures and showed negative values of $[\alpha]_D$ in tetrahydrofuran in comparison with the S,S-diastereomers. On the other hand, the R,R-enantiomers of the free dihydrodiols showed positive values of $[\alpha]_D$, except in cases showing a marked preference for the pseudodiaxial conformation (usually associated with steric crowding, e.g. a bay region). These empirical criteria should be employed with caution in making stereochemical assignments, since significant exceptions may exist.

The NMR coupling patterns of the methylene hydrogens of the $OCOCH_2O$ group in the MAA diesters of the K-region dihydrodiols were also found to be diagnostic of their absolute configuration. This observation was based on the earlier finding that the degree of magnetic nonequivalence between the methylene hydrogens of the MAA esters of the trans-bromo-hydrins of tetrahydro polyarenes is related to the chirality of the oxygen-bearing ring carbon atoms (Balani *et al.*, 1983). In general, the pairs of signals for the methylene protons are found to be equivalent or very nearly equivalent for the R,R-isomers (shown as a singlet or relatively simple splitting pattern in the NMR spectrum), whereas the analogous protons are magnetically nonequivalent for the S,S-isomers, resulting in a much more complex pattern. This same relationship has been found to hold for the MAA diesters of the non-K-region dihydrodiols and tetrahydrodiols. However, the experimental findings are not always clearcut. In the case of the MAA diester of DMBA *trans*-5,6-dihydrodiol, only a small amount of splitting was observed for one of the methylene signals in the R,R-isomer and no splitting was observed for one of the signals of the S,S-isomer (Balani *et al.*, 1986). Also, the NMR spectrum of the MAA ester of the bromohydrin derivative of tetrahydrobenzo[e]pyrene failed to reveal any significant differences in the splitting pattern of the exocyclic methylene protons that could be correlated with the absolute configurations of the individual diastereomers (Lee & Harvey, 1984).

Chiral shift reagents have also been employed to determine directly the absolute configuration of arene oxides and the ratios of enantiomers in mixtures (Yeh *et al.*, 1986). The addition of tris[3-(trifluorome-thylhydroxymethylene)-(+)-camphorato]europium(III) [Eu(tfc)$_3$] to solutions of K-region arene oxides induced downfield shifts of the oxirane ring proton signals which differed in magnitude for each enantiomer. The absolute configurations could be correlated with the induced shifts. On the basis of the results with eleven oxiranes of known stereochemistry, it appears that [Eu(tfc)$_3$] may be used to predict the absolute configurations of other K-region arene oxides.

Finally, the absolute configurations of several K-region arene oxides have been determined by conversion to their monomethylether derivatives and comparison of their CD spectra with those of enantiomeric monomethyl ether derivatives derived from *trans*-dihydrodiol enantiomers of known absolute configuration (Weems *et al.*, 1987).

12.2.6   Polycyclic imines

K-region imines are synthetically accessible from the corresponding arene oxides by reaction with sodium azide and treatment of the resulting mixture of isomeric *trans*-azido alcohols with tri-*n*-butylphosphine (Blum *et al.*, 1979; Yona & Blum, 1981) (Fig. 12.17). The K-region imines of BA, 7-methyl-BA, DBA, BaP, and 3-MC were prepared by this procedure. However, transformation of the azido alcohols derived from the 5,6-oxides of DMBA and benzo[c]phenanthrene were not successful. Several *N*-alkylated K-region imine derivatives of phenanthrene 9,10-imine were prepared from the 9,10-oxide by addition of the appropriate amine followed by cyclodehydration with PPh$_3$–CCl$_4$ reagent (Ittah *et al.*, 1978).

BA 8,9-imine is apparently the only non-K-region imine known. It was synthesized from BA 8,9-oxide by sequential reaction with sodium azide and tri-*n*-butylphosphine (Blum & Ben-Shoshan, 1983).

12.3   Chemical properties and reactivity

Investigations into the chemistry of the polyarene oxides must take into account the facility of their rearrangements to phenols and/or oxepins and their relative ease of hydrolysis. These are likely to be competing reactions under most conditions. Obviously, acidic media and elevated temperatures are to be avoided. Similar considerations apply to the polyarene imines which are converted into aromatic amines by thermolysis or by treatment with protic acids.

12.3.1   Solvolysis

Since the metabolic reactions of arene oxides occur in aqueous media, solvolysis studies may provide useful insight into the reactions taking place under these conditions. Investigations of the solvolysis of the isomeric oxides of phenanthrene reveal significant differences in the chemistry of the K-region and non-K-region isomers (Bruice & Bruice, 1976; Bruice *et al.*, 1976).

In the solvolysis of the K-region phenanthrene 9,10-oxide, H_3O^+-catalyzed opening of the oxide ring (k_2) to yield the carbonium ion (**21**) is the predominant pathway between pH 2 and 5 (Fig. 12.18). Between pH 5 and 7, H_2O-catalyzed ring-opening (k_1) becomes important. The carbonium ion intermediate **21** can undergo rearrangement with NIH shift to form 9-phenanthrol (k_3) or be trapped by water to yield the *cis*- and *trans*-dihydrodiols (k_4). In the pH range 5 to 8.5 the disappearance of the oxide was found to be subject to general acid catalysis. The principle of microscopic reversibility requires that ring closure of **21** to reform the oxide ring be catalyzed by HO^- ion. As the pH increases, this reverse reaction (k_1-) begins to compete with k_3 and k_4, accounting for an observed decrease in

Fig. 12.17. K-region imines may be synthesized from K-region oxides in two steps.

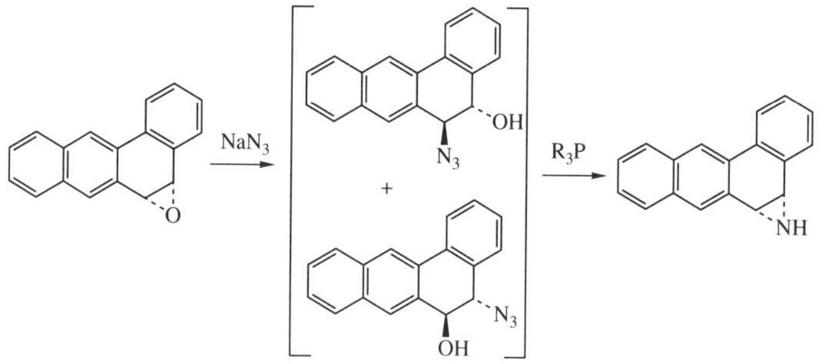

rate. Since the carbonium ion **21** is the dominant species in the lower pH range (2 to 8.5), the ratio of final products is constant in this region (75% phenol, 18% *trans*-diol, 7% *cis*-diol). Reactions at higher pH involve direct nucleophilic attack on the arene oxide by water and HO⁻ ion; this mechanism is consistent with the finding that the *trans*-dihydrodiol is virtually the sole product in the high pH range.

Studies of the solvolysis of the non-K-region 1,2- and 3,4-oxides of phenanthrene reveal a simpler picture. Below pH 6 they show general acid catalysis, while at higher pH the rate remains constant independent of pH. The major reaction path is ring-opening and subsequent NIH shift to give phenolic products. Dihydrodiol formation via nucleophilic attack on the oxide ring by water or hydroxyl ion does not occur to significant extent. The carbonium intermediates from the non-K-region oxides undergo more rapid intramolecular hydride transfer and proton elimination to yield phenols than does the K-region oxide.

Studies of the solvolysis of the K-oxides of the carcinogenic PAHs DMBA, BAP, and 3-MC reveal a similar, though somewhat more complex pattern of behavior (Keller & Heidelberger, 1976). In the pH range 3–6 these oxides produced 3:1 mixtures of the K-region phenols and dihydrodiols. The *cis/trans* dihydrodiol ratio varied from 20% for phenanthrene 9,10-oxide to 75% for 3-MC 11,12-oxide. The phenols were obtained as mixtures of the two possible positional isomers, the ratio of which varied markedly with the structure of the arene oxide.The results are consistent with a mechanism involving rate-limiting opening of the oxide ring, followed by competitive water attack on the intermediate benzylic carbocation or NIH shift to yield a phenol.

Substitution may strongly influence the course of solvolytic reaction. For example, solvolysis of 2- and 3-methoxyphenanthrene 9,10-oxide yields 2-methoxy-10-phenanthrol and 3-methoxy-9-phenanthrol, respectively

Fig. 12.18. Mechanism of solvolysis of arene oxides.

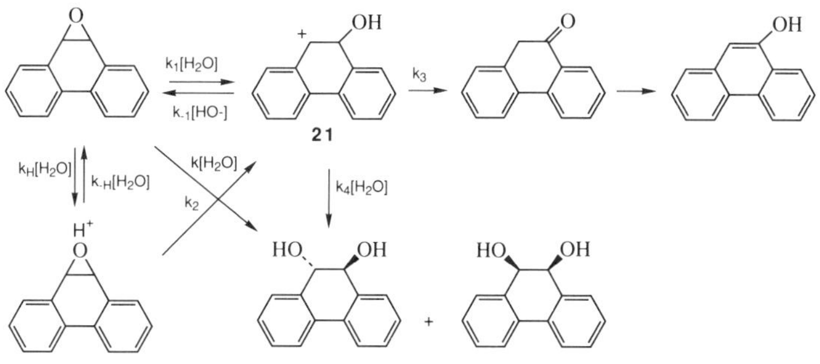

(Okamoto *et al.*, 1978); the alternative isomers are not detected. Carbomethoxy groups show contrary effects on the direction of ring opening.

12.3.2   Reactions with nucleophiles

The reactions of arene oxides with nucleophiles is of importance for mutagenicity and tumorigenicity, both of which are presumed to involve covalent binding to nucleic acids. Reactions with nucleophiles are also important for detoxification, known to involve reactions with glutathione and other cellular nucleophiles.

Detailed investigations of the mechanisms of the reactions of the isomeric arene oxides of phenanthrene with oxygen, nitrogen, and sulfur nucleophiles have been carried out by Bruice and coworkers (Bruice *et al.*, 1976a). The K-region oxide was found to undergo nucleophilic addition by oxygen bases, amines, and mercaptans. In general, oxygen bases are less reactive than amines, and tertiary amine bases such as trimethylamine exhibit enhanced nucleophilic reactivity. The second order rate constants for reaction of OH^-, CO_3^-, H_2O, and RNH_2 with phenanthrene 9,10-oxide and ethylene oxide are expressed by eq. 1. This relationship shows that the sensitivity of both oxides to the nature of the nucleophile is similar and that the arene oxide is more reactive than the aliphatic epoxide. On the other hand, for thiolate addition phenanthrene oxide is only one third as sensitive as ethylene oxide to the nucleophilicity of the thiol (eq. 2).

$$\log k_n[3] = 1.30 \log k_n[\text{ethylene oxide}] + 1.70 \qquad (1)$$

$$\log k_n[3] = 0.35 \log k_n[\text{ethylene oxide}] + 0.96 \qquad (2)$$

In the case of the non-K-region arene oxides, nucleophilic attack by amines and oxygen bases is insufficiently rapid to compete with spontaneous aromatization. Thiolate anions react with both K-region and non-K-region arene oxides, but the extent of reaction is considerably greater with the former. While phenanthrene 9,10-oxide is only slightly more reactive towards mercaptoethanol than are its 1,2- and 3,4-oxides, its lifetime is 100 times greater between pH 8.5 and 11.5. This is the major factor that determines the greater effectiveness of the 9,10-oxide in reacting with thiolate nucleophiles.

Tertiary amines catalyze the rearrangement of arene oxides to the corresponding phenols. The mechanism involves decomposition of the initial adducts via proton addition followed by general base-catalyzed (hydroxide and amine) elimination of the tertiary amine (Johnson & Bruice, 1975). It is likely that a similar process of aromatization occurs *in vivo* catalyzed by proteins, nucleic acids, and other cellular nucleophiles. This is expected to contribute to the detoxification of arene oxides and other reactive species formed metabolically.

An investigation of the reactions with *tert*-butylthiol of the K-oxides of higher polyarenes, including several potent carcinogens, was conducted by Beland & Harvey, 1976. *Tert*-butylthiolate was employed as a model sulfur nucleophile since the bulky *tert*-butyl group strongly favors the axial orientation, thereby locking the conformation of the adducts in this orientation and simplifying the interpretation of the NMR spectra of the products. The methyl protons of the *tert*-butyl group appear as a singlet at higher field than any of the ring hydrogen atoms. Reactions carried out in aqueous dioxane at basic pH gave the products of trans stereospecific addition, whereas similar reactions in THF furnished the *tert*-butylthio ether products arising from addition and subsequent dehydration. *For unsymmetrical arene oxides for which two isomeric adducts are possible, nucleophilic attack is predicted to take place preferentially at the site having the lowest Dewar reactivity number* (N_t) calculated by MO methods. In the case of benzo[c]phenanthrene oxide, comparison of the calculated reactivity of the two possible zwitterions **22a** and **22b** derived from the latter predict greater reactivity for **22b** ($N_t = 1.79$) than for **22a** ($N_t = 1.86$) (Fig. 12.19).

Consistent with this prediction, the product of reaction of *tert*-butylthiolate with benzo[c]phenanthrene oxide is exclusively the adduct formed from attack at the 6-position. The structures of the products formed with other K-oxides generally accord with the rule that initial nucleophilic attack occurs regioselectively at the most electrophilic center. It is worthy of note that the site of reaction may be influenced by a remote hydroxyl group. Thus, reaction of 9-hydroxy-BaP 4,5-oxide with ethanethiol takes place regiospecifically in the 5-position (Bochnitschek *et al.*, 1985), although BaP 4,5-oxide undergoes thiol addition less discriminately in both the 4- and 5-positions (Beland & Harvey, 1976).

While the structures of the arene oxide–thiol adducts are generally

Fig. 12.19. Nucleophilic attack is predicted to occur at the carbon atom of the epoxide ring with the lowest reactivity number in the corresponding zwitterion, i.e. **22b** ($N_t = 1.79$) rather than **22a** ($N_t = 1.86$).

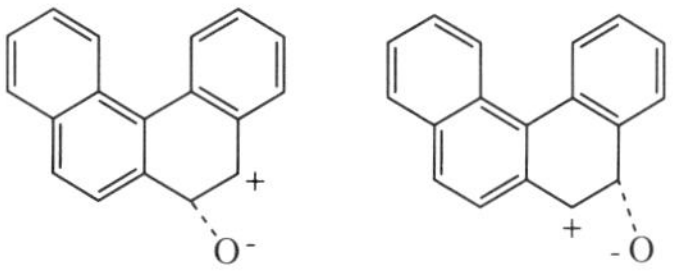

22a   22b

predictable, rearrangement may accompany their dehydration (Beland & Harvey, 1976). Thus, addition of *tert*-butyl thiolate to DMBA 5,6-oxide takes place preferentially at the 6-position in accord with MO prediction, but dehydration of the adduct occurs with migration of the sulfur group to the 5-position to furnish 5-*tert*-butyl-DMBA as the final product (Fig. 12.20). This rearrangement presumably proceeds via a sulfonium ion intermediate (**23**), and its driving forces are the steric interference between the 6-*tert*-butyl thiol group and the 7-methyl group and the greater stability of the carbonium ion at C-6 relative to C-5. Under acidic conditions of dehydration, sulfur migration occurs with considerably greater facility so that the same mixture of aryl alkyl thioethers is obtained upon reaction of either isomeric positional adduct, even for sterically uncrowded thiol–arene oxide adducts (Balani *et al.*, 1989). In some cases, acidic dehydration of thiol–arene oxide adducts has been shown to furnish variable amounts of the parent hydrocarbon as a secondary product. Thus, acid treatment of the adducts of benzo-[c]phenanthrene oxide with various thiols gave variable amounts of benzo[c]phenanthrene in addition to the expected thioether products (Balani *et al.*, 1989). A possible mechanism for hydrocarbon formation has been proposed that involves nucleophilic attack on sulfur in the sulfonium intermediate by the acidic counterion (e.g. Cl⁻ in the case of HCl).

Enzyme-catalyzed addition of glutathione to arene oxides is an important route for the detoxification of these metabolites. Synthetic preparation of the pure diastereomeric glutathione–arene oxide adducts is complicated by their relative facility of dehydration and decomposition. These difficulties may be minimized by the use of the *N*-trifluoroacetyl dimethyl ester of glutathione as the glutathione reagent (Hernandez & Gopinathan, 1984). The reactions of the K-oxides of phenanthrene, pyrene, and BaP with this reagent afforded the corresponding conjugates in good yield. The diastereomers were separated as their benzoate esters by HPLC methods. The isozymes of glutathione-S-transferase isolated from rat liver cytosol catalyze the addition of glutathione to K-oxides with variable efficiency and stereoselectivity (Cobb *et al.*, 1983).

Fig. 12.20. Dehydration of the adduct arising from attack of tert-butylthiolate on the 6-position of DMBA 5,6-oxide occurs with migration of sulfur via a sulfonium ion intermediate **23**.

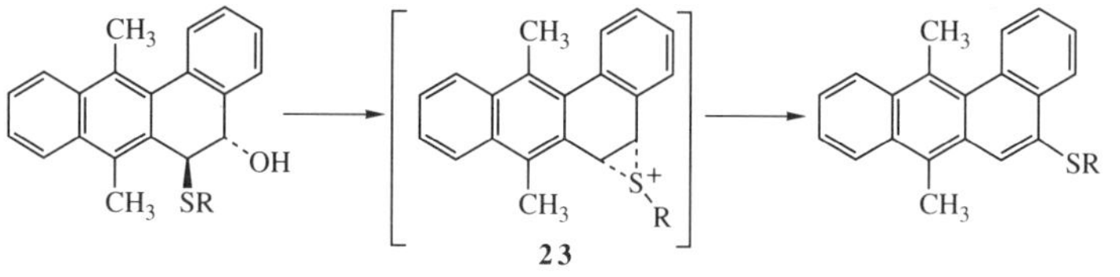

Isozyme C exhibits high stereoselectivity toward all substrates with predominant attack (> 95%) at the oxirane carbon of R absolute configuration to give the S,S product.

In other studies with sulfur nucleophiles, addition of sodium diethyldithiocarbamate (Et$_2$NCS$_2$Na) to phenanthrene 9,10-oxide is reported to yield a *trans* adduct (Stanior & Wiessler, 1984). The inhibitory effect of disulfiram on PAH carcinogenicity may be partially due to similar addition to reactive arene oxide metabolites.

Addition of oxygen nucleophiles to arene oxides often fails to compete favorably with isomerization to phenolic products. However, the addition of methoxide to naphthalene 1,2-oxide and phenanthrene 9,10-oxide is catalyzed by Woelm alumina to afford good yields of trans adducts (Posner & Rogers, 1977). The addition to naphthalene 1,2-oxide takes place exclusively in the 2-position. In other related studies, heating a mixture of phenanthrene 9,10-oxide with sodium phenoxide in DMF at 100 °C furnished 9-phenoxyphenanthrene (67%) and the trans addition product (19%) (Okamoto *et al.*, 1978). Similar results were obtained in analogous reactions with the sodium salts of *p*-cresol, and 1- and 2-naphthol.

The addition of nitrogen nucleophiles to arene oxides is of biological importance, since it is the principal mode of reaction of nucleic acids with PAH metabolites. Primary amines add to phenanthrene 9,10-oxide to yield *trans*-amino alcohol adducts (Dey & Neumeyer, 1974). These are useful intermediates for the preparation of the related *N*-alkylimines by treatment with trialkyl or triarylphosphine reagents (Ittah *et al.*, 1978). Reaction of sodium azide with K-region oxides gives *trans*-azido alcohols that may be converted to the corresponding K-region imines by treatment with Ph$_3$P (Fig. 12.17) (Blum *et al.*, 1979). Addition of sodium azide to naphthalene 1,2-oxide yields the trans adduct arising from attack at C-2 (Jeffrey *et al.*, 1974). Addition of nonpolarizable nitrogen nucleophiles to arene oxides is catalyzed by basic alumina (Posner & Rogers, 1977). In the presence of basic alumina, nucleophilic addition competes successfully with rearrangement to phenolic products, and both K- and non-K-region oxides yield *trans* adducts.

The reactions of polyarene imines with nucleophiles are relatively unexplored. The reactions of a series of substituted phenanthrene 9,10-imines with the model nucleophile N$_3^-$ afforded the corresponding *trans*-azido amines (Shtelzer *et al.*, 1988). The ratios of the isomeric azido amines from attack at C-9 and C-10 were virtually identical with the ratios of azido alcohols obtained from the analogous reactions of sodium azide with the corresponding phenanthrene 9,10-oxides. In both cases, the experimental findings showed excellent correlation with theoretical predictions based upon Huckel-type calculations of Wheland's π-localization energies.

12.3.3   Reduction and deoxygenation

K-region arene oxides are readily reduced with LiAlH4 to the corresponding alcohols. For example, treatment of phenanthrene 9,10-oxide with LiAlH4 gave 9-hydroxy-9,10-dihydrophenanthrene (Harvey *et al.*, 1976a), and analogous reaction of DMBA 5,6-oxide furnished 5-hydroxy-5,6-dihydro-DMBA accompanied by a trace of the 6-isomer (Harvey *et al.*, 1975).

Deoxygenation of phenanthrene 9,10-oxide and its substituted derivatives may be readily accomplished by treatment with various thione reagents, such as thiourea, *N*-methylbenzothiazole-2-thione, thioacetamide and thiosemicarbazone in organic solvents at room temperature (Griffin *et al.*, 1976). Pyrene 4,5-oxide also underwent deoxygenation under similar conditions. The reduction of arene oxides to the parent hydrocarbons may also be accomplished enzymatically (Booth *et al.*, 1975). Tetraphenylporphinatoiron(II) complex, a model complex for the reduced cytochrome P-450 enzyme, deoxygenates arene oxides (Miyata *et al.*, 1984). Yields were low (8–21%), so that this is not a synthetically useful reaction.

Finally, the polyarene imines are transformed into the parent hydrocarbons in high yield under nitrosating conditions (isoamyl nitrite and triethylamine) (Blum *et al.*, 1979).

12.4   References

Agarwal, S. A. & Van Duuren, B. L. (1977). Synthesis of 4,5:11,12-diepoxy-4,5,11,12-tetrahydrobenzo[a]pyrene and related compounds. *J. Org. Chem.* **42**, 2730–4.

Agarwal, S. C. & Van Duuren, B. L. (1975). Synthesis of diepoxides and diphenol ethers of pyrene and dibenz[a,h]anthracene. *J. Org. Chem.* **40**, 2307–10.

Agarwal, S. K., Boyd, D. R., Dunlop, R. & Jennings, W. B. (1988). Synthesis, spontaneous racemization, and photoisomerization of benz[e]pyrene 9,10-oxide. *J. Chem. Soc. Perkin I*, 3013–18.

Agarwal, S. K., Boyd, D. R. & Jennings, W. B. (1985). Synthesis of benzo[g]chrysene, benzo[g]chrysene 9,10-oxide and benzo[g]chrysene 1,2:9,10-dioxide. *J. Chem. Soc. Perkin I*, 857–60.

Agarwal, S. K., Boyd, D. R., Jennings, W. B., McGuckin, R. M. & O'Kane, G. A. (1989). General synthetic routes to diarene oxides of polycyclic aromatic hydrocarbons. *Tetrahedron Lett.* **30**, 123–6.

Aktar, M. N. & Boyd, D. R. (1975). Application of a new resolution method to chiral epoxides, arene oxides, and alcohols. *J. Chem. Soc. Chem. Commun.* 916–17.

Aktar, M. N., Boyd, D. R. & Hamilton, J. G. (1979). Synthesis of (+)- and (–)-naphthalene and anthracene 1,2-oxides. *J. Chem. Soc. Perkin I*, 2437–40.

Armstrong, R. N., Kedzierski, B., Levin, W. & Jerina, D. M. (1981). Enantioselectivity of microsomal epoxide hydrolase toward arene oxide metabolites. *J. Biol. Chem.* **256**, 4726–33.

Avnir, D., Grauer, A., Dinur, D. & Blum, J. (1975). Disubstituted 'K-region arene oxides'. *Tetrahedron*, **31**, 2547–59.

Balani, S. K., Boyd, D. R., Cassidy, E. S., Devine, D. G., Malone, J. F., McCombe, K. M., Sharma, N. D. & Jennings, J. W. (1983). A general method for the resolution of cyclic trans-bromohydrin enantiomers. Absolute configuration by crystal structure analysis of a 2-methoxy-2-phenyl-2-trifluoromethylacetate (MTPA) diastereomer. *J. Chem. Soc. Perkin I*, 2751–6.

Balani, S. K., Boyd, D. R., Greene, R. M. E. & Jerina, D. M. (1984). Synthesis and thermal racemization of the 3,4-oxide metabolite of benzo[c]phenanthrene. *J. Chem. Soc. Perkin I*, 1781–4.

Balani, S. K., Sayer, J. M. & Jerina, D. M. (1989). Rearrangements on acid-catalyzed dehydration of regioisomeric thiol adducts formed from K-region arene oxides. *J. Am. Chem. Soc.* **111**, 3290–5.

Balani, S. K., Van Bladeren, P. J., Cassidy, E. S., Boyd, D. R. & Jerina, D. M. (1987). Synthesis of the enantiomeric K-region arene 5,6-oxides derived from chrysene, 7,12-dimethylbenz[a]anthracene, and benzo[c]phenanthrene. *J. Org. Chem.* **52**, 137–44.

Balani, S. K., Van Bladeren, P. J., Shirai, N. & Jerina, D. M. (1986). Resolution and absolute configuration of K-region trans dihydrodiols from polycyclic aromatic hydrocarbons. *J. Org. Chem.* **51**, 1773–8.

Bartczak, A. W., Sangaiah, R., Ball, L. M., Warren, S. H. & Gold, A. (1987). Synthesis and bacterial mutagenicity of the cyclopenta oxides of the four cyclopenta-fused isomers of benzanthracene. *Mutagenesis*, **2**, 101–5.

Beland, F. A. & Harvey, R. G. (1976). Reactions of the K-region oxides of carcinogenic and related polycyclic hydrocarbons with nucleophiles: Stereochemistry and regio-selectivity. *J. Am. Chem. Soc.* **98**, 4963–70.

Bicker, U. & Fischer, W. (1974). Enzymatic aziridine synthesis from ß aminoalcohols-a new example of endogenous carcinogen formation. *Nature (Lond.)*, **249**, 344–5.

Blum, J. & Ben-Shoshan, S. (1983). 1a,11b-Dihydrobenz[5,6]anthra[1,2-b]azirine. A non K-region polycyclic arene imine. *J. Heterocyclic Chem.* **20**, 1461–4.

Blum, J., Yona, I., Tsaroom, S. & Sasson, Y. (1979). 'K-region' imines of some carcinogenic aromatic hydrocarbons. *J. Org. Chem.* **44**, 4178–82.

Bochnitschek, W., Seidel, A. & Kunz, H. (1985). Reactive metabolites of carcinogenic polycyclic hydrocarbons: Synthesis and trapping reaction of 9-hydroxybenzo[a]pyrene 4,5-oxide. *Angew. Chem. Int. Ed. Engl.* **24**, 699–700.

Booth, J., Hewer, A., Keysell, G. R. & Sims, P. (1975). Enzymatic reduction of aromatic hydrocarbon epoxides by the microsomal fraction of rat liver. *Xenobiotica*, **5**, 197–203.

Boyd, D. R., Agarwal, S. K., Balani, S. K., Dunlop, R., Gadaginamath, G. S., O'Kane, G. A., Sharma, N. D., Jennings, W. B., Yagi, H. & Jerina, D. M. (1987). Preparation of oxepins during direct chemical synthesis and facile oxygen walk reactions of arene oxides: Theoretical predictions and experimental evidence. *J. Chem. Soc. Chem. Commun.* 1633–5.

Boyd, D. R., Burnett, M. G. & Greene, R. M. E. (1983). Synthesis and thermal racemization of the predominant arene oxide metabolite of chrysene, (+)-(3S,4R)-chrysene 3,4-oxide. *J. Chem. Soc. Perkin I*, 595–9.

Boyd, D. R., Daly, J. W. & Jerina, D. M. (1972). Rearrangement of [1-^{2}H]- and [2-^{2}H]-naphthalene oxides to 1-naphthol. Mechanism of the NIH shift. *Biochemistry*, **11**, 1961–6.

Boyd, D. R., Dawson, K. A., Gadaginamath, G. S., Hamilton, J. G., Malone, J. F. & Sharma, N. A. (1981). Synthesis and absolute stereochemistry of (+)- and (–)-benz[a]anthracene 8,9-oxide and derived mammalian liver metabolites of benz[a]anthracene. *J. Chem. Soc. Perkin I*, 94–7.

Boyd, D. R., Gadaginamath, G. S., Kher, A., Malone, J. F., Yagi, H. & Jerina, D. M. (1980). (+)- and (-)-Benzo[a]pyrene 7,8-oxide: Synthesis, absolute stereochemistry, and stereochemical correlation with other mammalian metabolites of benzo[a]pyrene. *J. Chem. Soc. Perkin I*, 2112–6.

Boyd, D. R., Gadaginamath, G. S., Sharma, N. A., Drake, A. F., Mason, S. F. & Jerina, D. M. (1981a). The synthesis of chiral arene oxide metabolites of benz[a]anthracene: Optically active benz[a]anthracene 10,11- and 5,6-oxides. *J. Chem. Soc. Perkin I*, 2233–8.

Boyd, D. R. & Greene, R. M. E. (1982). Synthesis, resolution and racemization studies of 1,2-epoxy-1,2-dihydrochrysene. *J. Chem. Soc. Perkin I*, 1535–9.

Boyd, D. R., Kennedy, D. A., Malone, J. F. & O'Kane, G. A. (1987a). Synthesis of triphenylene 1,2-oxide (1,2-epoxy-1,2-dihydrotriphenylene) and absolute configuration of the trans-1,2-dihydro diol metabolite of triphenylene. Crystal structure of (−)-(1R,2R)-trans-2-bromo-1-menthyloxyacetoxy-1,2,3,4-tetrahydrotriphenylene. *J. Chem. Soc. Perkin I*, 369–75.

Boyd, D. R., Neill, J. D. & Stubbs, M. E. (1977). Chemical resolution and racemization of 1,2- and 3,4-epoxydihydrophenanthrene. *J. Chem. Soc. Chem. Commun.* 873–4.

Boyd, D. R. & O'Kane, G. A. (1987). Synthesis and oxygen-walk rearrangement of dibenz(a,c)anthracene 1,2-oxide. *Tetrahedron Lett.* **28**, 6395–6.

Boyd, D. R. & Sharma, N. A. (1984). Synthesis and spontaneous racemization of benz[a]anthracene 1,2-oxide. *J. Chem. Soc. Perkin I*, 839–41.

Boyd, D. R. & Stubbs, M. (1983). Arene oxide–oxepin isomerization. Theoretical predictions and experimental evidence. *J. Amer. Chem. Soc.* **105**, 2554–9.

Boyland, E. & Sims, P. (1965). The metabolism of benz[a]anthracene and dibenz[a,h]anthracene and their 5,6-epoxy-5,6-dihydro derivatives by rat-liver homogenates. *Biochem. J.* **97**, 7–16.

Boyland, E. & Sims, P. (1967). The carcinogenic activities in mice of compounds related to benz[a]anthracene. *Internat. J. Cancer*, **2**, 500–504.

Bruice, T. C. & Bruice, P. Y. (1976). Solution chemistry of arene oxides. *Acc. Chem. Res.* **9**, 378–84.

Bruice, T. C., Bruice, P. Y., Dansette, P. M., Selander, H. C., Yagi, H. & Jerina, D. M. (1976). Comparisons of the mechanisms of solvolysis and rearrangement of K-region vs. non-K-region arene oxides of phenanthrene. Comparative solvolytic rate constants of K-region and non-K-region arene oxides. *J. Amer. Chem. Soc.* **98**, 2965–72.

Bruice, T. C., Bruice, P. Y., Yagi, H. & Jerina, D. M. (1976a). Nucleophilic displacement on the arene oxides of phenanthrene. *J. Amer. Chem. Soc.* **98**, 2973–81.

Chang, R. L., Wood, A. W., Levin, W., Mah, H. D., Thakker, D. R., Jerina, D. M. & Conney, A. H. (1979). Differences in mutagenicity and cytotoxicity of (+)- and (−)-benzo(a)pyrene 4,5-oxide: A synergistic interaction of enantiomers. *Proc. Natl. Acad. Sci. USA.* **76**, 4280–84.

Cobb, D., Boehlert, C., Lewis, D. & Armstrong, R. N. (1983). Stereoselectivity of isozyme C of glutathione S-transferase toward arene and azaarene oxides. *Biochemistry*, **22**, 805–12.

Croisey-Delcey, M., Ittah, Y. & Jerina, D. M. (1979). Synthesis of benzo[c]phenanthrene dihydrodiols. *Tetrahedron Lett.* 2849–52.

Dansette, P. & Jerina, D. M. (1974). A facile synthesis of arene oxides at the K-regions of polycyclic hydrocarbons. *J. Amer. Chem. Soc.* **96**, 1224–5.

Dey, A. S. & Neumeyer, J. L. (1974). Synthesis and antimalarial evaluation of 9,10-dihydrophenanthrene amino alcohols. *J. Med. Chem.* **17**, 1095–1100.

Di Raddo, P. & Chan, T. H. (1982). Reactions at the K-region epoxides of polycyclic aromatic hydrocarbons with phosphodiesters. A potential detoxification reaction. *J. Org. Chem.* **47**, 1427–31.

Engel, J. F., Sankaran, V., McCaustland, D. J., Kolwyck, K. C., Ebert, D. A. & Duncan, W. P. (1978). Synthesis of carbon-13 labeled benzo[a]pyrene. *Polycyclic Hydrocarbons and Cancer*, 1, eds H. V. Gelboin & P. O. P. Ts'o, pp. 167–71, New York: Academic Press.

Fonouni, H. E., Krishnan, S., Kuhn, D. G. & Hamilton, G. A. (1983). Mechanism of epoxidations and chlorinations of hydrocarbons by inorganic hydrochloride in the presence of a phase-transfer catalyst. *J. Amer. Chem. Soc.* **105**, 7672–6.

Fu, P. P., Beland, F. & Yang, S. K. (1980). Cyclopenta polycyclic aromatic hydrocarbons: Potential carcinogens and mutagens. *Carcinogenesis*, **1**, 725–7.

Fu, P. P. & Harvey, R. G. (1977). [G-^{3}H]-7,12-Dimethylbenz[a]anthracene-5,6-oxide. *J. Label. Cpds. Radiopharm.* **13**, 619–21.

Fu, P. P., Harvey, R. G. & Beland, F. (1978). Molecular orbital theoretical prediction of the isomeric products formed from reactions of arene oxides and related metabolites of polycyclic aromatic hydrocarbons. *Tetrahedron*, **34**, 857–66.

Glatt, H., Ludewig, G., Platt, K. L., Waechter, F., Yona, I., Ben-Shoshan, S., Jerushalmy, P.,

Blum, J. & Oesch, F. (1985). Arene imines, a new class of exceptionally potent mutagens in bacterial and mammalian cells. *Cancer Res.* **45**, 2600–7.

Glatt, H., Shtelzer, S., Sheradsky, T., Blum, J. & Oesch, F. (1986). Mutagenicity of N-substituted phenanthrene 9,10-imines in *Salmonella typhimurium* and Chinese hamster V-79 cells. *Environ. Mutagen.* **8**, 829–37.

Glusker, J. (1985). X-ray analyses of polycyclic hydrocarbon metabolite structures. In *Polycyclic Hydrocarbons and Carcinogenesis.* ACS Symp. Vol. 283, ed. R. G. Harvey, pp.125–85. Washington, DC: American Chemical Society.

Gold, A., Brewster, J. & Eisenstadt, E. (1979). Synthesis of cyclopenta[cd]pyrene 3,4-epoxide, the ultimate mutagenic metabolite of the environmental carcinogen, cyclopenta[cd]pyrene. *J. Chem. Soc. Chem. Commun.* 903–4.

Griffin, G. W., Ishikawa, K. & Satra, S. K. (1976). Deoxygenation of arene oxides. Models for enzymatic deoxygenation. *J. Heterocyclic Chem.* **13**, 1369–70.

Griffin, G. W., Satra, S. K., Brightwell, N. E., Ishikawa, K. & Bhacca, N. S. (1976a). Synthesis and photorearrangement of substituted K-region arene oxides. *Tetrahedron Lett.* 1239–42.

Harada, N. & Nakanishi, K. (1972). The exciton chirality method and its application to configurational and conformational studies of natural products. *Acc. Chem. Res.* **5**, 257–63.

Harvey, R. G. (1986). Synthesis of oxidized metabolites of carcinogenic hydrocarbons. *Synthesis*, 605–19.

Harvey, R. G. & Cortez, C. (1983). K-region oxidized metabolites of 9-hydroxybenzo[a]pyrene. *Carcinogenesis*, **4**, 941–2.

Harvey, R. G. & Fu, P. (1976). Synthesis of high specific activity benzo[a]pyrene-6-*t* and its K-region oxidized derivatives. *J. Label. Cpds. Radiopharm*, **12**, 259–64.

Harvey, R. G., Fu, P. & Rabideau, P. W. (1976a). Stereochemistry of 1,3-cyclohexadienes. Conformational preferences in 9-substituted 9,10-dihydrophenanthrenes. *J. Org. Chem.* **41**, 3722–5.

Harvey, R. G., Goh, S. H. & Cortez, C. (1975). 'K-region' arene oxides and related oxidized metabolites of carcinogenic aromatic hydrocarbons. *J. Amer. Chem. Soc.* **97**, 3468–79.

Hernandez, O. & Gopinathan, M. B. (1984). Synthesis of glutathione adducts of K-region arene oxides. *J. Chem. Soc. Chem. Commun.* 1491–2.

Hylarides, M. D., Lyle, T. A., Daub, G. H. & Jagt, D. L. V. (1979). Carbon-13 nuclear magnetic resonance study of nucleophilic additions to benzo[a]pyrene 4,5-oxide and of its acid-catalyzed rearrangement. *J. Org. Chem.* **44**, 4652–7.

Ishikawa, K., Charles, H. C. & Griffin, G. W. (1977). Direct peracid oxidation of polynuclear hydrocarbons to arene oxides. *Tetrahedron Lett.* 427–30.

Ittah, Y., Shahak, I. & Blum, J. (1978). Stable arene imines. *J. Org. Chem.* **43**, 397–402.

Jeffrey, A. M., Yeh, H. J., Jerina, D. M., Marinis, R. M., Foster, C. H., Piccolo, D. E. & Berchtold, G. A. (1974). Stereochemical course in reactions between nucleophiles and arene oxides. *J. Amer. Chem. Soc.* **96**, 6229–37.

Jeyaraman, R. & Murray, R. W. (1984). Production of arene oxides by the caroate–acetone system (dimethyldioxirane). *J. Amer. Chem. Soc.* **106**, 2462–3.

Johnson, D. M. & Bruice, T. C. (1975). Nucleophilic catalysis of the aromatization of an arene oxide. The reaction of trimethylamine with 4-carbo-*tert*-butoxylbenzene oxide. *J. Am. Chem. Soc.* **97**, 6901–3.

Kedzierski, B., Thakker, D. R., Armstrong, R. N. & Jerina, D. M. (1981). Absolute configuration of the K-region 4,5-dihydrodiols and 4,5-oxide of benzo[a]pyrene. *Tetrahedron Lett.* 405–8.

Keller, J. W. & Heidelberger, C. (1976). Polycyclic K-region arene oxides. Products and kinetics of solvolysis. *J. Amer. Chem. Soc.* **98**, 2328–36.

Kinstle, T. H. & Ihrig, P. J. (1970). Acenaphthylene oxide. *J. Org. Chem.* **35**, 257–8.

Kolwyck, K. C., Duncan, W. P., Engel, J. F. & Selkirk, J. K. (1976). Labeled metabolites of polycyclic aromatic hydrocarbons. II. 4,5-Dihydrobenzo[a]pyrene-4,5-epoxide-G-^{3}H via cis-4,5-dihydrobenzo[a]pyrene-4,5-diol-G-^{3}H. *J. Label. Cpds. Radiopharm.* **12**, 153–8.

304 *Arene oxides and imines*

Konieczny, M. & Harvey, R. G. (1982). Oxidized metabolites of 7-methylbenzo[a]pyrene. *Carcinogenesis*, **3**, 573–5.

Krishnan, S., Kuhn, D. G. & Hamilton, G. A. (1977). Direct oxidation in high yield of some polycyclic aromatic compounds to arene oxides using hypochlorite and phase transfer catalysts. *J. Amer. Chem. Soc.* **99**, 8121–3.

Krishnan, S., Kuhn, D. G. & Hamilton, G. A. (1977a). The formation of arene oxides by direct oxidation of arenes using carbodimides and hydrogen peroxide. *Tetrahedron Lett.* 1369–72.

Kuroda, R. & Neidle, S. (1983). Molecular structure of (±)-3,4-epoxycyclopenta[cd]pyrene; and X-ray crystallographic study. *Carcinogenesis*, **4**, 217–19.

Lee, H. & Harvey, R. G. (1984). The absolute configuration of the 9,10-epoxides of 9,10,11,12-tetrahydrobenzo[e]pyrene: Application of the exciton chirality rule to a *p*-menthoxybenzoate of a bromohydrin. *J. Org. Chem.* **49**, 1114–17.

McCaustland, D. J., Ruehle, P. H. & Wiley, J. C. Jr (1980). Synthesis of cyclopenta[cd]pyrene-3,4-oxide, the suspected ultimate carcinogenic metabolite of cyclopenta[cd]pyrene. *J. Chem. Soc. Chem. Commun.* 93–4.

Miyata, N., Santa, T. & Hirobe, M. (1984). Deoxygenation of tertiary amine *N*-oxides and arene oxides by iron(II) porphyrin as a model of cytochrome P-450 dependent reduction. *Chem. Pharm. Bull.* **32**, 377–80.

Moriarity, R. M., Dansette, P. & Jerina, D. M. (1975). Pyrene derivatives oxygenated at both K-regions. Synthesis of a bis-arene oxide. *Tetrahedron Lett.* 2257–60.

Mushtaq, M., Weems, H. B. & Yang, S. K. (1984). Resolution and absolute configuration of 7,12-dimethylbenz[a]anthracene 5,6-oxide enantiomers. *Biochem. Biophys. Res. Commun.* **125**, 539–45.

Nagano, T., Yohoohji, K. & Hirobe, M. (1983). Direct epoxidation of polycyclic aromatic compounds by superoxide in the presence of phosgene dimer. *Tetrahedron Lett.* 3481–4.

Newman, M. S. & Blum, S. (1964). A new cyclization reaction leading to epoxides of aromatic hydrocarbons. *J. Amer. Chem. Soc.* **86**, 5598–600.

Okamoto, T., Shudo, K., Miyata, N., Kitahara, Y. & Nagata, S. (1978). Reactions of K-region oxides of carcinogenic and noncarcinogenic aromatic hydrocarbons. Comparative studies on reactions with nucleophiles and acid-catalyzed reactions. *Chem. Pharm. Bull.* **26**, 2014–26.

Platt, K. L. & Oesch, F. (1982). K-region trans-dihydrodiols of polycyclic arenes; an efficient and convenient preparation from *o*-quinones and *o*-diphenols by reduction with sodium borohydride in the presence of oxygen. *Synthesis*, 459–61.

Platt, K. L., Frank, H. & Oesch, F. (1982). Synthesis of the non-K-region arene oxides and tetrahydro epoxides of dibenz[a,h]anthracene. *J. Chem. Soc. Perkin I*, 2229–33.

Posner, G. H. & Rogers, D. Z. (1977). Organic reactions at alumina surfaces. Mild and selective opening of arene and related oxides by weak oxygen and nitrogen nucleophiles. *J. Amer. Chem. Soc.* **99**, 8214–18.

Rice, J. E., Coleman, D. T., Hosted T. J. Jr., LaVoie, E. J., McCaustland, D. J. & Wiley, J. C. Jr. (1985). Identification of mutagenic metabolites of indeno[1,2,3-cd]pyrene formed in vitro with rat liver enzymes. *Cancer Res.* **45**, 5421–5.

Robinson, P. L., Barry, C. N., Kelly, J. W. & Evans, S. A. J. (1985). Diethoxytriphenyl-phosphorane: A mild, regioselective cyclodehydrating reagent for the conversion of diols to cyclic ethers. Stereochemistry, synthetic utility, and scope. *J. Amer. Chem. Soc.* **107**, 5210–19.

Sangaiah, R. & Gold, A. (1985). A short and convenient synthesis of cyclopenta[cd]pyrene and its oxygenated derivatives. *Polynuclear Aromatic Hydrocarbons.* 8th Internat. Symp., eds M. Cooke & A. J. Dennis, pp. 1145–1150, Columbus, OH: Battelle.

Sayer, J. M., van Bladeren, P. J., Yeh, H. J. C. & Jerina, D. M. (1986). Absolute configuration of benzo[c]phenanthrene 5,6-oxide and other K-region derivatives. *J. Org. Chem.* **51**, 452–6.

Shtelzer, S., Meyer, A. Y., Sheradsky, T. & Blum, J. (1988). Regioselectivity of nucleophilic ring opening in substituted phenanthrene 9,10-imine and 9,10-oxide. Molecular orbital theoretical predictions and experimental results. *J. Org. Chem.* **53**, 161–6.

Silverman, I. R., Daub, G. & Jagt, D. L. V. (1985). Methoxybenzo[a]pyrene 4,5-oxides labeled with carbon-13: Electronic effects in the NIH shift. *J. Org. Chem.* **50**, 5550–6.

Sims, P. (1971). Epoxy derivatives of aromatic polycyclic hydrocarbons. The preparation of benz[a]anthracene 8,9-oxide and 10,11-dihydrobenz[a]anthracene 8,9-oxide and their metabolism by rat liver preparations. *Biochem. J.* **125**, 159–68.

Sims, P. (1972). Epoxy derivatives of aromatic polycyclic hydrocarbons. The synthesis of dibenz[a,c]anthracene 10,11-oxide and its metabolism by rat liver preparations. *Biochem. J.* **130**, 27–35.

Stanior, U. & Wiessler, M. (1984). Reaction of aromatic epoxides with sodium diethyl-dithiocarbamate. *Arch. Pharm. (Weinheim. Ger.)*, **317**, 1042–7.

Van Bladeren, P. J. & Jerina, D. M. (1983). Facile synthesis of K-region arene oxides. *Tetrahedron Lett.* **24**, 4903–6.

Van Duuren, B. L., Witz, G. & Agarwal, S. C. (1974). Synthesis and photorearrangement of 4,5-epoxy-4,5-dihydropyrene. *J. Org. Chem.* **39**, 1032–5.

Vogel, E. & Klarner, F. G. (1968). 1,2-Naphthalene oxide. *Angew. Chem. Int. Ed. Engl.* **7**, 374–5.

Waterfall, J. F. & Sims, P. (1972). Epoxy derivatives of aromatic polycyclic hydrocarbons. The preparation and metabolism of epoxides related to benzo[a]pyrene and to 7,8- and 9,10-dihydrobenzo[a]pyrene. *Biochem. J.* **128**, 265–77.

Weems, H. B., Mushtaq, M. & Yang, S. K. (1985). Resolution of epoxide enantiomers of polycyclic aromatic hydrocarbons by chiral stationary-phase high-performance liquid chromatography. *Anal. Biochem.* **148**, 328–38.

Weems, H. B., Mushtaq, M. & Yang, S. K. (1987). Absolute configurations of K-region epoxide enantiomers of 3-methylcholanthrene, benz[a]anthracene, and benzo[a]pyrene. *Anal. Chem.* **59**, 2679–88.

Yagi, H., Dansette, P. & Jerina, D. M. (1976). Specifically tritiated arene oxides. *J. Label. Cpds. Radiopharm.* **12**, 127–32.

Yagi, H. & Jerina, D. M. (1975). A general synthetic method for non-K-region arene oxides. *J. Amer. Chem. Soc.* **97**, 3185–92.

Yang, S. K. & Bao, Z. (1987). Stereoselective formations of K-region and non-K-region epoxides in the metabolism of chrysene by rat liver microsomal cytochrome P-450 isozymes. *Mol. Pharmacol.* **32**, 73–80.

Yang, S. K. & Chiu, P. (1985). Cytochrome P-450-catalyzed stereoselective epoxidation at the K-region of benz[a]anthracene and benzo[a]pyrene. *Arch. Biochem. Biophys.* **240**, 546–52.

Yang, S. K. & Weems, H. B. (1984). Direct enantiomeric resolution of some 7,12-dimethylbenz[a]anthracene derivatives by high-performance liquid chromatography with ionically and covalently bonded chiral stationary phases. *Anal. Chem.* **1984**, 2658–62.

Yeh, H. J. C., Balani, S. K., Yagi, H., Greene, R. M. E., Sharma, N. D., Boyd, D. R. & Jerina, D. M. (1986). Use of chiral lanthanide shift reagents in the determination of enantiomer composition and absolute configuration of epoxides and arene oxides. *J. Org. Chem.* **51**, 5439–43.

Yona, I. & Blum, J. (1981). A general synthesis of unsubstituted polycyclic arene imines. 3-Methylcholanthrene 11,12-imine. *Org. Prep. Proc. Int.* **13**, 109–12.

13

Dihydrodiols

Dihydrodiols are important secondary metabolites of PAHs produced by the hydration, enzymatic or nonenzymatic, of the primary arene oxides. This chapter surveys their structural and stereochemical properties, methods of synthesis, and chemical reactivity. It is based partially on earlier reviews of the synthesis (Harvey, 1986) and stereochemistry (Harvey, 1989) of polyarene dihydrodiol metabolites. Since the methods of synthesis and chemical properties of dihydrodiols are dependent upon their structural type, the various classes of dihydrodiols, K-region, bay region, etc., are discussed separately.

13.1   K-region dihydrodiols
13.1.1   Structure and stereochemistry
Dihydrodiols of this class may exist as *cis* or *trans* stereoisomers dependent upon whether the hydroxyl groups are on the same or the opposite faces of the molecule. For each of these diastereomers there are two possible conformers existing in dynamic equilibrium (Fig. 13.1). The hydroxyl groups of the *trans*-dihydrodiols may be oriented diaxially or diequatorially, while those of the corresponding *cis* isomers may equilibrate between axial–equatorial or equatorial–axial. Moreover, both the *cis* and *trans* isomers may also exist as pairs of optically active enantiomers, depending upon molecular symmetry.

K-region *trans*-dihydrodiols unsubstituted in the adjacent *peri* aromatic ring positions tend to exist predominantly in the diequatorial conformation in solution in aprotic solvents (Harvey, 1989). Thus, the ^{1}H NMR coupling constants between the carbinol protons of a series of such dihydrodiols are relatively large (9.9 – 10.3 Hz), indicative of a preferred diequatorial conformation (Harvey *et al.*, 1976). However, the position of the conformational equilibrium is solvent dependent. In aprotic solvents, such as acetone and chloroform, the diequatorial conformer is stabilized by hydrogen bonding between the hydroxyl groups. In protic solvents this effect is markedly diminished, allowing the equilibrium to shift in the direction of the diaxial conformer. The importance of intramolecular hydrogen-bonding in aprotic solvents is supported by the earlier observation that 9-hydroxy-9,10-dihydrophenanthrene, with only a single hydroxyl group, exists predominantly (94%) in the diaxial conformation in chloroform (Harvey *et al.*, 1976). In the biological milieux, it is likely that the hydroxyl groups of the K-region *trans*-dihydrodiols are associated with water molecules, favoring the diaxial conformation. It should be emphasized that the energies for conformational interconversion are relatively low so that the position of the conformational equilibrium may be readily shifted to favor the less stable conformer by interactions with solvents, nucleic acids, or other molecules.

The position of the conformational equilibria in aprotic solvents may be calculated from the relationship: $J_{obs} = xJ_{ee} + (1 - x)J_{aa}$, where J_{obs} is the observed coupling for the benzylic protons and J_{aa} and J_{ee} are the coupling constants for these protons in the conformations in which the hydroxyl groups are diaxial and diequatorial, respectively. Using the values of $J_{aa} = 16$ and $J_{ee} = 2$ Hz employed previously for the 9,10-dihydrophenanthrenes (Harvey *et al.*, 1976), the fraction (x) of the diequatorial conformers are calculated to be 57–60% for the unsubstituted K-region dihydrodiols of BA, BaP, and DBA (Harvey, 1989).

Esterification of the *trans*-dihydrodiols generally shifts the equilibrium strongly in favor of the diaxial conformer due to the greater steric requirement of the ester functions and the loss of intramolecular hydrogen-bonding. This effect is clearly evident in the lower values of the coupling

Fig. 13.1. The conformational equilibrium between the *trans*-diequatorial and *trans*-diaxial conformers of K-region dihydrodiols favors the former in aprotic solvents due to internal H-bonding. In protic solvents, such as water, it is likely that the latter predominates.

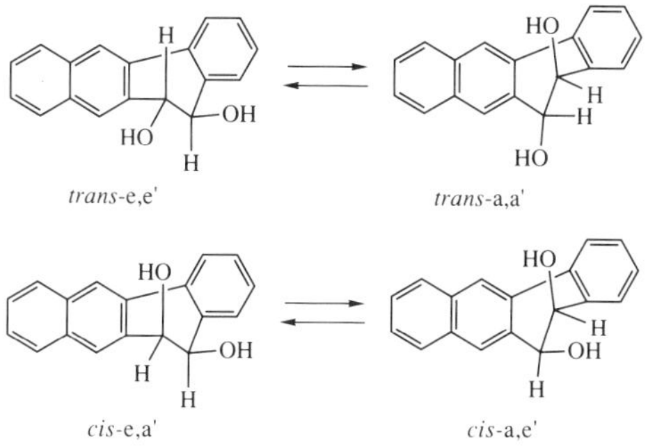

constants of the benzylic protons which are generally in the range of 1–2 Hz (Harvey, 1989). The position of the conformational equilibrium may also be affected by steric interaction with groups in the adjacent peri positions. Thus, the *trans*-5,6-dihydrodiol of DMBA exists in a preferred *trans*-a,a' conformation (Jeffrey *et al.*, 1976). This is consistent with the relatively low value of the coupling constant of its K-region benzylic protons ($J_{5,6} = 3.2 \pm 0.5$ Hz). The 4-methyl-, 7-methyl-, 7-bromo-, and 7-fluoro-derivatives of the *trans*-5,6-dihydrodiols of BA also exhibit small coupling constants (2.6 – 3.2 Hz), indicating that they also exist preferentially in the *trans*-a,a' conformation (Fu *et al.*, 1983).

For the corresponding *cis*-dihydrodiols, the conformational equilibrium is relatively independent of solvent effects, but steric interaction with groups in the peri positions shifts the equilibrium in favor of the conformer having an axially oriented hydroxyl group in the adjacent benzylic position. X-ray analysis of the crystal structure of the DMBA *cis*-5,6-dihydrodiol shows that the 6-hydroxyl group is axial and the 5-hydroxyl group is equatorial (Zacharias *et al.*, 1977). The ring system is also severely distorted from planarity as a consequence of the steric interaction between the 12-methyl group and the benzo ring. The coupling constant of the K-region benzylic protons ($J_{5,6} = 3.4 \pm 0.5$ Hz) of the DMBA *cis*-5,6-dihydrodiol was similar to that of the *trans* diastereomer, indicating that assignment of stereo-chemistry on the basis of ^{1}H-NMR data alone is unsafe (Jeffrey *et al.*, 1976). The *cis*-5,6-dihydrodiol of 7-methyl-BA also had $J_{5,6} = 3.4$ Hz, consistent with its existence in a similar conformation (Yang & Fu, 1984).

13.1.2   Synthesis and reactivity

K-region *cis*-dihydrodiols are directly accessible from the parent polyarenes by reaction with osmium tetroxide. This reagent reacts with the electron-rich K-region bonds regiospecifically (Cook & Schoental, 1948). Although the crude *cis*-dihydrodiol products tend to decompose in air, they are readily purified by diacetylation, followed by column chromatography and regeneration by treatment with methanolic ammonia (Harvey *et al.*, 1975). K-region *cis*-dihydrodiols synthesized by this method include the derivatives of BA (Cook & Schoental, 1948; Harvey *et al.*, 1975), 1-methyl-BA (Cook & Schoental, 1948), 7-methyl-BA (Newman & Blum, 1964; Sims, 1967), 12-methyl-BA (Sims, 1967), DMBA (Harvey *et al.*, 1975), 3-MC (Sims, 1966), chrysene (Cook & Schoental, 1948), benzo[c]phenanthrene (Balani *et al.*, 1987); pyrene (Cook & Schoental, 1948), BaP (Harvey *et al.*, 1975), 7-methyl-BaP (Konieczny & Harvey, 1980), 9-methoxy-BaP (Harvey & Cortez, 1983; Bochnitschek *et al.*, 1985), BeP (Lehr *et al.*, 1978; Lee *et al.*, 1981), and DBa,hA (Cook & Schoental, 1948; Harvey *et al.*, 1975). This method has also been employed to synthesize ^{3}H-labeled derivatives of the *cis*-4,5-dihydrodiol of BaP, the *cis*-5,6-dihydrodiol of BA, and the *cis*-9,10-dihydrodiol of phenanthrene (Harvey & Fu, 1976; Kolwyck *et al.*, 1976; Yagi *et al.*, 1976). 4,5-Dihydro-BaP reacts with OsO$_4$ on both the 11,12-bond and on the substituted 5a,6-bond to yield the corresponding *cis*-dihydrodiols (**1** and **2**) (Silverton *et al.*, 1976). An exception to the rule that reactions of OsO$_4$ afford the products of *cis*-addition is the reaction of this reagent with dibenzo[a,e]fluoranthene which furnishes the 5,5a-*trans*-dihydrodiol **3** (Jacquignon *et al.*, 1975).

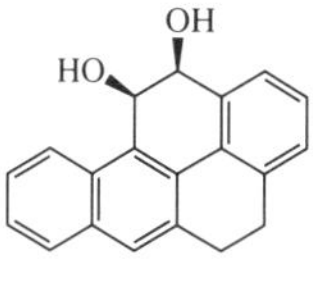

The K-region *trans*-dihydrodiols are readily accessible by reduction of the corresponding quinones with metal hydride reagents. LiAlH$_4$ was the reagent most commonly used in the early studies of this reaction (Harvey *et al.*, 1975). Optimum yields are obtained with the use of a Soxhlet apparatus to extract the poorly soluble polycyclic aromatic quinones into an ether suspension of the hydride reagent. Lower yields are obtained with the use of more efficient solvents or more soluble hydride reagents, and the air-sensitive hydroquinone is the major product. While the reduction of most K-region quinones with LiAlH$_4$ is *trans*-stereospecific, the reduction of the sterically hindered 7-methyl-BA- and DMBA-quinones affords a mixture of *trans*- and *cis*-dihydrodiols (Harvey *et al.*, 1975; Sims, 1967). K-region *trans*-dihydrodiols synthesized via the LiAlH$_4$ route include the derivatives of phenanthrene, pyrene, BA, chrysene, 7-methyl-BA, 12-methyl-BA, DMBA, DBA, 3-MC, BeP, BaP, and its 7-methyl- and 9-hydroxy-derivatives (for specific references see Harvey, 1986).

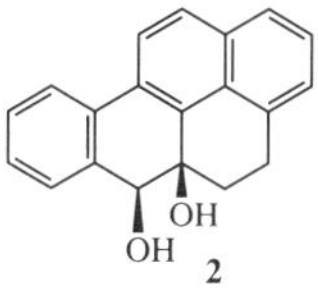

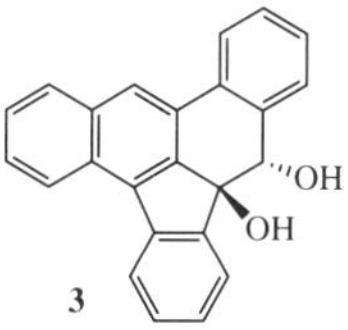

More recently it has been found that K-region quinones can be reduced to *trans*-dihydrodiols efficiently with NaBH$_4$ in ethanol by conducting the reduction in the presence of O$_2$ (Platt & Oesch, 1982). It is assumed that the O$_2$ serves to reoxidize hydroquinone intermediates (formed by base-catalyzed isomerization of partially reduced products) back to quinones (Harvey *et al.*, 1975). This method has been employed to synthesize the K-region *trans*-dihydrodiols of phenanthrene, BA, pyrene, BaP, BeP, DBA, DMBA, and 3-MC (Platt & Oesch, 1982). Other metal hydride reagents have been employed with variable success. The K-region *trans*-dihydrodiols of BeP (Lehr *et al.*, 1978), benzo[c]phenanthrene (Croisy-Delcey *et al.*, 1979), and benzo[g]chrysene (Bushman *et al.*, 1989) were prepared by reduction of the corresponding quinones with KBH_4.

The principal reactions of the K-region dihydrodiols are dehydration, esterification, oxidation, and ether formation. Dehydration may take place on heating or on treatment with mild acids. For this reason, it is not advisable to carry out chromatographic purification of dihydrodiols on mildly acidic adsorbants, such as silica gel. Dehydration is useful as a method of phenol synthesis. Although formation of a mixture of isomers is often possible, dehydration is frequently regioselective, affording mainly a single phenol isomer. The favored isomer is theoretically predictable from the relative stabilities of the carbonium ion intermediates (Fu *et al.*, 1978) (Chap. 15). Oxidation of K-region *cis*-dihydrodiols is the principal synthetic route to the corresponding K-region quinones. The choice of oxidants is limited by the necessity to avoid acidic conditions. The first reagent developed for this purpose was dimethyl sulfoxide–pyridine–SO_3 (Harvey *et al.*, 1975). However, its reactions are sometimes difficult to reproduce due to the necessity for scrupulously anhydrous conditions. The most useful alternative reagent is DDQ (Lehr *et al.*, 1978; Platt & Oesch, 1982).

13.2   Bay region dihydrodiols

13.2.1   *Structure and stereochemistry*

The conformational properties of the bay region dihydrodiol isomers are largely determined by steric crowding in this molecular region. Both the *cis*- and *trans*-isomers tend to favor a conformation in which the benzylic hydroxyl group is oriented axially in order to relieve the potentially strong steric interaction with the hydrogen atom of the adjacent aromatic ring (Fig. 13.2). For example, the hydroxyl groups of *trans*-1,2-dihydroxy-1,2-dihydro-BA were shown by X-ray crystallographic and NMR analysis to be diaxial in both the crystal lattice and in solution (Zacharias *et al.*, 1979). The observed coupling constant for the carbinol hydrogens ($J_{1,2} = 1.7$ Hz) is in good

Fig. 13.2.   Preferred conformations of the 1,2-dihydrodiols of benz[a]anthracene.

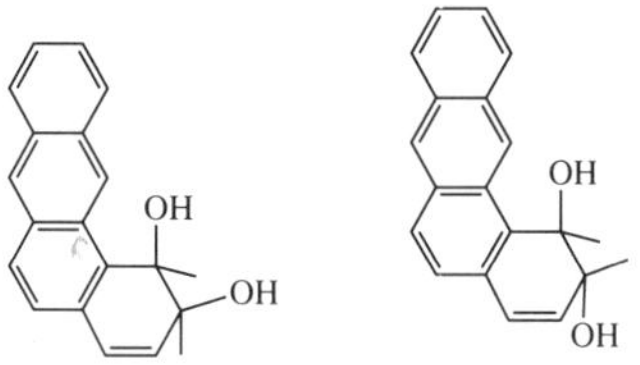

cis (axial–equatorial)   *trans* (diaxial)

agreement with the value calculated from the Karplus relationship as modified by Bothner-By ($J_{1,2}$ = 2.0 Hz) (Bothner-By, 1965) using the average torsion angle derived from the X-ray data. Esterification of this dihydrodiol has only minimal effect on the coupling constant, indicating that the diester derivatives also exist exclusively in the diaxial conformation. NMR coupling constant data for other bay region *trans*-dihydrodiols and diesters are generally close to the calculated value of 2.0 Hz, ranging from 1.0 to 2.0 Hz (Harvey, 1989; Zacharias *et al.*, 1979) (Fig. 13.3), consistent with their existence in the diaxial conformation. Since a fjord region is more sterically crowded than a bay region, the *trans*-1,2-dihydrodiol of benzo[c]-phenanthrene may also be expected to be diaxial. In agreement with this expectation, $J_{1,2}$ = 2.3 Hz.

Fig. 13.3. Bay region dihydrodiols and diesters (NMR coupling constants in Hz of the carbinol protons are given in parentheses; Ac = diacetate, Bz = dibenzoate). [a]Lehr *et al.*, 1977; [b]Fu & Harvey, 1979; [c]Karle *et al.*, 1977; [d]Zacharias *et al.*, 1979; [e]Harvey *et al.*, 1979; [f]Platt & Oesch, 1983; [g]Lee & Harvey, 1980; [h]Utermoehlen *et al.*, 1987; [i]Yang et al., 1987; [j]Croisy-Delcey *et al.*, 1979. The fjord region dihydrodiol of benzo[c]phenanthrene is included as the last entry.

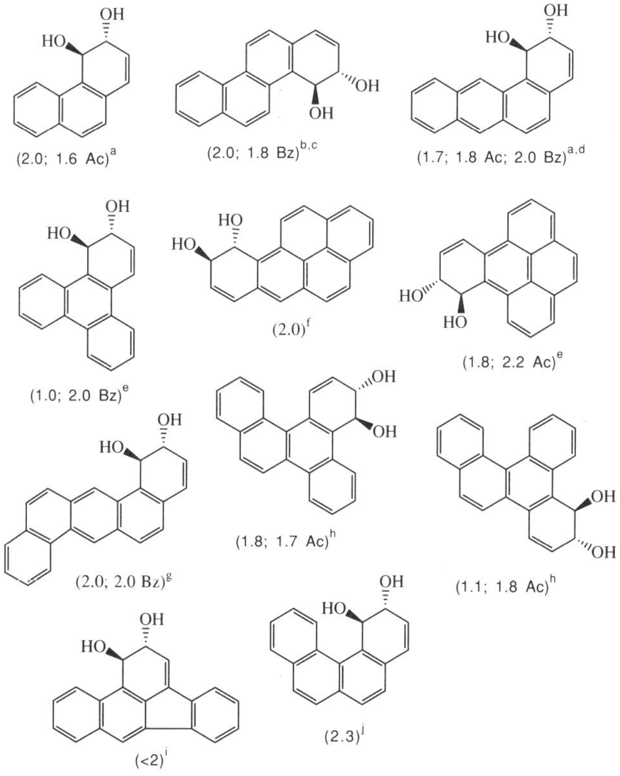

It may be inferred that the bay region *cis*-dihydrodiols also adopt a conformation in which the benzylic hydroxyl group is oriented axially. However, X-ray crystal structure data is lacking and NMR analysis is not useful in this regard, since the coupling constants for the carbinol hydrogens of both conformers are expected to be closely similar. The coupling constants for the carbinol protons of *cis*-1,2-dihydroxy-1,2-dihydro-BA and *cis*-9,10-dihydroxy-9,10-dihydro-BaP are $J_{1,2}$ = 5.4 Hz and $J_{1,2}$ = 5.2 Hz, respectively (Jerina *et al.*, 1984; Gibson *et al.*, 1975). The couplings for the analogous protons of the *cis*-1,2- and *cis*-3,4-dihydrodiols of dibenz[a,c]anthracene are $J_{1,2}$ = 4.7 Hz and $J_{3,4}$ = 5 Hz, respectively (Kole *et al.*, 1989). All of these values are in the range expected for axial–equatorial coupling.

13.2.2   *Synthesis and reactivity*

Bay region and other non-K-region dihydrodiols are synthetically accessible by methods based on dihydroarene or phenol precursors (Fig. 13.4) . Method **I**, the first approach to be developed, entails Prévost reaction of the appropriate dihydroarene with silver benzoate and iodine followed by dehydrogenation with DDQ (or by bromination with *N*-bromosuccinimide

Fig. 13.4. Methods for the synthesis of non-K-region dihydrodiols.

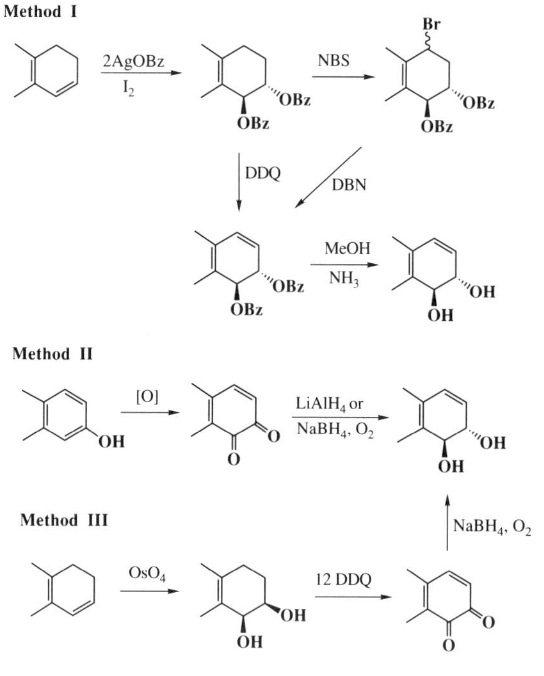

and basic dehydrobromination) (McCaustland & Engel, 1975; Harvey & Fu, 1978). It has been superseded for most applications by Method **II**, a two step procedure that entails oxidation of a phenolic precursor with Fremy's salt (or phenylselenenic anhydride) followed by reduction of the resulting quinone with a metal hydride reagent. Method **III** involves synthesis of quinone intermediates from dihydroarenes by reaction with osmium tetroxide followed by reaction of the resulting *cis*-tetrahydrodiol with DDQ (12 equiv.) in refluxing dioxane (Platt & Oesch, 1982). This approach suffers from the disadvantages that it requires more steps and employs relatively expensive and hazardous reagents.

The dihydroarenes required as starting compounds for Method **I** may be prepared from PAHs with one less ring by the Haworth synthesis with succinic anhydride and AlCl₃, followed by reduction of the resulting cyclic ketone with LiAlH₄ or NaBH₄, and acid-catalyzed dehydration (Fig. 13.5). They are also accessible by regioselective hydrogenation of the parent PAH in the appropriate benzo ring followed by dehydrogenation with DDQ (Fu *et al.*, 1978, 1980; Harvey, 1985). For example, low pressure hydrogenation of BA over a platinum catalyst provides 8,9,10,11-tetrahydro-BA which on treatment with DDQ yields 8,9- and 10,11-dihydro-BA in 4:1 ratio. It is advantageous that both isomeric olefins are obtained in the same reaction, because both are generally required for conversion to the corresponding dihydrodiols for metabolism and other biological studies. An alternative dihydroarene synthesis that involves controlled reduction of the PAH with Li/NH₃ followed by base-catalyzed isomerization (Harvey & Sukumaran, 1977) of the olefinic bond of the 1,4-dihydroaromatic ring into conjugation has also been employed. Reduction of BA with a small excess of Li in liquid NH₃ gives 1,4,7,12-tetrahydro-BA which undergoes base-catalyzed isomerization to yield both conjugated isomers. Although separation of the olefinic isomers is difficult, the diol dibenzoates obtained from the Prévost reaction of the mixture, are readily separable by chromatography.

Prévost reaction of the conjugated dihydroarenes occurs *trans*-stereospec-

Fig. 13.5. Synthetic routes to dihydroarene.

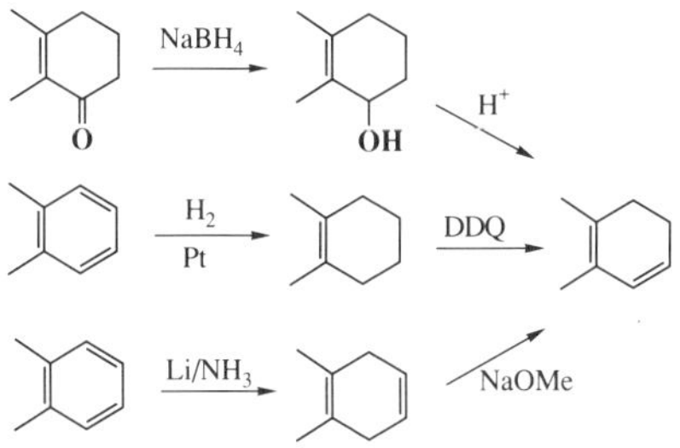

ifically to furnish the corresponding tetrahydrodiol diesters (Fig. 13.4). The diester functions protect the diol groups from oxidation in the subsequent dehydrogenation step. Introduction of the double bond was accomplished in the early studies by bromination with NBS and thermal or base-catalyzed dehydrobromination (Harvey & Fu, 1978). However, the yields tend to be erratic and difficult to reproduce and purification of the products is hampered by the presence of secondary products, including phenol esters, dibromo derivatives, and the monobromo olefin formed from the latter. Dehydrogenation using DDQ is operationally simpler and generally affords superior yields and purer products (Fu & Harvey, 1977). On the other hand, the DDQ method is not effective with some tetrahydrodiol diesters, such as the 1,2-dioldibenzoate of 1,2,3,4-tetrahydro-BA, that are readily dehydrogenated by the bromination–dehydrobromination method. Therefore, the two methods are complementary.

Bay region *trans*-dihydrodiols synthesized by Method I include the derivatives of phenanthrene (Lehr *et al.*, 1977), BA (Lehr *et al.*, 1977; Harvey & Fu, 1978), 7-methyl-BA (Lee & Harvey, 1979), BaP (Harvey & Fu, 1978; Yagi *et al.*, 1977), chrysene (Fu & Harvey, 1979; Karle *et al.*, 1977), BeP (Lehr *et al.*, 1978; Harvey *et al.*, 1979), triphenylene (Harvey *et al.*, 1979), DBA (Lee & Harvey, 1980; Karle *et al.*, 1977), and benzo[g]chrysene (Utermoehlen *et al.*, 1987).

The synthetic route to dihydrodiols from phenols (Fig. 13.4: Method II) is not useful for the synthesis of bay region dihydrodiols, because oxidation of the appropriate phenols fails to afford the desired quinone intermediates. Thus, attempted oxidation of 3-phenanthrol with Fremy's salt gave only recovered phenol, while oxidation with phenylseleninic anhydride furnished 2,2-dihydroxybenz[e]indan-1,3-dione (**4**) (Sukumaran & Harvey, 1980).

However, Method III has been successfully utilized for the preparation of bay region dihydrodiols. Its use is dependent upon the availability of a method for the efficient reduction of the *o*-quinone intermediates. The yields obtained in earlier studies of the reduction of non-K-region quinones by metal hydride reagents were in the range of 1–5%. For example, reduction of the phenanthrene 1,2- and 3,4-diones with LiAlH$_4$ furnished the corresponding *trans*-dihydrodiols in yields of 4% and 1%, respectively (Jerina *et al.*, 1976). The principal coproducts were hydroquinones (catechols), *cis*-dihydrodiols, and tetrahydrodiols. Substantially improved yields (15–66%) were obtained by an improved experimental procedure introduced by Sukumaran & Harvey, 1980. However, the most significant advance was the finding that *o*-quinones undergo efficient reduction to *trans*-dihydrodiols on treatment with $NaBH_4$ in ethanol in the presence of O_2 (Platt & Oesch, 1983; Pataki *et al.*, 1983; Jacobs *et al.*, 1983). The oxygen serves to reoxidize the hydroquinone byproducts back to quinones; hydroquinones arise from isomerization of the ketol intermediates formed initially by partial reduction. As discussed in the preceding section, these reductions generally proceed *trans*-stereospecifically for quinones that are not hindered sterically, both K-region and non-K-region. However, even the relatively hindered bay region quinones undergo reduction with high stereoselectivity. Thus, the reaction of BaP 9,10-dione with $NaBH_4$ furnished a 4:1 mixture of the *cis*- and *trans*-9,10-dihydrodiols (Platt & Oesch, 1983). The remarkable *trans* stereoselectivity of these reductions is most readily understood as due to delivery of the second hydrogen atom from the metal hydride–ketol complex formed in the reduction of the first carbonyl function to the same face of the molecule (Harvey *et al.*, 1975). It is notable that attempts to prepare the BaP *trans*-9,10-dihydrodiol by Method I were unsuccessful, so that metal hydride reduction provides the only synthetic access to this compound.

Bay region *trans*-dihydrodiols synthesized via reduction of *o*-quinones include the derivatives of phenanthrene (Jerina *et al.*, 1976; Sukumaran & Harvey, 1980; Platt & Oesch, 1983), BA (Platt & Oesch, 1983), triphenylene (Platt & Oesch, 1983), BaP (Platt & Oesch, 1983), and BeP (Platt & Oesch, 1983).

There has been relatively little interest in the corresponding *cis* stereoisomers, since they are not products of mammalian cell metabolism. The *cis*-9,10-dihydrodiol of BaP was synthesized from 7,8-dihydro-BaP by reaction with OsO_4 followed by acetylation and dehydrogenation (Gibson *et al.*, 1975).

Bay region dihydrodiols enter into all of the same reactions as the K-region dihydrodiols. These include dehydration, esterification, oxidation to quinones, and ether formation. Dehydration takes place with relative facility on treatment with acids. The phenol isomers obtained are theoretically predictable from the calculated relative stabilities of the two possible carbonium ion intermediates (Fu *et al.*, 1978). In addition, bay region dihydrodiols may react with peracids on the olefinic bond to yield the corresponding diol epoxides (Chap. 14).

13.3 Proximate and terminal ring dihydrodiols

13.3.1 Structure and stereochemistry

The most important class of dihydrodiols from the standpoint of biological activity are those that give rise to the bay region diol epoxides. These are potential 'proximate carcinogens', since they are metabolic precursors of the the diol epoxides that are the 'ultimate carcinogens'. These dihydrodiols, some examples of which are shown in Figs 13.6 and 13.7, occur in the nonbay region sites of benzo rings. They will be referred to as

Fig. 13.6. Proximate dihydrodiols and diesters (NMR coupling constants in Hz of the carbinol protons are given in parentheses; Ac = diacetate, Bz = dibenzoate). [a]Lehr *et al.*, 1977; [b]Sukumaran & Harvey *et al.*, 1980; [c]Harvey *et al.*, 1986; [d]Chiu *et al.*, 1985; [e]Lee & Harvey, 1980; [f]Harvey *et al.*, 1988; [g]Bushman *et al.*, 1989; [h]Pataki *et al.*, 1989; [i]Croisy-Delcey *et al.*, 1979; [j]Lehr *et al.*, 1979; [k]Amin *et al.*, 1981; [l]Harvey *et al.*, 1988a.

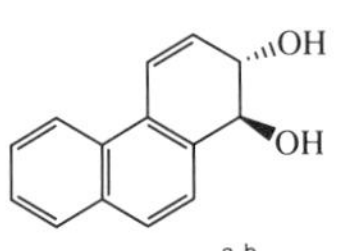
(11.3; 5.6 Ac)[a,b]

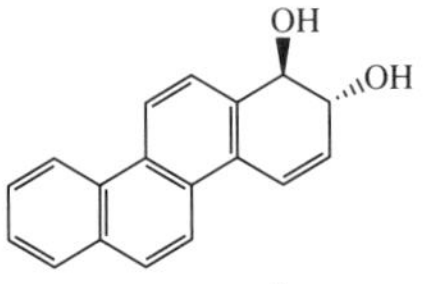
(10.8; 6.5 Ac)[c]

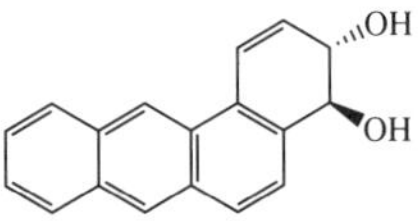
(11.5; 6.1 Ac)[a]

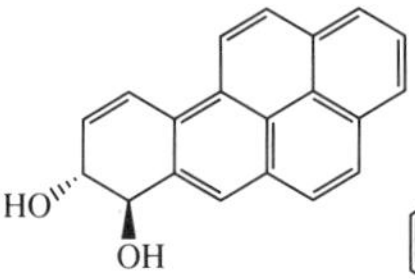
5 (10.0; 6.9 Ac)[d]

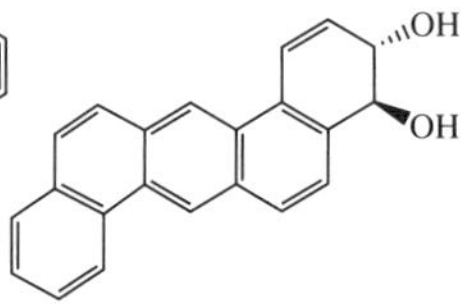
6 (11; 5.8 Ac; 7 Bz)[e]

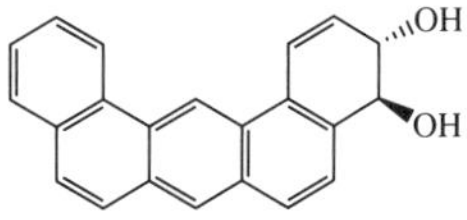
(10.8; 4.9 Ac)[f]

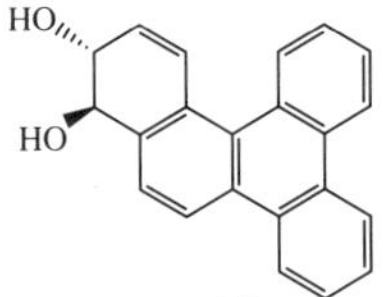
(11.6)[g]

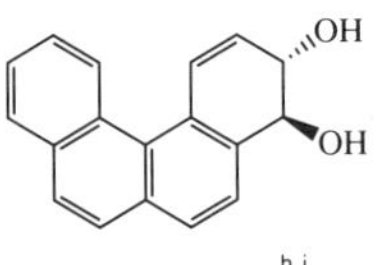
(11.1; 6.1 Ac)[h,i]

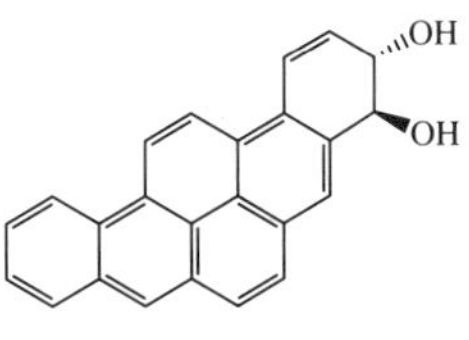
(10.5; 6 Ac)[j]

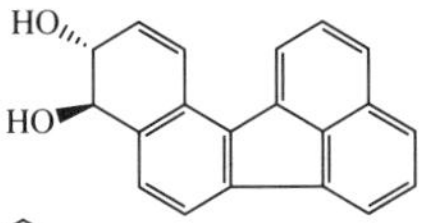
(10)[k]

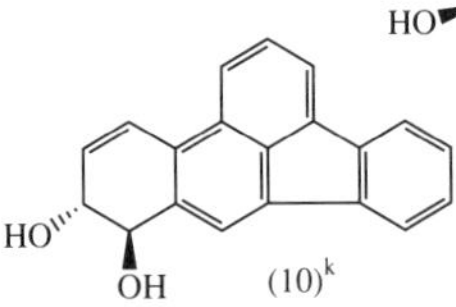
(10)[k]

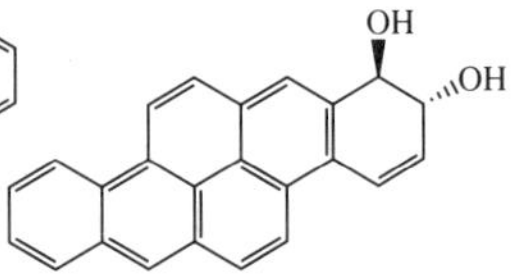
(11; 6 Ac)[j]

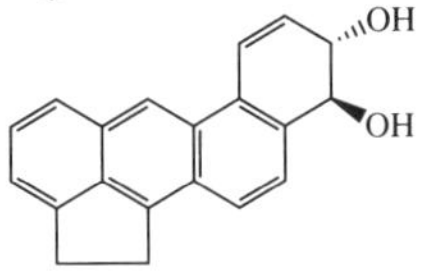
(5.7 Ac)[l]

proximate dihydrodiols. The remaining classes of dihydrodiols are the terminal ring derivatives of linearly fused regions of PAHs, such as anthracene *trans*-1,2-dihydrodiol and BA *trans*-8,9-dihydrodiol, and the derivatives of nonalternant hydrocarbons in which the substituted ring is also fused to a five-membered ring, such as the fluoranthene *trans*-2,3-dihydrodiol (**8**). Examples of both of these types are given in Fig. 13.8. The former will be referred to as *terminal ring dihydrodiols*.

The *trans*-dihydrodiols of the proximate and terminal dihydrodiols exist preferentially in the diequatorial conformation in the absence of steric or other effects. X-ray analysis of BaP *trans*-7,8-dihydrodiol (**5**) and BA *trans*-9,10-dihydrodiol (**7**) show that the aromatic ring systems of both are essentially planar and the hydroxyl groups are oriented diequatorially (Neidle *et al.*, 1981; Zacharias *et al.*, 1979). These findings are in accord with NMR spectral analysis. The coupling constant for the carbinol hydrogens of **7** was calculated to be $J_{10,11} = 12.7 \pm 0.2$ Hz using the average torsion angles from the X-ray data. Experimentally determined values were 9.5 Hz in dimethyl sulfoxide and 10.0 Hz in acetone indicating that this dihydrodiol exists in solution as a mixture of conformers in dynamic equilibrium. On the assumption that the observed couplings represent a weighted average, the percentage of the diequatorial conformer of **7** in solution in these solvents is

Fig. 13.7. Methyl-substituted proximate dihydrodiols (NMR coupling constants in Hz of the carbinol protons are given in parentheses). [a]Harvey *et al.*, 1988a; [b]Lee & Harvey, 1986; [c]Jacobs *et al.*, 1983; [d]Harvey *et al.*, 1986; [e]Harvey *et al.*, 1988.

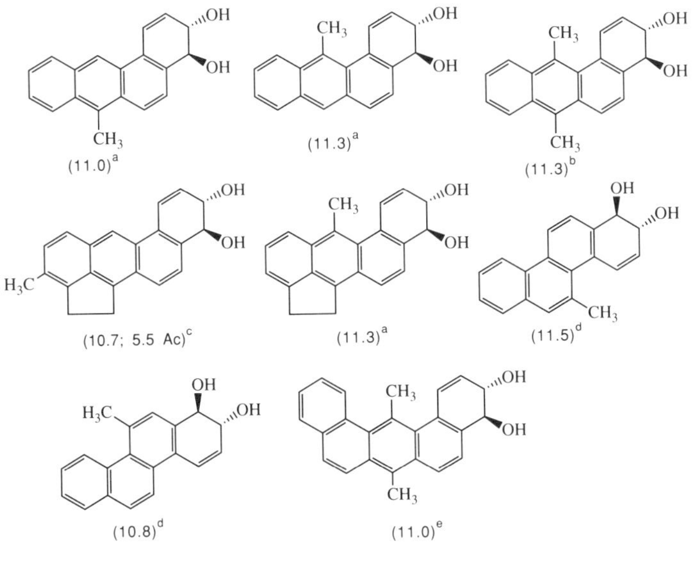

calculated to be 70–75% at ambient temperature. Similarly for **5**, for which $J_{7,8} = 10$ Hz is observed (Chiu *et al.*, 1985), the percentage of the diequatorial conformer in solution is calculated to be 75%. The dihydrodiol derivatives of nonalternant PAHs fused to a five-membered ring (Fig. 13.8) are part of a relatively rigid ring system that offers less freedom for conformational interconversion.

Esterification tends to shift the conformational equilibrium in favor of the diaxial structure. In agreement, esterification of **5** and **7** resulted in a decrease in the coupling of the carbinol hydrogens; $J_{10,11} = 6.3$ Hz for **7** dibenzoate and $J_{7,8} = 6.9$ Hz for **5** diacetate. Based on these values, the calculated ratios of the diaxial conformers of the diesters of **5** and **7** in solution are 70% and 65%, respectively. This shift in favor of the diaxial conformer on esterification is a consequence of loss of intramolecular hydrogen bonding and steric interaction between the more bulky ester groups. NMR data for other structurally related dihydrodiols and their diesters are generally consistent with similar conformational differences (Fig. 13.7). The coupling constants for the carbinol C-H protons of the *proximate trans*-dihydrodiols of PAHs unsubstituted in the *peri* positions fall in the range of 10–12 Hz. When

Fig. 13.8. Terminal ring and other dihydrodiols and their diesters (NMR coupling constants of Hz of the carbinol protons are given in parentheses). [a]Sukumaran & Harvey, 1980; [b]Lehr *et al.*, 1977; [c]Amin *et al.*, 1981; [d]Harvey & Fu, 1980; [e]Rastetter *et al.*, 1982; [f]Rice *et al.*, 1987.

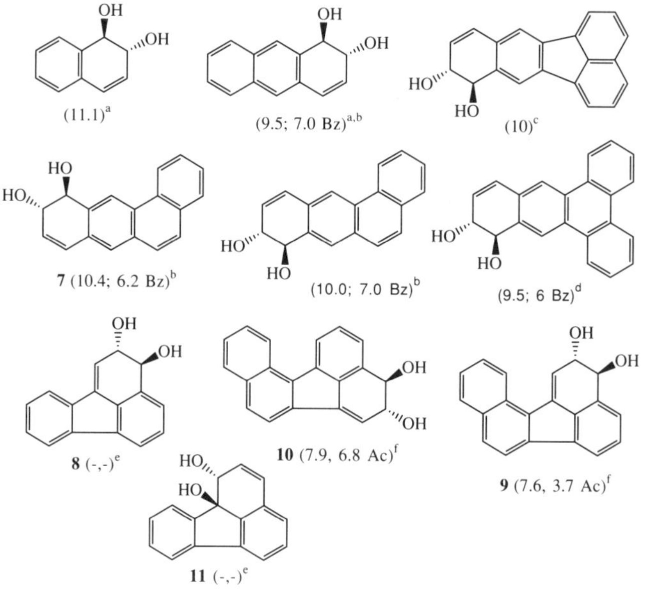

large groups are located in the *peri* positions, the conformational equilibrium is shifted in favor of the diaxial conformer. Thus, while **5** has $J_{7,8} = 10.0$ Hz and is diequatorial, the dihydrodiols of 6-bromo- and 6-methyl-BaP have $J_{7,8} = 1.7–1.8$ Hz and are diaxial (Chiu *et al.*, 1985). The coupling constants for the carbinol protons of the diesters of the *proximate trans*-dihydrodiols of PAHs fall in the range of 5–7 Hz, consistent with predominance of the diaxial conformers. The carbinol couplings for *terminal ring* dihydrodiols and diesters (Fig. 13.8) are in essentially the same range as those of the *proximate* dihydrodiols, indicative of similar conformational preferences. There is only minimal coupling constant data available on the dihydrodiols of nonalternant PAHs fused to a five-membered ring. However, it is interesting that $J_{2,3}$ of the diacetate of benzo[j]fluoranthene 2,3-dihydrodiol (**9**) is lower (3.7 Hz) than that of the free dihydrodiol (7.6 Hz), indicating that in this case esterification can change the conformation to a pseudodiaxial form.

13.3.2 *Synthesis and reactivity*

Dihydrodiols of these classes are synthetically accessible from dihydroarene or phenol precursors by the methods in Fig. 13.4. Method II is particularly advantageous for this purpose. The requisite phenols are commonly obtained from the corresponding ketones which may be efficiently converted to phenols by formation of enol acetates and dehydrogenation with o-chloranil or DDQ (Fu *et al.*, 1979). The yields obtained via this route are generally superior to those obtained by dehydrogenation with sulfur or catalytically which often result in considerable deoxygenation. In early studies, the ketones obtained from the Haworth synthesis were employed for this purpose. In more recent studies, the requisite ketones have been obtained by a novel synthesis that involves formation of α- or β-ketones as products of polycyclic ring construction. For example, alkylation of the lithium salt of 1,4-dimethoxycyclohexadiene by 2-(1-naphthyl)ethyl iodide, acid-catalyzed cyclization, and dehydrogenation

Fig. 13.9. Synthetic route to phenols by the method of Harvey *et al.*, 1986.

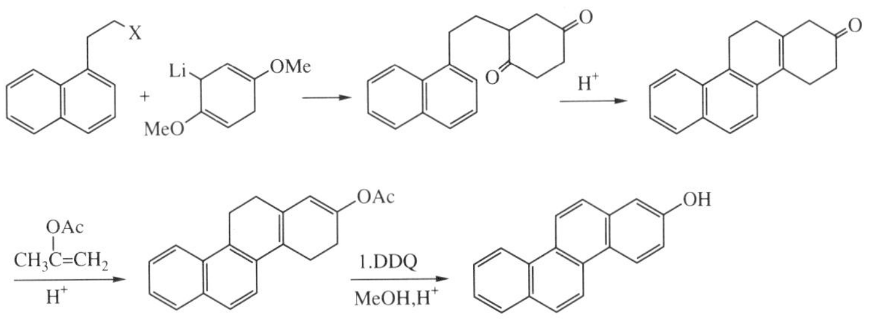

affords a partially saturated ketone derivative of chrysene that is readily converted to the corresponding phenol by formation of the enol acetate and dehydrogenation with DDQ (Fig. 13.9) (Harvey *et al.*, 1986). This approach entails fewer overall steps than alternative methods of phenol synthesis.

Proximate and terminal *trans*-dihydrodiols synthesized by Methods II and III include (Figs 13.6–13.8) the dihydrodiol derivatives of anthracene (Sukumaran & Harvey, 1980; Platt & Oesch, 1983), phenanthrene (Sukumaran & Harvey, 1980; Platt & Oesch, 1983), BA (Harvey *et al.*, 1988a; Platt & Oesch, 1983; Sukumaran & Harvey, 1980), 7-methyl-BA (Harvey *et al.*, 1988a; Lee & Harvey, 1979), 12-methyl-BA (Harvey *et al.*, 1988a), DMBA (Lee & Harvey, 1986), cholanthrene (Harvey *et al.*, 1988a), 3-MC (Jacobs *et al.*, 1983), 6-MC (Harvey *et al.*, 1988a), benzo[c]phen-anthrene (Pataki *et al.*, 1989), chrysene (Harvey *et al.*, 1986), 5-methylchry-sene (Harvey *et al.*, 1986), DBA (Platt & Oesch, 1983), BaP (Sukumaran & Harvey, 1980; Platt & Oesch, 1983), 1- and 3-hydroxy-BaP (Kumar *et al.*, 1989), 1-isopropyl-BaP (Pataki & Harvey, 1987), dibenz[a,j]anthracene (Harvey *et al.*, 1988), and 7,14-dimethyldibenz[a,j]anthracene (Harvey *et al.*, 1988). The 5-ethyl- and 5-propylchrysene *trans*-1,2-dihydrodiols (not shown in Fig. 13.7) have also been synthesized by Method II (Amin *et al.*, 1988).

Proximate *trans*-dihydrodiols synthesized via Method I (Fig. 13.8) include the derivatives of phenanthrene (Lehr *et al.*, 1977), BA (Harvey & Sukumaran, 1977; Harvey & Fu, 1978; Lehr *et al.*, 1977), BaP (Harvey & Fu, 1978; Yagi *et al.*, 1977a), chrysene (Fu & Harvey, 1979; Karle *et al.*, 1977), DBA (Lee & Harvey, 1980; Karle *et al.*, 1977), dibenzo[a,h]pyrene (Lehr *et al.*, 1979), dibenzo[a,i]pyrene (Lehr *et al.*, 1979), benzo[b]- and benzo[j]fluoranthene (Amin *et al.*, 1981), and benzo[g]chrysene (Bushman *et al.*, 1989). The G-^{3}H-, 7-^{13}C-, 10-^{13}C, and 7-^{14}C-labeled derivatives of **5** were also prepared by suitable modification of this procedure (Engel *et al.*, 1978; McCaustland *et al.*, 1976, 1976a). A number of terminal ring dihydrodiols have been synthesized from dihydroarenes by similar procedures. These include the dihydrodiol derivatives of anthracene (Lehr *et al.*, 1977), BA (Harvey & Fu, 1978; Lehr *et al.*, 1977), dibenz[a,c]anthracene (Harvey & Fu, 1980), and benzo[j]fluoranthene (Amin *et al.*, 1981). The dihydrodiol derivatives of the nonalternant polyarenes fluoranthene (**8**) and benzo[j]fluoranthene (**9, 10**) have also been synthesized by similar proced-ures (Rastetter *et al.*, 1982; Rice *et al.*, 1987).

The unusual fluoranthene 1,10b-dihydrodiol (**11**), which was unobtainable by Method I due to failure of the Prévost reaction, was synthesized from 2,3-dihydrofluoranthene by an alternative route (Fig. 13.10) (Rastetter *et al.*, 1982).

Prior to the development of more efficient synthetic approaches, a few *trans*-dihydrodiols have been synthesized by other methods. Thus, treatment of DBA 3,4-dione with bromine gave the 1,2-dibromo derivative which on further reaction with $NaBH_4$ in ethanol furnished a mixture of the *trans*-dihydrodiol (**6**) and the *cis* isomer (Kundu, 1979). Also, an ascorbic acid–ferrous sulfate–EDTA system was utilized to oxidize 3-MC, DMBA, and other PAHs to yield mixtures of products from which low yields (< 0.3%) of dihydrodiols could be isolated by HPLC or TLC (Hewer *et al.*, 1979).

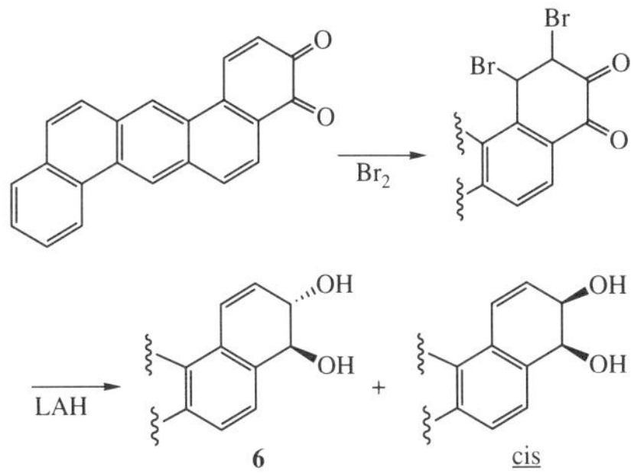

Only relatively few *cis*-dihydrodiol isomers of proximate and terminal dihydrodiols have been synthesized. They are readily synthetically accessible through the reaction of osmium tetroxide with dihydroarenes followed by dehydrogenation with DDQ or NBS. *cis*-7,8-Dihydroxy-7,8-dihydro-BaP (Harvey & Fu, 1978) and its 7-methyl (Fu *et al.*, 1981) and 8-methyl (Lee *et al.*, 1983) derivatives were prepared via this method. *cis*-9,10-Dihydroxy-9,10-dihydro-BaP (Gibson *et al.*, 1975) and *cis*-8,9-dihydroxy-8,9-dihydro-BA (Sims, 1971) were obtained via a similar route.

The types of reactions undergone by the proximate and terminal dihydro-

Fig. 13.10. Synthesis of the fluoranthene *trans*-1,10b-dihydrodiol.

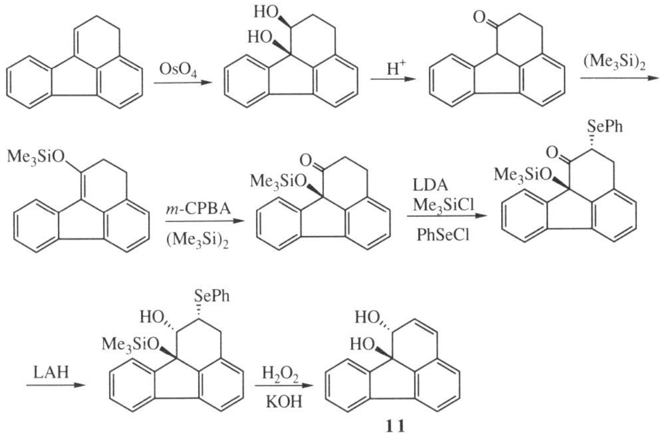

diols are the same as those of the bay region dihydrodiols. The most important of these from the viewpoint of carcinogenesis is oxidation to the corresponding *anti* and *syn* diol epoxides (Chap. 14). Other common reactions include esterification, dehydration, and oxidation to quinones. Dehydration generally affords the phenol isomer arising from the most stable of the two possible carbonium ion intermediates (Fu *et al.*, 1978).

13.4   Resolution of optically active dihydrodiols

Since enzymatic formation of dihydrodiols is highly stereoselective, resolution of the racemic dihydrodiol enantiomers obtained from synthesis is of considerable importance. This may be accomplished either by chromatographic separation of the mixtures of their diastereomeric derivatives or by direct resolution of racemic dihydrodiols on Pirkle-type chiral columns.

Resolution of the mixed enantiomers of (±)-*trans*-7,8-dihydroxy-7,8-dihydro-BaP was first achieved by HPLC separation of their diastereomeric (–)-dimenthoxyacetate (Harvey & Cho, 1977; Yang *et al.*, 1977) and bis(–)-α-methoxy-α-trifluoromethylphenylacetate (Thakker *et al.*, 1977) diesters. The absolute configuration of the BaP (–)-7,8-dihydrodiol was assigned as 7R,8S by application of the exciton chirality dichroism method (Harada & Nakanishi, 1972) to its 7,8-bis-*p*-dimethylaminobenzoate derivative (Nakanishi *et al.*, 1977; Yagi *et al.*, 1977a). This methodology has subsequently been utilized for the resolution and absolute stereochemical assignment of numerous dihydrodiol enantiomers.

Yang and his colleagues were the first to achieve the direct resolution of racemic dihydrodiols by HPLC separation of the enantiomers on chiral stationary phase columns. Their initial report (Weems & Yang, 1982) described resolution of dihydrodiol enantiomers of BaP, BA and 11-methyl-BA on a column of (R)-*N*-(3,5-dinitrobenzoyl)phenylglycine ionically bonded to γ-aminopropyl silanised silica developed by Pirkle (Pirkle & Finn, 1981). This methodology has subsequently been extended to other PAHs using commercially available ionically- and covalently-bonded phenyl-glycine- and leucine-based columns.

The absolute stereochemistries of PAH dihydrodiols may be assigned by application of the exciton chirality dichroism method to the appropriate derivative of the dihydrodiol, or in cases where the former is unstable, to the related tetrahydrodiol. In other cases, the absolute configurations can be assigned by relating a dihydrodiol enantiomer to an alcohol of known stereo-chemistry. For example, the absolute configuration of the naphthalene (+)-*cis*-1,2-dihydrodiol was assigned as 1R,2S by hydrogenolysis of its diacetate and hydrolysis to yield optically pure (–)-2S-hydroxy-1,2,3,4-

tetrahydronaphthalene of known configuration (Jeffrey *et al.*, 1975). The stereochemistries of substituted dihydrodiols, such as the 11-methyl-substituted BA-dihydrodiols, may conveniently be assigned by comparison of their CD spectra with those of the parent hydrocarbon whose configuration has been previously assigned (Yang, 1982). Tentative assignments of absolute configurations may also be made on the basis of the relative order of elution of the resolved dihydrodiol enantiomers on chiral columns. Yang and coworkers have shown that the *R,R* enantiomers of diequatorial *trans*-dihydrodiols are more strongly retained on ionically-bonded (*R*)-N-(3,5-dinitrobenzoyl)phenylglycine than the *S,S* enantiomers (Yang *et al.*, 1986). In contrast, the *S,S* enantiomers of diaxial *trans*-dihydrodiols are more strongly retained than the corresponding *R,R* enantiomers on columns of this type. It has been suggested by Jerina and coworkers (Balani *et al.*, 1986; Yagi *et al.*, 1982) that the NMR coupling patterns of the $OCOCH_2O$ hydrogens in the bis(menthoxyacetates) of dihydrodiols are diagnostic of their absolute configuration. The empirical rule that the less polar diastereomer with the larger negative optical rotation and minor magnetic nonequivalence of the methylene protons has the *R,R* configuration appears to be valid for most of the compounds investigated. Assignments of absolute configuration on the basis of the NMR method or the order of elution on chiral columns are empirical and should be used with appropriate caution.

The resolution and absolute stereochemical assignments of a large number *cis*- and *trans*-dihydrodiols have been accomplished to date. These include the derivatives of naphthalene (Muira *et al.*, 1968), anthracene (Aktar *et al.*, 1975), phenanthrene (Muira *et al.*, 1968; Koreeda *et al.*, 1978; Vyas *et al.*, 1982; Nordquist *et al.*, 1981), BA (Chou *et al.*, 1983; Yagi *et al.*, 1982; Thakker *et al.*, 1979; Levin *et al.*, 1978), 7-methyl-BA (Yang & Fu, 1984), DMBA (Yang & Fu, 1984a; Yang & Weems, 1984), chrysene (Nordquist *et al.*, 1981; Yagi *et al.*, 1982; Weems *et al.*, 1986; Balani *et al.*, 1986), 5-methylchrysene (Amin *et al.*, 1987), benzo[c]phenanthrene (Yagi *et al.*, 1983; Balani *et al.*, 1986), pyrene (Balani *et al.*, 1986), BaP (Harvey & Cho, 1977; Yang *et al.*, 1977; Thakker *et al.*, 1977; Kedzierski *et al.*, 1981), 7-methyl-BaP (Chiu *et al.*, 1983; Yang & Fu, 1984), DBA (Schollmeier *et al.*, 1986), benzo[g]chrysene (Bushman *et al.*, 1989), benzo[b]fluoranthene (Yang *et al.*, 1987), triphenylene (Boyd *et al.*, 1987), and 3-MC (Yang *et al.*, 1986). The foregoing list is not intended to be exhaustive. Many additional substituted dihydrodiol derivatives of BA, BaP, and phenanthrene have been resolved by HPLC on chiral stationary phase columns (Yang *et al.*, 1984; Weems *et al.*, 1986; Yang *et al.*, 1986).

13. 5 References

Akhtar, M. N., Boyd, D. R., Thompson, N. J., Koreeda, M., Gibson, D. T., Mahadevan, V. & Jerina, D. M. (1975). Absolute stereochemistry of the dihydroanthracene-*cis*- and -*trans*-1,2-diols produced from anthracene by mammals and bacteria. *J. Chem. Soc. Perkin I*, 2506–11.

Amin, S., Bedenko, V., LaVoie, E., Hecht, S. S. & Hoffmann, D. (1981). Synthesis of dihydrodiols as potential proximate carcinogens of benzofluoranthenes. *J. Org. Chem.* **46**, 2573–8.

Amin, S., Huie, K., Balanikas, G. & Hecht, S. S. (1988). Synthesis and mutagenicity of 5-alkyl-substituted chrysene-1,2-diol-3,4-epoxides. *Carcinogenesis,* **9**, 2305–8.

Amin, S., Huie, K., Balanikas, G., Hecht, S. S., Pataki, J. & Harvey, R. G. (1987). High stereoselectivity in mouse skin metabolic activation of methylchrysenes to tumorigenic dihydrodiols. *Cancer Res.* **47**, 3613–17.

Balani, S. K., Bladeren, P. J. v., Cassidy, E. S., Boyd, D. R. & Jerina, D. M. (1987). Synthesis of the enantiomeric K-region arene 5,6-oxides derived from chrysene, 7,12-dimethylbenz[a]anthracene, and benzo[c]phenanthrene. *J. Org. Chem.* **52**, 137–44.

Balani, S. K., Bladeren, P. J. v., Shirai, N. & Jerina, D. M. (1986). Resolution and absolute configuration of K-region trans dihydrodiols from polycyclic aromatic hydrocarbons. *J. Org. Chem.* **51**, 1773–8.

Bochnitschek, W., Seidel, A., Kunz, H. & Oesch, F. (1985). Reactive metabolites of carcinogenic polycyclic hydrocarbons: Synthesis and trapping reaction of 9-hydroxy-benzo[a]pyrene. *Angew. Chem. Int. Ed. Engl.* **24**, 699–700.

Bothner-By, A. A. (1965). Geminal and vicinal proton coupling constants in organic compounds. *Adv. Magn. Resn.* **1**, 195–316.

Boyd, D. R., Kennedy, D. A., Malone, J. F., O'Kane, G. A., Thakker, D. T., Yagi, H. & Jerina, D. M. (1987). Synthesis of triphenylene 1,2-oxides (1,2-epoxy-1,2-dihydrophenylene) and absolute configuration of the trans-1,2-dihydro diol metabolite of triphenylene. Crystal structure of (–)-(1R,2R)-trans-2-bromo-1-menthyloxyacetoxy-1,2,3,4-tetrahydrotriphenylene. *J. Chem. Soc. Perkin I*, 369–75.

Bushman, D. R., Grossman, S. J., Jerina, D. M. & Lehr, R. E. (1989). Synthesis of optically active fjord-region 11,12-diol 13,14-epoxides and the K-region 9,10-oxide of the carcinogen benzo[g]chrysene. *J. Org. Chem.* **54**, 3533–44.

Chiu, P., Fu, P. P., Weems, H. B. & Yang, S. K. (1985). Absolute configuration of *trans*-7,8-dihydroxy-7,8-dihydro-7-methylbenzo[a]pyrene enantiomer and the unusual quasidiequatorial conformation of the diacetate and dimenthoxyacetate derivatives. *Chem.–Biol. Interact.* **52**, 265–77.

Chiu, P., Weems, H. B., Wong, T. K., Fu, P. P. & Yang, S. K. (1983). Stereoselective metabolism of benzo[a]pyrene and 7-methylbenzo[a]pyrene by liver microsomes from Sprague–Dawley rats pretreated with polychlorinated biphenyls. *Chem.–Biol. Interact.* **44**, 155–68.

Chou, M. W., Chiu, P., Fu, P. P. & Yang, S. K. (1983). The effect of enzyme induction on the stereoselective metabolism of optically pure (–)1R,2R- and (+)1S,2S-dihydroxy-1,2-dihydrobenz[a]anthracenes to vicinal 1,2-dihydrodiol 3,4-epoxides by rat liver microsomes. *Carcinogenesis,* **4**, 629–38.

Cook, J. W. & Schoental, R. (1948). Oxidation of carcinogenic hydrocarbons by osmium tetroxide. *J. Chem. Soc.* 170–3.

Croisy-Delcey, M., Ittah, Y. & Jerina, D. M. (1979). Synthesis of benzo[c]phenanthrene dihydrodiols. *Tetrahedron Lett.* 2849–52.

Engel, J. F., Sankaran, V., McCaustland, D. J., Kolwyck, K. C., Ebert, D. A. & Duncan, W. P. (1978). Synthesis of carbon-13-labeled benzo[a]pyrene. *Polycyclic Hydrocarbons and Cancer*, Vol. 1, eds H. V. Gelboin & P. O. P. Ts'o, 167–71, New York: Academic.

Fu, P. P., Cortez, C., Sukumaran, K. & Harvey, R. G. (1979). Synthesis of isomeric phenols of benz[a]anthracene from benz[a]anthracene. *J. Org. Chem.* **44**, 4265–71.

Fu, P. P., Evans, F. E., Miller, D. W., Chou, M. W. & Yang, S. K. (1983). Conformation of K-region *trans*-dihydrodiols of polycyclic aromatic hydrocarbons. *J. Chem. Res. (S).* **1**, 158–9.

Fu, P. P. & Harvey, R. G. (1977). Synthesis of the diols and diolepoxides of carcinogenic hydrocarbons. *Tetrahedron Lett.* 2059–62.

Fu, P. P. & Harvey, R. G. (1979). Synthesis of the dihydro diols and diol epoxides of chrysene from chrysene. *J. Org. Chem.* **44**, 3778–84.

Fu, P. P., Harvey, R. G. & Beland, F. (1978). Molecular orbital theoretical prediction of the isomeric products formed from reactions of arene oxides and related metabolites of polycyclic aromatic hydrocarbons. *Tetrahedron,* **34**, 857–66.

Fu, P. P., Lai, C. & Yang, S. K. (1981). Synthesis of *cis-* and *trans*-7,8-dihydrodiols of 7-methylbenzo[a]pyrene. *J. Org. Chem.* **46**, 220–2.

Fu, P. P., Lee, H. M. & Harvey, R. G. (1978). Novel synthesis of the dihydroarene precursors of carcinogenic arene dihydrodiols and diolepoxides. *Tetrahedron Lett.* 5514.

Fu, P. P., Lee, H. M. & Harvey, R. G. (1980). Regioselective catalytic hydrogenation of polycyclic aromatic hydrocarbons under mild conditions. *J. Org. Chem.* **45**, 2797–803.

Gibson, D. T., Mahadevan, V., Jerina, D. M., Yagi, H. & Yeh, H. J. C. (1975). Oxidation of the carcinogens benzo[a]pyrene and benz[a]anthracene to dihydrodiols by a bacterium. *Science,* **189**, 295–7.

Harada, N. & Nakanishi, K. (1972). The exciton chirality method and its application to the configurational and conformational studies of natural products. *Acc. Chem. Res.* **5**, 257–63.

Harvey, R. G. (1985). Synthesis of the dihydrodiol and diol epoxide metabolites of carcinogenic polycyclic hydrocarbons. *Polycyclic Hydrocarbons and Carcinogenesis,* Symp. Series No. 283, ed. R. G. Harvey, 35–62, Washington, DC: American Chemical Society.

Harvey, R. G. (1986). Synthesis of oxidized metabolites of polycyclic aromatic hydrocarbons. *Synthesis,* 605–19.

Harvey, R. G. (1989). Conformational analysis of hydroaromatic metabolites of carcinogenic hydrocarbons and the relation of conformation to biological activity. *The Conformational Analysis of Cyclohexenes, Cyclohexadienes, and Related Hydroaromatics,* ed. P. W. Rabideau, pp. 267–98, New York: VCH.

Harvey, R. G. & Cho, H. (1977). Efficient resolution of the dihydrodiol derivatives of benzo[a]pyrene by high pressure liquid chromatography of the related (+)-dimenthoxyacetates. *Anal. Biochem.* **80**, 540–6.

Harvey, R. G. & Cortez, C. (1983). K-region oxidized metabolites of 9-hydroxybenzo[a]pyrene. *Carcinogenesis,* **4**, 941–42.

Harvey, R. G., Cortez, C., Sawyer, T. W. & DiGiovanni, J. (1988). Synthesis of the tumorigenic 3,4-dihydrodiol metabolites of dibenz[a,j]anthracene and 7,14-dimethyldibenz[a,j]anthracene. *J. Medic. Chem.* **31**, 1308–12.

Harvey, R. G., Cortez, C., Sugiyama, T., Ito, Y., Sawyer, T. W. & DiGiovanni, J. (1988a). Biologically active metabolites of polycyclic aromatic hydrocarbons structurally related to the potent carcinogenic hydrocarbon 7,12-dimethylbenz[a]anthracene. *J. Medic. Chem.* **31**, 154–9.

Harvey, R. G. & Fu, P. P. (1976). Synthesis of high specific activity benzo[a]pyrene-6-*t* and its K-region oxidized derivatives. *J. Label. Cpds. Radiopharm.* **12**, 259–64.

Harvey, R. G. & Fu, P. P. (1978). Synthesis and reactions of diolepoxides and related metabolites of carcinogenic hydrocarbons. *Polycyclic Hydrocarbons and Cancer: Environment, Chemistry, and Metabolism,* 1, eds H. V. Gelboin & P. O. P. Ts'o, 133–65, New York: Academic Press.

Harvey, R. G. & Fu, P. P. (1980). Synthesis of oxidized metabolites of dibenz[a,c]anthracene. *J. Org. Chem.* **45**, 169–71.

Harvey, R. G., Fu, P. P. & Rabideau, P. W. (1976). Stereochemistry of 1,3-cyclohexadienes: Conformational preferences in 9-substituted 9,10-dihydrophenanthrenes. *J. Org. Chem.* **41**, 3722–5.

Harvey, R. G., Goh, S. H. & Cortez, C. (1975). 'K-region' oxides and related oxidized metabolites of carcinogenic aromatic hydrocarbons. *J. Am. Chem. Soc.* **97**, 3468–79.

Harvey, R. G., Lee, H. L. & Shyamasundar, N. (1979). Synthesis of the dihydrodiols and diol epoxides of benzo[e]pyrene and triphenylene. *J. Org. Chem.* **44**, 78–83, 5006.

Harvey, R. G., Pataki, J. & Lee, H. (1986). Synthesis of the dihydrodiol and diol epoxide metabolites of chrysene and 5-methylchrysene. *J. Org. Chem.* **51**, 1407–12.

Harvey, R. G. & Sukumaran, K. (1977). Synthesis of the A-ring dihydrodiols and *anti*-diolepoxides of benz[a]anthracene. *Tetrahedron Lett.* 2387–90.

Hewer, A., Ribeiro, O., Walsh, C., Grover, P. L. & Sims, P. (1979). The formation of dihydrodiols from benzo[a]pyrene by oxidation with an ascorbic acid/ferrous sulphate/EDTA system. *Chem.–Biol. Interact.* **26**, 147–54.

Jacobs, S. A., Cortez, C. & Harvey, R. G. (1983). Synthesis of potential proximate and ultimate carcinogenic metabolites of 3-methylcholanthrene. *Carcinogenesis*, **4**, 519–22.

Jacquignon, P., Perin-Roussel, O., Perin, F., Chalvet, O., Lhoste, J. M., Mathieu, A., Saperas, B., Viallet, P. & Zajdela, F. (1975). Oxidation of dibenzo[a,e]fluoranthene by osmium tetroxide. *Can. J. Chem.* **53**, 1670–76.

Jeffery, A. M., Yeh, H. J., Jerina, D. M., Patel, T. R., Davey, J. F. & Gibson, D. T. (1975). Initial reactions in the oxidation of naphthalene by *Pseudomonas putida*. *Biochemistry*, **14**, 575–84.

Jeffrey, A., Blobstein, S. H., Weinstein, I. B., Beland, F. A., Harvey, R. G., Kasai, H. & Nakanishi, K. (1976). Structure of 7,12-dimethylbenz[a]anthracene guanosine conjugates. *Proc. Natl. Acad. Sci. USA*, **73**, 2311–5.

Jerina, D. M., van Bladeren, P. J., Yagi, H., Gibson, D. T., Mahadevan, V., Neese, A. S., Koreeda, M., Sharma, N. D. & Boyd, D. R. (1984). Synthesis and absolute configuration of the bacterial *cis*-1,2-, *cis*-8,9-, and *cis*-10,11-dihydrodiol metabolites of benz[a]anthracene formed by a strain of Beijerinckia. *J. Org. Chem.* **49**, 3621–8.

Jerina, D. M., Selander, H., Yagi, H., Wells, M. C., Davey, J. F., Mahadevan, V. & Gibson, D. T. (1976). Dihydrodiols from anthracene and phenanthrene. *J. Am. Chem. Soc.* **98**, 5988–96.

Karle, J. M., Mah, H. D., Jerina, D. M. & Yagi, H. (1977). Synthesis of dihydrodiols from chrysene and dibenzo[a,h]anthracene. *Tetrahedron Lett.* 4021–4.

Kedzierski, B., Thakker, D. R., Armstrong, R. N. & Jerina, D. M. (1981). Absolute configuration of the K-region 4,5-dihydrodiols and 4,5-oxide of benzo[a]pyrene. *Tetrahedron Lett.* **22**, 405–8.

Kole, P. L., Dubey, S. K. & Kumar, S. (1989). Synthesis of isomeric *cis*-dihydrodiols and phenols of highly mutagenic dibenz[a,c]anthracene. *J. Org. Chem.* **54**, 845–9.

Kolwyck, K. C., Duncan, W. P., Engel, J. F. & Selkirk, J. K. (1976). Labeled metabolites of polycyclic aromatic hydrocarbons. II. 4,5-Dihydrobenzo[a]pyrene-4,5-epoxide-G-^{3}H via *cis* 4,5-dihydrobenzo[a]pyrene-4,5-diol-G-^{3}H. *J. Labelled Compd. Radiopharm.* **12**, 153–8.

Konieczny, M. & Harvey, R. G. (1980). Reductive methylation of polycyclic aromatic quinones. *J. Org. Chem.* **45**, 1308–10.

Koreeda, M., Akhtar, M. N., Boyd, D. R., Neill, J. D., Gibson, D. T. & Jerina, D. M. (1978). Absolute stereochemistry of *cis*-1,2-, *trans*-1,2-, and *cis*-3,4-dihydrodiol metabolites of phenanthrene. *J. Org. Chem.* **43**, 1023–7.

Kumar, S., Kole, P. L. & Sehgal, R. K. (1989). Synthesis of the phenolic derivatives of highly tumorigenic *trans*-7,8-dihydroxy-7,8-dihydrobenzo[a]pyrene. *J. Org. Chem.* **54**, 5272–7.

Kundu, N. G. (1979). Convenient method for the reduction of *ortho*-quinones to dihydrodiols. *J. Chem. Soc. Chem. Commun.* 564–5.

Lee, H. & Harvey, R. H. (1986). Synthesis of the active diol epoxide metabolites of the potent carcinogenic hydrocarbon 7,12-dimethylbenz[a]anthracene. *J. Org. Chem.* **51**, 3502–7.

Lee, H., Sheth, J. & Harvey, R. G. (1983). Synthesis of putative oxidized metabolites of 8-methylbenzo[a]pyrene. *Carcinogenesis*, **4**, 1297–9.

Lee, H., Shyamasundar, N. & Harvey, R. G. (1981). Isomeric phenols of benzo[e]pyrene. *J. Org. Chem.* **46**, 2889–95.

Lee, H. M. & Harvey, R. G. (1979). Synthesis of biologically active metabolites of 7-methylbenz[a]anthracene. *J. Org. Chem.* **44**, 4948–53.

Lee, H. M. & Harvey, R. G. (1980). Synthesis of biologically active metabolites of dibenz[a,h]anthracene. *J. Org. Chem.* **45**, 588–92.

Lehr, R. E., Kumar, S., Cohenour, P. T. & Jerina, D. M. (1979). Dihydrodiols and diol epoxides of dibenzo[a,i]- and dibenzo[a,h]pyrene. *Tetrahedron Lett.* 3819–22.

Lehr, R. E., Schaefer-Ridder, M. & Jerina, D. M. (1977). Synthesis and properties of the vicinal *trans* dihydrodiols of anthracene, phenanthrene, and benzo[a]anthracene. *J. Org. Chem.* **42**, 736–44.

Lehr, R. E., Taylor, C. W., Kumar, S., Mah, H. D. & Jerina, D. M. (1978). Synthesis of the non-K-region and K-region *trans*-dihydrodiols of benzo[e]pyrene. *J. Org. Chem.* **43**, 3462–6.

Levin, W., Thakker, D. R., Wood, A. W., Chang, R. L., Lehr, R. E., Jerina, D. M. & Conney, A. H. (1978). Evidence that benzo[a]anthracene 3,4-diol-1,2-epoxide is an ultimate carcinogen on mouse skin. *Cancer Res.* **38**, 1705–10.

McCaustland, D. J., Duncan, W. P. & Engel, J. F. (1976). Labeled metabolites of polycyclic aromatic hydrocarbons. V. *Trans*-7,8-dihydrobenzo[a]pyrene-7,8-diol-7-^{14}C and (±)-7α,8ß-dihydroxy-9ß,10ß-epoxy-7,8,9,10-tetrahydrobenzo[a]pyrene-7-^{14}C. *J. Labelled Compd. Radiopharm.* **12**, 443–8.

McCaustland, D. J. & Engel, J. F. (1975). Metabolites of polycyclic hydrocarbons. II. Synthesis of 7,8-dihydrobenzo[a]pyrene-7,8-diol and 7,8-dihydrobenzo[a]pyrene-7,8-epoxide. *Tetrahedron Lett.* 2549–52.

McCaustland, D. J., Fischer, D. L., Duncan, W., Ogilvie, E. J. & Engel, J. F. (1976a). Labeled metabolites of polycyclic aromatic hydrocarbons. V. *Trans*-7,8-dihydrobenzo[a]pyrene-7,8-diol-G-^{3}H and (±)-7α,8ß-dihydroxy-9ß,10ß-epoxy-7,8,9,10-tetrahydrobenzo[a]pyrene-G-^{3}H. *J. Labelled Compd. Radiopharm.* **12**, 583–90.

Miura, R., Honmaru, S. & Nakazaki, M. (1968). The absolute configurations of the metabolites of naphthalene and phenanthrene in mammalian systems. *Tetrahedron Lett.* 5271–4.

Nakanishi, K., Kasai, H., Cho, H., Harvey, R. G., Jeffery, A. M., Jennette, K. W. & Weinstein, I. B. (1977). Absolute configuration of an RNA adduct formed *in vivo* by metabolism of benzo[a]pyrene. *J. Am. Chem. Soc.* **99**, 258–60.

Neidle, S., Subbiah, A. & Osborne, M. (1981). The molecular structure of (±)-7α,8ß-dihydroxy-7,8-dihydrobenzo[a]pyrene, an early metabolite of benzo[a]pyrene. *Carcinogenesis*, **2**, 533–6.

Newman, M. S. & Blum, S. (1964). A new cyclization reaction leading to epoxides of aromatic hydrocarbons. *J. Am. Chem. Soc.* **86**, 5598–600.

Nordqvist, M., Thakker, D. R., Vyas, K. P., Yagi, H., Levin, W., Ryan, D. E., Thomas, P. E., Conney, A. H. & Jerina, D. M. (1981). Metabolism of chrysene and phenanthrene to bay-region diol epoxides by rat liver enzymes. *Mol. Pharmacol.* **19**, 168–78.

Pataki, J. & Harvey, R. G. (1987). Synthesis of a sterically impeded analog of the carcinogenic *anti*-diol epoxide of benzo[a]pyrene. *J. Org. Chem.* **52**, 2226–30.

Pataki, J., Lee, H. & Harvey, R. G. (1983). Carcinogenic metabolites of 5-methylchrysene. *Carcinogenesis*, **4**, 399–402.

Pataki, J., Raddo, P. D. & Harvey, R. G. (1989). An efficient synthesis of the highly tumorigenic *anti* diol epoxide derivative of benzo[c]phenanthrene. *J. Org. Chem.* **54**, 840–4.

Pirkle, W. H. & Finn, J. M. (1981). Chiral high-pressure liquid chromatographic stationary phases. 3. General resolution of arylalkylcarbinols. *J. Org. Chem.* **46**, 2935–8.

Platt, K. & Oesch, F. (1982). K-region *trans*-dihydrodiols of polycyclic arenes; and efficient and convenient preparation from o-quinones or o-diphenols by reduction with sodium borohydride in the presence of oxygen. *Synthesis*, 459–61.

Platt, K. L. & Oesch, F. (1982a). Synthesis of non-K-region *ortho*-quinones of polycyclic aromatic hydrocarbons from cyclic ketones. *Tetrahedron Lett.* **23**, 163–6.

Platt, K. L. & Oesch, F. (1983). Efficient synthesis of non-K-region *trans*-dihydrodiols of polycyclic aromatic hydrocarbons from o-quinones and catechols. *J. Org. Chem.* **48**, 265–8.

Rastetter, W. H., Nachbar, R. B. Jr., Russo-Rodriguez, S., Wattley, R. V., Thilly, W. G., Andon, B. M., Jorgensen, W. L. & Ibrahim, M. (1982). Fluoranthene synthesis and mutagenicity of four diol epoxides. *J. Org. Chem.* **47**, 4873–8.

Rice, J. E., Shih, H., Hussain, N. & LaVoie, E. J. (1987). Synthesis of the major metabolic dihydrodiols of benz[j]fluoranthene. *J. Org. Chem.* **52**, 849–55.

Schollmeier, M., Frank, H., Oesch, F. & Platt, K. L. (1986). Assignment of absolute configuration to metabolically formed *trans*-dihydrodiols of dibenz[a,h]anthracene by two distinct spectroscopic methods. *J. Org. Chem.* **51**, 5368–72.

Silverton, J. V., Dansette, P. M. & Jerina, D. M. (1976). Oxidation of 4,5-dihydrobenzo[a]pyrene with osmium tetroxide. Stereochemistry of a substituted K-region diol. *Tetrahedron Lett.* 1557–60.

Sims, P. (1966). The metabolism of 3-methylcholanthrene and some related compounds by rat-liver homogenates. *Biochem. J.* **98**, 215–28.

Sims, P. (1967). The metabolism of 7- and 12-methylbenz[a]anthracene and their derivatives. *Biochem. J.* **105**, 591–8.

Sims, P. (1971). Epoxy derivatives of aromatic polycyclic hydrocarbons. The preparation of benz[a]anthracene 8,9-oxide and 10,11-dihydrobenz[a]anthracene 8,9-oxide and their metabolism by rat liver preparations. *Biochem.* **125**, 159–68.

Sukumaran, K. B. & Harvey, R. G. (1980). Synthesis of *o*-quinones and dihydrodiols of polycyclic aromatic hydrocarbons from the corresponding phenols. *J. Org. Chem.* **45**, 4407–13.

Thakker, D. R., Levin, W., Yagi, H., Turujman, S., Kapadia, D., Conney, A. H. & Jerina, D. M. (1979). Absolute stereochemistry of the *trans*-dihydrodiols formed from benzo[a]anthracene by liver microsomes. *Chem.–Biol. Interact.* **27**, 145–61.

Thakker, D. R., Yagi, H., Akagi, H., Koreeda, M., Lu, A. Y. H., Levin, W., Wood, A. W., Conney, A. H. & Jerina, D. M. (1977). Metabolism of benzo[a]pyrene VI. Stereoselective metabolism of benzo[a]pyrene and benzo[a]pyrene 7,8-dihydrodiol to diol epoxides. *Chem.–Biol. Interact.* **16**, 281–300.

Utermoehlen, C. M., Singh, M. & Lehr, R. E. (1987). Fjord region 3,4-diol 1,2-epoxides and other derivatives in the 1,2,3,4- and 5,6,7,8-benzo rings of the carcinogen benzo[g]chrysene. *J. Org. Chem.* **52**, 5574–82.

Vyas, K. P., Thakker, D. R., Levin, W., Yagi, H., Conney, A. H. & Jerina, D. M. (1982). Stereoselective metabolism of the optical isomers of *trans*-1,2-dihydroxy-1,2-dihydrophenanthrene to bay-region diol epoxides by rat liver microsomes. *Chem.–Biol. Interact.* **38**, 203–13.

Weems, H., Fu, P. P. & Yang, S. K. (1986). Stereoselective metabolism of chrysene by rat liver microsomes. Direct resolution of diol enantiomers by chiral stationary phase h.p.l.c. *Carcinogenesis*, **7**, 1221–30.

Weems, H. B., Mushtaq, M., Fu, P. P. & Yang, S. K. (1986). Direct separation of non-K-region mono-ol and diol enantiomers of phenanthrene, benz[a]anthracene, and chrysene by high-performance liquid chromatography with chiral stationary phases. *J. Chromatog.* **371**, 211–25.

Weems, H. B. & Yang, S. K. (1982). Resolution of optical isomers by chiral high performance chromatography: separation of dihydrodiols and tetrahydrodiols of benzo[a]pyrene and benz[a]anthracene. *Anal. Biochem.* **125**, 156–61.

Yagi, H., Akagi, H., Thakker, D. R., Mah, H. D., Koreeda, M. & Jerina, D. M. (1977a). Absolute stereochemistries of the highly mutagenic 7,8-diol 9,10-epoxides derived from the potent carcinogen *trans*-7,8-dihydroxy-7,8-dihydrobenzo[a]pyrene. *J. Am. Chem. Soc.* **99**, 2358–59.

Yagi, H., Dansette, P. & Jerina, D. M. (1976). Specifically tritiated arene oxides. *J. Labelled Compd. Radiopharm.* **12**, 127–32.

Yagi, H., Thakker, D. R., Hernandez, O., Koreeda, M. & Jerina, D. M. (1977). Synthesis and reactions of the highly mutagenic 7,8-diol 9,10-epoxides of the carcinogen benzo[a]pyrene. *J. Am. Chem. Soc.* **99**, 1604–11.

Yagi, H., Thakker, D. R., Ittah, Y., Croisy-Delcey, M. & Jerina, D. M. (1983). Synthesis and assignment of absolute configuration to the *trans* 3,4-dihydrodiols and 3,4-diol epoxides of benzo[c]phenanthrene. *Tetrahedron Lett.* **24**, 1349–52.

Yagi, H., Vyas, K. P., Tada, M., Thakker, D. R. & Jerina, D. M. (1982). Synthesis of the enantiomeric bay-region diol epoxides of benz[a]anthracene and chrysene. *J. Org. Chem.* **47**, 1110–17.

Yang, S. K. (1982). The absolute stereochemistry of the major *trans*-dihydrodiol enantiomers formed from 11-methylbenz[a]anthracene by rat liver microsomes. *Drug Metab. Dispos.* **10**, 205–11.

Yang, S. K. & Fu, P. P. (1984). Stereoselective metabolism of 7-methylbenz[a]anthracene: Absolute configuration of five dihydrodiol metabolites and the effect of dihydrodiol conformation on circular dichroism spectra. *Chem.–Biol. Interact.* **49**, 71–88.

Yang, S. K. & Fu, P. P. (1984a). The effect of the bay-region 12-methyl group on the stereoselective metabolism at the K-region of 7,12-dimethylbenz[a]anthracene by rat liver microsomes. *Biochem. J.* **223**, 775–82.

Yang, S. K., Gelboin, H. V., Weber, J. D., Sankaran, V., Fischer, D. L. & Engel, J. F. (1977). Resolution of optical isomers by high-pressure liquid chromatography. *Anal. Biochem.* **78**, 520–6.

Yang, S. K. & Mushtaq, M. (1986). Elution order-absolute configuration relationship of K-region dihydrodiol enantiomers of benz[a]anthracene derivatives in chiral stationary phase high-performance liquid chromatography. *J. Chromatog.* **371**, 195–209.

Yang, S. K., Mushtaq, M. & Kan, L. (1987). Absolute configurations of 1,2-dihydro-benzo[b]fluoranthene-*trans*-1,2-diols and diastereomeric 1,2,3,3a-tetrahydrobenzo-[b]fluoranthene-*trans*-1,2-diols. *J. Org. Chem.* **52**, 125–9.

Yang, S. K. & Weems, H. B. (1984). Direct enantiomeric resolution of some 7,12-dimethylbenz[a]anthracene derivatives by high-performance liquid chromatography with ionically and covalently bonded chiral stationary phases. *Anal. Chem.* **56**, 2658–62.

Yang, S. K., Weems, H. B., Mushtaq, M. & Fu, P. P. (1984). Direct resolution of mono- and diol enantiomers of unsubstituted and methyl-substituted benz[a]anthracene and benzo[a]pyrene by high-performance liquid chromatagraphy with a chiral stationary phase. *J. Chromatog.* **316**, 569–84.

Zacharias, D. E., Glusker, J. P., Fu, P. P. & Harvey, R. G. (1979). Molecular structures of the dihydrodiols and diol epoxides of carcinogenic polycyclic aromatic hydrocarbons. X-ray crystallographic and NMR analysis. *J. Am. Chem. Soc.* **101**, 4043–51.

Zacharias, D. E., Glusker, J. P., Harvey, R. G. & Fu, P. P. (1977). Molecular structure of the K-region *cis*-dihydrodiol of 7,12-dimethylbenz[a]anthracene. *Cancer Res.* **37**, 775–82.

14

Diol epoxides

Diol epoxides have been identified as the principal active metabolites of carcinogenic polyarenes that bind covalently to nucleic acids, leading to mutation and neoplastic growth. The development of methods for the synthesis of diol epoxides stimulated an outpouring of research directed towards elucidation of the mechanisms of carcinogenesis of polyarenes at the molecular-genetic level. This chapter reviews the chemistry of the PAH diol epoxides, with emphasis on methods for their synthesis and their structural and chemical properties. Some aspects of these topics were touched upon in earlier reviews by the author (Harvey, 1985, 1989; Harvey & Fu, 1978).

Investigations of the chemical and biological properties of diol epoxides have focused mainly on the isomers that contain an epoxide ring in a bay region. The bay region diol epoxides are implicated as the principal active forms of carcinogenic PAHs. The best known and most intensively investigated bay region diol epoxides are the benzo[a]pyrene *anti* and *syn* diol epoxides (*anti*- and *syn*-BPDE) (Fig. 14.1).

14.1   Structure and stereochemistry

The conformational properties of PAH diol epoxides may be expected *a priori* to resemble those of the parent dihydrodiols. However, a potential significant difference is the contribution of hydrogen bonding

Fig. 14.1. The bay region diol epoxide isomers of benzo[a]pyrene.

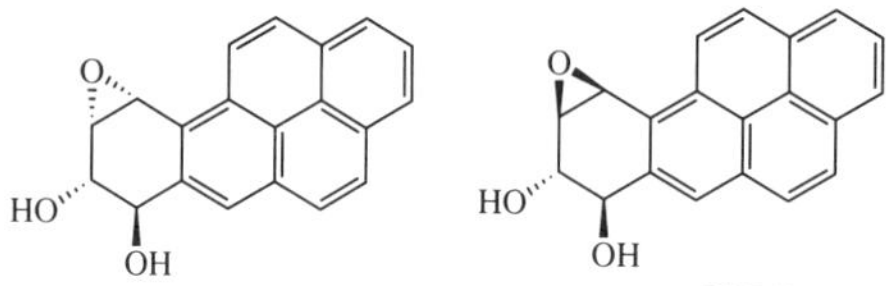

anti-BPDE   syn-BPDE

between the benzylic hydroxyl group and the epoxide oxygen of the *syn*-isomer. Molecular orbital theoretical studies on *anti*-BPDE predict its diequatorial conformer to be more stable than its diaxial conformer (Yeh *et al.*, 1978; Kikuchi *et al.*, 1979; Klopman *et al.*, 1979). CNDO/2 calculations on *syn*-BPDE indicate that transannular hydrogen-bonding is not energetically favored in the semi-chair conformation of the saturated ring but is favored in an alternative more puckered diaxial conformation (Yeh *et al.*, 1978). CNDO/2L and MINDO/3 calculations also support an internally hydrogen-bonded diaxial conformation for *syn*-BPDE. The relevance of these theoretical findings to biological events is uncertain, since in the biological milieux the hydroxyl groups of the diol epoxide molecules are likely to be associated with water molecules, considerably decreasing the likelihood of intramolecular hydrogen bonding.

X-ray crystallographic analysis of *anti*- and *syn*-BPDE show that both isomers exist exclusively in diequatorial conformations in the crystal lattice (Neidle *et al.*, 1980; Neidle & Cutbush, 1983). However, the saturated ring of the *syn*-isomer is more puckered than that of the *anti*-isomer as a consequence of the steric interaction between the C-8 hydrogen atom and the oxygen atom of the epoxide ring. The angle between the plane of the epoxide ring and the aromatic ring system of *anti*-BPDE is 83°, whereas in the *syn*-isomer this angle is splayed out to 118°. X-ray studies of the *anti*-diol epoxide derivative of naphthalene indicate that its structure is closely similar (Klein & Stevens, 1984).

NMR analysis of BPDE in solution indicates that both diastereomers exist as rapidly equilibrating mixtures of conformers. The percentage of the diequatorial conformer of *anti*-BPDE in solution in dimethyl sulfoxide at room temperature is calculated to be 58–65% (Harvey, 1989) based on the coupling of the carbinol hydrogens $J_{7,8} = 8.25–9.0$ Hz. This value is closely similar to that of its dihydrodiol precursor for which $J_{7,8} = 9.0$ Hz. *syn*-BPDE exhibits a smaller coupling constant ($J_{7,8} = 6.0$ Hz), indicative of a lower percentage of the diequatorial conformer (~62%) under the same conditions. The diequatorial conformer of *syn*-BPDE is disfavored by steric interaction between the nonbenzylic carbinol hydrogen atom and the epoxide oxygen atom as well as by eclipsing between the 8-hydroxyl group and the 9-hydrogen atom. This is partially counterbalanced by the interaction between the benzylic oxiranyl hydrogen atom and the aromatic proton in the adjacent bay region site in the diaxial conformer.

In comparison, the analogous couplings of the *anti*- and *syn*-diol·epoxides of naphthalene were $J_{1,2} = 9.0$ and 3.0 Hz, respectively. These findings indicate that the conformation of the *anti*-isomer is essentially identical with that of *anti*- BPDE, while the *syn*-isomer shows a considerably higher ratio of the diaxial conformer (~90%). The coupling constants of the dimethyl ethers of the *anti-* and *syn*-diol epoxides of naphthalene were very similar ($J_{1,2}$ = 8.8 and 2.8 Hz, respectively) to those of the unmethylated compounds. This suggests that intramolecular hydrogen bonding may be less important in determining conformational preferences than is usually assumed.

NMR data on the *anti*-diol epoxides of other proximate dihydrodiols reveal a relatively narrow range of values for the coupling constants of the carbinol hydrogens (Figs 14.2 and 14.3). For molecules free to adopt the diequatorial orientation, the values of J_{diol} lie between 8 and 9 Hz, indicative of a small preference for this conformation. More sterically restricted bay

Fig. 14.2. Bay region *anti*-diol epoxide derivatives (NMR coupling constants in Hz of the carbinol protons of the *anti-* and *syn*-isomers, respectively, are given in parentheses). [a]Lehr *et al.*, 1977; [b]Pataki *et al.*, 1989; [c]Sayer *et al.*, 1981; [d]Yagi *et al.*, 1979; [e]Harvey *et al.*, 1986; [f]Beland & Harvey, 1976; [g]Yagi *et al.*, 1975; [h]Lee & Harvey, 1980; [i]Harvey *et al.*, 1988; [j]Utermoehlen *et al.*, 1987; [k]Bushman *et al.*, 1989; [l]Lehr *et al.*, 1979; [m]Geddie *et al.*, 1987.

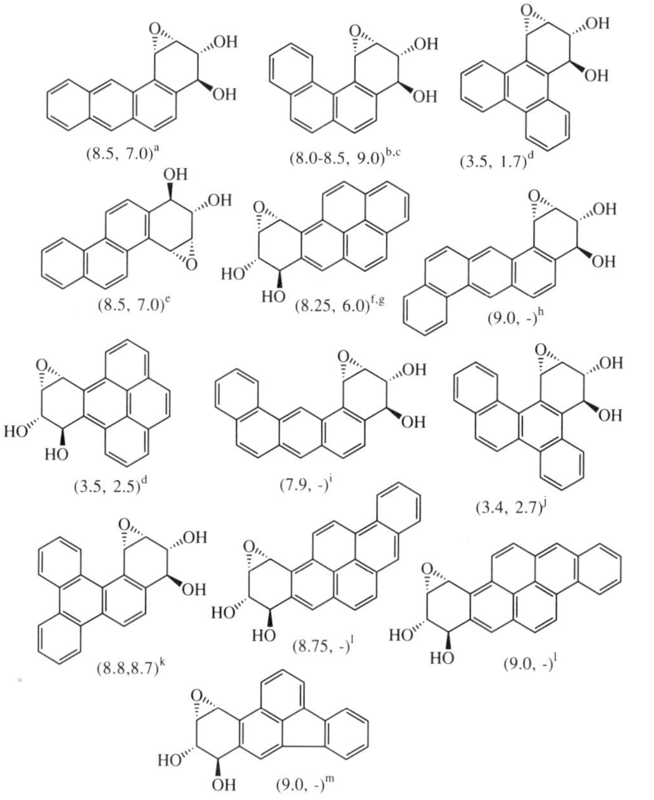

region *anti*-diol epoxides in which the diol function is also in a bay region, such as the diol epoxide derivatives of triphenylene, BeP, and benzo[g]chrysene 3,4-diol-1,2-epoxide, or in which the diol function is sterically hindered by a peri group, such as 6-fluoro-BaP, exhibit lower values of J_{diol} (3.4–5.5 Hz) consistent with a diaxial conformation.

The *syn*-diol epoxide derivatives of the proximate dihydrodiols (Figs 14.2 and 14.3) exhibit a wider range of values for J_{diol}. Molecules free to adopt the diequatorial conformation have values of J_{diol} in the range of 6–9.6 Hz, indicative of only a small preference for one or the other conformation. The 3-MC *syn*-diol epoxide, for which J_{diol} is 3.0 Hz, is an exception for which there is no obvious explanation. Sterically hindered bay region *syn*-diol epoxides, such as the derivatives of triphenylene, BeP, 6-fluoro-BaP, and benzo[g]chrysene 3,4-diol-1,2-epoxide, exhibit lower values of J_{diol} (1.7–2.7 Hz), confirming their existence exclusively in the diaxial conformation. It is also of some interest that the *syn*-diol epoxides in which the epoxide oxygen atom is exceptionally crowded, e.g. in a fjord region, such as the benzo[c]-phenanthrene, or that have a bay region methyl group, such as 5-methylchrysene, tend to exhibit higher values of J_{diol} consistent with a preferred diequatorial conformation. It is probably significant that these diol epoxides and/or the parent hydrocarbons tend to exhibit the highest carcino-

Fig. 14.3. Substituted bay region *anti*-diol epoxides (NMR couplings in Hz of the carbinol protons of the *anti*- and *syn*-isomers are given in parentheses). [a]Lee & Harvey, 1979; [b]Lee & Harvey, 1986; [c]Harvey *et al.*, 1988a; [d]Jacobs *et al.*, 1983; [e]Harvey *et al.*, 1986; [f]Amin *et al.*, 1986; [g]Yagi *et al.*, 1987.

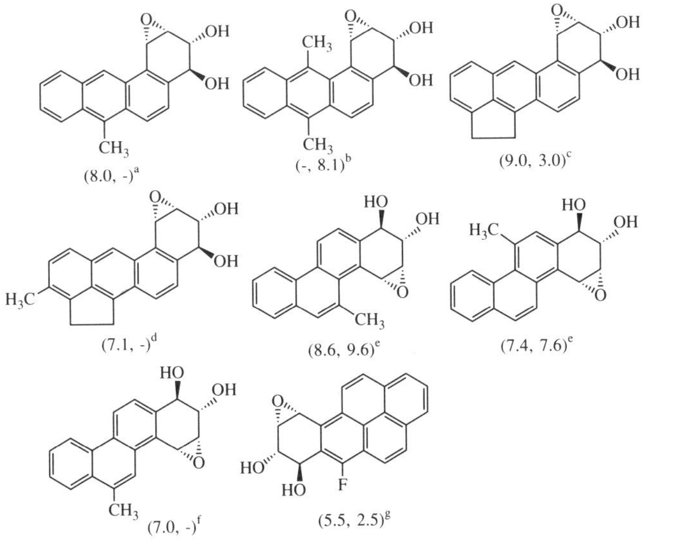

genic potency. Although solvent effects have been ignored in the preceding discussion, they may also play a significant role in conformation. Thus, the NMR spectrum of the benzo[g]chrysene *syn*-11,12-diol-13,14-epoxide exhibited $J_{11,12} = 8.7$ Hz in DMSO-d_6, but this value dropped to 3.3 Hz in CDCl$_3$, indicative of a change in preferred conformation from diequatorial to diaxial. This difference is likely due to the hydrogen bonding with the solvent in DMSO-d_6 and internal hydrogen bonding between the benzylic hydroxyl group and the epoxide ring in CDCl$_3$.

It should be emphasized that the energy for conformational inter-conversion of the bay region diol epoxide isomers is normally low in the absence of steric effects. Consequently, the ratio of conformers in equil-ibrium may be expected to shift readily with changes in experimental conditions and during reaction. The position of the conformational equili-brium may also be expected to be readily altered by association with hydrogen-bonding solvents or with DNA and other cellular macromolecules. For these reasons, it is unsafe to assume that the reactions of these diol epoxide isomers involve the conformer that happens to be most favored by the unreacting molecule in solution or in the crystal lattice.

Various types of nonbay region diol epoxides are also known (Fig. 14.4). These include terminal ring diol epoxides, the diol epoxide derivatives of bay region dihydrodiols, and the unusual diol epoxide derivatives of fluoranthene that contain a diol epoxide ring fused to both a benzo ring and a five-membered ring. Both possible pairs of *anti* and *syn* diastereomers of the

Fig. 14. 4. Nonbay region *anti*-diol epoxides (NMR couplings in Hz of the carbinol protons of the *anti*- and *syn*-isomers are given in parentheses). [a]Lehr *et al.*, 1977; [b]Harvey & Sukumaran, 1977; [c]Yagi *et al.*, 1987; [d]Lee & Harvey, 1980; [e]Lee & Harvey, 1981; [f]Harvey & Fu, 1980; [g]Rastetter *et al.*, 1982.

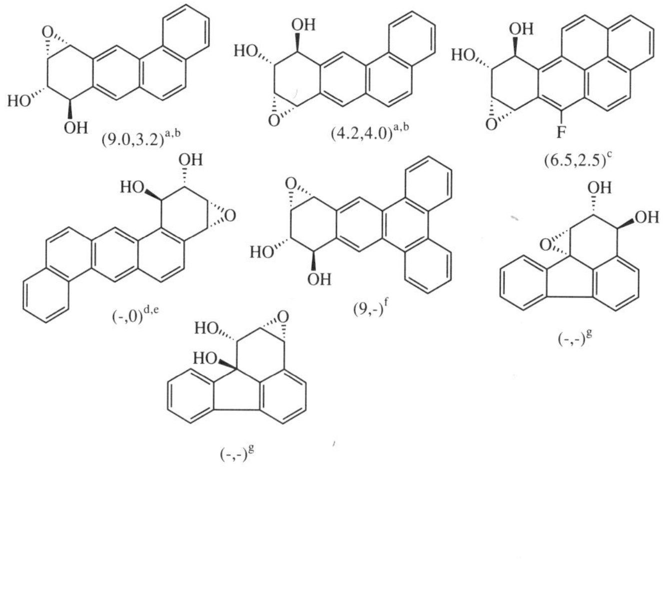

latter, one in which the epoxide ring is bonded to a tertiary carbon atom, and the other in which the benzylic hydroxyl group is attached to the trisubstituted carbon atom, have been synthesized (Rastetter *et al.*, 1982). These diol epoxides may presumably exist in fixed conformation because of the constraints of the relatively rigid ring system. However, there is no information available on the structural properties of the fluoranthene diol epoxide isomers.

14.2   Synthesis

The synthesis of polyarene diol epoxides presents a special challenge because of their exceptional reactivity and susceptibility to decomposition by several modes. The problem is compounded by the necessity to obtain the diol epoxides in a highly pure state for mutation studies and other biological investigations.

The *anti*- and *syn*-diol epoxide derivatives of benzo[a]pyrene were the first to be synthesized and their chemical and biological properties have been the subjects of intensive subsequent investigations. The benzo[a]pyrene *anti*-diol epoxide (*anti*-BPDE) is synthetically accessible from BaP *trans*-7,8-dihydro-diol by reaction with *m*-chloroperbenzoic acid at room temperature (Harvey & Fu, 1978; Yagi *et al.*, 1977; Beland & Harvey, 1976) (Fig. 14.5). The stereospecificity of the epoxidation reaction with *m*-CPBA is believed to be controlled by association of the reagent with the allylic 8-hydroxyl group, forming an intermediate complex that delivers the peracid oxygen atom from the same face of the molecule (Fig. 14.6). A large excess of *m*-CPBA is generally employed in order to keep reaction time relatively short and

Fig. 14.5. Stereospecific syntheses of *trans*-7α,8β-dihydroxy-*anti*-8ß,10ß-epoxy-7,8,9,10-tetrahydrobenzo[a]pyrene (*anti*-BPDE) and *trans*-7α,8β-dihydroxy-*syn*-9α,10α-epoxy-7,8,9,10-tetrahydrobenzo[a]pyrene (*syn*-BPDE).

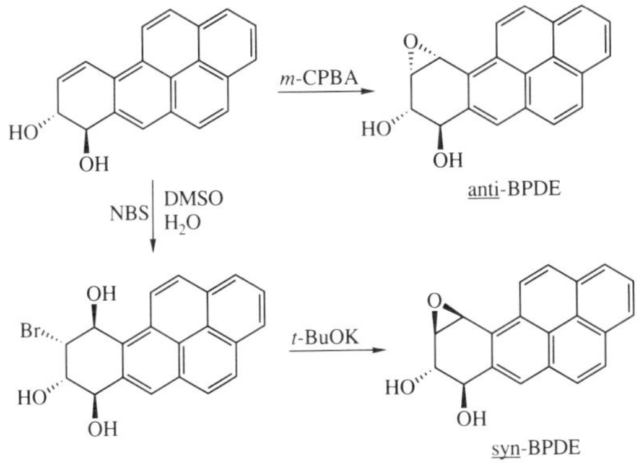

minimize secondary reaction of *anti*-BPDE with byproduct benzoic acid. For the same reason, and because *anti*-BPDE is also susceptible to acid-catalyzed hydrolysis, reactions are generally worked up as rapidly as possible by partition between ethyl ether and cold 10% aqueous NaOH. The ether extracts are then dried and concentrated *in vacuo* avoiding heating which also may cause decomposition. Final purification is usually accomplished by column chromatography on deactivated activity IV alumina, keeping column residence time to a minimum. Higher activity adsorbants or mildly acidic adsorbants, such as silical gel, cannot be employed because substantial decomposition takes place on columns of these types. Product purity is usually verified by HPLC and NMR analysis. Further purification, although usually not necessary, can be accomplished in most cases by HPLC methods. Samples of pure, dry *anti*-BPDE may be stored for prolonged periods in the freezer without significant decomposition. Conversely, less pure samples, or samples from which traces of moisture have not been excluded, may decompose rapidly. For a more detailed description of the recommended experimental procedure for the synthesis of *anti*-BPDE see Harvey & Fu, 1978.

Stereospecific synthesis of *syn*-BPDE is accomplished in two steps by reaction of BaP *trans*-7,8-dihydrodiol with N-bromosuccinimide in moist dimethylsulfoxide, or with N-bromoacetamide, to generate the corresponding bromohydrin followed by base-catalyzed cyclization with potassium tert-butoxide (or Amberlite IRA-400 resin, OH form) (Harvey & Fu, 1978; Yagi *et al.*, 1977; Beland & Harvey, 1976) (Fig. 14.5). The bromination reaction occurs *trans*-stereospecifically to furnish the bromohydrin isomer in which the bromine atom is on the same face of the molecule as the 8-hydroxyl group. This steric preference is explicable as due to initial formation of a bromonium ion intermediate on the same face of the molecule as favored by epoxidation (Fig. 14.6). Attack on the opposite face is disfavored by steric interaction between the large bromine atom and the hydrated 7-hydroxyl

Fig. 14.6. The stereospecificity of *anti*- and *syn*-diol epoxide synthesis is a consequence of hydrogen-bonding and steric factors in the respective intermediate complexes A and B. The aromatic ring systems are omitted for simplicity.

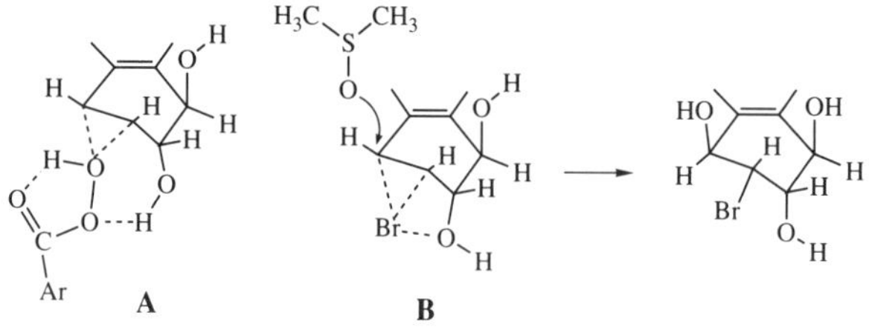

group anticipated to be oriented predominantly axially in the partially aqueous medium (rather than the equatorial orientation favored in non-hydrogen bonding organic solvents). Attack of the bromine atom on the same face of the molecule as the 8-hydroxyl group may also be aided by partial bonding of the bromonium ion with this hydroxyl group. Backside attack by the oxygen atom of DMSO on the benzylic carbon of the bromonium ion intermediate (Dalton & Jones, 1967) followed by hydrolysis affords the bromohydrin isomer in which the 10-hydroxyl group is *cis* to the 7-hydroxyl group. With NBA as the brominating reagent in the absence of DMSO, water is the probable source of the hydroxyl group of the bromohydrin. On treatment of the bromohydrin with an appropriate base it undergoes *trans*-elimination to furnish the *syn*-diol epoxide. Since *syn*-BPDE like its *anti*-isomer is a highly reactive molecule, similar precautions must be taken during its preparation and purification to avoid loss by decomposition.

The isomeric structures of the *anti* and *syn* diastereomers were un-equivocally assigned by Beland & Harvey, 1976 on the basis of NMR spectral and chemical evidence. Thus, the reactions of both *anti*- and *syn*-BPDE with the strong nucleophilic reagent sodium *tert*-butylthiolate in aqueous dioxane furnished the products of *trans*-stereospecific S_N2 addition (**1a** and **1b**) which on acetylation gave the corresponding triacetates (**2a** and **2b**) (Fig. 14.7). Acetylation simplified interpretation of the NMR spectra by abolishing the hydroxyl proton couplings and locking the conformation into one in which the bulky *tert*-butyl group adopts the more comfortable axial orientation in the sterically crowded bay region. Analysis of the couplings of

Fig. 14.7. Addition of *tert*-butylthiolate to *anti*- and *syn*-BPDE yields adducts in which the bulky group is in the bay region where it must adopt the pseudoaxial conformation due to steric restriction. Chemical tests confirm the presence of vicinal *cis*-hydroxyl groups in **1a** but not in **1b**, and NMR analysis of the diacetates **2a** and **2b** provides proof of the assignment of the diol epoxide diastereomers.

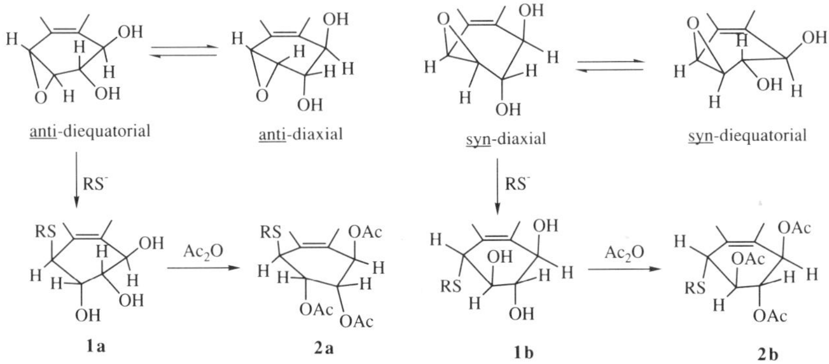

anti-diequatorial   anti-diaxial   syn-diaxial   syn-diequatorial

1a   2a   1b   2b

the remaining nonaromatic protons permitted assignment of the structures of the acetylated adducts as those depicted in Fig. 14.7. These structures were also consistent with the observations that the adduct **1a** gave a precipitate with Criegee's potassium triacetylosmate reagent and reacted with acetone in the presence of acid to furnish an acetonide, characteristic reactions of *cis*-hydroxyl groups, confirming the *cis* relationship between the 8- and 9-hydroxyl groups. The isomer **1b** failed to undergo either reaction, consistent with its lack of *cis*- hydroxyl groups. These structural assignments of *anti*- and *syn*-BPDE agree with those proposed by Yagi *et al.*, 1975 on the basis of NMR analysis and the presumed analogy of the epoxidation reaction with some reported examples of stereoselective epoxidation of cyclohexenols. These assignments are also supported by aqueous solvolysis studies (Keller *et al.*, 1976; Yagi *et al.*, 1977; Yang *et al.*, 1977) reviewed in Section 14.4.

The methods devised for the synthesis of *anti*- and *syn*-BPDE were utilized subsequently with appropriate modification for the synthesis of the diol epoxide derivatives of numerous polyarenes representing a wide range of carcinogenic activities. These syntheses were conducted principally in the author's laboratory or by Jerina, Lehr and their associates. While the same general methodology is effective for virtually all the PAHs studied to date, the diol epoxide derivatives of various PAHs vary markedly in their relative stability. In particular, the bay region diol epoxide derivatives of the most potent carcinogenic hydrocarbons, particularly those that contain a methyl group in a nonbenzo bay region position such as the DMBA 1,2-diol-3,4-diol epoxide, tend to be highly reactive and difficult to obtain in a pure state (Lee & Harvey, 1986). Nevertheless, even in these cases it is frequently possible, by utilizing mild conditions and working rapidly, to isolate the pure diol epoxides and conduct limited biological studies with them. In Figs 14.2–14.3 are listed the bay region *anti*- and *syn*-diol epoxide derivatives of polyarenes whose syntheses have been reported to date.

The directing effect of the allylic hydroxyl group, used to advantage for the stereospecific syntheses of *anti*-BPDE, is not always so effective. Lower stereoselectivity is generally observed in the peracid oxidation of bay-region and other dihydrodiols in which the conformation of the allylic hydroxyl group is restricted to the axial orientation. Thus, epoxidation of the bay region dihydrodiols of triphenylene and BeP affords a mixture of *anti*- and *syn*-diol epoxides in which the former predominates (Yagi *et al.*, 1975), and epoxidation of the bay region dihydrodiols of 7-methyl-BA and DBA is actually *syn*-stereoselective (Lee & Harvey, 1981). The latter finding has been interpreted as due to exertion of steric control over epoxidation by the axial benzylic hydroxyl groups. Similar effects have been observed in the epoxidation of the 9,10-dihydrodiol of BaP (Thakker *et al.*, 1978) and the

7,8-dihydrodiol of 6-fluoro-BaP (Yagi *et al.*, 1987) both of which exist preferentially in the diaxial conformation.

Similar lack of stereospecificity was observed in the peracid oxidation of fluoranthene 1,10b-dihydrodiol (Fig. 14.8: **3a**) in which the benzylic hydroxyl group is attached to a fluorene ring (Rastetter *et al.*, 1982). However, the stereoselective synthesis of the corresponding *anti*- and *syn*-diol epoxides was achieved by a modified strategy. Epoxidation of the TMS-protected dihydrodiol **3b** with *tert*-BuOOH/VO (acac)₂ and desilylation gave the *anti*-diol epoxide, while epoxidation of the monoacetate **3c** with this reagent and deacetylation afforded the *syn*-diol epoxide isomer. The latter observation provides further evidence that axial benzylic hydroxyl groups may exert steric control over the direction of epoxidation, favoring *syn* addition.

14.3   Optically active diol epoxides

While direct resolution of the optical isomers of *anti*- and *syn*-diol epoxides is generally impractical due to their instability, the (+) and (−) enantiomers may be obtained by epoxidation of the optically pure dihydrodiol enantiomers which are readily accessible by HPLC methods (Chap. 13). In Fig. 14.9 are listed the absolute configurations of the enantiomers of the *anti*- and *syn*-diol epoxide derivatives of the polyarenes that have been assigned to date. Omitted from this list are the diol epoxides of smaller ring systems, such as naphthalene, anthracene, and phenanthrene, that are of less interest in carcinogenesis research. In general, the *anti*-isomers exist as R,S,S,R and S,R,R,S pairs, and the *syn*-isomers occur as R,S,R,S and S,R,S,R pairs. Only one enantiomer of each pair is shown in Fig. 14.9.

Fig. 14.8. Stereospecific syntheses of the *anti*- and *syn*-diol epoxides of fluoranthene.

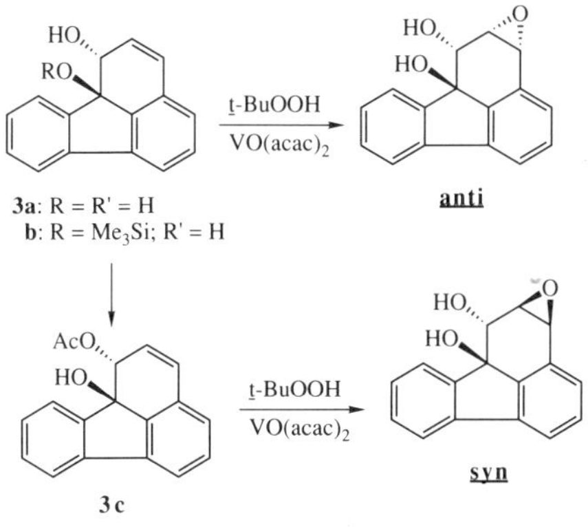

3a: R = R' = H
  b: R = Me₃Si; R' = H

3c

The stereoselectivity of the metabolism of dihydrodiols to diol epoxides is outside the scope of this volume. This topic has been reviewed by Yang *et al.*, 1985.

14.4   Reactions of diol epoxides

Diol epoxides, like other active carcinogenic metabolites, are electrophilic reagents, and their most important reactions are with nucleophiles. As a consequence of their relatively high reactivity, they

Fig. 14.9. The absolute configurations of these diol epoxides are assigned as shown: [a]Yagi *et al.*, 1983; [b]Hecht *et al.*, 1987; [c]Nakanishi *et al.*, 1977; [d]Yagi *et al.*, 1977; [e]Yagi & Jerina, 1982; [f]Yagi *et al.*, 1982; [g]Bushman *et al.*, 1989.

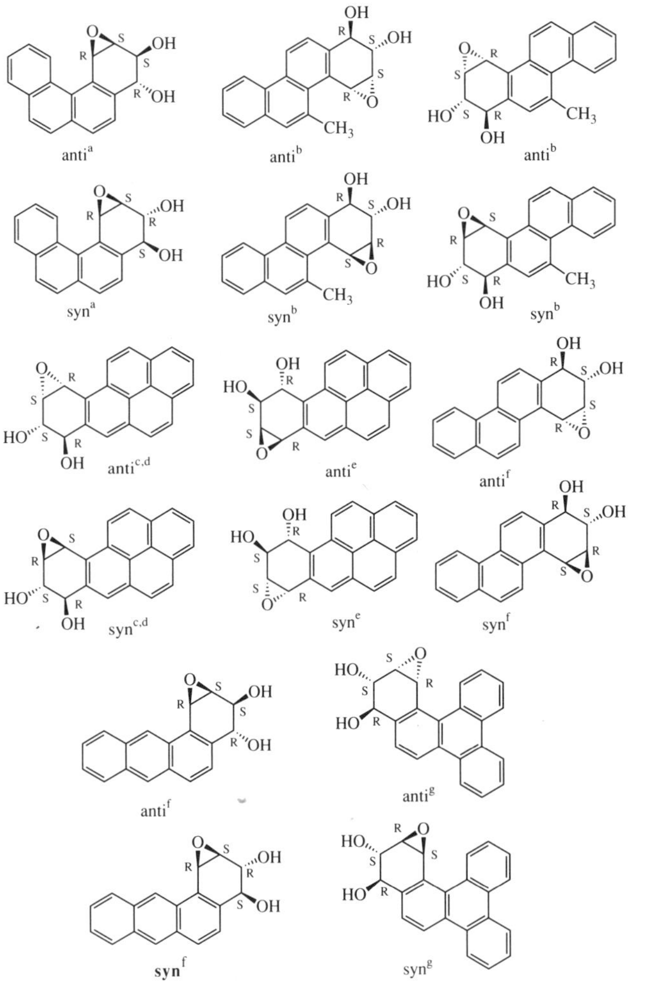

readily enter into reactions with even relatively weak nucleophiles, such as water.

14.4.1 Hydrolysis

Hydrolysis of diol epoxides at neutral pH is sufficiently rapid to necessitate special precautions to minimize this mode of decomposition during the isolation and purification of the synthetic compounds. In most cases, these precautions suffice to allow isolation and characterization of the pure diol epoxides. However, some highly reactive diol epoxide isomers, such as the *anti*-diol epoxide derivative of DMBA, require extreme precautions for their isolation and must be used immediately to minimize their decomposition (Lee & Harvey, 1986). Others, such as the analogous bay region diol epoxide derivatives of 7,14-dimethyldibenz[a,j]anthracene, are so reactive that attempts to obtain them synthetically have not yet been successful.

The stabilities of the isomeric diol epoxides in aqueous solutions is dependent upon experimental conditions and sample purity. Less pure samples tend to decompose more rapidly than very pure samples. The half-lives of *anti*- and *syn*-BPDE in tissue culture medium were reported to be ~8 min and ~0.5 min, respectively (Yagi *et al.*, 1977). On the other hand, considerably longer half-lives, > 120 min and 30 min, respectively, are commonly observed for these diol epoxides in aqueous solutions at neutral pH (e.g. Jennette *et al.*, 1977). It is likely that polyarene diol epoxides are absorbed into the lipid membranes of cells where they may have relatively long half-lives. Indeed, *anti*-BPDE was found to be still present in cells an hour after treatment (Kootstra, 1982). There is also evidence that diol epoxides are stabilized by association with proteins in solution (Roche *et al.*, 1985, Busbee *et al.*, 1982). Therefore, it is likely that these reactive metabolites may be transported in the serum from a tissue where they are formed to a remote target site.

The aqueous solvolysis of the isomeric BaP diol epoxides affords mixtures of tetraols arising from the *cis* and *trans* addition of water to the epoxide function (Keller *et al.*, 1977; Yagi *et al.*, 1977; Yang *et al.*, 1977) (Fig. 14.10). The rates of hydrolysis of the *syn*- and *anti*-BPDE isomers and the ratios of the isomeric tetraols produced are pH dependent. At low pH values (1 to 9) the *syn*-isomer is hydrated mainly by *cis* addition of water to form the corresponding tetraol **4a**, but between pH 9 to 12 the percentage of the *trans* tetraol **4b** increases from 15 to 33%. In contrast, hydration of the *anti*-isomer occurs predominantly *trans* to yield the tetraol **5a** throughout the entire pH range, decreasing from 87% at pH 1 to ~60% at pH 5 where it levels off and remains approximately constant between pH 5 to 12. The stereochemical findings are consistent with regiospecific or highly regioselective attack of water at the more reactive benzylic carbon atom of the epoxide ring. Thus, the tetraol isomer **4b** expected to arise from *trans*-specific attack of water at C-9 of *anti*-BPDE is generally not detected as a product of its hydration, and the tetraol **5a** expected from *trans*-specific attack of water at C-9 of *syn*-BPDE is either not detected or is only a minor product of its reaction. Aqueous solvolysis of *syn*-BPDE at higher pHs (5 to 11) leads under some conditions to formation of significant amounts of the isomeric ketone, *trans*-7,8-dihydroxy-9-keto-7,8,9,10-tetrahydro-BaP (Yagi *et al.*, 1977); this product is not detected under more acidic conditions. The relatively high level of *cis* addition to the *syn*-isomer was partially attributed to intramolecular hydrogen bonding between the benzylic hydroxyl group and the oxirane ring in the transition state.

Kinetic studies of these reactions reveal significant differences in the relative rates of the reactions of the *syn*- and *anti*-BPDE isomers toward water, the former isomer being ~30-fold more reactive at neutral to alkaline pH. The findings indicate that these hydrolyses are specific- and general-acid-catalyzed and involve the intermediacy of a benzylic carbocation species. General acid catalysts include phenol, phosphate ion, acetic acid, and Tris buffer. There is evidence for formation of BaP triol-phenoxide, -phosphate, and similar adducts as byproducts of these reactions (Yang *et al.*, 1977; Whalen *et al.*, 1979). Koreeda *et al.* (1976) found that 15% of *syn*-BPDE added to a phosphate buffer could not be extracted with an organic solvent, indicating covalent reaction with phosphate ions had taken place. On the other hand, Gamper *et al.* (1980) found that reaction of *anti*-BPDE with dibutyl phosphate gave only a small amount of the triester.

Fig. 14.10. Hydrolysis of *syn*-BPDE is *cis*-stereoselective giving **4a** as the principal product, while *anti*-BPDE exhibits *trans*-stereoselectivity yielding mainly **5a**.

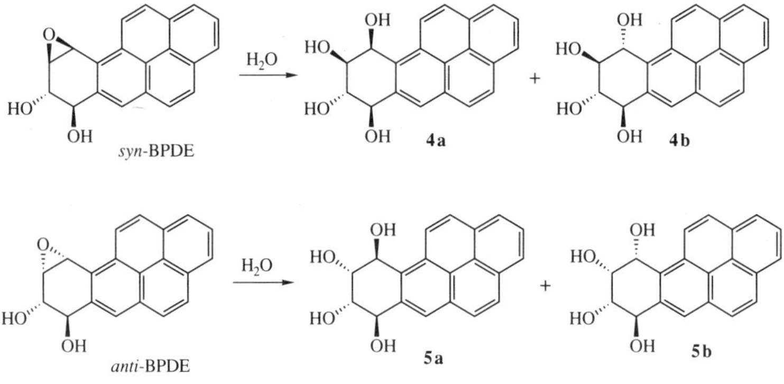

Solvolysis studies of the analogous bay region diol epoxides of chrysene and phenanthrene and the corresponding bay region epoxides lacking the hydroxyl groups provide additional insight (Whalen *et al.*, 1978). The rates of these hydrolyses, like those of the BaP diol epoxides, were found to fit the equation: $k_{obsd} = k_{H^+}a_{H^+} + k_0$ where k_{H^+} and k_0 are the rate constants for acid-catalyzed and spontaneous hydrolysis, respectively. The ratio of *cis* to *trans* hydrolysis of the epoxides without hydroxyl groups were found to increase in parallel with the theoretically calculated ease of carbonium ion formation at the benzylic positions. This is consistent with the previous findings that aryl substituents that favor carbonium ion formation tend to enhance the ratio of *cis* to *trans* hydrolysis products from 1-arylcyclohexene oxide. Moreover, the rates of hydrolysis of the tetrahydroepoxides were generally considerably higher than those of the related bay region diol epoxides. This difference was attributed to a combination of stereoelectronic factors and polar substituent effects. Molecular models indicate that a severe nonbonding interaction exists between H_{10} and H_{11} in the bay region of conformation **6a** of the tetrahydroepoxide of BaP, but this is substantially relieved in its alternative conformation **7a** (Fig. 14.11). In the latter conformation the benzylic C-O bond of the protonated epoxide bond that breaks in the hydrolysis reaction is nearly colinear with the p orbital of the aromatic ring system, an arrangement that allows maximum stabilization of the developing positive charge in the transition state. However, in the related diol epoxide *anti*-BPDE, NMR evidence indicates that the more stable conformation corresponds to **6b** in which the dihedral angle between the benzylic C-O bond and the planar aromatic ring system is ~60°. A similar conformation is preferred by *syn*-BPDE. Since this geometry does not contribute to stabilization of the developing positive charge at the benzylic site, hydrolysis must take place from this less favorable conformation or reorientation of the intermediate must occur prior to addition of water. In either case, reduced reactivity toward hydrolysis is be expected, consistent with the experimental finding. Additional evidence in support of this mechanism is provided by solvolysis experiments with the conformationally

Fig. 14.11. Conformation **7a** (R = H) of the BaP tetrahydroepoxide is favored by severe steric interaction between the bay region hydrogens in structure **6a**. On the other hand, the more stable conformation of the related *anti*-diol epoxide corresponds to **6b** (R = OH).

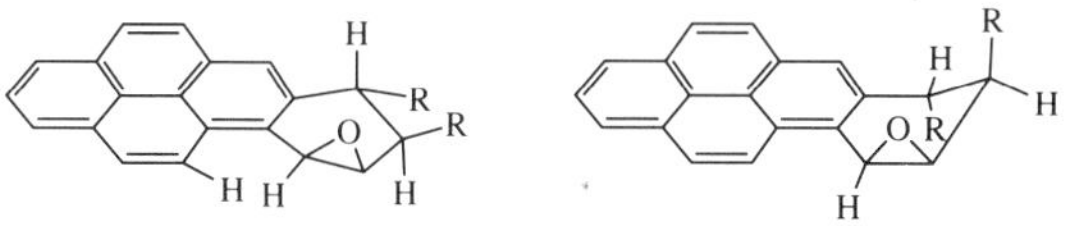

rigid, diastereomeric 9,10-oxides derived from hexahydrophenanthrene (**8** and **9**) as models for the more flexible BaP diol epoxides (Sayer *et al.*, 1982).

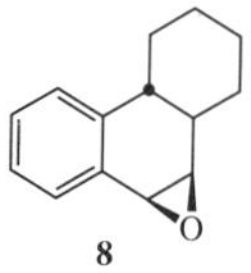

8 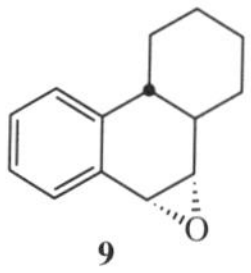   9

Conformational effects in the hydrolyses of several additional diol epoxides have also been investigated and the findings utilized as the basis of a set of rules to predict the relative rates and stereochemistries of hydrolysis of diol epoxides derived from polyarenes (Sayer *et al.*, 1984). For this purpose diol epoxides are divided into two categories, type A in which a major fraction exists as the *aligned conformer* at equilibrium and type N in which the epoxide exists predominantly as the *nonaligned conformer*. For type A diol epoxide isomers, pH independent hydrolysis (k_0) occurs more rapidly via this conformer, resulting in a relatively fast rate and a high percentage of *cis*-tetraol and/or keto diol products. Acid-catalyzed hydrolysis (k_{H^+}) of type A epoxides yields mixtures of *cis* and *trans* diols. For type N diol epoxide isomers, pH independent hydrolysis (k_0) is relatively slow, and gives predominantly or exclusively the *trans* diol product and no keto diol product. Hydrolysis of type N epoxides under acidic conditions also furnishes preferentially the *trans* diol product.

Hydrolysis of diol epoxides is catalyzed by DNA and nucleotides, but nucleosides have only a very minor effect (Geacintov *et al.*, 1982; Gupta *et al.*, 1982, 1987). In the presence of native DNA the hydrolysis of *anti*- BPDE is markedly accelerated by a factor of up to ~80. Denatured DNA is less effective with a pseudo-first-order rate constant that is smaller by a factor of ~3. Nucleotides and nucleosides increase the rate relative to DNA by factors of 3–10 and 1–2, respectively, dependent upon the purine or pyrimidine base and other experimental factors. Addition of magnesium ions (known to decrease intercalative binding of planar aromatic molecules to DNA) reduces these rate enhancements. The results suggest, but do not prove, that DNA-catalyzed hydrolysis involves an intercalated diol epoxide intermediate.

14.4.2   *Reactions with simple nucleophiles*

The reactions of diol epoxides with nucleophiles generally take place regiospecifically at the benzylic site of the oxirane ring. Reaction at this site is strongly favored by stabilization by the polycyclic aromatic ring system of the incipient positive charge formed on opening the epoxide ring. The reactions of the strong nucleophile *tert*-butylthiolate with *anti*- and *syn*-

BPDE were utilized initially to aid in the stereochemical assignments of these isomers (Beland & Harvey, 1976). The geometries of the resulting adducts resembles that of cyclohexene, which can adopt either a half-chair or a flattened boat conformation (Fig. 14.12). As a consequence of the steric crowding in the bay region, the bulky *tert*-butylthiol is constrained to attack the benzylic carbon from the axial direction to afford adducts in which this group is axially oriented. Consistent with this expectation, the observed couplings of the benzylic protons of the acetylated *trans*-adducts of *tert*-

Fig. 14.12. Conformational equilibria for the adducts formed by the addition of nucleophiles (N) to isomeric diol epoxides of benzo[a]pyrene followed by acetylation.

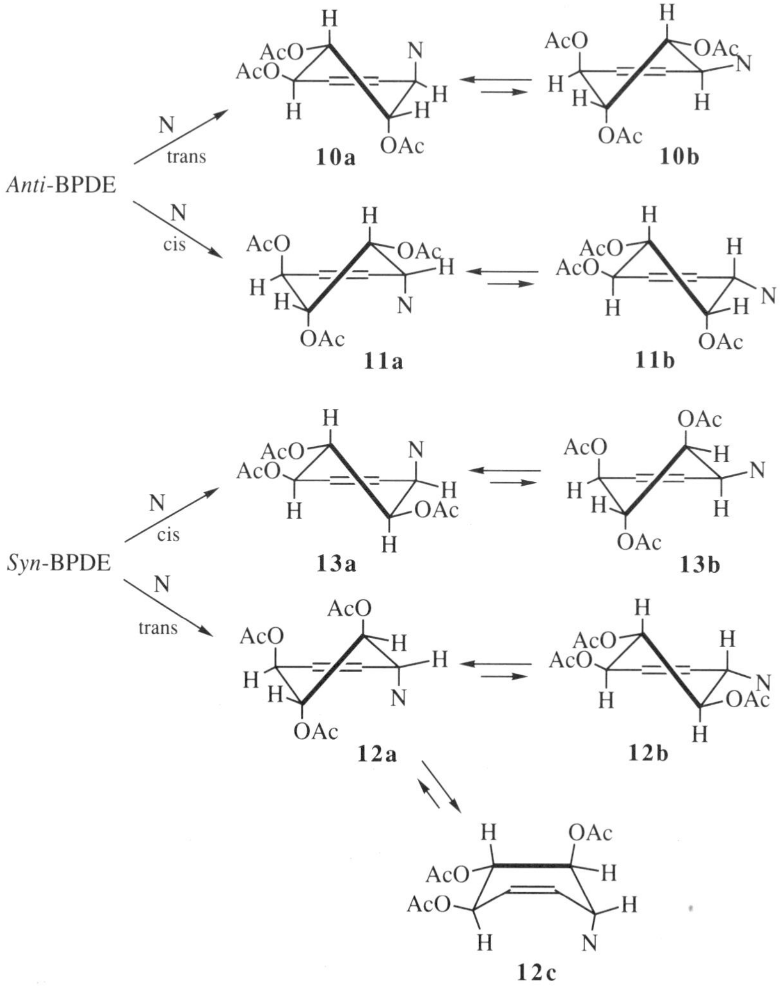

Table 14.1. *NMR coupling constants of the acetates of the adducts from* cis *and* trans *addition of nucleophiles to* anti *and* syn-*BPDE*[a]

N	*anti*-BPDE			*syn*-BPDE		
	$J_{7,8}$	$J_{8,9}$	$J_{9,10}$	$J_{7,8}$	$J_{8,9}$	$J_{9,10}$
trans adducts						
OH	8.8	2.5	3.6	8.0	5.0	3.5
OMe	9.0	2.5	3.6	8.8	3.8	3.8
$SC_6H_4NO_2$	9.0	2.5	3.5	8.0	2.8	2.0
NHC_6H_5	9.0	2.5	2.5	4.5	4.0	4.0
OC_6H_5				7.4	3.6	3.6
cis adducts						
OH	3.5	2.5	4.6	8.0	11.5	3.5
OC_6H_5	4.5	2.5	5.0	7.8	11.3	3.3

[a]Data are from Yagi *et al.* (1977); spectra were taken in $CDCl_3$ at 100 or 200 MHz, and coupling constants are in hertz.

butylthiolate with *anti-* and *syn*-BPDE were $J_{9,10}$ = 4.0 and 2.0 Hz, respectively. For the *anti*-BPDE adduct, the observed large coupling for $J_{7,8}$ = 10.0 Hz and small coupling for $J_{8,9}$ = 2.8 Hz are most compatible with conformer **10a** in which the hydroxyl groups are diequatorial. For the *syn*-BPDE adduct, the relatively large coupling for $J_{7,8}$ = 8.25 Hz is inconsistent with conformer **12a** which is also unlikely because of the expected serious steric interaction of the four axial substituents. Consequently, the alternative flattened boat conformation **12c**, which does not suffer from this deficiency and is consistent with the NMR data, has been assigned to this isomer.

The reactions of these diol epoxides with a variety of other sulfur and nitrogen nucleophiles were also examined (Yagi *et al.*, 1977) and the stereochemistries of the adducts were assigned on the basis of NMR analysis of their acetylated derivatives (Table 14.1). All the nucleophiles studied exhibited regiospecific attack at the benzylic carbon atom. This was confirmed by characteristic downfield shifts of the signals for the C-10 benzylic hydrogen atoms. *Trans*-stereospecific addition was observed for all nucleophiles except phenol and water, which gave significant amounts of *cis*-adducts. The conformational preferences of the adducts are expected to be dependent upon the steric interactions between the substituent groups on the saturated ring and the interactions of the benzylic groups with the aromatic *peri* and bay-region protons i.e. H_6 and H_{11}. For the *trans*-adducts of *anti*- and *syn*-BPDE, the values of $J_{9,10}$ were generally small ($J_{9,10}$ = 2.5–3.6 and 2.0–4.0 Hz, respectively) consistent with the expected axial orientation of the benzylic groups. For the *trans*-adducts of *anti*-BPDE, the large couplings for $J_{7,8}$ = 9 Hz and small couplings for $J_{8,9}$ = 2.5 Hz allow assignment as conformer **10a**. For the *trans*-adducts of *syn*-BPDE, a flattened boat conformation **12c**, like the *tert*-butylthiolate *trans*-adduct, is favored due to the presence of serious interactions in the two chair forms **12a** and **12b**. The relatively large values for $J_{7,8}$ ~8 Hz and the unusual coupling for $J_{8,9}$ = 2.8–5 Hz are consistent with this assignment. An exception is the aniline adduct for which all three couplings are small. The data are compatible with a somewhat distorted conformer **12a** in which all four substituents are pseudoaxially oriented. Hydrogen bonding between the amine hydrogen and the acetate carbonyl may contribute to stabilization of this unusual conformation.

The adducts formed by *cis* addition to *anti*-BPDE were assigned the half-chair conformation **11a** in which the acetoxy group at C-9 is equatorial and the other substituents are axial. This is consistent with the small values of the pertinent coupling constants. For the *cis*-adducts of *syn*-BPDE, the observed couplings are most compatible with the half-chair conformation **13a** in which the nucleophilic substituent in the bay region is axial and the remaining three groups are equatorial.

The sulfhydryl reagent 2-mercaptoethanol reacts rapidly with *anti*-BPDE and has been employed in studies of DNA binding to stop reaction of the diol epoxide with DNA (Gamper *et al.*, 1980). The adducts formed have not been characterized.

14.4.3 *Reactions with nucleic acids and related compounds*

The most biologically significant reaction pathway of polyarene diol epoxide metabolites is their covalent binding to nucleic acids. The mechanisms of these reactions and the structures of the covalent DNA adducts were discussed in Chapter 4. The major products formed by the reactions of *anti*- and *syn*-BPDE with DNA and RNA have been shown to be guanine adducts. The adducts from reactions with polyguanylic acid were hydrolyzed to ribonucleosides, derivatized, and their structures determined by NMR, CD, and mass spectral techniques (Jeffrey *et al.*, 1976). The NMR and mass spectral data on the major adduct of *anti*-BPDE showed it to be the product of *trans* addition of the 2-amino group of guanine to the C-10 benzylic position of the epoxide ring. Its NMR chemical shift and coupling constant data were closely similar to those of the analogous *trans*-adducts formed by the addition of other nucleophiles to *anti*-BPDE (Table 14.1), allowing assignment of its conformer structure as **10a**. Its absolute configuration was assigned by the exciton chirality method (Fig. 14.13) and shown to be identical with that of the major adduct formed by binding of *anti*-BPDE to RNA *in vivo*. Analogous reaction of *syn*-BPDE yielded products of both *cis* and *trans* addition to the 2-amino group of guanine (Koreeda *et al.*, 1976). For the *trans*-adduct, the coupling constants were relatively small ($J_{7,8} = 5.2$, $J_{8,9} = 5.4$, $J_{9,10} = 5.4$ Hz), resembling those of the adduct formed by aniline with *syn*-BPDE (Table 14.1), allowing its assignment as conformation **12a**. For the *cis*-adduct, the coupling constant pattern ($J_{7,8} = 8.0$, $J_{8,9} = 12$, $J_{9,10} = 4.0$ Hz) matched more closely that of the *cis*-adduct of phenol, allowing its assignment as conformer **13a**. The reaction of ($\pm$)-*anti*-BPDE with polyadenylic acid gave *trans*-7R-N^6-dA, *cis*-7S-N^6-dA, *cis*-7R-N^6-dA, and *trans*-7S-N^6-dA in the ratio of 3:3:1:1 (Jeffrey *et al.*, 1979). Therefore, there was no enantiomeric preference in the reactions of the diol epoxide isomers with these synthetic RNAs.

The major products formed by the reactions of *anti*- and *syn*-BPDE with DNA are the related N^2-deoxyguanosine adducts. These account for 90% of the products with double-stranded DNA, but only 30% with single-stranded DNA (Meehan & Straub, 1979). Reaction also occurs to significant extent at adenine residues to yield principally *trans*-adducts covalently attached to the

Fig. 14.13. The principal adduct formed in the covalent binding of *anti*-BPDE with DNA is the N^2-dG adduct. It is generally accompanied by lesser amounts of the N^6-dA adduct. The unstable N^7-G and O^6-dG adducts are only detected when appropriate precautions are taken to minimize their decomposition in the workup. Similar adducts are formed in the covalent binding of *anti*-BPDE with RNA.

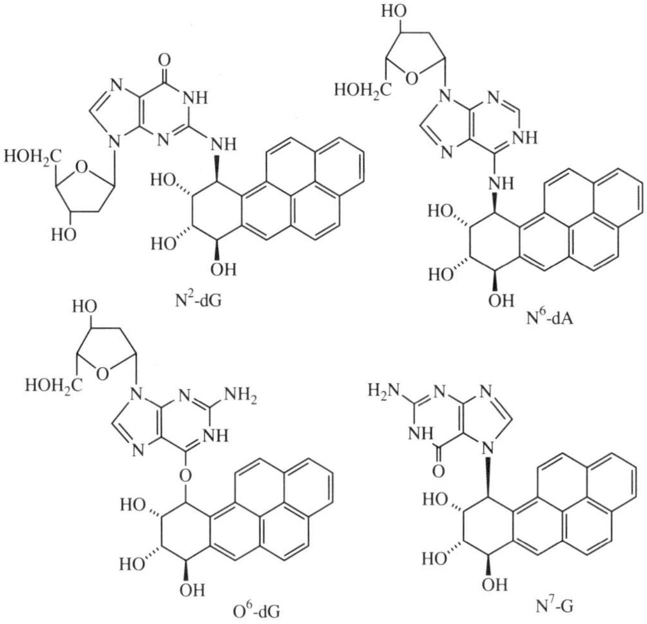

6-amino function (Fig. 14.13) (Jeffrey *et al.*, 1979; Meehan & Straub, 1979). Minor amounts of adducts of deoxycytidine are also formed; it is likely that they are substituted on the amino group, but this has not been proven. The enantiomers of *anti*-BPDE exhibit remarkably different selectivities (Osborne *et al.*, 1981). The 7R-enantiomer affords virtually exclusively the N^2-dG adduct (91%) with only 2% each of N^6-dA and N^7-G adducts, whereas the 7S-enantiomer yields 45% of the N^2-dG adduct accompanied by an O^6-dG adduct (31%), an N^7-G adduct (18%), and an N^6-dA adduct (6%). The identifications of the O^6-dG and N^7-G adducts have not been confirmed by other workers, and variations in product profiles have been reported from different laboratories. These discrepancies appear to be largely a function of experimental differences. Thus, the O^6-dG adducts are acid-labile, and would be lost by the acid treatment of products usually employed in the isolation of adducts. DNA treated with *anti*-BPDE on incubation for several hours after treatment undergoes some depurination due to loss of N^7-G residues (Osborne *et al.*, 1981). The (–)-*anti*-BPDE–DNA adducts also undergo photodissociation to form tetraols in the presence of laboratory fluorescence lights (Zinger *et al.*, 1987). The conformations of the adducts produced by the reactions of the BPDE isomers with DNA are essentially similar to those previously assigned for the adducts obtained from reaction with RNA (Cheng *et al.*, 1989).

The reaction of *syn*-BPDE with synthetic oligonucleotides and DNA has been less thoroughly studied. The major adducts formed by reaction with polyguanylic acid are the corresponding *cis* and *trans* N^2-dG adducts (Koreeda *et al.*, 1976). Evidence was also obtained for alkylation of the phosphodiester linkages of the poly-G to produce labile phosphotriesters. Alkylation of DNA with *syn*-BPDE also affords mainly *cis* and *trans* N^2-dG adducts, but N^6-dA adducts have also been detected.

The alkylation of DNA by BaP diol epoxides also produces a low level of strand scission (Gamper *et al.*, 1977). This is catalyzed by alkali and inhibited by counterions. Mechanisms for nicking based upon the hydrolysis of phosphotriesters rendered unstable by the presence of β-hydroxyl groups on the attached hydrocarbon moieties (Gamper *et al.*, 1977) and depurination of N^7-dG adducts (Shooter *et al.*, 1977) have been proposed. However, no direct evidence could be obtained for nicking occurring through phosphotriester hydrolysis (Gamper *et al.*, 1980), and it is highly likely that nicking proceeds through depurination/depyrimidination.

The products of reaction with DNA of the diol epoxide derivatives of several additional polyarenes have subsequently been characterized using similar methods. These include the bay region diol epoxides of 5-methylchrysene (Melikian *et al.*, 1984; Reardon *et al.*, 1987), DMBA (Cheng *et al.*, 1988), dibenz[a,j]anthracene (Chadha *et al.*, 1989; Nair *et al.*, 1989), 7-methyldibenz[a,j]anthracene (Nair *et al.*, 1989), and the fjord region diol epoxide of benzo[c]phenanthrene (Agarwal *et al.*, 1987).

In the case of 5-methylchrysene, the major adduct from the (±)-*anti*-1,2-diol-3,4-epoxide was shown to arise from *trans* addition of the 2-amino group of deoxyguanosine to the benzylic position of the epoxide ring of the (+)-enantiomer. A minor product formed by analogous reaction of the (−)-enantiomer was also detected. In addition, two diastereomeric products arising from *trans* addition of the 6-amino group of adenosine to the epoxide ring and an adduct formed by *cis* addition of adenosine to one enantiomer were also characterized. In all cases the NMR data for the acetylated derivatives of these adducts is consistent with a conformation in which the purine base ligand is axially oriented. The *trans*-adducts were assigned the half-chair conformation **10a** on the basis of the large couplings observed for $J_{1,2} = 9.0$–9.4 Hz. The *cis*-adducts exhibited relatively small values of all coupling constants ($J_{1,2} = 6.0$–6.7, $J_{2,3} \sim 2$, $J_{3,4} \sim 4.0$ Hz), paralleling those of the *cis*-adducts of *anti*-BPDE assigned as conformer **11a**.

Characterization of the DNA adducts of the potent carcinogen DMBA was hampered initially by the difficulty of synthesis of the unstable diol epoxide isomers. Following development of satisfactory methods for their synthesis (Lee & Harvey, 1986), the relatively more stable *syn*-DMBA diol epoxide was employed to identify the adducts formed by reaction with DNA of the DMBA diol epoxides *in vivo* and *in vitro* (Cheng *et al.*, 1988, 1988a). This carcinogen is unusual in that three of the four major adducts formed with DNA in mouse skin derive from reaction of the *syn*-diol epoxide isomer with adenosine; the fourth adduct is formed from guanosine. NMR and mass spectral analyses of the acetate derivatives of these adducts allowed their assignment as *cis* and *trans* N^6-dA adducts covalently attached to the benzylic C-1 position. Although the adducts formed by the reaction of *syn*-DMBA diol epoxide with poly-dA were mainly *cis*, the adducts formed by reaction with DNA in cells were principally *trans*-adducts. The selective formation of dA adducts in mouse epidermis by the *syn*-DMBA diol epoxide could provide a rational basis for the observation of AT → TA transitions with this carcinogen (Bizub *et al.*, 1986). An N^6-dA adduct and an N^2-dG adduct are formed in roughly equal amounts by the *anti*-DMBA diol epoxide (Dipple *et al.*, 1983).

Chemical characterization of 16 principal adducts formed by reaction of both pairs of enantiomeric *anti*- and *syn*-benzo[c]phenanthrene diol epoxides with the dA and dG residues of DNA has also been reported (Agarwal *et al.*, 1987). The site of covalent attachment of the diol epoxide moiety to the nucleoside residue was in all cases the exocyclic amino group. Although the parent hydrocarbon is not carcinogenic, its diol epoxide derivatives are highly active tumor initiators on mouse skin. Unlike *anti-* and *syn-*BPDE, but like the diol epoxide metabolites of the more potent carcinogen DMBA, benzo[c]phenanthrene diol epoxides react extensively with dA residues in DNA. *Trans-*adducts are the major products from reaction on both dG and dA sites.

Structural characterizations of the DNA adducts derived from reaction of the racemic bay region *anti-* and *syn-*diol epoxides of dibenz[a,j]anthracene (Chadha *et al.*, 1989; Nair *et al.*, 1989) and the *anti-*diol epoxide of 7-methyldibenz[a,j]anthracene (Nair *et al.*, 1989) have also been carried out. The major dG and dA adducts in DNA were found to arise from *trans* addition of the exocyclic amino group to the (+)-enantiomer of either diol epoxide at the C-1 position. In contrast, the major dG adducts from reaction of either of these diol epoxides with individual deoxyribonucleotides was formed by *trans* addition to the (−)-enantiomer. Moreover, significant proportions of *cis-*adducts were produced in the reactions utilizing individual deoxyribonucleotides, but negligible amounts of the products of *cis* addition were detected in the corresponding reactions with DNA. In all cases, the products derived from *trans* addition of purines to the diol epoxides were formed in major amounts. This finding is consistent with other studies using the diol epoxides derived from other polyarenes. Analysis of the NMR data for the *anti-*DBa,jA diol epoxide adducts indicates a preferred half-chair conformation with the C-1 substituent axially oriented. In the acetylated *cis-*adducts, the preferred conformation (**11a**) has the 3,4-acetoxy groups also axial. In the acetylated *trans* adducts, these groups are oriented predominantly equatorially (**10a**). The conformations of these adducts closely resemble those of the analogous adducts of other diol epoxides, such as *anti-*BPDE. For the *trans* adducts derived from the *syn-*diol epoxide isomer, the axially oriented purine moiety at C-1 forces the saturated benzo ring to adopt a chair conformation in which all the acetoxy substituents are also axial (Fig. 14.12: **12a**). In this respect, it differs from the corresponding *trans-*adduct of *syn-*benzo[c]phenanthrene diol epoxide which favors a more boat-like conformation (**12c**). Analogously, the *cis-*adducts from the *syn-*DBa,jA diol epoxide isomer also exist predominantly in a half-chair conformation in which the 3,4-acetoxy groups are diequatorial (**13a**). The conformations of these adducts closely resemble those of the analogous *syn-*BPDE adducts.

14.4.4   *Reactions with glutathione*

Although the spontaneous reaction of glutathione with diol epoxides takes place only very slowly under physiological conditions, enzyme-catalyzed conjugation appears to be an important pathway for detoxification of *anti*-BPDE, at least in liver cells which are rich in glutathione transferases (Jernstrom *et al.*, 1984; Ho & Fahl, 1984). *Anti*-BPDE is a substrate for six well-characterized GSH transferases of the soluble supernatant fraction of the rat liver (Jernstrom *et al.*, 1985). In normal rat cytosol, the rate of enzymic conjugation is estimated to be ~500 times the non-enzymic rate. The efficient detoxification of *anti*-BPDE by the rat liver GSH transferases probably contributes importantly to ensuring that BaP is not a hepatocarcinogen in this species. The human acidic and near neutral GSH transferases have also been shown to efficiently conjugate *anti*-BPDE, particularly the more carcinogenic (+)-enantiomer (Robertson *et al.*, 1986). Information on the structures of the glutathione adducts is unavailable.

14.4.5   *Reactions with proteins*

While it has been known for some years that metabolites of carcinogenic polyarenes bind covalently to proteins in mammalian cells, elucidation of the nature of the products has received relatively little attention and the role of PAH–protein adducts in chemical carcinogenesis has remained obscure. Early work established generalized binding of polyarene metabolites to proteins *in vivo* and identified specific proteins with a high affinity for protein binding (for leading references see MacLeod *et al.*, 1981). In hamster embryo cells exposed to [^{3}H]-benzo[a]pyrene a significant level of binding occurs to specific proteins in nuclei (MacLeod *et al.*, 1981). Core histones H3 and H2A are heavily labeled, while other histones of the nucleosome core are devoid of radioactivity. Similar regiospecific binding mediated by diol epoxide metabolites also occurs in mouse cells and human cells. Recent findings indicate that a short histidine-containing C-terminal peptide is the principal target site for covalent binding of *anti*-BPDE to H2A histones (Kurokawa & MacLeod, 1988). However, the specific base site of attachment has not been elucidated. In other recent studies, it has been shown that binding of microsomally activated fluoranthene to rat hemoglobin involves principal covalent linkage between *syn* and *anti* isomers of the *trans*-2,3-dihydrodiol-1,10b-epoxide metabolites and β-cysteine-125 (Hutchins *et al.*, 1988). A minor class of adducts appeared to involve the binding of an unidentified metabolite to the same cysteine residue. It has been proposed that these adducts may serve as markers for exposure to polyarenes.

14.4.6   *Reactions with ellagic acid*

The naturally occurring plant phenol ellagic acid enters into facile reaction with *anti*-BPDE and exhibits exceptionally high activity as an inhibitor of its mutagenic activity (Sayer *et al.*, 1982a). The predominant products are mixtures of the *cis-* and *trans-* adducts **14** and **15** (Fig. 14.14). The unstable **14** undergoes facile hydrolysis to tetraols. Ellagic acid also reportedly exerts a protective effect against carcinogenesis induced by 3-MC and other polycyclic hydrocarbons (Mukhtar *et al.*, 1986; Chang *et al.*, 1985) and is a potent inhibitor of BaP metabolism and its subsequent glucuronidation, sulfation, and covalent binding to DNA (Mukhtar *et al.*, 1986). However, other investigators (Smart *et al.*, 1986) report that ellagic acid does not inhibit 3-MC-induced skin tumors in BALB/c or CD-1 mice, and is not effective in inhibiting BaP–DNA adduct formation in mouse skin and lung. The reason for these discrepancies is not at present clear.

Fig. 14.14. *anti-*and *syn*-BPDE react with ellagic acid to yield mixtures of the *cis-* and *trans*-adducts **14** and **15**.

ellagic acid

14   **15**

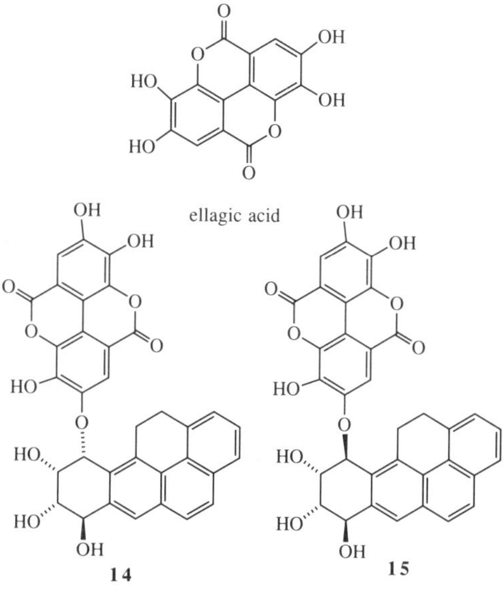

Fig. 14.15. Reduction of *anti-* and *syn*-BPDE with NADPH affords stereoselectivity the triols **16** and **17**, respectively.

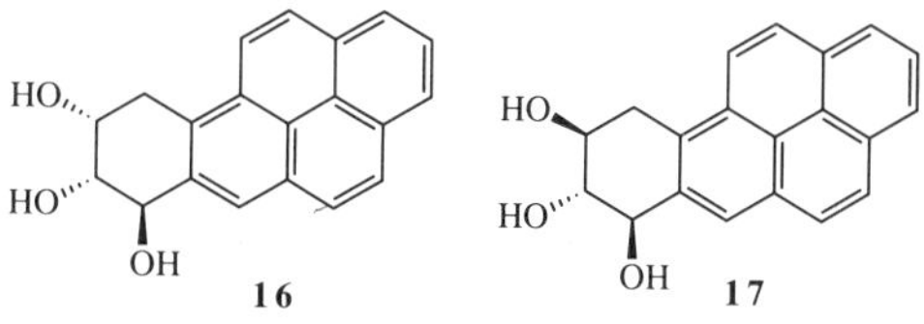

16   **17**

14.4.7   *Reduction with NADPH*

anti- and *syn-*BPDE undergo stereoselective *trans*-reduction with NADPH to the corresponding triols (Yang & Gelboin, 1976) (Fig. 14.15). This reduction, which requires no additional cofactors, may play a role in reducing the extent of binding to DNA of PAH diol epoxides formed *in vivo.*

14.5   References

Agarwal, S. K., Sayer, J. M., Yeh, H. J. C., Pannell, L. K., Hilton, B. D., Pigott, M. A., Dipple, A., Yagi, H. & Jerina, D. M. (1987). Chemical characterization of DNA adducts derived from the configurationally isomeric benzo[c]phenanthrene 3,4-diol 1,2-epoxides. *J. Am. Chem. Soc.* **109**, 2497–505.

Amin, S., Huie, K., Hecht, S. S. & Harvey, R. G. (1986). Synthesis of 6-methylchrysene-1,2-dihydrodiol-3,4-epoxides and comparison of their mutagenicity to 5-methylchrysene-1,2-dihydrodiol-3,4-epoxides. *Carcinogenesis*, **7**, 2067–70.

Beland, F. A. & Harvey, R. G. (1976). The isomeric 9,10-oxides of *trans*-7,8-dihydroxy-7,8-dihydrobenzo[a]pyrene. *J. Chem. Soc. Chem. Commun.* 84–5.

Bizub, D., Wood, A. W. & Skalka, A. M. (1986). Mutagenesis of the Ha-*ras* oncogene in mouse skin tumors induced by polycyclic aromatic hydrocarbons. *Proc. Natl. Acad. Sci. USA.* **83**, 6048–52.

Busbee, D. L., Rankin, P. W., Payne, D. M. & Jasheway, D. W. (1982). Binding of benzo-(a)pyrene and intracellular transport of a bound electrophilic benzo(a)pyrene metabolite by lipoproteins. *Carcinogenesis*, **3**, 1107–12.

Bushman, D. R., Grossman, S. J., Jerina, D. M. & Lehr, R. E. (1989). Synthesis of optically active fjord-region 11,12-diol 13,14-epoxides and the K-region 9,10-oxide of the carcinogen benzo[g]chrysene. *J. Org. Chem.* **54**, 3533–44.

Chadha, A., Sayer, J. M., Yeh, H. J. C., Yagi, H., Cheh, A. M., Pannell, L. K. & Jerina, D. M. (1989). Structures of covalent nucleoside adducts formed from adenine, guanine, and cytosine bases of DNA and the optically active bay-region 3,4-diol 1,2-epoxides of dibenz[a,j]anthracene. *J. Am. Chem. Soc.* **111**, 5456–63.

Chang, R. L., Huang, M. T., Wood, A. W., Wong, C. Q., Newmark, H. L., Yagi, H., Sayer, J. M., Jerina, D. M. & Conney, A. H. (1985). Effect of ellagic acid and hydroxylated flavonoids on the tumorigenicity of benzo(a)pyrene and (±)-7ß,8α-dihydroxy-9α,10α-epoxy-7,8,9,10-tetrahydrobenzo(a)pyrene on mouse skin and in the newborn mouse. *Carcinogenesis*, **6**, 1127–33.

Cheng, S. C., Hilton, B. D., Roman, J. M. & Dipple, A. (1989). DNA adducts from carcinogenic and non-carcinogenic enantiomers of benzo[a]pyrene dihydrodiol epoxide. *Chem. Res. Toxicol.* **2**, 334–40.

Cheng, S. C., Prakash, A. S., Pigott, M. A., Hilton, B. D., Lee, H., Harvey, R. G. & Dipple, A. (1988). A metabolite of the carcinogen 7,12-dimethylbenz[a]anthracene that reacts predominantly with adenine residues in DNA. *Carcinogenesis*, **9**, 1721–3.

Cheng, S. C., Prakash, A. S., Pigott, M. A., Hilton, B. D., Roman, J. M., Lee, H., Harvey, R. G. & Dipple, A. (1988a). Characterization of 7,12-dimethylbenz[a]anthracene–adenine nucleoside adducts. *Chem. Res. Toxicol.* **1**, 216–21.

Dalton, D. R. & Jones, D. G. (1967). Halohydrin formation in dimethyl sulfoxide. *Tetrahedron Lett.* 2875–8.

Dipple, A., Pigott, M. A., Moschel, R. C. & Costantino, J. (1983). Evidence that binding of 7,12-dimethylbenz[a]anthracene to DNA in mouse cell cultures results in extensive substitution of both adenine and guanine residues. *Cancer Res.* **43**, 4132–5.

Gamper, H. B., Bartholomew, J. C. & Calvin, M. (1980). Mechanism of benzo[a]pyrene diol epoxide induced DNA strand scission. *Biochemistry,* **19**, 3948–56.

Gamper, H. B., Tung, A. S., Straub, K., Bartholomew, J. & Calvin, M. (1977). DNA strand scission by benzo[a]pyrene diol epoxides. *Science,* **197**, 671–3.

Geacintov, N. E., Yoshida, H. & Harvey, R. G. (1982). Noncovalent binding of 7β,8α-dihydroxy-9α,10α-epoxytetrahydrobenzo[a]pyrene to deoxyribonucleic acid and its catalytic effect on the hydrolysis of the diol epoxide to tetrol. *Biochemistry,* **21**, 1864–9.

Geddie, J. E., Amin, S., Huie, K. & Hecht, S. S. (1987). Formation and tumorigenicity of benzo[b]fluoranthene metabolites in mouse epidermis. *Carcinogenesis,* **8**, 1579–1784.

Gupta, S. C., Islam, N. B., Whalen, D. L., Yagi, H. & Jerina, D. M. (1987). Bifunctional catalysis in the nucleotide-catalyzed hydrolysis of (±)-7β,8α-dihydroxy-9α,10α-epoxy-7,8,9,10-tetrahydrobenzo[a]pyrene. *J. Org. Chem.* **52**, 3812–5.

Gupta, S. C., Pohl, T. M., Friedman, S. L., Whalen, D. L., Yagi, H. & Jerina, D. M. (1982). Guanosine 5'-monophosphate catalyzed hydrolysis of diastereomeric benzo[a]pyrene-7,8-diol 9,10-epoxides. *J. Am. Chem. Soc.* **104**, 3101–4.

Harvey, R. G. (1985). Synthesis of the dihydrodiol and diol epoxide metabolites of carcinogenic polycyclic hydrocarbons. *Polycyclic Hydrocarbons and Carcinogenesis,* Symp. Series No. 283. ed. R. G. Harvey, pp. 35–62. Washington, DC: American Chemical Society

Harvey, R. G. (1989). Conformational analysis of hydroaromatic metabolites of carcinogenic hydrocarbons and the relation of conformation to biological activity. *The Conformational Analysis of Cyclohexenes, Cyclohexadienes, and Related Hydroaromatics,* ed. P. W. Rabideau, pp. 67–298. New York: VCH.

Harvey, R. G., Cortez, C., Sawyer, T. W. & DiGiovanni, J. (1988). Synthesis of the tumorigenic 3,4-dihydrodiol metabolites of dibenz[a,j]anthracene and 7,14-dimethyldibenz[a,j]anthracene. *J. Medic. Chem.* **31**, 1308–12.

Harvey, R. G., Cortez, C., Sugiyama, T., Ito, Y., Sawyer, T. W. & DiGiovanni, J. (1988a). Biologically active metabolites of polycyclic aromatic hydrocarbons structurally related to the potent carcinogenic hydrocarbon 7,12-dimethylbenz[a]anthracene. *J. Medic. Chem.* **31**, 154–9.

Harvey, R. G. & Fu, P. P. (1980). Synthesis of oxidized metabolites of dibenz[a,c]anthracene. *J. Org. Chem.* **45**, 169–71.

Harvey, R. G., Pataki, J. & Lee, H. (1986). Synthesis of the dihydrodiol and diol epoxide metabolites of chrysene and 5-methylchrysene. *J. Org. Chem.* **51**, 1407–12.

Harvey, R. G. & Sukumaran, K. (1977). Synthesis of the A-ring dihydrodiols and *anti*-diol epoxides of benz[a]anthracene. *Tetrahedron Lett.* 2387–90.

Hecht, S. S., Amin, S., Huie, K., Melikian, A. A. & Harvey, R. G. (1987). Enhancing effect of a bay region methyl group on tumorigenicity in newborn mice and mouse skin of enantiomeric bay region diol epoxides formed stereoselectively from methylchrysenes in mouse epidermis. *Cancer Res.* **47**, 5310–15.

Ho, D. & Fahl, W. E. (1984). Quantitative significance of glutathione and glutathione-S-transferase in regulating benzo[a]pyrene *anti* diol-epoxide level in reconstituted C3H 10T1/2 cell lysates, and comparison to rat liver. *Carcinogenesis,* **5**, 143–8.

Hutchins, D. A., Skipper, P. L., Naylor, S. & Tannenbaum, S. R. (1988). Isolation and characterization of the major fluoranthene–hemoglobin adducts formed *in vivo* in the rat. *Cancer Res.* **48**, 4756–61.

Jacobs, S. A., Cortez, C. & Harvey, R. G. (1983). Synthesis of potential proximate and ultimate carcinogenic metabolites of 3-methylcholanthrene. *Carcinogenesis,* **4**, 519–22.

Jeffrey, A. M., Grzeskowiak, K., Weinstein, I. B., Nakanishi, K., Roller, P. & Harvey, R. G. (1979). Benzo[a]pyrene-7,8-dihydrodiol-9,10-oxide-adenosine and deoxy–adenosine adducts: Structure and stereochemistry. *Science,* **206**, 1309–11.

Jeffrey, A. M., Jennette, K. W., Blobstein, S. H., Weinstein, I. B., Beland, F. A., Harvey, R. G., Kasai, H., Miura, I. & Nakanishi, K. (1976). Benzo[a]pyrene–nucleic acid derivative found *in vivo*: Structure of a benzo[a]pyrenetetrahydrodiol epoxide guanosine adduct. *J. Am. Chem. Soc.* **98**, 5714–16.

Jennette, K., Jeffrey, A. M., Blobstein, S. H., Beland, F. A., Harvey, R. G. & Weinstein, I. B. (1977). Characterization of nucleoside adducts from the *in vitro* reaction of benzo[a]pyrene-7,8-dihydrodiol-9,10-oxide or benzo[a]pyrene-4,5-oxide with nucleic acids. *Biochemistry*, **16**, 932–93.

Jernstrom, B., Martinez, M., Meyer, D. J. & Ketterer, B. (1985). Glutathione conjugation of the carcinogenic and mutagenic electrophile (±)-7β,8α-dihydroxy-9α,10α-oxy-7,8,9,10-tetrahydrobenzo[a]pyrene catalyzed by purified rat liver glutathione transferases. *Carcinogenesis.* **6**, 85–9.

Jernstrom, B., Martinez, M., Svensson, S. A. & Dock, L. (1984). Metabolism of benzo[a]pyrene-7,8-dihydrodiol and benzo[a]pyrene-7,8-dihydrodiol-9,10-epoxide to protein binding products and glutathione conjugates in isolated rat hepatocytes. *Carcinogenesis*, **5**, 1079–85.

Keller, J. W., Heidelberger, C., Beland, F. A. & Harvey, R. G. (1976). Hydrolysis of *syn*- and *anti*-benzo[a]pyrene diol epoxides: Stereochemistry, kinetics, and the effect of an intramolecular hydrogen bond on the rate of *syn*-diol epoxide solvolysis. *J. Am. Chem. Soc.* **98**, 8276–7.

Kikuchi, O., Hopfinger, A. J. & Klopman, G. (1979). Electronic structure and reactivity of four stereoisomers of benzo[a]pyrene 7,8-diol-9,10-epoxide. *Cancer Biochem. Biophys.* **4**, 1–8.

Klein, C. L. & Stevens, E. D. (1984). Molecular structure of *anti*-3,4-dihydroxy-1,2,3,4-tetrahydronaphthalene 1,2-oxide. *Cancer Res.* **44**, 1523–6.

Klopman, G., Gringerg, H. & Hopfinger, A. J. (1979). MINDO/3 calculations of the conformation and carcinogenicity of epoxy-metabolites of aromatic hydrocarbons; 7,8-dihydroxy-9,10-oxy-7,8,9,10-tetrahydrobenzo[a]pyrene. *J. Theor. Biol.* **79**, 355–66.

Kootstra, A. (1982). Formation and removal of BaP diol epoxide–DNA adducts in human fibroblasts. *Carcinogenesis*, 3953–5.

Koreeda, M., Moore, P. D., Yagi, H., Yeh, H. J. & Jerina, D. M. (1976). Reaction of polyguanylic acid at the 2-amino group and phosphate by the potent mutagen (±)7β,8α-dihydroxy-9β,10β-epoxy-7,8,9,10-tetrahydrobenzo[a]pyrene. *J. Am. Chem. Soc.* **98**, 6720–2.

Kurokawa, M. & MacLeod, M. (1988). Comparison of benzo[a]pyrene-diol-epoxide binding to histone H2A with different carboxy-terminal regions. *Carcinogenesis*, **9**, 419–25.

Lee, H. & Harvey, R. G. (1981). Stereoselective *syn* epoxidation of the dihydrodiols of dibenz[a,h]anthracene and 7-methylbenz[a]anthracene. *Tetrahedron Lett.* **22**, 1657–60.

Lee, H. & Harvey, R. G. (1986). Synthesis of the active diol epoxide metabolites of the potent carcinogenic hydrocarbon 7,12-dimethylbenz[a]anthracene. *J. Org. Chem.* **51**, 3502–7.

Lee, H. M. & Harvey, R. G. (1979). Synthesis of biologically active metabolites of 7-methylbenz[a]anthracene. *J. Org. Chem.* **44**, 4948–53.

Lee, H. M. & Harvey, R. G. (1980). Synthesis of biologically active metabolites of dibenz[a,h]anthracene. *J. Org. Chem.* **45**, 588–92.

Lehr, R. E., Kumar, S., Cohenour, P. T. & Jerina, D. M. (1979). Dihydrodiols and diol epoxides of dibenzo[a,i]- and dibenzo[a,h]pyrene. *Tetrahedron Lett.* 3819–22

Lehr, R. E., Schaefer-Ridder, M. & Jerina, D. M. (1977). Synthesis and reactivity of diol epoxides derived from non-K-region *trans*-dihydrodiols of benzo[a]anthracene. *Tetrahedron Lett.* 539–42.

MacLeod, M. C., Kootstra, A., Mansfield, B. K., Slaga, T. J. & Selkirk, J. K. (1981). Binding of benzo(a)pyrene derivatives to specific proteins in nuclei of intact hamster embryo cells. *Cancer Res.* **41**, 4080–6.

Meehan, T. & Straub, K. (1979). The covalent binding of enantiomeric benzo[a]pyrene diol epoxides to double stranded DNA is stereoselective. *Nature (Lond.)*, **277**, 410–2.

Melikan, A. A., Amin, S., Hecht, S. S., Hoffmann, D., Pataki, J. & Harvey, R. G. (1984). Identification of the major adducts formed by reaction of 5-methylchrysene *anti*-dihydrodiol epoxides with DNA. *Cancer Res.* **44**, 2524–9.

Mukhtar, H., Das, M. & Bickers, D. R. (1986). Inhibition of 3-methylcholanthrene-induced skin tumorigenicity in BALB/c mice by chronic oral feeding of trace amounts of ellagic acid in drinking water. *Cancer Res.* **46**, 2262–5.

Mukhtar, H., DelTito, B. J. J., Marcelo, C. L., Das, M. & Bickers, D. (1984). Ellagic acid: a potent naturally occurring inhibitor of benzo(a)pyrene metabolism and its subsequent glucuronidation, sulfation and covalent binding to DNA in cultured BALB/c mouse keratinocytes. *Carcinogenesis*, **5**, 1565–72.

Nair, R. V., Gill, R. D., Cortez, C., Harvey, R. G. & DiGiovanni, J. (1989). Characterization of DNA adducts derived from (±)-*trans*-3,4-dihydroxy-*anti*-1,2-epoxy-1,2,3,4-tetrahydrodibenz-[a,j]anthracene and (±)-7-methyl-*trans*-3,4-dihydroxy-*anti*-1,2-epoxy-1,2,3,4-tetrahydro-dibenz[a,j]anthracene. *Chem. Res. Toxicol.* **2**, 341–8.

Nakanishi, K., Kasai, H., Cho, H., Harvey, R. G., Jeffery, A. M., Jennette, K. W. & Weinstein, I. B. (1977). Absolute configuration of an RNA adduct formed in vivo by metabolism of benzo[a]pyrene. *J. Am. Chem. Soc.* **99**, 258–60.

Neidle, S. & Cutbush, S. D. (1983). X-ray crystallographic analysis of (±)-7β,8α-dihydroxy-9β,10β-epoxy-7,8,9,10-tetrahydrobenzo[a]pyrene: molecular structure of a '*syn*' diol epoxide. *Carcinogenesis*, **4**, 415–18.

Neidle, S., Subbiah, A., Cooper, C. S. & Ribeiro, O. (1980). Molecular structure of (±)-7α,8β-dihydroxy 9β,10β-epoxy-7,8,9,10-tetrahydrobenzo[a]pyrene; an X-ray crystallographic study. *Carcinogenesis*, **1**, 249–54.

Osborne, M. R., Jacobs, S., Harvey, R. G. & Brookes, P. (1981). Minor products from the reaction of (+) and (-) benzo[a]pyrene *anti*-diol epoxide with DNA. *Carcinogenesis*, **2**, 553–8.

Pataki, J., DiRaddo, P. & Harvey, R. G. (1989). An efficient synthesis of the highly tumorigenic *anti*-diol epoxide derivative of benzo[c]phenanthrene. *J. Org. Chem.* **54**, 840–4.

Pruess-Schwartz, D., Mauthe, R. J. & Baird, W. M. (1988). Instability of 7β,8α-dihydroxy-9β,10β-epoxytetrahydrobenzo[a]pyrene (*syn*-BPDE)-DNA adducts formed in benzo[a]pyrene-treated Wistar rat embryo cell cultures. *Carcinogenesis*, **9**, 1863–8.

Rastetter, W. H., Nachbar, R. B. Jr., Russo-Rodriguez, S., Wattley, R. V., Thilly, W. G., Andon, B. M., Jorgensen, W. L. & Ibrahim, M. (1982). Fluoranthene synthesis and mutagenicity of four diol epoxides. *J. Org. Chem.* **47**, 4873-8.

Reardon, D., Prakash, A. S., Hilton, B. D., Roman, J. M., Pataki, J. & Harvey, R. G. (1987). Characterization of 5-methylchrysene-1,2-dihydrodiol-3,4-epoxide–DNA adducts. *Carcinogenesis*. **8**, 1317–22.

Robertson, I. G., Guthenberg, C., Mannervik, B. & Jerstrom, B. (1986). Differences in stereoselectivity and catalytic efficiency of three human glutathione transferases in the conjugation of glutathione with 7β,8α-dihydroxy-9α,10α-oxy-7,8,9,10 tetrahydro-benzo(a)pyrene. *Cancer Res.* **46**, 2220–4.

Roche, C. J., Zinger, D., Geacintov, N. E. & Harvey, R. G. (1985). Enhancement of stability of 7β,8α-dihydroxy-9α,10α-epoxybenzo(a)pyrene by complex formation with serum albumin. *Cancer Biochem. Biophys.* **8**, 35–40.

Sayer, J. M., Whalen, D. L., Friedman, S. L., Paik, A., Yagi, H., Vyas, K. P. & Jerina, D. M. (1984). Conformational effects in the hydrolyses of benzo-ring diol epoxides that have bay-region diol groups. *J. Am. Chem. Soc.* **106**, 226–33.

Sayer, J. M., Yagi, H., Croisy-Delcey, M. & Jerina, D. M. (1981). Novel bay-region diol epoxides from benzo[c]phenanthrene. *J. Am. Chem. Soc.* **103**, 4970–2.

Sayer, J. M., Yagi, H., Silverton, J. V., Friedman, S. L., Whalen, D. L. & Jerina, D. M. (1982a). Conformational effects in the hydrolyses of rigid benzylic epoxides: Implications for diol epoxides of polycyclic hydrocarbons. *J. Am. Chem. Soc.* **104**, 1972–8.

Sayer, J. M., Yagi, H., Wood, A. W., Conney, A. H. & Jerina, D. M. (1982b). Extremely facile reaction between the ultimate carcinogen benzo[a]pyrene-7,8-diol 9,10-epoxide and ellagic acid. *J. Am. Chem. Soc.* **104**, 5562–4.

Shooter, K. V., Osborne, M. R. & Harvey, R. G. (1977). The interaction of the 7,8-dihydrodiol-9,10-oxides of benzo[a]pyrene with bacteriophages R17 and T7. *Chem.–Biol. Interact.* **19**, 215–33.

Smart, R. C., Huang, M., Chang, R. L., Sayer, J. M., Jerina, D. M., Wood, A. W. & Conney, A. H. (1986). Effect of ellagic acid and 3-*o*-decylellagic acid on the formation of benzo[a]pyrene-derived DNA adducts *in vivo* and on the tumorigenicity of 3-methylcholanthrene in mice. *Carcinogenesis,* **7**, 1669–75.

Thakker, D. R., Yagi, H., Lehr, R. E., Levin, W., Buening, M., Lu, A. Y. H., Chang, R. L., Wood, A. W., Conney, A. H. & Jerina, D. M. (1978). Metabolism of *trans*-9,10-dihydroxy-9,10-dihydrobenzo[a]pyrene occurs primarily by arylhydroxylation rather than formation of a diol epoxide. *Mol. Pharm.* **14**, 502–13.

Utermoehlen, C. M., Singh, M. & Lehr, R. E. (1987). Fjord region 3,4-diol 1,2-epoxides and other derivatives in the 1,2,3,4- and 5,6,7,8-benzo rings of the carcinogen benzo[g]chrysene. *J. Org. Chem.* **52**, 5574–82.

Whalen, D. L., Ross, A. M., Montemarano, J. A., Thakker, D. R., Yagi, H. & Jerina, D. M. (1979). General acid catalysis in the hydrolysis of benzo[a]pyrene 7,8-diol 9,10-epoxides. *J. Am. Chem. Soc.* **101**, 5086–8.

Whalen, D. L., Ross, A. M., Yagi, H., Karle, J. M. & Jerina, D. M. (1978). Stereoelectronic factors in the solvolysis of bay region diol epoxides of polycyclic aromatic hydrocarbons. *J. Am. Chem. Soc.* **100**, 5218–21.

Yagi, H., Hernandez, O. & Jerina, D. M. (1975). Synthesis of (±)-7ß,8α-dihydroxy-9ß,10ß-epoxy-7,8,9,10-tetrahydrobenzo[a]pyrene, a potential metabolite of the carcinogen benzo[a]pyrene with stereochemistry related to the antileukemic triptolides. *J. Am. Chem. Soc.* **97**, 6881–3.

Yagi, H. & Jerina, D. M. (1982). Absolute configuration of the *trans*-9,10-dihydrodiol metabolite of the carcinogen benzo[a]pyrene. *J. Am. Chem. Soc.* **104**, 4026–7.

Yagi, H., Sayer, J. M., Thakker, D. R., Levin, W. & Jerina, D. M. (1987). Effects of 6-fluoro substituent on the solvolytic properties of the diastereomeric 7,8-diol 9,10-oxides of the carcinogen benzo[a]pyrene. *J. Am. Chem. Soc.* **109**, 838–84.

Yagi, H., Thakker, D. R., Hernandez, O., Koreeda, M. & Jerina, D. M. (1977). Synthesis and reactions of the highly mutagenic 7,8-diol 9,10-epoxides of the carcinogen benzo[a]pyrene. *J. Am. Chem. Soc.* **99**, 1604–11.

Yagi, H., Thakker, D. R., Ittah, Y., Croisy-Delcey, M. & Jerina, D. M. (1983). Synthesis and assignment of absolute configuration to the *trans* 3,4-dihydrodiols and 3,4-diol-1,2-epoxides of benzo[c]phenanthrene. *Tetrahedron Lett.* **24**, 1349–52.

Yagi, H., Thakker, D. R., Lehr, R. E. & Jerina, D. M. (1979). Benzo-ring diol epoxides of benzo[e]pyrene and triphenylene. *J. Org. Chem.* **44**, 3439–42.

Yagi, H., Vyas, K. P., Tada, M., Thakker, D. R. & Jerina, D. M. (1982). Synthesis of the enantiomeric bay-region diol epoxides of benz[a]anthracene and chrysene. *J. Org. Chem.* **47**, 1110–17.

Yang, S. K. & Gelboin, H. V. (1976). Nonenzymatic reduction of benzo(a)pyrene diol-epoxides to trihydroxypentahydrobenzo(a)pyrenes by reduced nicotinamide adenine dinucleotide phosphate. *Cancer Res.* **36**, 4185–9.

Yang, S. K., McCourt, D. M., Gelboin, H. V., Miller, J. R. & Roller, P. P. (1977). Stereochemistry of the hydrolysis products and their acetonides of two stereoisomeric benzo[a]pyrene 7,8-diol-9,10-epoxides. *J. Am. Chem. Soc.* **99**, 5124–30.

Yang, S. K., Mushtaq, M. & Chiu, P. (1985). Stereoselective metabolism and activations of polycyclic aromatic hydrocarbons. *Polycyclic Hydrocarbons and Carcinogenesis*, ACS Monograph No. 283. ed. R. G. Harvey, pp. 19-34. Washington, DC: American Chemical Society.

Yeh, C. Y., Fu, P. P., Beland, F. A. & Harvey, R. G. (1978). Application of CNDO-2 theoretical calculations to interpretation of the chemical reactivity and biological activity of the *syn* and *anti* diolepoxides of benzo[a]pyrene. *Bioorg. Chem.* **7**, 497–6.

Zinger, D., Geacintov, N. E. & Harvey, R. G. (1987). Conformations and selective photo-dissociation of heterogeneous benzo[a]pyrene diol epoxide enantiomer-DNA adducts. *Biophys. Chem.* **27**, 131–8.

15

Other oxidized metabolites

This chapter surveys the structural properties, methods of synthesis, and chemical reactivities of polycyclic phenols, quinones, and other oxidized metabolites of polyarenes not covered in previous chapters.

15.1   Phenols and their ketone tautomers

Phenols are important not only as major metabolites of PAHs but also as key intermediates in the synthesis of quinones, dihydrodiols, and other oxidized derivatives. As metabolites, phenols occur both free and in esterified form as glucuronides, sulfates, and other conjugates.

Phenols may potentially exist in tautomeric equilibrium with the corresponding ketones (Fig. 15.1). For phenol itself and other simple benzenoid phenols, equilibrium strongly favors the hydroxylated structures, since ketone formation entails substantial loss of resonance energy. However, as the number of fused rings increases, this energy difference tends to diminish. For L-region phenols, such as 9-anthrol, the keto form generally predominates; the percentage of anthrone in equilibrium with 9-anthrol at room temperature is 89%. With higher acenes this percentage increases. The

Fig. 15.1.   The keto-phenol tautomeric equilibrium shifts to favor the former with increasing annelation of L-region phenols.

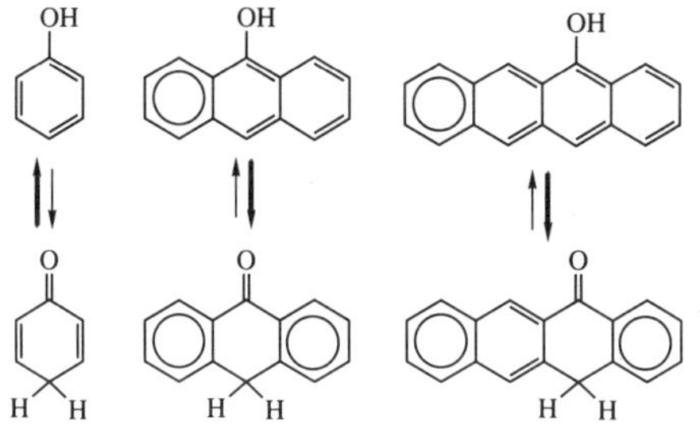

enol form of 5-hydroxytetracene is unstable and cannot be isolated in a pure state (Fieser, 1930), and pentacenone apparently cannot be enolized to hydroxypentacene. Formation of the keto structures breaks up the aromaticity of the acene ring system into two essentially independent regions. This decrease in aromatic character is partially compensated energetically by the gain of a conjugated carbonyl function. In the case of the L-region phenols, the keto form is also favored according to Clar's annelation rule (Chap. 5.1) by the net gain of an aromatic sextet.

For K-region phenols, ketonization does not lead to an increase in the number of aromatic sextets. The K-region phenols of benz[a]anthracene, benzo[a]pyrene, benzo[e]pyrene, benzo[c]phenanthrene, and other common PAHs appear to exist exclusively in the phenolic form as evidenced by the absence of the expected methylene protons in their proton NMR spectra and/or the lack of a carbonyl absorption in their IR spectra (Harvey *et al.*, 1975; Lee *et al.*, 1981; Newman & Blum, 1964). Newman and coworkers (Newman *et al.*, 1976) evaluated the tendency of phenolic compounds to exist or react as their ketonic tautomers on the basis of three criteria: the presence of a ketone band near 6.0 μ in the IR spectrum, the formation of a 2,4-dinitrophenylhydrazone, and the extent of formation of a methyl ether at room temperature under standardized conditions. Of all the phenolic compounds investigated, only the K-region phenolic derivatives of 12-methyl- and 7,12-dimethylbenz[a]anthracene showed an IR band near 6.0 μ indicative of the presence of the ketonic form. The presence of the ketonic forms in these instances was ascribed to the steric strain introduced by the 12-methyl group. The observed phenol/ketone ratios for 5-hydroxy-12-MBA and 5-hydroxy-7,12-DMBA were 0.42 and 0.8, respectively, while those for 6-hydroxy-12-MBA and 6-hydroxy-7,12-DMBA were 0.25 and 0, respectively. These concentrations do not necessarily represent equilibrium concentrations. 5-Hydroxy-BA and 5-hydroxy-7-MBA were entirely in the phenolic form as shown by the absence of the IR band near 6.0 μ. Newman suggested that the keto tautomers of phenols may be involved in the covalent binding of carcinogenic PAHs to biopolymers (Newman *et al.*, 1976). However, the 5- and 6-keto derivatives of DMBA were found to exhibit no carcinogenic activity in mice in comparison with DMBA itself (Dipple *et al.*, 1975).

The phenols for which ketonic tautomers were detectable by IR readily formed 2,4-dinitrophenylhydrazones. However, 5-hydroxy-BA, 5-hydroxy-7-MBA, 6-hydroxy-7,12-DMBA, and 9-phenanthrol also formed similar derivatives in high yield after long standing. This suggests that the free energy barrier for keto–enol tautomerism is low for these compounds. In contrast, 1- and 2-naphthol and phenol failed to form similar derivatives even on long standing.

The formation of methyl ethers from phenols by treatment with acidic methanol is assumed to involve reaction of the keto form with methanol to form a hemiketal which loses water to yield the methyl ether. The most strained BA phenolic derivatives that contain a 12-methyl group readily form methyl ethers under these conditions. However, so do 5-hydroxy-BA and 5-hydroxy-7-MBA which are not particularly strained, and anthrone which exists predominantly in the keto form fails to give a methyl ether. Thus, formation of methyl ethers by polycyclic phenols is unreliable as an indicator of the relative ease of formation of ketonic intermediates.

For polycyclic phenols other than the K- and L-region derivatives, the available evidence indicates that the phenolic tautomers are strongly favored. All of the isomeric phenol derivatives of BA, BaP, BeP, DMBA, and benzo[c]phenanthrene are known (Fu & Harvey, 1983; Harvey *et al.*, 1975; Lee *et al.*, 1981; Newman *et al.*, 1976, 1978; Yagi *et al.*, 1976), and the published NMR spectral data and other evidence is consistent with their existence exclusively as the phenolic tautomers.

15.2   Synthesis of phenols

Although the phenolic derivatives of PAHs are synthetically accessible from the parent hydrocarbons by substitution, direct or indirect, this route is of practical utility for only a small fraction of the possible isomers. The remainder are obtainable mainly by total synthesis methods, or in some cases by dehydration of dihydrodiols or rearrangement of arene oxides.

Methods for the synthesis of polycyclic phenols via substitution include: (i) reaction with lead tetraacetate, (ii) sulfonation and alkali fusion, (iii) halogenation followed by displacement with sodium methoxide or conversion to the Grignard derivative followed by reaction with diborane and oxidation with alkaline peroxide, and (iv) Baeyer–Villiger oxidation of acetylated derivatives (Fig. 15.2).

Acetoxylation with Pb(OAc)$_4$ in acetic acid was used to prepare 9-hydroxyanthracene, 7-hydroxy-BA, 6-hydroxy-BaP, and 4-hydroxyfluoranthene in 40–80% yields (Fieser & Hershberg, 1938; Shenbor & Cheban, 1969). However, DBA failed to react with Pb(OAc)$_4$ even under forcing conditions. This may be a consequence of steric hindrance in the reactive meso region of this molecule. Acetoxylation with Pb(OAc)$_4$ is limited by the relative facility of further reaction of the primary oxidized products, e.g. to quinones (Fieser & Putnam, 1947), and by competitive oxidation elsewhere in the molecule, particularly on any alkyl groups present. For example, reaction of 7-methyl-BA with this reagent furnished 7-acetoxymethyl-BA as the principal product (Fieser & Hershberg, 1938). Similar reaction of 12-

methyl-BA gave both 12-acetoxymethyl-BA and 7-acetoxy-12-MBA (Sims, 1967), and reaction of 3-MC yielded 1-acetoxy-3-MC as the principal oxidized product (Fieser & Hershberg, 1938a). Although reactions with $Pb(OAc)_4$ tend to occur predominantly in the molecular sites most susceptible to electrophilic attack, this method may be extended to the synthesis of other phenol isomers by the use of halogen blocking groups. Thus, reaction of 6-chloro- or 6-bromo-BaP with this reagent furnished the corresponding 1-acetoxy derivative which was converted to 1-hydroxy-BaP by treatment with *n*-butyllithium (Harvey & Cho, 1975).

Oxidative conversion of polyarenes to phenols has also been accomplished by reaction with benzoyl peroxide in chlorobenzene (Roit & Waters, 1952). Reaction of this reagent with anthracene, BA, and BaP gave products analogous to those obtained from oxidation with $Pb(OAc)_4$, namely 9-benzoyloxyanthracene, 7-benzoyloxy-BA, and 6-benzoyloxy-BaP, albeit in lower yield.

Aryl halides are the most convenient starting compounds for the introduction of hydroxyl groups at specific sites in large polycyclic aromatic ring systems. The usual method entails conversion of an aryl bromide to the corresponding Grignard reagent or aryllithium compound followed by reaction of the latter with diborane or trimethylborate and oxidation of the arylboron intermediate with alkaline peroxide. This method has been employed to synthesize 1-hydroxypyrene, 9-hydroxyphenanthrene, 6-methoxy-2-naphthol, and 3-hydroxy-BaP in yields of 74–90% (Lee *et al.*, 1981; Kidwell *et al.*, 1973). Although bromination of pyrene occurs essentially exclusively in the 1-position, 2-hydroxypyrene was obtained by a modification of this procedure involving bromination of 4,5,9,10-tetrahydropyrene which took place preferentially in the 2-position (Harvey *et*

Fig. 15.2. Synthetic routes to polycyclic phenols from the parent hydrocarbons. These methods provide the phenolic isomers formed by electrophilic substitution in the most reactive ring positions.

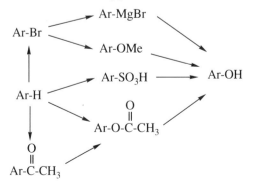

al., 1988). The conversion of aryl halides to phenols by direct displacement has also been described. 1-Hydroxypyrene was prepared from 1-bromo-pyrene by reaction with NaOH in the presence of copper bronze at 280 °C in a pressure reaction vessel (Gumprecht, 1973). More recently, it has been discovered that even aryl chlorides undergo smooth displacement with NaOMe in the polar solvent hexamethylphosphoramide (HMPA) under mild conditions (Shaw *et al.*, 1976). This method was utilized to synthesize 1-hydroxy-BeP from BeP via bromination to 3,6-dibromo-BeP followed by chlorination to 1,8-dichloro-3,6-dibromo-BeP and debromination of the latter to yield 1,8-dichloro-BeP (**1**: Fig. 15.3). Reaction of **1** with NaOMe in HMPA furnished 1-chloro-8-methoxy-BeP which was dechlorinated with n-BuLi and demethylated with NaSEt to provide 1-hydroxy-BeP (Lee *et al.*, 1981). This synthetic strategy is potentially applicable to the synthesis of other phenol derivatives of polyarenes that are not otherwise easily accessible.

Baeyer–Villiger oxidation of ketones also provides synthetic access to phenols. Recently, it has been shown that simple aromatic ketones, such as acetophenone, undergo efficient oxidation with sodium perborate in trifluoroactic acid at room temperature to the corresponding phenol ester derivatives (McKillop & Tarbin, 1987). This method was recently employed in the author's laboratory to prepare 1-hydroxypyrene from 1-acetylpyrene and found to be superior to the synthesis from 1-bromopyrene (Harvey *et al.*, 1990). In another recent study, oxidation of 12-acetylindeno[1,2,3-cd]pyrene with *m*-chloroperbenzoic acid gave the corresponding phenol acetate in low yield (Minabe *et al.*, 1989). Although Baeyer–Villiger oxidation has been only minimally utilized, the McKillop modification appears to be a potentially generally useful method for the synthesis of polyarene phenols.

One of the older established methods of phenol synthesis is sulfonation

Fig. 15.3. Synthesis of 1-hydroxy-BeP illustrates the use of bromine blocking groups to direct chlorination to the less reactive 1,8-positions and conversion of chlorinated product to the 1-phenol by reaction with NaOMe in HMPA.

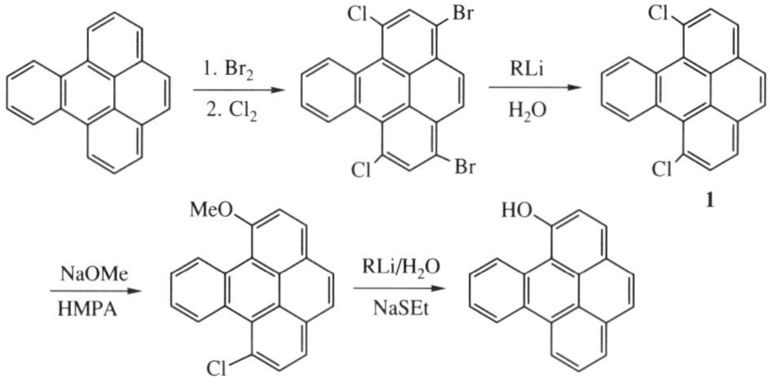

with fuming sulfuric acid followed by fusion of the arene sulfonic acid with KOH. A typical procedure is described for the synthesis of the 2- and 3-phenols of phenanthrene (Fieser, 1943). This method has, however, seen little application to polycyclic phenols.

Some polycyclic phenol isomers that are not synthetically accessible by direct substitution are obtainable from dihydrodiols via dehydration or from arene oxides by acidic rearrangement. The dehydration method is most commonly employed for K-region phenol isomers. Although loss of water occurs on heating dihydrodiols, cleaner products result from treatment with acids under mild anhydrous conditions. Dehydration is frequently regioselective affording predominantly one isomer. The preferred isomer is predictable theoretically from the calculated relative stabilities of the two potential carbonium ion intermediates. Reactions of this type have been reviewed (Fu *et al.*, 1978). Athough acidic rearrangement of arene oxides readily affords phenols, the method is of limited synthetic utility because direct dehydration of the dihydrodiols that are the usual synthetic precursors of the arene oxides is more convenient. The regioselectivity of acidic rearrangement of arene oxide is also predictable theoretically by comparison of carbonium ion stabilities calculated by quantum mechanical methods.

Polycyclic phenol isomers that are not otherwise readily available are most commonly obtained by total synthesis from smaller structural components. For example, K-region phenols may be obtained by acid-catalyzed cyclization of bay region acetic acid derivatives. Thus, 4- and 5-hydroxy-BaP were synthesized by cyclodehydration of the corresponding acetic acid derivatives of chrysene (Fieser & Johnson, 1940; Fu & Harvey, 1983) (Fig. 15.4). 11- and 12-hydroxy-BaP were similarly synthesized from the corresponding acetic acid derivatives of BaP (Fieser & Heymann, 1941; Fu & Harvey, 1981). In these cases, the acetic acid precursors were obtained either through Reformatski reaction of the appropriate ketones or from the corresponding methyl derivatives via bromination, reaction with cyanide, and hydrolysis.

The most frequently employed total synthesis methods are based upon

Fig. 15.4. Synthesis of K-region phenols via cyclodehydration.

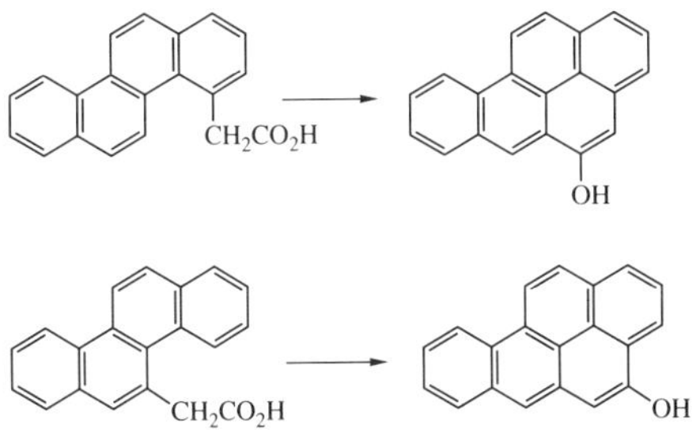

ketonic intermediates (Fig. 15.5). Thus, α-type ketones (e.g. **2**) can be transformed directly to phenols by dehydrogenation catalytically or by heating with sulfur at elevated temperatures. Deoxygenation is often a significant secondary reaction. This transformation may be accomplished under milder conditions and without loss of oxygen by conversion of the ketones to their enol ester derivatives (e.g. **3**) followed by dehydrogenation with *o*-chloranil or DDQ (Fu *et al.*, 1979; Harvey & Fu, 1982; Kole *et al.*, 1989). This modification also affords superior yields. That the phenols are obtained as esters is advantageous, since many polycyclic phenols are air sensitive and are more easily purified in protected form, e.g. by chromatography. The requisite α-type ketones are readily obtainable from the Haworth synthesis (Chap. 7), by oxidation of partially saturated PAHs with DDQ in moist acetic acid (Lee & Harvey, 1988), or through cyclization of alkylated 1,3-cyclohexadiones (Fig. 15.6). An example of the DDQ method is oxidation of 7,8,9,10-tetrahydro-BaP with this reagent to the 10-keto derivative (**4**) which is readily converted to 10-acetoxy-BaP via its enol acetate derivative. The cyclohexadione cyclization method is illustrated by the synthesis of the ketone **5** from an alkylated diketone precursor by acidic cyclization (Harvey & Lee, 1986). Polycyclic phenols synthesized by dehydrogenation of enol acetate intermediates include the 1-, 2-, 3-, 8-, 9-, and 11-phenols of BA (Fu *et al.*, 1979), 9-hydroxy-BeP (Lee *et al.*, 1981), 7-hydroxy-BaP (Harvey & Fu, 1982), benzo[c]phenanthren-4-ol (Pataki & Harvey, 1982), and 2-chrysenol (Harvey *et al.*, 1986).

The synthetic routes to α-phenols are equally effective with β-phenols. Direct conversion of β-type-ketones to phenols may also be achieved by treatment with trityl trifluoroacetate (Fu *et al.*, 1979). Although this method has only been employed to synthesize 2- and 3-hydroxy-BA, the yields were good, and the method is potentially applicable to other phenols.

Fig. 15.5. Synthesis of phenols from ketonic intermediates. Similar methods are effective for both α- and β-ketones.

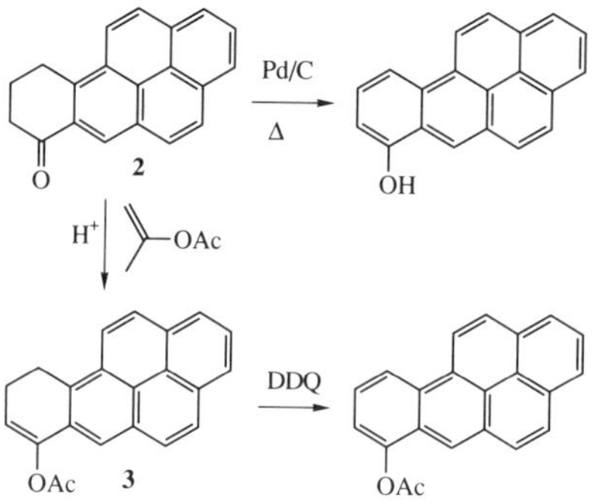

Transposition of α-type ketones to β-type ketones may be accomplished by reduction to the alcohol, acidic dehydration, epoxidation and acidic rearrangement (Fu *et al.*, 1979) (Fig. 15.7). β-Type ketones are also synthetically accessible by dehydration of tetrahydrodiols (Fig. 15.7) and by cyclization of alkylated 1,4-cyclohexadione intermediates (Harvey *et al.*, 1986) (Fig. 15.6). Another convenient route to β-phenols entails acid-catalyzed elimination of tetrahydrodiol diesters to β-enol esters followed by dehydrogenation and de-esterification. Phenols synthesized by this latter route include 10-hydroxy-BA (Fu *et al.*, 1979), 10-hydroxy-BeP (Lee *et al.*, 1981), 3-hydroxy-DBA (Lee & Harvey, 1980), 2- and 3-hydroxydibenz-[a,c]anthracene (Kole *et al.*, 1989), 2- and 3-hydroxy-7-methyl-BA (Lee & Harvey, 1979), 5-methylchrysen-8-ol (Harvey *et al.*, 1986), and 1-isopropyl-8-hydroxy-BaP (Pataki & Harvey, 1987).

One of the oldest methods of phenol synthesis is from precursors with fewer rings one of which contains an oxygen function, usually a methoxy group, at an appropriate site. For example, this approach has been employed by Newman and coworkers for the synthesis of the isomeric phenols of

Fig. 15.6. Synthetic routes to α- and β-type ketones that complement the Haworth synthesis.

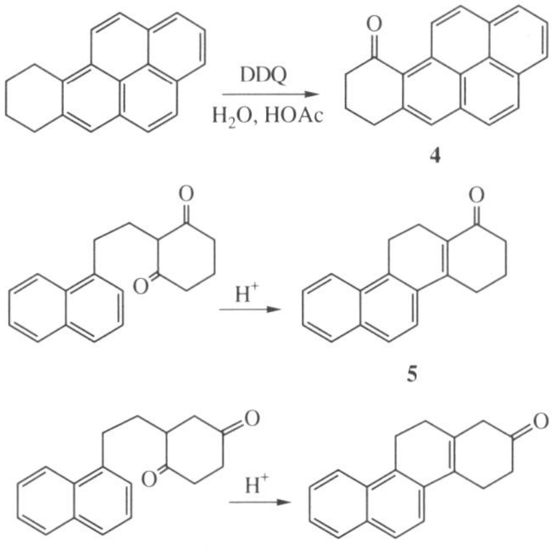

Fig. 15.7. Conversion of α-type ketones to β-type ketones.

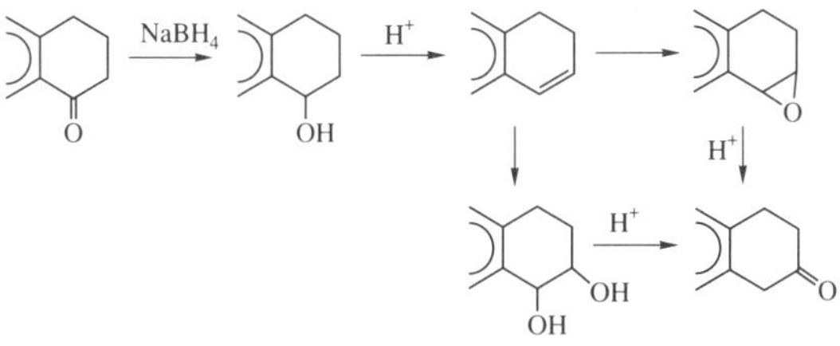

DMBA (Newman *et al.*, 1976, 1978) and benzo[c]phenanthrene (Newman & Blum, 1964) and by Harvey and coworkers for the synthesis of 3-hydroxy-DMBA (Lee & Harvey, 1986), 7-methyl- and 12-methyl-3-hydroxy-BA (Harvey *et al.*, 1987), 9-hydroxycholanthrene (Harvey *et al.*, 1987), 3-hydroxydibenz[a,j]anthracene and its 7,14-dimethyl derivative (Harvey *et al.*, 1988), and benzo[c]phenanthren-3-ol (Pataki *et al.*, 1989). Numerous additional examples may be found in the literature.

The Diels–Alder reaction has been frequently employed for the synthesis of phenol derivatives of polyarenes. For example, the Diels–Alder reaction between 1,4-naphthoquinone and methoxy-substituted styrenes produced the corresponding 1-, 2-, 3-, 4-, and 5-methoxy-BA 7,12-diones which could be converted to the related BA phenols (Fig. 15.8) (Muschik *et al.*, 1979). These quinones were also utilized for the synthesis of the 1-, 2-, 3-, 4-, and 5-phenols of DMBA. An analogous approach was employed to synthesize the 8-, 9-, 10-, and 11-phenols of BA and DMBA (Manning *et al.*, 1979) as well as phenolic derivatives of DBa,hA and DBa,jA (Muschik *et al.*, 1982). Diels–Alder cycloaddition has also been used for the synthesis of the phenol derivatives of several polycyclic fluoranthenes. Thus, Diels–Alder reaction of cyclopenta[c,d]pyrene with 2-(trimethylsilyloxy)butadiene furnished a mixture of two isomeric adducts which on hydrolysis and dehydrogenation gave a mixture of 8- and 9-hydroxyindeno[1,2,3-cd]pyrene separable by HPLC (Fig. 15.9) (Rice *et al.*, 1986). Cyclopenta[c,d]pyrene also underwent Diels–Alder reaction with 1-acetoxybutadiene to give a mixture of adducts which on hydrolysis and oxidation with pyridinium chlorochromate furnished 7- and 10-hydroxyindeno[1,2,3-cd]pyrene. However, the yields of all of these phenolic derivatives were very poor. More satisfactory results were obtained from the Diels–Alder reaction of acephenanthrylene with 1-acetoxybutadiene; aromatization of the adducts and hydrolysis provided a

Fig. 15.8. Syntheses of phenolic derivatives of BA and DMBA utilizing Diels–Alder reactions.

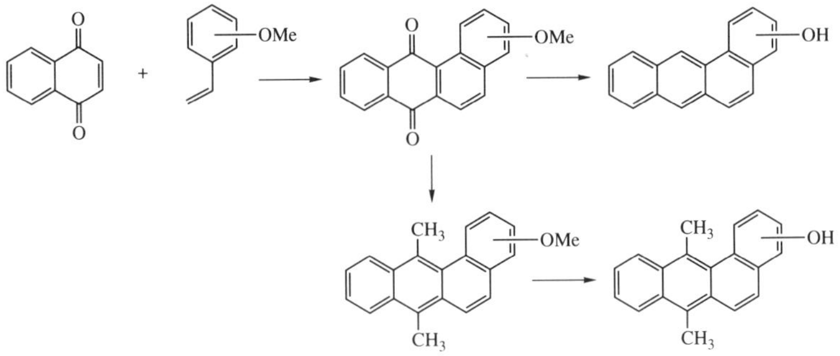

Table 15.1. *Phenol isomers of benz[a]anthracene*

Isomer	mp (°C)	UV	NMR	Reference
1	169–70		+	a,b,c
2	193–94		+	a,c,d
3	209–10		+	a,c
4	225		+	b
5	202–4	+	+	e,f
6	139–40	+	+	f
7	154.5–5.5		+	g
8	217–18	+	+	a,h,i,j
9	205–6.5	+	+	a,h,j
10	218–22		+	a,j
11	120–4		+	a,j

[a]Fu *et al.*, 1979; [b]Schoental, 1952; [c]Muschik *et al.*, 1979;
[d]Fieser & Fieser, 1933; [e]Fieser & Dietz, 1929; [f]McCaustland
et al., 1976; [g]Fieser & Hershberg, 1937; [h]Sims, 1971;
[i]Cook & Schoental, 1952; [j]Manning *et al.*, 1982 report the
methyl ether derivatives of these phenols.

mixture of 4- and 7-hydroxybenzo[b]fluoranthene in good overall yield
(Amin *et al.*, 1986). Similar methods were employed for the synthesis of 7-
and 8-hydroxyfluoranthene from acenaphthylene (Rice *et al.*, 1983).

Published information on the synthesis and properties of the phenol
isomers of the most studied PAHs in the 4–6 ring range is summarized in
Tables 15.1 – 15.9.

Fig. 15.9. Synthesis of 7-, 8-, 9-, and 10-hydroxyindeno[1,2,3-cd]pyrene
(R = OH, R' = H or vice versa) via Diels–Alder cycloaddition to
cyclopenta[c,d]pyrene.

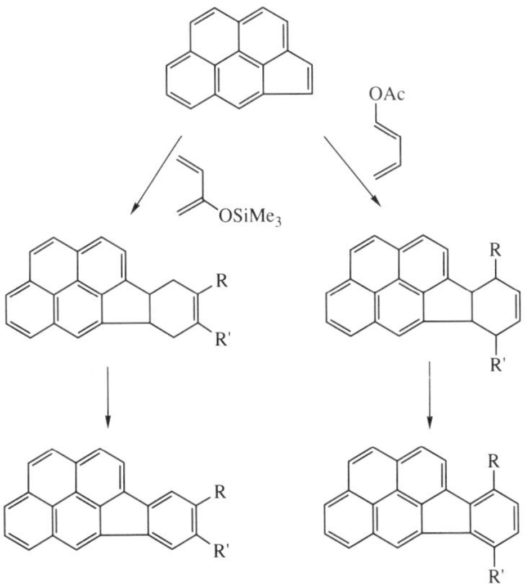

Table 15.2. *Phenol isomers of chrysene*

Isomer	mp (°C)	UV	NMR	Reference
1	281–3	+		a
2	273–5			a,b
3	271–3	+		c
4	152–3			a
5	208–9	+		a
6	248–50			d,e

[a]Cook & Schoental, 1945; [b]Harvey *et al.*, 1986; [c]Wilds & Shunk, 1943; [d]Newman & Cathcart, 1940; [e]Harvey *et al.*, 1975.

Table 15.3. *Phenol isomers of benzo[a]pyrene*

Isomer	mp (°C)	UV	NMR	Reference
1	(dec.)	+	+	a,b
2	227–8	+	+	a
3	226–7	+	+	a,c
4	225–7	+	+	a,d
5	195–6	+	+	a,e
6	207–9	+	+	a,f
7	218–19	+	+	a,g,h
8	228	+	+	a,i
9	196	+	+	a,i
10	200–1	+	+	a
11	220	+	+	a,j
12	230–1	+	+	a,k

[a]Yagi *et al.*, 1976; [b]Harvey & Cho, 1975; [c]Cook *et al.*, 1950; [d]Fu & Harvey, 1983; [e]Fieser & Johnson, 1940; [f]Fieser & Hershberg, 1939; [g]Fieser *et al.*, 1937; Harvey & Fu, 1982; [i]Sims, 1968; [j]Fieser & Heymann, 1941; [k]Fu & Harvey, 1981.

Table 15.4. *Phenol isomers of benzo[e]pyrene*

Isomer	mp (°C)	UV	NMR	Reference
1	180–1	+	+	a
2	229–30	+	+	a
3	246–8	+	+	a
4	242–3	+	+	a
9	210	+	+	a
10	239–40	+	+	a

[a]Lee *et al.*, 1981

Table 15.5. *Phenol isomers of benzo[c]phenanthrene*

Isomer	mp (°C)	UV	NMR	Reference
1	125–26	+		a
2	116.0–17.5	+		a
3	112–113	+		a,b
4	112.5–113	+		a,c
5	133–34	+		a
6	158.5–159.5	+		a

[a]Newman & Blum, 1964; [b]Pataki *et al.*, 1989; [c]Pataki & Harvey, 1982.

Table 15.6. *Phenol isomers of dibenz[a,h] anthracene*

Isomer	mp (°C)	UV	NMR	Reference
1	277–8	+	+	a
2	281–2	+	+	a,b
3	288–9	+	+	a–c
4	305–7	+	+	a,b
5	263–4	+	+	a
6	258–9	+	+	a
7	254–6	+	+	a

[a]Platt & Oesch, 1982a; [b]Muschik *et al.*, 1982; [c]Lee & Harvey, 1980.

Table 15.7. *Phenol isomers of dibenz[a,j]anthracene*

Isomer	mp (°C)	UV	NMR	Reference
1	233–6		+	a
2	215–35		+	a
3	221–32		+	a
4	220–32		+	a
7	255–6	+	+	b

[a]Muschik *et al*, 1982; [b]Snatzke *et al.*, 1973 report data on the acetate ester only.

Table 15.8. *Phenol isomers of DMBA*

Isomer	mp (°C)	UV	NMR	Reference
1	hygroscopic	+		a,b
2	122–4	+		a,b
3	167–8	+	+	a–c
4	164–5	+		a,b,d
5	(dec.)			e
6	(dec.)			e
9	197–8			a
10	133–04			a

[a]Newman *et al.*, 1978; [b]Muschik *et al.*, 1975; [c]Lee & Harvey, 1986; [d]Flesher *et al.*, 1967; [e]Newman *et al.*, 1976.

Table 15.9. *Phenol isomers of benzo[b]fluoranthene*

Isomer	mp (°C)	UV	NMR	Reference
1	235–6	+	+	a
2	221–2	+	+	a
3	248–9	+	+	a
4		+	+	a
5		+	+	a
6	232–3	+	+	a
7		+	+	a
8	209–10	+	+	a
9	221–2	+	+	a
10	229–30	+	+	a
11	215–16	+	+	a
12	214–15	+	+	a

[a]Amin *et al.*, 1986

15.3   Diphenols

Few diphenolic derivatives of polyarenes are known. Since they tend to undergo relatively facile air oxidation, they are usually isolated in protected form as dimethyl ethers or diacetates. They are conveniently synthesized by reduction of the corresponding quinones with $NaBH_4$ in dimethylformamide (Cho & Harvey, 1976). PAH diphenol diacetates synthesized by this means include 9,10-diacetoxyphenanthrene, 9,10-diacetoxyanthracene, 5,6-diacetoxychrysene, 1,6-, 1,8-, and 4,5-diacetoxy-pyrene, 5,6- and 7,12-diacetoxy-BA, 1,6-, 3,6-, and 4,5-diacetoxy-benzo[a]pyrene, and 5,6-diacetoxydibenz[a,h]anthracene.

15.4   Quinones

15.4.1   K-region quinones

Some polycyclic K-region quinones are synthetically accessible from the parent polyarenes by direct oxidation. The K-region quinones of phenanthrene, chrysene, and benzo[c]phenanthrene were prepared by direct oxidation with chromic acid (Lee, 1969; Wendland & LaLonde, 1963; Graebe & Honigsberger, 1900). However, the majority of PAHs undergo oxidation predominantly in other molecular regions. These PAHs may be transformed to K-region quinones via the corresponding *cis*-dihydrodiols obtained from reaction with OsO4 or via the K-region dihydro derivatives obtained from hydrogenation over a Pd catalyst (Fu *et al.*, 1980). Oxidation of the *cis*-dihydrodiols to quinones may be accomplished by treatment with SO3/pyridine in dimethyl sulfoxide, CrO3, MnO2, or DDQ (Harvey *et al.*, 1975; Boyland & Sims, 1964; Rice *et al.*, 1986; Lehr *et al.*, 1978). In the author's experience, the most reproducible results are given by DDQ. The SO3/pyridine–DMSO reagent also gives excellent results, but extremely dry DMSO is necessary. Quinones synthesized via the *cis*-dihydrodiol route include pyrene-4,5-dione (Harvey *et al.*, 1975), BA-5,6-dione (Harvey *et al.*, 1975), 7-methyl-BA-5,6-dione (Sims, 1967), 12-methyl-BA-5,6-dione (Sims, 1967), DMBA-5,6-dione (Harvey *et al.*, 1975), BaP-4,5-dione (Harvey *et al.*, 1975), 7-methyl-BaP-4,5-dione (Konieczny & Harvey, 1980), 6-^{3}H-BaP-4,5-dione (Harvey & Fu, 1976), BeP-4,5-dione (Lee *et al.*, 1981; Platt & Oesch, 1982), DBahA-5,6-dione (Harvey *et al.*, 1975), and 3-MC-11,12-dione (McCaustland *et al.*, 1976; Platt & Oesch, 1982).

The synthesis of quinones from K-region dihydroarenes, although the yields are only moderate, avoids the use of the hazardous OsO4 reagent, is operationally simple, and is adaptable to preparation on any scale. Oxidation of the K-region dihydroarenes to quinones is accomplished by treatment with sodium dichromate in acetic acid–ethyl acetate (Cho & Harvey, 1974). Pyrene-4,5-dione, BA-5,6-dione, and BaP-4,5-dione have been synthesized by this route.

Oxidation of K-region phenols provides another route to K-region quinones. This approach offers little practical advantage in cases where the phenols are obtained from dehydration of the *cis*-dihydrodiols since the latter may be oxidized directly to quinones. BA-5,6-dione (Yang & Trie, 1982), and 4,5- and 7,12-^{13}C-BaP-4,5-dione (Bodine *et al.*, 1978) have been prepared by oxidation of phenols with Fremy's salt. Benzo[k]fluoranthene-1,2-dione was obtained by oxidation of 1-hydroxybenzo[k]fluoranthene with ceric ammonium sulfate (Balanikas *et al.*, 1988).

15.4.2 *Non-K-region o-quinones*

Non-K-region *ortho*-quinones are most conveniently synthesized by oxidation of phenolic precursors by Fremy's salt or phenylseleninic anhydride (Sukumaran & Harvey, 1980). Oxidation of β-phenols, such as 3-hydroxy-BA, with these reagents yields the corresponding *o*-quinones, whereas analogous oxidation of α-phenols, such as 4-hydroxy-BA, affords principally *p*-quinones (Fig. 15.10). However, sterically hindered bay region phenols tend to be resistant to oxidation by either of these reagents. Thus, oxidation of 3-hydroxyphenanthrene with Fremy's salt furnished 2,2-dihydroxybenz[e]indan-1,3-dione (**6**), while attempted oxidation of this phenol with (PhSeO)$_2$ gave no reaction. This reagent also failed to react with 3-hydroxydibenz[a,c]anthracene (Harvey *et al.*, 1983). On the other hand, oxidation of 1-hydroxybenzo[b]fluoranthene with ceric ammonium sulfate furnished the corresponding *o*-quinone **7** in 30% yield (Balanikas *et al.*, 1988).

The resistance to oxidation in sterically crowded regions may be used to advantage to direct oxidation of an α-phenol to the *ortho* rather than to the

Fig. 15.10. Oxidation of α- and β-phenols with (i) Fremy's salt, (ii) phenylseleninic anhydride, and (iii) ceric ammonium sulfate.

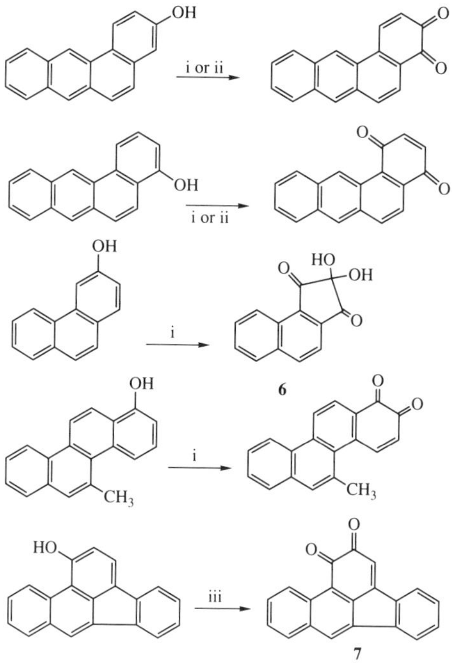

para position. Thus, oxidation of 1-hydroxy-5-methylchrysene with Fremy's reagent furnished 5-methylchrysene-1,2-dione rather than the sterically crowded 5-methylchrysene-1,4-dione (Pataki *et al.*, 1983). *o*-Quinones synthesized via oxidation of phenolic precursors include anthracene-1,2-dione (Sukumaran & Harvey, 1980), phenanthrene-1,2-dione (Sukumaran & Harvey, 1980), BA-3,4-dione (Harvey *et al.*, 1988; Sukumaran & Harvey, 1980), 7-methyl-BA-3,4-dione (Harvey *et al.*, 1987), 12-methyl-BA-3,4-dione (Harvey *et al.*, 1987), DMBA-3,4-dione (Lee & Harvey, 1986), cholanthrene-9,10-dione (Harvey *et al.*, 1988), 3-MC-9,10-dione (Jacobs *et al.*, 1983), 6-methylcholanthrene-9,10-dione (Harvey *et al.*, 1988), benzo[c]-phenanthrene-3,4-dione (Pataki *et al.*, 1989), chrysene-1,2-dione (Harvey *et al.*, 1986), 5-methylchrysene-1,2-dione (Harvey *et al.*, 1986), BaP-7,8-dione (Sukumaran & Harvey, 1980), 1-isopropyl-BaP-7,8-dione (Pataki & Harvey, 1987), DBajA-3,4-dione (Harvey *et al.*, 1988), and 7,14-dimethyl-DBajA-3,4-dione (Harvey *et al.*, 1988).

Non-K-region *ortho*-quinones are also synthetically accessible by oxidation of *cis*-tetrahydrodiols with DDQ (Fig. 15.11) (Platt & Oesch, 1982). The *cis*-tetrahydrodiols are most conveniently obtained from the corresponding dihydroarenes by reaction with OsO4. *o*-Quinones synthesized by this method include the phenanthrene-1,2- and -3,4-diones, the BA-1,2- and 8,9-diones, triphenylene-1,2-dione, the BaP-7,8- and 9,10-diones, BeP-9,10-dione, and DBa,hA-3,4-dione.

Oxidation of *o*-aminophenols provides a useful alternative synthetic route that allows the preparation of *o*-quinones in sterically crowded bay regions, e.g. phenanthrene-3,4-dione (Fig. 15.12). Chromic acid and FeCl3 have been employed as oxidants for this purpose. *o*-Aminophenols may be obtained from β-phenols by coupling with a diazonium salt followed by reduction of the diazo compound with SnCl2 or sodium hyposulfite. The *o*-quinone derivatives of naphthalene (Fieser, 1943a), anthracene (Lagodzinski, 1905), and phenanthrene (Fieser, 1929a,b) were first synthesized by this method.

Oxidation of *o*-diphenols (i.e. catechols) also provides synthetic access to *o*-quinones. Although seldom employed for this purpose, it has important application in the oxidative recycling of the *o*-diphenolic byproducts

Fig. 15.11. Synthesis of *o*-quinones from dihydroarenes via *cis*-dihydrodiol intermediates.

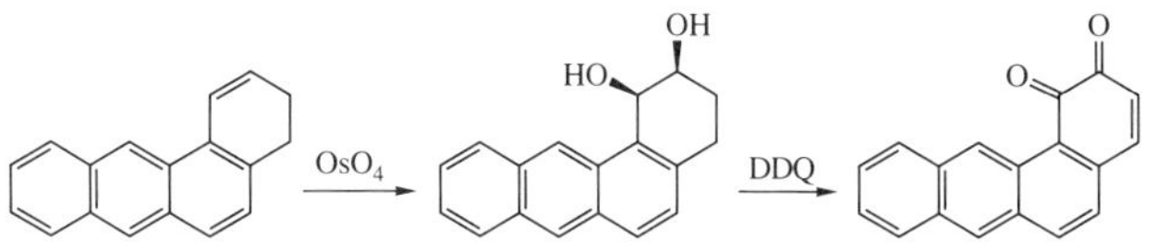

obtained in the reduction of *o*-quinones to *trans*-dihydrodiols by metal hydrides (Platt & Oesch, 1983). This method was employed to synthesize DBa,hA-3,4-dione (Kundu, 1979).

15.4.3 Other quinones

While quinone derivatives of PAHs in which the carbonyl functions are *para* or further removed from one another are well known, these are not commonly detected as metabolites of intact mammalian cells. They are, however, sometimes found as products of microsomal oxidation. Thus, the 1,6-, 3,6- and 6,12-diones of BaP have been identified among the metabolites of BaP formed by rat liver microsomes (Gelboin, 1980). Oxidation of BaP by sodium dichromate or aqueous chromic acid affords the same quinones (Cho & Harvey, 1976; Vollmann *et al.*, 1900). Similar oxidation of pyrene affords the analogous 1,6-, 3,6- and 6,12-diones.

The most common quinone derivatives of polyarenes with three or more linearly fused aromatic rings are the meso-region *para*-quinones. The reactions of anthracene, BA, DBA, and other similar PAHs, with strong oxidants such as chromic acid, generally takes place preferentially in this molecular region to yield the corresponding *para*-quinones (Clar, 1964). Oxidation of the corresponding meso-region dihydroaromatic derivatives of these PAHs also occurs predominantly in this molecular site (Harvey & Cortez, 1986). Quinones of this type are also readily available as intermediates in the construction of polycyclic ring systems. One of the most common methods entails cyclization of keto-acid intermediates. For example, synthesis of 3-hydroxy-DMBA, a key intermediate in the synthesis of the DMBA diol epoxide, was accomplished in relatively few steps by the sequence shown (Fig. 15.13). Cyclization of the keto-acid **8** took place readily in methanesulfonic acid to generate the quinone intermediate **9**.

Fig. 15.12. Synthesis of a sterically hindered bay region quinone from a phenol via diazonium coupling, conversion to an aminophenol, and oxidation with chromic acid.

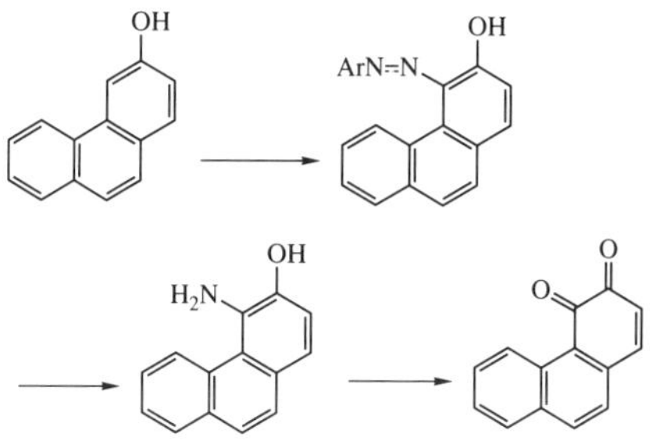

Quinones are also formed as products of the Diels–Alder cycloaddition of dienes to quinones, e.g. in the synthesis of substituted BAs and DMBAs (Fig. 15.8). Quinones of this type are also obtained from the oxidation of meso-region phenols. For example, 3-methoxy-12-acetoxy-BA obtained from the cyclization of **11** with ZnCl$_2$ in Ac$_2$O/HOAc undergoes direct conversion to the quinone **9** on treatment with sodium dichromate in acetic acid.

The main importance of the meso-region *para*-quinones is as synthetic intermediates. Their reduction provides the corresponding polycyclic aromatic compounds, e.g. reduction with HI of BA-7,12-dione provides convenient access to BA (Konieczny & Harvey, 1990). They also undergo ready conversion to the dialkyl derivatives by the addition of organolithium or Grignard reagents followed by reduction. For example, addition of methyllithium to **9** followed by treatment of the adduct with the TiCl$_3$·LiAlH$_4$ furnished smoothly 3-methoxy-DMBA. Deoxygenation of the adduct **10** was also achieved by a modification of the method of Newman (Newman *et al.*, 1978) through reaction with HCl to form 3-methoxy-7-chloromethyl-12-methyl-BA followed by reduction with NaBH$_4$ (Fig. 15.13), rather than SnCl$_2$, HCl as employed in the original Newman procedure.

Polycyclic quinones of all types may also be reduced under appropriate conditions to the corresponding hydroquinones. The most generally useful reagent for this purpose is NaBH$_4$ in dimethylformamide (Cho & Harvey, 1976).

15.5 Hydroxyalkyl and keto derivatives

Oxidative metabolism of methyl and other alkyl substituents on polyarenes leads to formation of hydroxyalkyl and keto derivatives. The most studied example is 3-MC whose metabolites include the 1-, 2-, and 3-

Fig. 15.13. Synthesis of 3-methoxy-DMBA proceeds via a quinone intermediate.

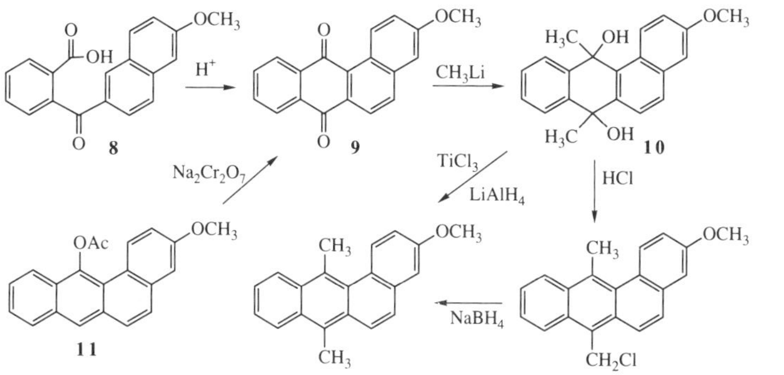

hydroxy derivatives and the 1- and 2-keto derivatives (Sims & Grover, 1981). There is also evidence that hydroxymethyl derivatives of BaP, BA, and other polyarenes are formed by hydroxymethylation of the parent hydrocarbons by reaction with S-adenosyl-L-methionine (Flesher *et al.*, 1982, 1986). The hydroxyalkyl and keto derivatives of polyarenes are generally synthetically accessible from the parent polyarenes by direct oxidation with lead tetraacetate, DDQ in moist acetic acid, one electron oxidants, or other chemical oxidants. Thus, oxidation of DMBA with lead tetraacetate affords the 7-acetoxymethyl, 12-acetoxymethyl, and 7-12-diacetoxymethyl, derivatives as well as other oxidized products (Boyland & Sims, 1965). However, because of the complexity of the products often produced by oxidation with lead tetraacetate or one electron oxidants, such as ceric ammonium nitrate (Fried & Schumm, 1967), other methods are generally preferred. 7-Hydroxymethyl-DMBA is more conveniently obtained by reaction of 7-iodomethyl-DMBA with alkaline silver carbonate solution (Flesher *et al.*, 1967). The new method of PAH oxidation using DDQ in moist acetic acid is particularly promising from a synthetic standpoint. Thus, oxidation of 7-methyl-BA and 3-MC with this reagent affords 7-formyl-BA and 1-keto-3-MC, respectively, in good yield (Lee & Harvey, 1988). These compounds are reduced readily with NaBH4 to the corresponding hydroxy derivatives (Lee & Harvey, 1988a). 7-Formyl-14-methyldibenz[a,j]-anthracene and 7-hydroxymethyl-14-methyldibenz[a,j]anthracene have also recently been synthesized in good overall yield by this route in the author's laboratory. The oxidized derivatives of 3-MC in the 1-, 2-, and 3-positions

Fig. 15.14. Synthetic routes to the 1-, 2-, and 3-oxygenated metabolites of 3-MC.

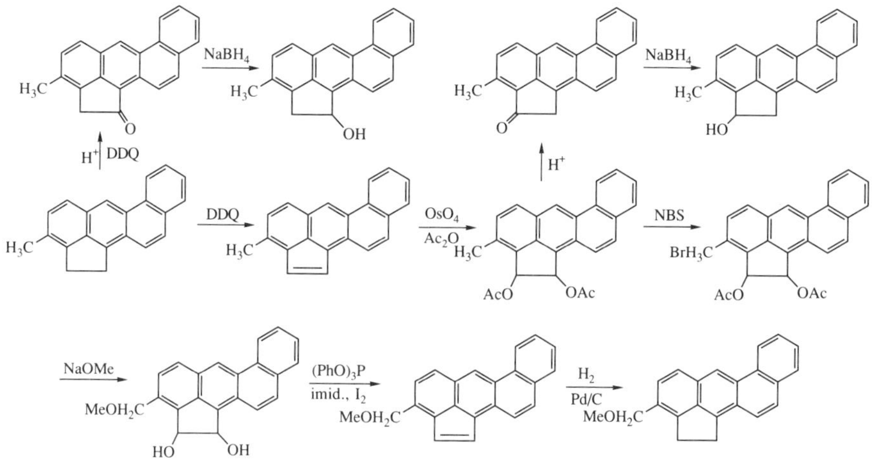

are conveniently prepared from 3-MC via the route depicted in Fig. 15.14 (Lee & Harvey, 1988a).

15.6   References

Amin, S., Huie, K., Hussain, N., Balanikas, G., Carmella, S. G. & Hecht, S. S. (1986). Synthesis of potential phenolic metabolites of benz[b]fluoranthene. *J. Org. Chem.* **51**, 1206–11.

Balanikas, G., Hussain, N., Amin, S. & Hecht, S. S. (1988). Oxidation of polynuclear aromatic hydrocarbons with ceric ammonium sulfate: Preparation of quinones and lactones. *J. Org. Chem.* **53**, 1007–10.

Bodine, R. S., Hylarides, M., Daub, G. & VanderJagt, D. L. (1978). ^{13}C-Labeled benzo[a]pyrene and derivatives. 1. Efficient pathways to labeling the 4,5,11, and 12 positions. *J. Org. Chem.* **43**, 4025–8.

Boyland, E. & Sims, P. (1964). Metabolism of polycyclic compounds. 24. The metabolism of benz[a]anthracene. *Biochem. J.* **91**, 493–506.

Boyland, E. & Sims, P. (1965). Metabolism of polycyclic compounds. The metabolism of 7,12-dimethylbenz[a]anthracene by rat-liver homogenates. *Biochem. J.* **95**, 780–7.

Cho, H. & Harvey, R. G. (1974). Synthesis of 'K-region' quinones and arene oxides of polycyclic aromatic hydrocarbons. *Tetrahedron Lett.* 1491–4.

Cho, H. & Harvey, R. G. (1976). Synthesis of hydroquinone diacetates from polycyclic aromatic quinones. *J. Chem. Soc. Perkin I*, 836–9.

Cook, J. W., Ludwiczak, R. S. & Schoental, R. (1950). Polycyclic aromatic hydrocarbons. Part XXXVI. Synthesis of the metabolic oxidation products of 3:4-benzpyrene. *J. Chem. Soc.* 1112–21.

Cook, J. W. & Schoental, R. (1945). Polycyclic aromatic hydrocarbons. Part XXX. Synthesis of chrysenols. *J. Chem. Soc.* 288–93.

Cook, J. W. & Schoental, R. (1952). 5-Hydroxy-1:2-benzanthracene and 1'-hydroxy-1:2-5:6-dibenzanthracene. *J. Chem. Soc.* 9–11.

Dipple, A., Levy, L. S. & Iype, T. P. (1975). Investigation of the possible involvement of ketonic derivatives of polycyclic hydrocarbons in hydrocarbon carcinogenesis. *Cancer Res.* **35**, 652–7.

Fieser, L. F. (1929a). Some derivatives of 3,4-phenanthrenequinone. *J. Am. Chem. Soc.* **51**, 940–52.

Fieser, L. F. (1929b). 1,2-Phenanthrenequinone. *J. Am. Chem. Soc.* **51**, 1896–1906.

Fieser, L. F. (1943). 2- and 3-Phenanthrenesulfonic acid. *Org. Syn.* Coll. Vol. II, 482–5.

Fieser, L. F. (1943a). 1,2-Naphthoquinone. *Org. Syn.* Coll. Vol. II, 430–2.

Fieser, L. F. & Dietz, E. M. (1929). 1,2-Benz-3,4-anthraquinone. *J. Am. Chem. Soc.* **51**, 3141–8.

Fieser, L. F. & Fieser, M. (1933). The conversion of phthaloylnaphthalenes and naphthoyl-2-benzoic acids into benzanthraquinone. *J. Am. Chem. Soc.* **55**, 3342–52.

Fieser, L. F. & Hershberg, E. B. (1937). 10-Substituted 1,2-benzanthracene derivatives. *J. Am. Chem. Soc.* **59**, 1028–35.

Fieser, L. F. & Hershberg, E. B. (1938). Substitution reactions and meso derivatives of 1,2-benzanthracene. *J. Am. Chem. Soc.* **60**, 1893–6.

Fieser, L. F. & Hershberg, E. B. (1938a). The oxidation of methylcholanthrene and 3,4-benzpyrene with lead tetraacetate; further derivatives of 3,4-benzpyrene. *J. Am. Chem. Soc.* **60**, 2542–7.

Fieser, L. F. & Hershberg, E. B. (1939). The orientation of 3,4-benzpyrene in substitution reactions. *J. Am. Chem. Soc.* **61**, 1565–74.

Fieser, L. F., Hershberg, E. B., Long Jr, L. & Newman, M. S. (1937). Hydroxy derivatives of 3,4-benzpyrene and 1,2-benzanthracene. *J. Am. Chem. Soc.* **59**, 475–8.

Fieser, L. F. & Heymann, H. (1941a). Synthesis of 2-hydroxy-3,4-benzpyrene and 2-methyl-3,4-benzpyrene. *J. Am. Chem. Soc.* **63**, 2333–40.

Fieser, L. F. & Heymann, H. (1941b). Synthesis of 2-hydroxy-3,4-benzpyrene and 2-methyl-3,4-benzpyrene. *J. Am. Chem. Soc.* **63**, 2333–40.

Fieser, L. F. & Johnson, W. S. (1940). Synthesis of 6-hydroxy-3,4-benzpyrene and 8-isopropyl-1,2-benzanthracene from 9,10-dihydrophenanthrene. *J. Am. Chem. Soc.* **62**, 575–7.

Fieser, L. F. & Putnam, S. T. (1947). Mechanism of the oxidation of anthracene with lead tetraacetate. *J. Am. Chem. Soc.* **69**, 1038–46.

Flesher, J. W., Myers, S. R. & Blake, J. W. (1986). Bioalkylation of polynuclear aromatic hydrocarbons: a predictor of carcinogenic activity. *Polynuclear Aromatic Hydrocarbons: Chemistry, Characterization, and Carcinogenesis*, eds M. Cooke & A. J. Dennis, pp. 271–84. Columbus, OH: Battelle.

Flesher, J. W., Soedigdo, S. & Kelley, D. R. (1967). Syntheses of metabolites of 7,12-dimethylbenz[a]anthracene, 4-hydroxy-7,12-dimethylbenz[a]anthracene, 7-hydroxymethyl-7,12-dimethylbenz[a]anthracene, their methyl ethers, and acetoxy derivatives. *J. Medic. Chem.*, **10**, 932–6.

Flesher, J. W., Stanbury, K. H. & Sydnor, K. L. (1982). S-Adenosyl-1-methionine is a carbon donor in the conversion of benzo[a]pyrene to 6-hydroxymethylbenzo[a]pyrene by rat liver S-9. *Cancer Lett.*, **16**, 91–2.

Fried, J. & Schumm, D. E. (1967). One electron transfer oxidation of 7,12-dimethyl-benz[a]anthracene, a model for the metabolic activation of carcinogenic hydrocarbons. *J. Am. Chem. Soc.*, **89**, 5508–9.

Fu, P. P., Cortez, C., Sukumaran, K. B. & Harvey, R. G. (1979). Synthesis of the isomeric phenols of benz[a]anthracene from benz[a]anthracene. *J. Org. Chem.* **44**, 4265–71.

Fu, P. P. & Harvey, R. G. (1981). Synthesis of benzo[a]pyren-12-ol. *Org. Proc. Prep. Internat.* **13**, 152–5.

Fu, P. P. & Harvey, R. G. (1983). Synthesis of 4-hydroxybenzo[a]pyrene. *J. Org. Chem.* **48**, 1534–6.

Fu, P. P., Harvey, R. G. & Beland, F. A. (1978). Molecular orbital theoretical prediction of the isomeric products formed from the reactions of arene oxides and related metabolites of polycyclic aromatic hydrocarbons. *Tetrahedron*, **34**, 857–66.

Gelboin, H. V. (1980). Benzo[a]pyrene metabolism, activation and carcinogenesis: role and regulation of mixed-function oxidases and related enzymes. *Physiol. Rev.* **50**, 1107–66.

Graebe, C. & Honigsberger, F. (1900). Products of oxidation of chrysene. *Liebigs Ann. Chem.* **311**, 257–75.

Gumprecht, W. H. (1973). 3-Hydroxypyrene. *Org. Syn.* Coll. Vol. V, 632–5.

Harvey, R. G. & Cho, H. (1975). Improved synthesis of benzo[a]pyren-1-ol and isolation of a covalent benzo[a]pyrene lead compound. *J. Chem. Soc. Chem. Commun.* 373–4.

Harvey, R. G. & Cortez, C. (1986). Synthesis of 7,12-dimethylbenz[a]anthracene and its 1,2,3,4-tetrahydro derivative. *J. Org. Chem.* **51**, 5023–4.

Harvey, R. G., Cortez, C., Sawyer, T. W. & DiGiovanni, J. (1988). Synthesis of the tumorigenic 3,4-dihydrodiol metabolites of dibenz[a,j]anthracene and 7,14-dimethyldibenz[a,j]anthracene. *J. Medic. Chem.* **31**, 1308–12.

Harvey, R. G., Cortez, C., Sugiyama, T., Ito, Y., Sawyer, T. W. & DiGiovanni, J. (1987). Biologically active dihydrodiol metabolites of polycyclic aromatic hydrocarbons structurally related to the potent carcinogenic hydrocarbon 7,12-dimethylbenz[a]anthracene. *J. Medic. Chem.* **31**, 154–9.

Harvey, R. G. & Fu, P. P. (1976). Synthesis of high specific activity benzo[a]pyrene-6-t and its K-region oxidized derivatives. *J. Label. Cpds. Radiopharm.* **12**, 259–64.

Harvey, R. G. & Fu, P. P. (1982). Synthesis of 7-hydroxybenzo[a]pyrene. *Org. Prep. Proc. Internat.* **14**, 414–7.

Harvey, R. G., Goh, S. H. & Cortez, C. (1975). 'K-Region' oxides and related oxidized metabolites of carcinogenic aromatic hydrocarbons. *J. Am. Chem. Soc.* **97**, 3468–79.

Harvey, R. G., Hahn, J.-T. Bukowska, M. & Harvey, R. G. (1990). A new chromone and flavone synthesis and its utilization for the synthesis of potentially antitumorigenic polycyclic chromones and flavones. *J. Org. Chem.* **55**, 6161–6.

Harvey, R. G., Pataki, J. & Lee, H. (1986). Synthesis of the dihydrodiol and diol epoxide metabolites of chrysene and 5-methylchrysene. *J. Org. Chem.* **51**, 1407–12.

Harvey, R. G., Ray, J. K. & Sukumaran, K. B. (1983). Synthesis of 3-hydroxydibenz-[a,c]anthracene. *Org. Prep. Proc. Internat.* **15**, 335–40.

Harvey, R. G., Schmolka, S., Cortez, C. & Lee, H. (1988). Syntheses of 2-bromopyrene and 2-hydroxypyrene. *Syn. Commun.* **18**, 2207–9.

Jacobs, S. A., Cortez, C. & Harvey, R. G. (1983). Synthesis of potential proximate and ultimate carcinogenic metabolites of 3-methylcholanthrene. *Carcinogenesis*, **4**, 519–22.

Kidwell, R. L., Murphy, M. & Darling, S. D. (1973). Phenols: 6-methoxy-2-naphthol. *Org. Syn* Coll. Vol. V, 918–20.

Kole, P. L., Dubey, S. K. & Kumar, S. (1989). Synthesis of isomeric *cis*-dihydrodiols and phenols of highly mutagenic dibenz[a,c]anthrancene. *J. Org. Chem.* **54**, 845–9.

Konieczny, M. & Harvey, R. G. (1980). Reductive methylation of polycyclic aromatic quinones. *J. Org. Chem.* **45**, 1308–10.

Konieczny, M. & Harvey, R. G. (1990). Reduction of quinones with hydroiodic acid: Benz[a]-anthracene. *Org. Syn.* Coll. Vol. VII, 18–20.

Kundu, N. (1979). Synthesis of some non-K-region derivatives of dibenz[a,h]anthracene. *J. Org. Chem.* **44**, 3086–8.

Lagodzinski, K. (1905). 1,2-Anthraquinone. *Liebigs Ann. Chem.* **342**, 59–89.

Lee, D. G. (1969). Hydrocarbon oxidation using transition metal compounds. *Oxidation*, 1. ed. R. L. Augustine, 1–47. New York: Marcel Dekker.

Lee, H. & Harvey, R. G. (1979). Synthesis of biologically active metabolites of 7-methylbenz[a]anthracene. *J. Org. Chem.* **44**, 4948–53.

Lee, H. & Harvey, R. G. (1980). Synthesis of biologically active metabolites of dibenz[a,h]anthracene. *J. Org. Chem.* **45**, 588–92.

Lee, H. & Harvey, R. G. (1986). Synthesis of the active diol epoxide metabolites of the potent carcinogenic hydrocarbon 7,12-dimethylbenz[a]anthracene. *J. Org. Chem.* **51**, 3502–7.

Lee, H. & Harvey, R. G. (1988). 2,3-Dichloro-5,6-dicyano-1,4-benzoquinone (DDQ) in aqueous acetic acid, a useful new reagent for the synthesis of aryl ketones and aldehydes via benzylic oxidation. *J. Org. Chem.* **53**, 4587–9.

Lee, H. & Harvey, R. G. (1988a). Syntheses of oxygenated derivatives of 3-methylcholanthrene. *Org. Prep. Proc. Internat.* **20**, 123–8.

Lee, H. M., Shyamasundar, N. & Harvey, R. G. (1981). Isomeric phenols of benzo[e]pyrene. *J. Org. Chem.* **46**, 2889–95.

Lehr, R. E., Taylor, C. M., Kumar, S., Mah, H. D. & Jerina, D. M. (1978). Synthesis of the non-K-region and K-region *trans*-dihydrodiols of benzo[e]pyrene. *J. Org. Chem.* **43**, 3462–6.

Manning, W. B., Muschik, G. M. & Tomaszewski, J. E. (1979). Preparation of derivatives of 8-, 9-, 10-, and 11-hydroxybenz[a]anthracene-7-12-diones, benz[a]anthracenes, and 7,12-dimethylbenz[a]anthracenes. *J. Org. Chem.* **44**, 699–702.

McCaustland, D. J., Fischer, D. L., Kolwyck, K. C., Duncan, W. P., Wiley Jr, J. C., Menon, C. S., Engel, J. F., Selkirk, J. K. & Roller, P. P. (1976). Polycyclic aromatic hydrocarbon derivatives: Synthesis and physicochemical characterization. *Carcinogenesis*, **1**. R. I. Freudenthal & P. W. Jones, 349–411. New York: Raven Press.

Minabe, M., Cho, B. P. & Harvey, R. G. (1989). Electrophilic substitution of polycyclic fluoranthene hydrocarbons. *J. Am. Chem. Soc.* **111**, 3809–12.

Muschik, G. M., Kelly, T. P. & Manning, W. B. (1982). Simple synthesis of 1-, 2-, 3-, and 4-hydroxydibenz[a,j]anthracenes and 2-, 3-, and 4-hydroxydibenz[a,h]anthracenes. *J. Org. Chem.* **47**, 4709–12.

Newman, M. S. & Blum, J. (1964). The synthesis and ionization constants of the six hydroxybenzo[c]phenanthrenes. *J. Am. Chem. Soc.* **86**, 503–7.

Newman, M. S. & Cathcart, J. A. (1940). The orientation of chrysene. *J. Org. Chem.* **5**, 618–22.

Newman, M. S., Khanna, J. M., Kanakarajan, K. & Kumar, S. (1978). Syntheses of 1-, 2-, 3-, 4-, 6-, 9-, and 10-hydroxy-7,12-dimethylbenz[a]anthracenes. *J. Org. Chem.* **43**, 2553–7.

Newman, M. S., Sankaran, V. & Olson, D. R. (1976). Phenolic and ketonic tautomers in polycyclic aromatic hydrocarbons. *J. Am. Chem. Soc.* **98**, 3237–42.

Pataki, J. & Harvey, R. G. (1982). Benzo[c]phenanthrene and its oxidized metabolites. *J. Org. Chem.* **47**, 20–2.

Pataki, J. & Harvey, R. G. (1987). Synthesis of a sterically impeded analogue of the carcinogenic *anti*-diol epoxide of benzo[a]pyrene. *J. Org. Chem.* **52**, 2226–30.

Pataki, J., Lee, H. & Harvey, R. G. (1983). Carcinogenic metabolites of 5-methylchrysene. *Carcinogenesis*, **4**, 399–402.

Pataki, J., Raddo, P. D. & Harvey, R. G. (1989). An efficient synthesis of the highly tumorigenic *anti*-diol epoxide derivative of benzo[c]phenanthrene. *J. Org. Chem.* **54**, 840–4.

Platt, K. L. & Oesch, F. (1982a). Synthesis and properties of the seven isomeric phenols of dibenz[a,h]anthracene. *J. Org. Chem.* **47**, 5321–6.

Platt, K. L. & Oesch, F. (1982b). Synthesis of non-K-region *ortho*-quinones of polycyclic aromatic hydrocarbons from cyclic ketones. *Tetrahedron Lett.* **23**, 263–6.

Platt, K. L. & Oesch, F. (1983). Efficient synthesis of non-K-region *trans*-dihydrodiols of polycyclic aromatic hydrocarbons from o-quinones and catechols. *J. Org. Chem.* **48**, 265–8.

Rice, J. E., LaVoie, E. J., McCaustland, D. J., Fischer, D. L. & Wiley Jr, J. C. (1986). Synthesis of oxygenated metabolites of indeno[1,2,3-cd]pyrene. *J. Org. Chem.* **51**, 2428–34.

Roitt, I. M. & Waters, W. A. (1952). The action of benzoyl peroxide on polycyclic aromatic hydrocarbons. *J. Chem. Soc.* 2695–705.

Schoental, R. (1952). Friedel–Crafts succinoylation of anthracene. Synthesis of 1'- and 4'-hydroxy-1:2-benzanthracene. *J. Chem. Soc.* 4403–6.

Shaw, J. E., Kunerth, D. C. & Swanson, S. B. (1976). Nucleophilic aromatic substitution reactions of unactivated chlorides with methoxide ion in hexamethylphosphoramide. *J. Org. Chem.* **41**, 732–3.

Shenbor, M. I. & Cheban, G. A. (1969). Preparation of 3-fluoranthenol by the action of lead tetraacetate on fluoranthene. *Zh. Org. Khim.* **5**, 143–4.

Sims, P. (1967). The metabolism of 7- and 12-methylbenz[a]anthracene and their derivatives. *Biochem. J.* **105**, 591–8.

Sims, P. (1968). The synthesis of 8- and 9-hydroxybenzo[a]pyrene and the role of the products in benzo[a]pyrene metabolism. *J. Chem. Soc. (C)*. 32–4.

Sims, P. (1971). Epoxy derivatives of aromatic polycyclic hydrocarbons. *Biochem. J.* **125**, 159–68.

Sims, P. & Grover, P. L. (1981). Involvement of dihydrodiols and diol epoxides in the metabolic activation of polycyclic hydrocarbons other than benzo[a]pyrene. *Polycyclic Hydrocarbons and Cancer*, eds H. V. Gelboin & P. O. P. Ts'o, pp. 117–81. Academic: New York.

Sukumaran, K. B. & Harvey, R. G. (1980). Synthesis of o-quinones and dihydrodiols of polycyclic aromatic hydrocarbons from the corresponding phenols. *J. Org. Chem.* **45**, 4407–13.

Wendland, R. & LaLonde, J. (1963). Phenanthrenequinone. *Org. Syn.* Coll. Vol. IV, 757–9.

Wilds, A. L. & Shunk, C. H. (1943). The preparation of derivatives of chrysene by means of the Robinson–Mannich base synthesis of unsaturated ketones. *J. Am. Chem. Soc.* **65**, 469–75.

Yagi, H., Holder, G. M., Dansette, P. M., Hernandez, O., Yeh, H. J. C., LeMahieu, R. A. & Jerina, D. M. (1976). Synthesis and spectral properties of the isomeric hydroxy-benzo[a]pyrenes. *J. Org. Chem.* **41**, 977–85.

Yang, D. T. C. & Trie, W. M. (1982). Synthesis of benz[a]anthracene-5,6-dione. *Org. Prep. Proc. Internat.* **14**, 202–3.

Index